SECOND
EDITION

# Consultation in Internal Medicine

SECOND EDITION

# Consultation in Internal Medicine

**John T. Harrington, M.D.**
Dean for Academic Affairs,
Dean ad interim,
Professor of Medicine,
Tufts University School of Medicine,
Boston, Massachusetts

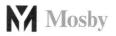
Mosby

St. Louis   Baltimore   Boston
Carlsbad   Chicago   Naples   New York   Philadelphia   Portland
London   Madrid   Mexico City   Singapore   Sydney   Tokyo   Toronto   Wiesbaden

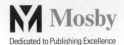

**Mosby**

Dedicated to Publishing Excellence

A Times Mirror
Company

*Vice President and Publisher:* Anne S. Patterson
*Executive Editor:* James Shanahan
*Developmental Editor:* Laura Berendson
*Project Manager:* Dana Peick
*Project Specialist:* Catherine Albright
*Production Editors:* Carl Masthay, Catherine Albright
*Cover Designer:* Janis Giger
*Designer:* Amy Buxton
*Manufacturing Manager:* J. A. McAllister

SECOND EDITON
Copyright © 1997 by Mosby-Year Book, Inc.

Previous editions copyrighted 1990 by B.C. Decker, Inc.

Printed in the United States of America

Composition by TCSystems, Inc.

Project Management by Spectrum Publisher Services, Inc.

Printing and binding by R. R. Donnelley & Sons

Mosby-Year Book, Inc.
11830 Westline Industrial Drive
St. Louis, Missouri 63146

**Library of Congress Cataloging-in-Publication Data**

Consultation in internal medicine / [edited by] John T. Harrington—
    2nd ed.
        p.        cm.
    Includes bibliographical references and index.
    ISBN 0-8151-4164-5 (alk. paper)
    1. Internal medicine—Handbooks, manuals, etc.   2. Medical
consultation—Handbooks, manuals, etc.   I. Harrington, John T.
(John Tolan), 1936-   .
    [DNLM:   1. Clinical Medicine—handbooks.   2. Referral and
Consultation—handbooks.   WB 39 C758 1997]
    RC55.C59   1997
    616—dc20
    DNLM/DLC
    for Library of Congress                                  96-19077
                                                                    CIP

98 99 00 01 02  /  9 8 7 6 5 4 3 2 1

# Contributors

**PIERRE ABI HANNA, M.D.**
Chief Medical Resident,
Carney Hospital,
Boston, Massachusetts

**FREDERICK R. ARONSON, M.D., M.P.H.**
Oncologist
Portland, Maine

**SANJEEV ARORA, M.D.**
Associate Professor of Medicine,
University of New Mexico School of Medicine,
Albuquerque, New Mexico;
Section Chief, Division of Gastroenterology,
University of New Mexico Health Sciences Center

**RONALD L. CIUBOTARU, M.D.**
Clinical Fellow,
Tufts University School of Medicine;
Research Fellow in Pulmonary and Critical Care Medicine,
New England Medical Center,
Boston, Massachusetts

**JENNIFER DALEY, M.D.**
Director, Health Services Research and Development,
Brockton/West Roxbury Veterans Affairs Medical Center;
Staff Physician, Beth Israel Hospital,
Harvard Medical School,
Boston, Massachusetts

**SCOTT K. EPSTEIN, M.D.**
Associate Director, Medical Intensive Care Unit,
Pulmonary and Critical Care Division,
New England Medical Center;
Assistant Professor of Medicine,
Tufts University School of Medicine,
Boston, Massachusetts

**N.A. MARK ESTES III, M.D.**
Director, Cardiac Arrhythmia Service,
New England Medical Center;
Professor of Medicine,
Tufts University School of Medicine,
Boston, Massachusetts

**KARIM A. FAWAZ, M.D.**
Professor of Medicine,
Tufts University School of Medicine,
New England Medical Center,
Boston, Massachusetts

**CAROLINE B. FOOTE, M.D.**
Co-Director, Cardiac Arrhythmia Clinic,
New England Medical Center;
Assistant Professor of Medicine,
Tufts University School of Medicine,
Boston, Massachusetts

**NELSON M. GANTZ, M.D.**
Chairman, Department of Medicine;
Chief, Division of Infectious Diseases,
Pinnacle Health Hospitals,
Harrisburg, Pennsylvania;
Clinical Professor of Medicine,
Pennsylvania State University College of Medicine,
Hershey, Pennsylvania

**RICHARD A. GLECKMAN, M.D.**
Professor of Medicine,
Boston University School of Medicine;
Director of Medicine, Carney Hospital,
Boston, Massachusetts

**DON L. GOLDENBERG, M.D.**
Chief of Rheumatology,
Newton-Wellesley Hospital,
Newton, Massachusetts;
Professor of Medicine,
Tufts University School of Medicine,
Boston, Massachusetts

**JOHN T. HARRINGTON, M.D.**
Dean for Academic Affairs,
Dean ad interim,
Professor of Medicine,
Tufts University School of Medicine,
Boston, Massachusetts

**MUNTHER HOMOUD, M.D.**
Assistant Professor of Medicine,
Tufts University School of Medicine;
Co-Director, Cardiac Electrophysiology and Pacing Laboratory,
New England Medical Center,
Boston, Massachusetts

**JEFFREY M. ISNER, M.D.**
Chief, Cardiovascular Research,
St. Elizabeth's Medical Center;
Professor of Medicine and Pathology,
Tufts University School of Medicine,
Boston, Massachusetts

**CAREY D. KIMMELSTIEL, M.D.**
Associate Director, Cardiac Catheterization Laboratory,
New England Medical Center Hospital;
Assistant Professor of Medicine,
Tufts University School of Medicine,
Boston, Massachusetts

**MARVIN A. KONSTAM, M.D.**
Professor of Medicine and Radiology,
Tufts University School of Medicine;
Acting Chief of Cardiology,
New England Medical Center,
Boston, Massachusetts

**RICHARD A. LAFAYETTE, M.D.**
Co-Director, Renal Physiology,
Stanford University School of Medicine;
Director, In-Patient Dialysis Services,
Stanford University Medical Center;
Assistant Professor of Medicine,
Division of Nephrology,
Stanford University School of Medicine,
Stanford, California

**DAVID S. LAZARUS, M.D.**
Staff Physician,
Pulmonary and Critical Care Division,
New England Medical Center;
Assistant Professor,
Tufts University School of Medicine,
Boston, Massachusetts

**KENNETH B. MILLER, M.D.**
Associate Professor of Medicine,
Tufts University School of Medicine;
Director of Bone Marrow Transplant Program,
Director of Leukemia Service,
New England Medical Center,
Boston, Massachusetts

**DOUGLAS T. PHELPS, M.D.**
Associate Professor of Medicine,
Albany Medical College;
Staff Physician, Stratton VA Medical Center,
Albany, New York

**ROGER PLATT, M.D.**
Vice-President and Medical Director,
Phillips Ambulatory Care Center,
Beth Israel Medical Center,
New York, New York

**FRANCIS RENNA, M.D.**
Chief of Dermatology,
Newton-Wellesley Hospital,
Newton, Massachusetts;
Assistant Professor of Dermatology,
Tufts University School of Medicine,
Boston, Massachusetts

**RICHARD A. RUDDERS, M.D.**
Chief, Hematology/Oncology,
Boston Veterans Administration Medical Center;
Professor of Medicine and Pathology,
Boston University,
Boston, Massachusetts

**LEONARD SICILIAN, M.D.**
Director, Medical Intensive Care Unit,
New England Medical Center;
Associate Professor of Medicine,
Tufts University School of Medicine,
Boston, Massachusetts

**AYMAN O. SOUBANI, M.D.**
Pulmonary Fellow, New England Medical Center;
Instructor,
Tufts University School of Medicine,
Boston, Massachusetts

**PAUL J. WANG, M.D.**
Associate Director,
Cardiac Electrophysiology and Pacing Laboratory;
Director, Heart Station,
New England Medical Center;
Associate Professor of Medicine,
Tufts University School of Medicine,
Boston, Massachusetts

**ALEXANDER C. WHITE, M.B., M.R.C.P.I.**
Assistant Professor of Medicine,
Tufts University School of Medicine;
Assistant Physician,
Pulmonary and Critical Care Division,
New England Medical Center,
Boston, Massachusetts

# Preface

This second edition of our highly successful pocket medical text hews to the same course utilized in the first edition. Each and every chapter in this edition has been reviewed carefully and revised as necessary, and references have been brought up to date. I again have asked a small group of professional colleagues, most affiliated with Tufts University School of Medicine or the New England Medical Center Hospital, and all sophisticated clinicians, to tell our readers how they approach the major, important symptom complexes in their own subspecialty of internal medicine. The contributors have covered nine topics each in infectious diseases, gastroenterology, and hematology with oncology, and seven topics each in cardiovascular medicine, nephrology, and pulmonary disease. A major endocrinology problem, diabetes mellitus, and a major rheumatologic problem, polyarthritis, are covered in the chronic disease section. Dr. Richard Lafayette has replaced Dr. Andrew Levey as the major author for the renal disease section. Moreover, several new chapters, which replace chapters that appeared in the first edition, have been added, including Dr. Karim Fawaz's chapter on ascites, Dr. Don Goldenberg's chapter on polyarthritis, and Dr. Leonard Sicilian's chapter on active tuberculosis. The authors have emphasized the practical aspects of diagnosis and treatment, weaving into their chapters the relevant underlying pathophysiology. Cost-effective approaches are utilized throughout, especially important in this day and age. I thank all of them for their diligence and their thoughtful contributions.

I also wish to thank my secretary Ms. Irene V. Deychman for her expert secretarial and managerial support over the last year, and Mrs. Laura Berendson at Mosby–Year Book for her superb editorial efforts. To each of our industrious readers, *carpe diem!*

**John T. Harrington, M.D.**

# Preface to the First Edition

The art and science of performing a consultation in internal medicine is often neglected in traditional internal medicine teaching, both in medical schools and in residency programs. In this text, *Consultation in Internal Medicine*, we have provided the systematic approach of a collegial group of clinicians to the clinical problems for which we are most often consulted. All the contributors have (or have had) appointments at the New England Medical Center and/or Tufts University School of Medicine.

In compiling the topics for our text, I asked the contributors to review the specific problems they were asked to address in inpatients. I estimate that more than 90 percent of the problems for which internists or internal medicine subspecialists are called to see patients are covered in this text. The contributors have covered eight topics in cardiovascular medicine, nine topics in infectious disease, gastroenterology, and hematology-oncology, seven topics in nephrology and pulmonary disease, and four topics in general medicine. Endocrinology and rheumatology sections deliberately were omitted because most of these patients currently are cared for as outpatients. Diabetes mellitus is reviewed in the general medicine section, as are other general medicine problems of chronic pain, hypertension, and noncompliance.

Who needs this text? The number of medical texts seems to increase exponentially. We have tried not to be responsible solely for chopping down more trees, but rather to provide a highly focused examination of the diagnosis and treatment of major, common problems. We have aimed the text at the young internist and surgeon who need precise answers to such pragmatic questions as "What do I do with an elderly patient who has fainted once?", "Should I treat every patient with a positive PPD?", "What tests should I order in my patient with dysphagia?", "How should I work up and treat acute bronchospasm? Pigmented skin lesions? Hyponatremia? Chronic pain?"

It is my belief that the thorough, pithy discussion of the problems covered in this handbook provides readily-available and invaluable information to young internists and surgeons. I believe that the systematic approach emphasized in this text also will provide sustenance to the seasoned internist in his or her daily practice. The text is designed to be carried in one's pocket for ready consultation at the bedside.

My thanks to our publisher, Brian Decker, for supporting this series; to the editor of the series, Dr. Jerome P. Kassirer, my long-time friend and colleague; and special thanks to Ms. Karen Coyne for her devotion to this task over the last year.

**John T. Harrington, M.D.**

# Contents

SECOND
EDITION

# Consultation in Internal Medicine

# Part 1

# Cardiovascular Disease

## Chapter 1

## Syncope

Caroline B. Foote
N.A. Mark Estes III

Syncope, defined as a sudden temporary loss of consciousness and postural tone accounts for 3% of all emergency room visits and up to 6% of all medical admissions. Although the causes for syncope are numerous and can be divided into noncardiac and cardiac (see the box on pp. 2 and 3), ultimately syncope is the result of systemic hypotension resulting in cerebral hypoperfusion. Despite careful history, physical examination, and screening electrocardiography, up to 50% of all patients with syncope defy diagnosis. Because the underlying cause of syncope determines prognosis and therapy, it is important to pursue a diagnosis with appropriate further testing as determined by the initial evaluation.

## HISTORY

The history elicited from the patient and from observers is essential to proper evaluation of syncope and frequently provides critical diagnostic

1

## Causes of Syncope

### CARDIAC

**Arrhythmias**

Bradyarrhythmia
  Sinus bradycardia
  Sinus arrest, asystole
  High-degree AV block
  Atrial fibrillation with slow ventricular response
Tachyarrhythmia
  Supraventricular tachycardia
  Ventricular tachycardia

**Anatomic**

Aortic stenosis
Hypertrophic cardiomyopathy
Pulmonary hypertension
Myocardial infarction
Atrial myxoma
Pulmonary embolism

### NONCARDIAC

Alteration of vasomotor tone
  Vasodepressor (vasovagal or neurally mediated)
  Orthostatic hypotension
  Carotid sinus hypersensitivity
  Cough, micturition, deglutition, defecation

### DRUG INDUCED

Hypotension
Tachycardia
Bradycardia
Overdose

### CEREBROVASCULAR DISEASE

Seizure
Hemorrhage
Cerebrovascular insufficiency

*continued*

*continued*

| METABOLIC |
|---|
| Hypoxia |
| Hypoglycemia |
| Hyperventilation |
| **PSYCHIATRIC** |
| Panic disorder |
| Major depression |
| Hysteria |

clues. Episodes of dizziness or light-headedness frequently precede episodes of true syncope and differ from loss of consciousness only in degree. This is called *near syncope*, or *presyncope*, and must be carefully differentiated from vertigo and functional symptoms.

Neurally mediated syncope (vasovagal syncope), the common "fainting spell," is a response enacted through the autonomic nervous system and occurs in patients with an exaggerated response to stressful circumstances. Two components exist; a vagally mediated cardioinhibitory component results in bradycardia, and a vasodepressor component causes hypotension. This syndrome should be suspected when syncope occurs after a triggering event, such as pain, fear, or other emotional stress. Most commonly, a prodrome of yawning, pallor, sweating, and nausea precedes the spell. Occasionally palpitations associated with the sinus tachycardia preceding syncope may also be described. During syncope, an astute observer may notice a weak, slow pulse. In elderly patients, vasovagal syncope may occur with a drop in blood pressure (the vasodepressor component) that is not accompanied by a decrease in heart rate (the cardioinhibitory component). Vasovagal syncope constitutes the most common cause of syncope in patients presenting to the emergency room after a single episode of loss of consciousness. A careful history usually is sufficient in making the diagnosis, though provocative testing is available if needed.

Orthostatic hypotension, defined as a drop in systolic blood pressure that is sufficient to cause cerebral hypoperfusion with assumption of an upright posture, is another common cause of syncope. Drugs that cause vasodilatation, reduce blood volume, or block the sympathetic nervous system often play a role in precipitating orthostatic hypotension. Orthostatic hypotension may be secondary to other factors, such as impaired vascular regulation by the autonomic nervous system or depletion of circulating blood volume, as with blood loss. One must question the patient in detail regarding any changes in posture that precede the episode of loss of consciousness.

Situational syncope associated with cough, micturition, deglutition, and defecation just before loss of consciousness, usually can be diagnosed by history. These situations are believed to trigger reflexes (usually vagally mediated) in individuals, resulting in hypotension and bradycardia. Postprandial hypotension has been described mostly in the elderly population.

Exertional syncope usually is more ominous and should alert the clinician to possible cardiac syncope. During exercise, patients with aortic stenosis often cannot meet the increased metabolic demands because the narrow valve causes a fixed cardiac output, which may result in hypotension and global ischemia; and tachyarrhythmias also can cause syncope in patients with aortic stenosis. An independent vasodepressor hypotensive reaction from uncertain mechanisms also can exist in patients with aortic stenosis. Likewise, hypertrophic cardiomyopathy may result in outflow obstruction, ischemia, or tachyarrhythmias during exercise, causing hypotension and syncope. Pulmonary hypertension and pulmonic stenosis also may cause effort syncope. Less commonly, left atrial myxomas or other large mobile intracardia masses result in mechanical blockade of the circulation with exertion. Finally, when a history of exertional loss of consciousness is obtained, one must consider the possibility of cardiac ischemia on the basis of significant coronary artery disease that induces either low cardiac output or a transient arrhythmia. Two hereditary conditions, a cardiomyopathy called *right ventricular dysplasia* (resulting from fat infiltration and fibrosis of the heart muscle) and congenital long QT syndrome (a primary electrical abnormality), can predispose the heart to ventricular tachyarrhythmias during exercise.

Syncope associated with shaving of the neck, with application of a tight collar or necktie, or with rotation of the head should raise the possibility of carotid sinus hypersensitivity. With this condition, stimulation of carotid sinus baroreceptors results in bradycardia or hypotension, or both. Patients with this syndrome often have some degree of intrinsic sinus node disease. A hyperactive reflex actually may be an indicator of hypersensitivity of the sinus node, rather than of excessive activity of the innervation of the sinus node.

Abrupt onset of loss of consciousness in which a patient "drops like a stone" is suggestive of a sudden loss of cardiac output, as is seen with Stokes-Adams attacks caused by heart block. By contrast, a period of presyncope, or dizziness, especially when associated with palpitations, is suggestive of a tachyarrhythmia. Symptoms of near syncope also may result from bradyarrhythmias, such as sinus bradycardia, sinus arrest, and sinus pauses after the termination of supraventricular tachycardia, or from atrial fibrillation with a slow ventricular response.

Generally, a diagnosis of seizure disorder can be made when loss of consciousness is noted to occur with tonic-clonic movements and postictal confusion, but it should be remembered that any cause for prolonged cerebral hypofusion may result in some tonic-clonic activity. Many young patients with long QT syndrome have been wrongly diagnosed with seizures. When recurrent spells diagnosed as seizures do not respond to standard antiepileptic therapy, the possibility of an arrhythmic cause should be considered and evaluated.

Syncope associated with diplopia, dysarthia, ataxia, and other brain-stem dysfunction may represent a transient ischemic attack of the vertebral-basilar system. Carotid artery disease, however, is rarely associated with syncope. External compression of the vertebral arteries should be suspected if syncope is induced by positional head changes, particularly hyperextension and lateral rotation. Syncope with arm exercise raises the possibility of subclavian steal syndrome.

Overwhelming anxiety or hyperventilation raises the possibility of anxiety attacks causing syncope, though more commonly these produce presyncope. Other psychiatric reasons for syncope include panic disorders and major depression. Finally, hysterical or psychogenic syncope should be considered in patients with a dramatic loss of consciousness in the presence of others without change in blood pressure or pulse.

## PHYSICAL EXAMINATION

Examination of the patient, an essential component of the initial evaluation, occasionally reveals findings diagnostic of the cause of syncope. A careful check for orthostatic hypotension is mandatory and is done by measurement of blood pressure and pulse in the supine and standing positions. Generally, a fall of 25 to 30 mm of mercury in systolic blood pressure is needed to make a diagnosis of orthostatic hypotension. However, some people develop symptoms with a lesser drop, and these individuals still should be classified as having orthostatic hypotension. Any drop in systolic blood pressure that leads to syncope is significant. Some normal elderly patients may have an asymptomatic drop in blood pressure of up to 40 mm Hg without central hypoperfusion. The diagnosis of orthostatic hypotension then is dependent on replication of symptoms during a postural drop in blood pressure, rather than on some arbitrary level of decline in the blood pressure. Many times orthostatic hypotension is transient, as after the use of vasodilators like nitroglycerin or an antihypertensive drug. Occasionally, a patient with reduced intravascular volume will have had rehydration by the time the blood pressure is measured, thus eliminating the prior orthostatic blood pressure drop.

The carotid and subclavian arteries should be examined to detect bruits that would indicate extracranial vascular disease. The presence of a transmitted cardiac murmur raises the possibility of some form of aortic outflow tract obstruction. The classic upstrokes in a patient with significant aortic stenosis are described as "parvus et tardus," thereby indicating a weak and late-peaking carotid upstroke. By contrast, patients with hypertrophic cardiomyopathy generally have bounding carotid upstrokes that are bisferious in quality. Careful cardiac examination may detect significant aortic stenosis, cardiomyopathy, left atrial myxoma, and pulmonary hypertension. Dilated cardiomyopathy may also be suspected by exam.

Carotid sinus massage is a diagnostic maneuver that should be performed to detect any abnormal slowing of the heart rhythm. This massage is contraindicated in the presence of a carotid bruit or of other signs of carotid disease because there is a risk of precipitating a neurologic deficit under these circumstances. Both the heart rhythm and blood pressure must be monitored during carotid sinus massage. Gentle massage should be applied to one carotid at the level of bifurcation for a period of approximately 5 seconds. If this does not result in any diagnostic abnormalities, the other carotid should be massaged in a similar fashion. A normal response manifests as a gradual slowing of the sinus rate. Any fall in blood pressure or in heart rate that results in presyncope or syncope is abnormal. Sinus pauses of 3 or more seconds or a fall in systolic blood pressure greater than 40 mm Hg also is diagnostic of carotid sinus hypersensitivity.

Other maneuvers that can be done include hyperventilation for 2 minutes with roughly 20 deep breaths per minute. Although many individuals will become light headed, true loss of consciousness with this maneuver usually indicates a psychiatric cause for syncope. Rapid arm flexions and extensions can be used to screen for subclavian steal syndrome, and hyperextension of the neck can be used to screen for vertebral basilar disease.

## DIAGNOSTIC TESTS

An electrocardiogram is essential in all patients who present with syncope. An ECG not only serves as a screening tool for any bradycardia or tachyarrhythmias, but also as an indicator of any underlying heart disease. Abnormalities of conduction systems, such as chronic bifascicular block, raise the possibility of an intermittent progression to a higher degree of block. Occasionally, ventricular preexcitation is noted, with a shortened PR interval accompanied by a delta wave. In patients with Wolff-Parkinson-White syndrome, there is a higher frequency of supraventricular tachycardia and of atrial fibrillation with a rapid ventricular response. Sinus pauses, sinus arrest, blocked atrial premature contractions and heart block or atrial fibrillation with a slow ventricular response are suggestive of bradycardia as the cause of syncope. Congenital or drug-induced long QT syndrome should be suspected if the QT interval is 440 milliseconds or greater.

Careful history and physical examination define the causes for syncope in most cases where a diagnosis is reached, but the majority of patients require diagnostic testing. Outpatient evaluation is suitable for most patients, but inpatient evaluation is preferable if syncope has caused significant injury or if a potentially life-threatening cause of syncope is suspected, such as ventricular tachycardia or myocardial ischemia.

If cardiac rhythm disturbances are suspected as the cause of syncope, a 24-hour Holter monitor should be performed to screen for bradyarrhythmias and malignant tachyarrhythmias. Occasionally, the ambulatory electrocardiogram does reveal an abnormality highly suggestive of a diagnosis. For example, runs of nonsustained ventricular tachycardia are presumptive evidence that ventricular arrhythmia contributed to syncope. Documentation of Mobitz type II block, complete heart block, or sinus pauses over 3 seconds frequently is adequate justification for placement of a permanent pacemaker. In most patients, however, no diagnostic abnormalities are present. Short episodes of supraventricular tachycardia and ventricular tachycardia are often asymptomatic or the patient fails to have symptoms of presyncope or syncope during the 24-hour Holter monitoring. Increasing monitoring times to 48 or 72 hours usually fails, but prolonged ambulatory monitoring with patient-activated transtelephonic loop monitors have been shown by us and others to have a considerable diagnostic yield in unexplained syncope. These "loop recorders" are digital or solid-state memory loops that can be activated after the syncopal episode and retrieve information about the cardiac rhythm during the preceding 4 minutes. The devices are small and reasonably unobtrusive, allowing the patient to wear them for weeks or months at a time until an episode of syncope occurs.

Signal-averaged electrocardiography (SA-ECG) recently has been reported to be useful in identifying individuals at risk for ventricular tachycardia as a cause of syncope. The SA-ECG is a noninvasive technique that records, amplifies, and filters the surface ECG such that low-amplitude, high-frequency signals (late potentials) at the terminal portion of the QRS complex can be detected. These late potentials represent delayed myocardial activation in areas of scar tissue, which may serve as the electrophysiologic substrate for ventricular arrhythmias. The predictive accuracy of SA-ECG is best in patients with coronary artery disease.

In patients with unexplained syncope or suspected neurally mediated syncope, head-up tilt test is a noninvasive procedure used to provoke vasovagal syncope. Although protocols vary, generally a patient is placed on a tilt table with a footboard for weight bearing, and the table is brought upright to a tilt of 60 to 80 degrees for up to 60 minutes. The patient also may receive an intravenous infusion of isoproterenol, especially if the base line study is negative. The upright tilt causes venous pooling with diminution of blood return to the heart and compensatory tachycardia. In patients with vasovagal syncope, it is believed that this results in stimulation of afferent C-fibers in the base of the left and right ventricle (cardiac mechanoreceptors) that triggers a neurally (vagally) mediated reflex that subsequently induces bradycardia or vasodilatation with resulting hypotension. Even prolonged asystole may be seen, requiring resuscitation with intravenous atropine and fluids. Although no standard exists for diagnosing neurally mediated syncope, this test is believed to be both relatively sensitive and relatively specific if it reproduces syncope.

A growing body of data has demonstrated that electrophysiologic testing plays an important role in identifying the cause of syncope and in guiding therapy in carefully selected patients. Patients with recurrent unexplained syncope who have been studied in the electrophysiology lab are selected based on the absence of identifiable causes for their syncope despite a thorough noninvasive evaluation that includes a history and physical examination (including testing for orthostatic hypotension and carotid sinus hypersensitivity), an ECG, and at least 24 hours of continuous ambulatory ECG monitoring. In many instances, exercise tests and echocardiograms also have been nondiagnostic. If there is evidence of structural heart disease, an invasive electrophysiology study may be justified, particularly if the syncope is recurrent. The likelihood of finding a significant abnormality during electrophysiologic testing is directly related to the presence or the absence of heart disease. Between 60% and 90% of patients with some form of heart disease and syncope with a nondiagnostic noninvasive evaluation have an abnormality identified in the electrophysiology laboratory. In the absence of structural heart disease, the yield from electrophysiologic testing is considerably lower, with only 10% to 50% of the patients having any abnormality found. Most commonly, ventricular tachycardia is found with programmed ventricular stimulation. Less commonly, supraventricular tachycardia (10% of patients), sinus node dysfunction (5% to 15% of patients), or His-Purkinje conduction defects (5% to 15% of patients) are found. Therapy based on the electrophysiologic abnormalities eliminates recurrent syncope in more than 80% of cases.

Other specialized diagnostic tests, such as electroencephalograms, skull films, and computerized tomography (CT) or MRI scans, have extremely low yields as screening tools, particularly if the neurologic examination is normal and the history is not suggestive of a seizure or of a focal neurologic event. Similarly, echocardiography and cardiac catheterization should be reserved for patients with physical findings suggestive of a significant cardiac abnormality and should not be used as screening tools. In patients with carotid bruits, carotid noninvasive studies can give a reliable indication of the degree of stenosis, but extracranial cerebrovascular disease rarely causes syncope. Intracranial Doppler studies also may be useful.

## THERAPY

The treatment of syncope must be directed by the underlying cause. The patient with neurally mediated syncope must be advised to avoid the trigger event as much as possible. With an acute episode, the patient should be advised to assume a supine position. Atropine and intravenous fluids may be necessary to treat a severe episode. It is extremely difficult to prevent recurrent episodes. Recently, several reports of successful therapy with beta-adrenergic receptor blockers have been published. Occasionally, long-term therapy with fludrocortisone (a salt-retaining steroid), aminophylline, or anticholinergic medication is successful in preventing or in minimizing the severity of these episodes, but these medications must be taken in doses such that side effects (such as dry mouth) are common. Permanent dual-chamber pacing may be indicated in patients with recurrent, severe episodes where medical therapy has failed.

Therapy of orthostatic hypotension is directed at the underlying cause of the syndrome. In patients with diabetic or alcoholic neuropathy, improvement in symptoms occasionally occurs with better control of the diabetes or with abstinence from alcohol. In instances where the orthostatic hypotension is caused by the use of drugs, alternative therapy should be instituted. Orthostatic hypotension can result from multiple medications being taken at one time; alteration in the medication schedule frequently obviates the problem. Volume repletion is the appropriate therapy for patients in whom intravascular volume is depleted by dehydration or blood loss.

Patients with orthostatic hypotension should be instructed to rise gradually from a supine to a sitting position and to spend several minutes in that position before standing slowly. In the event they feel dizzy, they should be instructed to sit down immediately. Elastic stockings or an elastic body garment are sometimes helpful to increase venous return and to minimize symptoms. Occasionally, liberalization of the intake of salt and fluids or treatment with fludrocortisone helps when other measures fail.

Patients with postprandial hypotension and syncope may improve with frequent, smaller meals as well as adequate hydration and salt intake. Paradoxically treatment of baseline hypertension has been shown useful in some patients. Others require caffeine or octreotide (a somatostatin analog) to control symptoms.

Pacemaker therapy frequently is necessary when carotid sinus hypersensitivity is documented. Experience with ventricular pacing in patients with carotid sinus hypersensitivity, however, indicates that a significant percentage of patients continue to have syncope. The vasodepressor response (with hypotension) can continue to cause syncope despite protection by the pacemaker against the cardioinhibitory response. An atrioventricular dual-chamber pacemaker generally is needed in patients with carotid sinus hypersensitivity. In refractory cases with severe symptoms, it may be necessary to attempt denervation of the carotid sinus.

Permanent pacemaker therapy is warranted when a clinically significant bradycardia is documented. The indications for permanent pacemaker therapy are listed in Table 1-1. Indications for permanent pacemakers have been grouped into three major operational classifications: Class I indications for pacing are those in which there is general agreement that a permanent pacemaker should be implanted. Class II indications are those indications for which permanent pacemakers are frequently used, but among experts there is a divergence of opinion regarding the necessity for their insertion. Class III indications are conditions for which there is a general agreement that pacemakers are unnecessary.

When supraventricular or ventricular tachycardia is the cause of syncope, initial therapy often consists in the selection of appropriate antiarrhythmic agents to suppress the spontaneous arrhythmia (or the arrhythmia induced in the electrophysiology laboratory). Catheter ablation therapy is indicated in patients with Wolff-Parkinson-White syndrome, especially if atrial fibrillation with rapid ventricular response is documented. Patients with documented or suspected life-threatening ventricular arrhythmias may be candidates for defibrillators, as well. Rarely, surgical therapy is necessary for cure of cardiac arrhythmias.

**Table 1-1.** *Indications for permanent pacemaker therapy*

| Dysrhythmia | Class I (indicated) | Class II (sometimes indicated) | Class III (not indicated) |
|---|:---:|:---:|:---:|
| FIRST-DEGREE AV BLOCK | | | × |
| SECOND-DEGREE AV BLOCK | | | |
| Type I (Wenckebach) | | | |
|   Asymptomatic | | | × |
|   Symptomatic | × | | |
| Type II (Mobitz II) | | | |
|   Asymptomatic | | × | |
|   Symptomatic | × | | |
| COMPLETE AV BLOCK | | | |
| Congenital | | | |
|   Asymptomatic | | × | |
|   Symptomatic | × | | |
| Acquired | | | |
|   Asymptomatic | | × | |
|   Symptomatic | × | | |
| CHRONIC BIFASCICULAR AND TRIFASCICULAR BLOCK | | | |
| Intermittent CHB with symptoms | × | | |
| Intermittent Mobitz type II without symptoms | × | | |
| With syncope not proved to be caused by CHB, but other causes not identifiable | | × | |
| No AV block or symptoms | | | × |
| With first degree AV block without symptoms | | | × |
| AV BLOCK ASSOCIATED WITH MI | | | |
| CHB | × | | |
| First degree AV block with new BBB | | | × |
| Transient advanced AV block and BBB | × | | |
| Transient AV block without BBB | | | × |
| Transient AV block with LAHB | | | × |
| Acquired LAHB without AV block | | | × |
| Acquired bifascicular BBB | | | × |

(*continued*)

**Table 1-1.** *Indications for permanent pacemaker therapy—cont'd*

| Dysrhythmia | Class I (indicated) | Class II (sometimes indicated) | Class III (not indicated) |
|---|---|---|---|
| **SINUS NODE DYSFUNCTION (SICK SINUS SYNDROME)** | | | |
| Symptomatic bradycardia | × | | |
| With heart rates <40 bpm without documented symptomatic bradycardia | | × | |
| Asymptomatic | | | × |
| **HYPERSENSITIVE CAROTID SINUS SYNDROME** | | | |
| Recurrent syncope associated with carotid sinus stimulation with >3 sec pauses with carotid sinus massage | × | | |
| Recurrent syncope without clear provocative event and with a hyperactive cardioinhibitory response | | × | |
| Asymptomatic | | | × |
| Syncope from vasodepressor response | | | × |
| **ATRIAL FIBRILLATION OR FLUTTER WITH SLOW VENTRICULAR RESPONSE** | | | |
| Asymptomatic | | | × |
| Symptomatic | × | | |
| **TACHYCARDIA PREVENTION** | | | |
| Associated with bradycardia | × | | |
| Associated with long QT syndrome Torsade de pointes | | × | |

*AV,* Atrioventricular; *BBB,* bundle branch block; *CHB,* complete heart block; *LAHB,* left anterior hemiblock; *MI,* myocardial infarction.

When cardiac syncope is caused by aortic stenosis, an echocardiogram and Doppler study can allow one to estimate the severity of the stenosis and assess left ventricular function. When patients lose consciousness because of aortic stenosis, cardiac catheterization is indicated to assess the severity of the aortic stenosis as well as left ventricular function and coronary artery anatomy. Aortic valve replacement (or percutaneous aortic valvuloplasty in inoperable patients) is indicated in patients with aortic stenosis and syncope.

An echocardiogram and Doppler study provides information regarding the magnitude of the outflow-tract gradient in patients in whom hypertrophic cardiomyopathy causes syncope. Medical therapy with beta-blockers, calcium-channel blockers, or other negative inotropes such as disopyramide reduces the aortic outflow-tract gradient. Recently dual-chamber pacing has been shown to decrease effectively the outflow-tract gradient and reduce symptoms in patients with hypertrophic cardiomyopathy. In an occasional patient, however, where repetitive episodes of syncope occur, surgical therapy with a myotomy or myectomy is mandated. Ventricular arrhythmias frequently occur in patients with hypertrophic cardiomyopathy, and the clinician should diligently search for an arrhythmia as the cause of syncope. Holter monitoring should be performed in this patient population.

Despite major advances in the diagnostic tests that enable the clinician to define the cause of syncope, approximately one half of all patients who present with syncope have no specific diagnosis found. Prospective studies have shown that the mortality is approximately 30% over the first year after an episode of syncope in patients with untreated cardiac cause of syncope. The mortality is considerably less, in the range of 5% to 10% per year, for patients who have a noncardiac cause of syncope or who have syncope of unknown origin. Therefore an individual who presents with an episode of syncope and who has heart disease needs a more extensive evaluation. By contrast, the prognosis is relatively good in patients who present with syncope, particularly a single episode, who have no evidence of heart disease by examination or by ECG.

A rational stepwise diagnostic approach begins with a careful history and physical examination with maneuvers. Selected use of noninvasive and invasive testing should follow as neccessary. Cardiac syncope has a high mortality compared to noncardiac syncope and unexplained syncope and thus mandates a more intensive evaluation.

## References

1. Kapoor WN, Karpf M, Wieand S, et al: A prospective evaluation and follow-up of patients with syncope, *N Engl J Med* 309(4):197-204, 1983.
2. Manolis AS, Linzer M, Salem DN, Estes NAM III: Syncope: current diagnostic evaluation and management, *Ann Intern Med* 112(11):850-863, 1990.
3. Linzer M, Varia L, Pontinen M, et al: Medically unexplained syncope: relationship to psychiatric illness, *Am J Med* 92:18-25, 1992.
4. Bachinsky W, Linzer M, Welds L, Estes NAM III: Usefulness of clinical characteristics in predicting the outcome of electrophysiologic studies in unexplained syncope, *Am J Cardiol* 69:1044-1049, 1992.
5. Jansen RWMM, Lipsitz LA: Postprandial hypotension: epidemiology, pathophysiology, and clinical management, *Ann Intern Med* 122(4):286-295, 1995.

## Chapter 2

# Cardiac Consultation in Patients Undergoing Noncardiac Surgery

Jeffrey M. Isner

Cardiac disease accounts for a significant proportion of perioperative complications, and management of cardiac problems in the perioperative period constitutes one of the most frequent reasons for medical consultations on surgical patients. The consultant providing perioperative care for the cardiac patients serves two distinct functions: (1) assessment of the degree to which a patient's cardiac disease increases the risk, that is, the morbidity and mortality, of the surgical procedure, and (2) the diagnosis and treatment of cardiac disorders in the perioperative period. I discuss risk assessment first and then the management of arrhythmias and conclude by reviewing the management of several common cardiac disorders in the preoperative period.

## AGE, TYPE OF SURGERY, AND CHOICE OF ANESTHETIC

Postoperative mortality from cardiac disease is significantly greater in older age groups; the risk becomes striking beyond 70 years of age. There is general agreement on the magnitude of this risk; the combined figure for all series is a mortality of nearly 14% for patients over 70. Although few studies have addressed the issue of mortality in patients over 60 but less than 70, selective analyses of these various series indicates that mortality in patients between 60 and 70 years of age may be only about one half that of patients over 70 (that is, about 7%). Intra-abdominal and thoracic surgery involve greater risk to the patient with cardiac disease than other surgical procedures. Emergency procedures increase fourfold the risk of postoperative myocardial infarction or cardiac death.

Although it has been suggested that the duration of surgery increases the risk in patients with cardiac disease, review of the available experience does not support this view. Specifically the duration of surgery does not influence the risk of perioperative myocardial infarction. Reports of increased risk associated with longer procedures appear to reflect differences in the type of surgical procedure. Although there is increased risk of perioperative congestive heart failure and noncardiac death in procedures lasting more than 5 hours, no effect on the incidence of infarction or cardiac death is seen even at this length of procedure.

All commonly used general anesthetics depress the mechanical performance of isolated heart muscle or decrease the cardiac output of experimental heart-lung preparations at concentrations that produce surgical anesthesia. With cyclopropane and ether, the cardiac depressant effect is offset by a simultaneous increase in sympathetic discharge; the net result is that the blood pressure tends to be maintained or is even slightly increased. Halothane, enflurane, and methoxyflurane do not cause the same increase in sympathetic tone; the systemic blood pressure therefore tends to fall as the level of anesthesia rises. Nitrous oxide may further compromise myocardial contractility in patients with impaired left ventricular function. Spinal and epidural anesthesia do not directly depress myocardial performance, though hypotension may occur as a result of blockade of sympathetic outflow. In general, there is no evidence that the choice of anesthetic agent or the route by which the anesthesia is delivered significantly affects cardiac morbidity or mortality.

Spinal or epidural anesthesia may be advantageous in terms of one cardiac complication. Spinal anesthesia rarely results in new or worsened congestive heart failure. In contrast, new congestive heart failure has been reported in 4.3% of patients receiving general anesthesia and worsened in 22% of the patients with preoperative failure. This consequence of general anesthesia is probably attributable to its direct myocardial depressant effects, which are not shared by the spinal anesthetics. Thus, although spinal anesthesia carries a risk of intraoperative hypotension and may not significantly alter cardiac mortality or infarction rate, it is probably preferable to general anesthesia in patients with a history of heart failure.

# RELATION OF CARDIAC FACTORS TO PERIOPERATIVE CARDIAC MORBIDITY AND MORTALITY

## Congestive heart failure

Congestive heart failure (CHF) may have a profound effect on a patient's intraoperative and postoperative course. It is essential that careful attention be given to its etiology, severity, and treatment.

Preoperative CHF increases surgical risk, and the increment in risk is proportional to the extent of hemodynamic compromise. Multivariate analysis of the signs and symptoms of CHF indicates that only two findings may correlate with increased surgical risk: increased systemic venous pressure (by clinical examination or central venous pressure measurement) and $S_3$ (ventricular) gallop sound on auscultatory examination. A past history of CHF without evidence of CHF at the time of surgery is not associated with a statistically significant increase in cardiac mortality.

The incidence of postoperative CHF varies from 0.02% to 5.8%, and its presence is associated with a mortality of 15% to 20%. Postoperative CHF associated with coronary artery disease has a higher mortality (25% to 79%) than CHF because of other cardiac disease (0 to 17%).

Several factors (such as chronic obstructive pulmonary disease, emergency surgery, thoracic or major intra-abdominal surgery, and valvular heart disease) have been found to increase the risk of developing postoperative CHF. Significant worsening of preoperative CHF has been commonly found in patients with the preoperative findings of an $S_3$ gallop heart sound (47%), jugular venous distension (35%), or history of pulmonary edema (32%), probably because of inappropriate fluid administration in the postoperative period.

## Hypotension

The patient with postoperative hypotension presents a challenge to the surgeon, anesthesiologist, and internist alike, because the cause may lie in any one of these three disciplines. Intraoperative blood loss or postoperative bleeding, gastrointestinal bleeding caused by stress ulceration, or hemorrhage secondary to invasive monitoring devices, such as central venous catheters, arterial lines, or the intra-aortic balloon, are common causes of perioperative hypotension. Pneumothorax, particularly in intubated patients ventilated under positive pressure, is another common cause for hypotension in the perioperative period. Reflex mechanisms may play a role in hypotension after intubation, carotid endarterectomy, and the thoracic or abdominal procedures in which the vagus nerve is stimulated; excess vagal tone with resultant hypotension may also occur during ocular surgery.

Medications administered intraoperatively and postoperatively must be considered as a potential cause of hypotension. These include anesthetic agents, morphine and other analgesics, antihypertensive or sympatholytic agents as well as anaphylactic reactions to drugs, blood products, or special substances such as the acrylic cement used in stabilizing orthopedic prosthetic devices.

Cardiac disorders that may result in hypotension include arrhythmias, primary depression of left ventricular pump function, and cardiac tamponade. Tamponade is often responsible for hypotension after thoracic procedures, in patients with anticoagulants, and in patients with neoplastic disease known to involve the mediastinum. Postoperative hypotension may be attributable to a variety of noncardiac causes. Among these is pulmonary embolism, whether caused by thrombus, fat, or amniotic fluid in the case of the obstetric patient treated by caesarean section, though only the last is likely to cause hypotension in the immediate postoperative period. Sepsis must always be considered in the differential diagnosis of postoperative hypotension. Although fever and leukocytosis may be clues to the presence of underlying infection, their absence certainly does not exclude septicemia. In the patient with either unrecognized myxedema or Addison's disease, the stress of surgery may precipitate acute crisis with hypotension or coma. Hypotension also may occur in patients receiving doses of steroids or patients who recently have received steroids. Adrenal hemorrhage with acute adrenal insufficiency may produce a similar clinical picture. Patients recently treated with oral steroids obviously should receive supplemental steroid coverage throughout the perioperative period.

# ARRHYTHMIAS IN THE SURGICAL PATIENT

Cardiac arrhythmias are not only the most common of all cardiac disorders, but also potentially the most lethal. The management of these diverse disorders is of paramount importance in caring for the surgical patient.

## Supraventricular arrhythmias: effect on risk

Supraventricular tachyarrhythmias are the most frequent type of cardiac rhythm disturbance noted in the surgical patient, even if sinus tachycardia is excluded. Supraventricular tachyarrhythmias in patients with ischemic, myopathic, or valvular heart disease may lead to loss of hemodynamic stability as a result of diminished duration of the diastolic filling period or the loss of active atrial contribution to ventricular filling. Furthermore, when atrial arrhythmias are associated with rapid heart rates, otherwise "normal" patients may experience a significant fall in cardiac output. Supraventricular tachyarrhythmias also may be the initial manifestation of serious medical complications such as myocardial infarction, pulmonary embolism, and sepsis.

Predictably, patients with preoperative supraventricular tachyarrhythmias have a vast increase (up to thirteenfold) in similar postoperative arrhythmias. Unfortunately, good data demonstrating a reduction in surgical mortality after treatment of preoperative supraventricular arrhythmias are not available.

## Supraventricular tachyarrhythmias: evaluation and management in the preoperative period

In evaluating the patient with atrial fibrillation or flutter preoperatively, a careful assessment for other cardiac disease is indicated. Certainly, fixed vulvular heart disease should be excluded. Less common disorders such as atrial septal defect, atrial myxoma, and hypertrophic cardiomyopathy should be looked for as well. Echocardiography provides a convenient screening test for these disorders and, in addition, allows accurate measurement of left atrial size. Thyrotoxicosis should also be considered, particularly in the elderly, because its clinical manifestations may be subtle. If atrial fibrillation is of recent onset, more acute problems (pulmonary embolus, infection, metabolic derangements, myocardial ischemia, pericarditis) should be sought.

Given the high perioperative mortality associated with atrial fibrillation, it is reasonable to question whether patients might benefit from preoperative cardioversion to normal sinus rhythm. Unfortunately, this question has not been well studied. Certainly, normal sinus rhythm after cardioversion is unlikely to persist in a patient with long-standing atrial fibrillation and massive left atrial enlargement. On the other hand, a patient with atrial fibrillation that is acute in onset may benefit from conversion to normal sinus rhythm and, if necessary, treatment with maintenance drug therapy designed to preserve sinus rhythm. In particular, when a potentially reversible cause for atrial fibrillation exists, postponement of the planned surgery should be seriously considered. Similar consideration should be given to patients in whom atrial fibrillation can be expected to be poorly tolerated (such as those with aortic stenosis, hypertrophic cardiomyopathy). The decision to proceed with cardioversion becomes more problematic in those patients in whom anticoagulation is indicated before conversion to prevent systemic embolization. Although the incidence of systemic embolization might be expected to be increased during the perioperative period, available studies fail to document such an increased risk.

Although data are not conclusive, it would seem reasonable to approach anticoagulation in patients with mitral valve disease and atrial fibrillation in the same manner as patients with valvular prostheses (see below). In patients with long-standing atrial fibrillation (caused by other types of disease) who are receiving therapy, anticoagulation can probably be stopped 3 to 5 days preoperatively and restarted 3 to 5 days postoperatively without adverse effects.

Two groups of patients with atrial fibrillation deserve additional comment. First, in patients with an inappropriately fast (greater than 150 beats per minute) ventricular response, underlying accessory conduction fibers (including Wolff-Parkinson-White) should be suspected. The fast ventricular response results from atrioventricular conduction across the specialized bypass fibers. Hemodynamic decompensation in these patients may occur abruptly. Furthermore, digitalis is contraindicated in such patients because it may enhance conduction across the bypass fibers. Instead, such patients should be treated with electrical cardioversion and subsequently, if necessary, with propranolol. Second, in patients with an inappropriately slow ventricular response (less than 90 beats per minute in the absence of digitalis therapy) underlying atrioventricular node disease should be suspected; this phenomenon may be one manifestation of the so-called sick-sinus syndrome. Patients with the sick-sinus syndrome present complicated management problems because of their inability to develop appropriate ventricular rates under the stress of surgery or, alternatively, because of associated tachyarrhythmias. Such patients require careful monitoring and, not infrequently, transvenous pacemaker (temporary or permanent) therapy.

Multifocal atrial tachycardia usually occurs in the setting of a compromised pulmonary status and may be associated with life-threatening ventricular ectopy. It is not likely to respond to digitalization; an all-out attack on respiratory tract secretion is often the only effective therapy. The excess surgical risk associated with all these disorders must, of course, be considered when one is assessing the need for surgical intervention.

## Supraventricular tachyarrhythmias: evaluation and management in the postoperative period

Atrial arrhythmias are quite common in the postoperative period. Atrial fibrillation and atrial flutter constitute 70% of reported postoperative arrhythmias; atrial tachycardia, supraventricular tachycardia, and nodal tachycardia account for another 18%. If the type of surgery being performed is a thoracotomy, the risk of developing a postoperative arrhythmia is substantially increased. In addition, some other factors appear to be related to an increased incidence of postoperative arrhythmias: 70 years of age or greater, congestive heart failure, chronic obstructive pulmonary disease, nondiagnostic ST-T wave changes, and intra-abdominal, thoracic, or major vascular procedures. There is a definite relationship between the occurrences of these arrhythmias and medical problems such as cardiac disorders infections, hypotension, anemia, and hypoxia. The mortality of patients with postoperative arrhythmias is not directly attributable to the arrhythmias themselves but rather to the underlying problem. Most of these arrhythmias revert to normal sinus rhythm without the use of antiarrhythmic agents.

Because atrial fibrillation constitutes the most frequently observed postoperative supraventricular tachyarrhythmia, preoperative (prophylactic) digitalization is often a consideration in certain high-risk patients. Previous investigations have identified several risk factors for the development of postoperative atrial fibrillation: advanced age, pulmonary resection, congestive heart failure, chronic obstructive pulmonary disease, preoperative pneumonia, or preoperative arrhythmias including atrial premature beats. The risk of developing atrial fibrillation to a patient with several of these factors is 10% to 15%. Furthermore, some studies have demonstrated a reduction in the incidence of postoperative atrial fibrillation in such patients when they are prophylactically digitalized. With respect to overall mortality, however, there appears to be little difference between the digitalized and nondigitalized groups. The decision to prophylactically digitalize such patients must also take into account the fact that many of the same factors that predispose to atrial fibrillation in these patients also predispose to the development of digitalis toxicity.

In summary, I believe that it is justifiable to recommend preoperative digitalization in a metabolically suitable patient who has more than one of the above-noted risk factors, provided that appropriate precautions are taken to avoid digitalis toxiocity. Although it is common practice at many institutions to withhold digitalis on the morning of surgery, there is no evidence to support the efficacy of this approach.

## Ventricular arrhythmias

The majority of ventricular arrhythmias seen in patients undergoing noncardiac surgery fall into the category of isolated ventricular ectopy in asymptomatic patients and do not require therapy. In critically ill patients, patients with underlying cardiac disorders, and patients with various forms of metabolic abnormalities, however, ventricular arrhythmias are much less likely to be benign.

## Ventricular ectopic activity

Five premature ventricular contractions per minute on any previous ECG increase the cardiac mortality from noncardiac surgery by a factor of 10.

Hypoxia and electrolyte abnormalities are the most common noncardiac causes of reversible ventricular arrhythmias and are generally more common in the postoperative rather than preoperative period. Patients with primary or secondary pulmonary disorders are particularly at risk for hypoxia-related ectopy, whereas patients with prolonged gastrointestinal disorders are at increased risk for electrolyte abnormalities that may precipitate ventricular ectopic activity. In addition, the use of more potent diuretic agents has greatly increased the incidence of these electrolyte disturbances. Patients with hypokalemia who do not respond to potassium replacement may have associated hypomagnesemia; in these patients, the arrhythmia generally resolves after magnesium replacement.

Often neglected as a source of cardiac ventricular arrhythmias is the displaced intravascular line, whether it be a Swan-Gantz catheter, central venous pressure tubing, pacemaker electrode, or a sheared indwelling peripheral venous catheter embolism. Ectopic activity resulting from such a foreign body is obviously an indication for immediate removal or repositioning of the mechanical irritant.

Finally, drugs commonly employed during the perioperative period, such as digitalis, adrenergic-stimulating agents, aminophylline, cyclopropane and chloroform anesthetics, psychotropic drugs, or injected radiopaque dyes need to be ruled out as a basis for ventricular ectopy.

In summary, ventricular arrhythmias may be attributable to a wide variety of causes. On the basis of published experience it is not possible to explicitly define which causes are specifically responsible for the increased perioperative risk in patients with ventricular ectopy. Nevertheless, on the basis of experience with nonoperative patients it would appear that high-grade ventricular ectopy, particularly in the patient with underlying ischemic heart disease, increases the risk of perioperative complications of ventricular ectopic activity. I recommend for this group in particular that it would seem prudent to recommend aggressive antiarrhythmic therapy in the perioperative period.

## Intraoperative cardiac arrest

The incidence of intraoperative cardiac arrest varies from 0.03% to 0.12% of all surgical procedures with a resultant mortality of 50% to 93% in patients sustaining an arrest. Fifty percent of cardiac arrests are asystolic, whereas the remainder are attributable to ventricular fibrillation; there is no difference in prognosis between the two groups. Cardiac arrests may occur at any point during the perioperative period, with 12% to 24% occurring during the induction of anesthesia, about 67% during the surgery itself, and 8% to 22% during the immediate postoperative period. Approximately 15% to 36% of intraoperative arrests are attributable to problems with anesthetic management and generally involve patients who were previously healthy. Another 5% to 25% of intraoperative arrests are primarily attributable to surgical problems such as excessive blood loss, whereas 13% to 22% have been observed in patients classified as poor operative risks for a variety of reasons. The remainder are attributable to a combination of these factors. Unfortunately, clearly identifiable risk factors for intraoperative cardiac arrest have not been defined.

## Cardiac conduction abnormalities

With the development of simple, reliable, and safe techniques for the insertion of both temporary and permanent pacemakers, treatment of conduction abnormalities has become an important aspect of the care of the perioperative patient.

First-degree heart block is usually a benign abnormality and results in no significant clinical impairment. Second-degree heart block of the Wenkebach (Mobitz type I) variety may be seen in otherwise "normal" hearts and is easily abolished by vagolytic agents such as atropine. Mobitz type II second-degree heart block is a more serious disorder, often appearing as a harbinger of complete heart block; pacemaker insertion is routinely recommended.

Acquired third-degree (complete) heart block is always an indication for pacemaker insertion. Although patients with bifascicular heart block have been noted to have increased surgical mortality, the excess mortality is attributable to the underlying cardiac disorder rather than the conduction abnormality itself.

Patients with an asymptomatic conduction disturbance that otherwise would not be an indication for pacemaker insertion may require such intervention when they develop ventricular irritability requiring antiarrhythmic therapy. Potent antiarrhythmic agents may suppress necessary escape mechanisms and in addition may theoretically exacerbate a preexisting conduction problem leading to the development of high-degree atrioventricular block.

In the patient with a conduction disturbance in whom transvenous pacing is not categorically indicated, external stand-by pacing may be a satisfactory contingency. As a final contingent, atropine, epinephrine, and isoproterenol are typically available for immediate use in the operating room for such patients.

Patients with permanent pacemakers pose special problems. Knowledge of the location, type, manufacturer, and age of the pacing unit is important in the management of such patients. Demand pacemakers may be temporarily "turned off" by electrical cautery, and caution must be taken in keeping cauterization units as far as possible from the pacing site. Patients must be monitored carefully while such devices are being used. A magnet for conversion of the pacemaker to fixed mode should be available for use should the demand pacer be suppressed by the cauterization unit. Although present-day pacemakers are said to be "protected" from the effects of defibrillation currents, initial attempts at defibrillation should be made with the axis of defibrillation perpendicular to the axis of the pacing wire.

# SPECIFIC CARDIAC DISORDERS IN THE GENERAL SURGICAL PATIENT

## Coronary heart disease

The combination of anesthetic agents and operative procedure place increased demands on the myocardium through both direct and indirect mechanisms, including pain, anxiety, increased metabolic requirements, catecholamine release, hypoxia, hemorrhage, fever with or without infection, and rapid fluctuations in intravascular volume. Superimposition of these factors on the patient with marginal ability to meet the demand of increased myocardial oxygen consumption, that is, the patient with coronary heart disease, results in a pronounced increase in surgical mortality. The magnitude of increased risk for patients with coronary heart disease varies from approximately two to four times that of noncoronary patients in individual series; in the overall compilation of data, surgical mortality is increased more than threefold.

## Myocardial infarction in the perioperative period

An ominous prognostic significance is associated with perioperative myocardial infarction: the combined results of 12 different series yields a mortality of 51.6% for patients with a perioperative myocardial infarction. The peak incidence of perioperative infarcts is on postoperative day 3, whereas nearly 40% of infarctions occur on days 4 to 6.

Because of the high incidence of clinically "silent" infarcts in the perioperative period, the diagnosis of myocardial infarction is often limited solely to evaluation of laboratory data. To interpret elevations of creatinine phosphokinase (CK), serum aspartate aminotransferase (ALT, formerly SGOT), and lactate dehydrogenase (LDH) caused by tissue trauma during surgery, determination of the isoenzyme fractions of CK and LDH for elevation of the cardiac-specific bands (CK and LDH, respectively) is essential. Postoperative technetium pyrophosphate scanning has also been used to detect postoperative infarctions with some success. Because of the high incidence of perioperative myocardial infarction on postoperative days 3 to 6, serial studies, including ECGs, serum isoenzymes, and radioisotope studies must be followed for up to 6 days postoperatively to document evolution of the majority of postoperative infarcts.

## Angina pectoris

Several studies have evaluated the extent to which a history of angina pectoris affects a patient's surgical risk. The overall surgical mortality varies from 0 to 16.2% for such patients, though the only study that segregated out cardiac mortality found it to be 4.0%. The overall mortality for the combined series is almost 9%. Most studies, however, do not comment on the stability of anginal pattern. Nevertheless, given the increased mortality of the inoperable patient with unstable angina, it would seem prudent to delay noncardiac surgery whenever possible in such patients.

Antianginal medicines should, in general, be continued in the patient with coronary heart disease during the perioperative period. When the patient is unable to take oral medication, either sublingual long-acting nitrates or nitroglycerin ointment may be substituted. In general, propranolol should be continued in the preoperative and postoperative periods.

## Previous myocardial infarction

A history of previous myocardial infarction denotes an increased risk of perioperative myocardial infarction. New perioperative infarction occurs in 6% to 7% of patients with evidence of previous myocardial infarction. Furthermore, the interval between a previous infarction and surgery appears to have a dramatic effect on the incidence of new perioperative infarction and mortality. In patients who experience an infarct less than 3 months before surgery, the incidence of perioperative infarction is 27% to 54% with a cardiac mortality of up to 70%. The perioperative infarction rate is reduced by at least 50% if the infarct occurred between 3 and 6 months before surgery. Most studies indicate that after 6 months, the risk of new perioperative infarction and mortality levels off at approximately 5%, a figure that is higher than that of the general population but comparable to patients with angina pectoris. The risk of noncardiac surgery in the first 3 months after infarction thus is prohibitive for all but "lifesaving" surgical procedures.

## Electrocardiographic evidence of ischemic heart disease in the asymptomatic patient

The finding of "nonspecific" ST-T wave changes in a preoperative patient remains problematic. "Nonspecific," or nonclassifiable, ST-segment changes and flat or inverted T waves are associated with an increased postoperative cardiac mortality by univariate and not multivariate analysis. In particular, ischemic-appearing ST-segment deviations are not associated with either a higher incidence of postoperative myocardial infarction or of cardiac death.

The finding of ECG signs of myocardial infarction of indeterminate age in the asymptomatic preoperative patient is another common problem. This may be a critical finding in view of the high risk associated with surgical procedures performed in the first 6 months after a myocardial infarction. A thorough search for old ECG tracings often yields important information. If no other tracings can be found and a reasonable likelihood exists that the patient has in fact sustained an unrecognized myocardial infarction at some point in the past, the conservative approach would be to delay elective surgery a minimum of 3 months. If more urgent surgery is indicated, the risks and benefits of early operation must be carefully analyzed. The cardiac risk of early operation under these circumstances, however, must be assumed to be in the 5% to 10% range.

## Previous coronary artery surgery

Available data indicate that the overall mortality from subsequent noncardiac surgery in patients who have previously undergone coronary artery bypass grafting, appears to be 1% to 2%, whereas the rate of myocardial infarction is about 1% and serious perioperative arrhythmias about 4%. Timing of the latter procedure appears to be critical: 75% of the deaths occur in patients undergoing the second procedure within 30 days of bypass surgery.

## Aortic stenosis

The risk of perioperative death in patients with clinically significant valvular heart disease appears to be 6% to 14%. This figure is highly dependent, however, on the location of the lesion, the degree of valvular dysfunction, and the extent of associated ventricular dysfunction. In one study, aortic stenosis was the only type of valvular heart disease associated with increased surgical mortality: cardiac mortality in patients with aortic stenosis was 13% versus an overall cardiac mortality of only 1.9%. A surgical mortality of 10% in all patients with aortic valve disease and mortality of 20% in patients undergoing intrathoracic or intra-abdominal surgery has been reported in patients with aortic stenosis.

## Mitral stenosis

The risk of surgery in patients with mitral stenosis is a function of the presence or absence of (1) atrial fibrillation and (2) pulmonary vascular congestion. The surgical mortality for all patients with mitral stenosis ranges from 5% to 7%. When mitral stenosis is complicated by atrial fibrillation, however, there is an 18% increase in mortality, as well as a 10% to 18% increase in nonfatal complications. The hemodynamic consequences associated with combined loss of diastolic filling time and active atrial contribution to ventricular filling presumably account for the powerful effect of atrial fibrillation on perioperative mortality.

The relationship between pulmonary vascular congestion and mitral stenosis is similar to that between atrial fibrillation and mitral stenosis: the perioperative risk is considerably higher in patients with mitral stenosis and pulmonary vascular congestion and approximates the mortality of patients with cardiac decompensation caused by other forms of cardiac disease. As well as representing a preoperative risk factor for cardiac mortality in noncardiac surgery, pulmonary vascular congestion is also a frequent postoperative complication of valvular heart disease of all types occurring in about 20% of patients with mitral regurgitation, mitral stenosis, aortic regurgitation, or aortic stenosis.

## Mitral valve prolapse

Mitral valve prolapse (MVP) usually occurs as an isolated finding but may occur in association with various cardiac or systemic disorders. MVP is relatively common, occurring in up to 10% of patients, male as well as female.

Although supraventricular, ventricular, and bradyarrhythmias have all been described in association with mitral valve prolapse, it is not clear whether arrhythmias associated with mitral valve prolapse syndrome have the same high surgical risk as arrhythmias from other causes. It would seem reasonable to approach both supraventricular and ventricular tachyarrhythmias in these patients at least as aggressively as outlined for the surgical patient in general, including perioperative propranolol therapy and continuous ECG monitoring for these patients with high-grade ventricular ectopy. Although the question of endocarditis prophylaxis for patients with mitral valve prolapse remains the subject of debate, evidence of significant mitral regurgitation secondary to mitral valve prolapse is an indication for bacterial endocarditis prophylaxis.

## Patients with valvular prostheses

Mortality in patients with valvular prostheses is generally related to hemostatic problems: patients in whom anticoagulants are discontinued 1 to 5 days preoperatively have a 5.7% mortality and complication rate, whereas patients in whom anticoagulation is continued perioperatively have an 11% mortality and a 44% complication rate.

It appears that a regimen of anticoagulation therapy maintained in the therapeutic range until 1 to 3 days before surgery and resumed 1 to 3 days postoperatively provides reasonable control of thromboembolic complications but results in an unavoidable incidence of hemorrhagic complications, a fact that must be taken into consideration in calculating the necessity for the planned surgical procedure.

An alternative approach to the problem of perioperative anticoagulation is to discontinue orally administered anticoagulants 3 to 5 days preoperatively (or reverse anticoagulation with vitamin K) and substitute full-dose heparin therapy by continuous infusion up to 6 hours preoperatively and beginning again 12 to 24 hours postoperatively. Oral anticoagulation can then be reinstituted when the patient is capable of taking medications by mouth; heparin infusion is discontinued when therapeutic prothrombin times have again been achieved by oral anticoagulation. This approach has considerable theoretical merits in terms of providing the fullest possible anticoagulation for the longest period of time while still ensuring adequate clotting capabilities during the critical immediate perioperative period.

The preoperative evaluation of the patient with prosthetic valves must also include evaluation of prosthetic dysfunction as well as the underlying functional status of the myocardium. Routine preoperative blood tests for bilirubin, lactate dehydrogenase, and reticulocyte count are useful in detecting occult hemolysis that might result from prosthetic dysfunction or a paravalvular leak. Echocardiography and fluoroscopy may be useful for the assessment of prosthetic function. Antibiotic prophylaxis is mandatory in patients with prosthetic valves. Rhythm monitoring and hemodynamic monitoring using a Swan-Ganz catheter during the perioperative period is recommended.

## Hypertrophic cardiomyopathy

Because intravascular volume depletion may result in diminution of left ventricular filling and thereby aggravate dynamic left ventricular outflow tract obstruction, careful fluid management is probably the single most important aspect of the perioperative care of patients with hypertrophic cardiomyopathy (HC). Preoperative insertion of a Swan-

Ganz catheter and intra-arterial monitoring line allows optimal management of these patients. Care must be used to avoid beta-adrenergic receptor stimulating agents such as isoproterenol, dopamine, and epinephrine, which may aggravate left ventricular outflow tract obstruction. If hypotension is refractory to treatment with volume replacement, pharmacologic therapy should be limited to alpha-adrenergic receptor stimulating agents such as phenylephrine HCl preparations (NeoSynephrine). Because of the decreased myocardial compliance in HC, supraventricular tachyarrhythmias may lead to considerable hemodynamic deterioration, and such arrhythmias generally require prompt treatment (including electrical cardioversion). Propanolol is the drug of choice for control of the ventricular response to refractory atrial fibrillation in patients with HC. Although no firm data are available on how atrial fibrillation in the setting of HC influences perioperative mortality in noncardiac surgery, one could reasonably assume that it would be at least as high as those in patients with atrial fibrillation from other causes.

# SPECIFIC TREATMENT OPTIONS IN PATIENTS WITH CARDIAC DISEASE UNDERGOING GENERAL SURGERY

## Digitalis therapy

The perioperative use of digitalis may be divided into two major categories: (1) continuation of a patient's maintenance regimen of digitalis in the perioperative period and (2) prophylactic digitalization before surgery.

Patients already receiving digitalis should continue to receive their medication during the perioperative period. Determination of the serum level of digitalis may be useful as a reference for subsequent perioperative therapy, as well as a screen for subtle digitalis excess. Since absorption of an oral dose of digoxin is less than 100%, it is recommended that parenteral maintenance doses be reduced to 85% of the oral dose.

Controversy exists regarding the role of prophylactic digitalization before surgery. The greatest potential value of such therapy concerns the group of patients who are at risk for the development of atrial fibrillation, a complication that, as mentioned previously, denotes a high incidence of postoperative complications. The majority of studies demonstrate a reduction in the rate of atrial fibrillation in prophylactically digitalized patients. With respect to overall mortality, however, there is little difference between prophylactically digitalized and nondigitalized groups. Several studies have shown increased incidence of bradyarrhythmias in perioperatively digitalized patients. Although it seems reasonable to digitalize prophylactically patients who appear to be at increased risk for the development of atrial fibrillation, rigid rules are difficult to support at present.

## Beta-blocking agents

With the widespread use of beta-adrenergic receptor blocking agents in the management of hypertension, coronary artery disease, cardiac arrhythmias, and hypertrophic cardiomyopathy, increasing attention has been devoted to the proper use of these agents in the perioperative period.

Theoretical concerns have been raised regarding the possible additive myocardial depressant effects of beta-adrenergic receptor blocking agents and general anesthetics. Some studies have demonstrated no significant difference in the frequency of perioperative hypotension, congestive heart failure, bradycardia, or mortality when propranolol was continued until just before surgery. In the only prospective randomized study of this problem, no significant difference in the postoperative incidence of myocardial infarction, hypotension, mortality, or requirement for prolonged intra-aortic balloon support was found when patients whose propranolol was stopped 48 hours before surgery were compared with patients who were given propranolol until 1 to 2 hours preoperatively.

With regard to the pharmacokinetics of propranolol withdrawal, it is now fairly clear that neither propranolol nor active metabolites are detectable in the blood or left atrial tissue 24 to 48 hours after its discontinuation. Although reports based on the use of noninvasive techniques have suggested that some degree of beta-blockade persists for 12 to 24 hours after the last dose of drug, beta-blockade measured in vitro by left atrial sensitivity to norepinephrine or isoprenaline is absent at this interval.

In summary, both the dangers of continuing propranolol perioperatively and the dangers of abrupt withdrawal probably have been exaggerated. Certainly, there is insufficient evidence to warrant discontinuation of propranolol in a patient receiving it for control of arrhythmias or hypertrophic cardiomyopathy. Similarly, in a patient with angina and good left ventricular function it is probably safer to continue the drug perioperatively. In the patient with severe angina or compromised left ventricular function, the decision is more difficult and the approach must be individualized. Should the decision be made to discontinue propranolol preoperatively, discontinuation at 48 hours preoperatively should be adequate to avoid the myocardial depressant effect of propranolol at the time of surgery.

## References

1. Goldman L, Caldera DL, Nussbaum SR, et al: Multifocal index of cardiac risk in noncardiac surgical procedures, *N Engl J Med* 297:845, 1977.
2. Mangano DT, Goldman L: Preoperative assessment of patients with known or suspected coronary disease, *N Engl J Med* 333:1750-1756, 1995.
3. Eagle KA, Coley CM, Newell JB: Combining clinical and thallium data optimizes preoperative assessment of cardiac risk before major vascular surgery, *Ann Intern Med* 110:859-866, 1989.
4. Leppo JA: Preoperative cardiac risk assessment for noncardiac surgery, *Am J Cardiol* 75:42D-51D, 1995.
5. Rihal CS, Eagle KA, Mickel MC, et al: Surgical therapy for coronary artery disease among patients with combined coronary artery and peripheral vascular vascular disease, *Circulation* 91:46-53, 1995.

# Chapter 3
## Ventricular Arrhythmias

Munther Homoud
N.A. Mark Estes III

The evaluation and treatment of patients with ventricular arrhythmias have undergone a remarkable evolution over the last decade. During this period many new agents were approved, the Cardiac Arrhythmia Suppression Trial results were reported, and one agent (encainide) was withdrawn from use. The results of prospective clinical trials have forced a serious reevaluation of the risks and benefits of suppression of ventricular arrhythmias in all patient populations. The potential benefits of antiarrhythmic drugs include reduction in the risk of sudden cardiac death or improvement in clinically important symptoms such as severe palpitations or syncope. The risks of antiarrhythmic agents include production of new arrhythmias, worsening of congestive heart failure, and noncardiac toxicity. Despite the release of numerous antiarrhythmic agents over the last decade, the patient population in whom therapy is recommended has narrowed considerably based on a reevaluation of the risk-benefit ratio of these drugs. Results of clinical investigations currently in progress will further refine future guidelines for therapy and clarify the utility of pharmacologic versus nonpharmacologic therapy such as the implantable cardioverter defibrillator (ICD) for ventricular tachycardia.

## CLASSIFICATION OF VENTRICULAR ARRHYTHMIAS

Multiple classification schemes for ventricular arrhythmias based on mechanism, morphology, frequency, associated clinical features, and prognosis have been proposed.[1-2] Ventricular premature beats (VPBs) are the most common type of ventricular arrhythmia and occur in individuals with normal hearts. Population surveys that utilize ambulatory electrocardiographic monitoring have demonstrated the presence of VPBs in 20% of men 35 to 48 years of age. The incidence increases steadily with aging: by 65 years approximately 70% of males have premature ventricular contractions. An association has been noted between frequent premature beats (more than 10 per hour, or 10 per

27

1000 QRS complexes) and males with some form of structural heart disease, most commonly coronary artery disease. In patients with ischemic heart disease, the frequency of VPBs increases with severity of coronary artery involvement and with impairment of left ventricular function. Ventricular premature beats occur in almost all patients with an acute myocardial infarction and in most patients with cardiomyopathy, myocarditis, valvular heart disease, coronary artery disease, or heart failure.

Ventricular premature beats are classified as uniform or unifocal when there is one morphology and as multiform or multifocal when there is more than one morphology. Repetitive forms include couplets (two VPBs in a row) and ventricular tachycardia (VT), three or more consecutive VPBs in a row at a rate of 120 bpm or faster. By definition, nonsustained ventricular tachycardia (NSVT) occurs when ventricular tachycardia self-terminates before 30 seconds and 100 beats. This form of VT becomes more frequent in patients with structural heart disease and advancing age but usually does not occur in patients with otherwise normal hearts. Sustained VT persists (by definition) for longer than 30 seconds or more than 100 beats, or requires termination because of hemodynamic compromise. Sustained VT is usually symptomatic and should be regarded as a life-threatening arrhythmia.

Distinguishing ventricular tachycardia from other wide-complex tachycardias such as supraventricular tachycardia with aberrancy or supraventricular arrhythmias with Wolff-Parkinson-White syndrome is important for appropriate therapy.[3] The presence of AV dissociation during a wide-complex tachycardia is diagnostic of ventricular tachycardia. Certain morphologic characteristics on the surface 12-lead ECG such as a QRS duration greater than 0.14 second and precordial concordance support the diagnosis of ventricular tachycardia. In any patient with underlying structural heart disease, particularly a history of myocardial infarction, the probability of ventricular tachycardia is very high, and agents such as verapamil should be avoided because of the risk of hemodynamic compromise.

When VPBs occur during ventricular repolarization (the R-on-T phenomenon), repetitive ventricular responses, ventricular tachycardia, or ventricular fibrillation can be initiated. Extrasystoles that occur during this vulnerable period, which corresponds to the peak of the T wave on the surface ECG, cause life-threatening arrhythmias such as ventricular tachycardia or fibrillation most commonly in the setting of acute ischemia, drug toxicity, or metabolic derangement.

Recently, a clinically useful classification scheme has been developed as a consideration of the nature of the ventricular arrhythmia, any underlying heart disease, and the likely prognosis (Table 3-1). This newer system, evolved from the proposals of Bigger and Morganroth, classifies arrhythmias into "benign," "potentially lethal," and "lethal."[1,2] Patients with "benign" ventricular arrhythmias generally have no structural heart disease. Population studies indicate that fewer than 5 VPBs per hour or fewer than 100 VPBs per day can be considered normal. Ventricular couplets and nonsustained ventricular tachycardia are rare but do occur in patients with no heart disease. Patients may

**Table 3-1.** *Clinical classification of ventricular arrhythmias*

| Class | Benign | Potentially lethal | Lethal |
|---|---|---|---|
| Risk of sudden death | Minimal | Moderate | Highest |
| Presentation | Palpitations | Screening* | Syncope† |
| | Routine examination | | Cardiac arrest |
| Serious hemodynamic compromise | No | No | Yes |
| Heart disease | None | Present | Present |
| Possible type of arrhythmia | VPBs | VPBs | VPBs |
| | NSVT | NSVT | NSVT |
| | | | SMVT |
| | | | VF |
| Treatment objective | Relieve symptoms | Possible sudden death prevention* | Sudden death prevention† |

*NSVT,* Nonsustained ventricular tachycardia; *SMVT,* sustained monomorphic ventricular tachycardia; *VF,* ventricular fibrillation; *VPBs,* ventricular premature beats.

*Modified from Bigger JT: *Am J Cardiol* 52(6):47-55, 1983, and †Morganroth J: *J Am Coll Cardiol* 252:673-676, 1984.

have palpitations with these benign ventricular arrhythmias, but they have no hemodynamic compromise (that is, with presyncope or syncope) and are at no increased risk for sudden cardiac death.

Patients with ventricular arrhythmias classified as "potentially lethal" usually have some type of structural heart disease, with coronary artery disease being the most common. The ventricular arrhythmias range from VPBs to ventricular couplets and nonsustained ventricular tachycardia. Serious hemodynamic consequences from these arrhythmias are usually absent, but symptoms such as palpitations or presyncope may occur. The risk for these patients ranges from moderate to high.

The third group in this classification scheme includes patients with malignant or "lethal" ventricular arrhythmias. Many already have experienced out-of-hospital cardiac arrest or episodes of sustained ventricular tachycardia. Most commonly, coronary artery disease with left ventricular dysfunction is present. Ventricular arrhythmias seen in these patients include sustained ventricular tachycardia, polymorphic ventricular tachycardia, and ventricular fibrillation. These patients carry a high risk of sudden cardiac death.

Lethal ventricular arrhythmias occur in 5% to 10% of the total population of patients who have ventricular arrhythmias detected. By contrast, approximately one third of these patients have benign arrhythmias.

This leaves approximately 60% of these patients with potentially lethal arrhythmias.

# EVALUATION OF VENTRICULAR ARRHYTHMIAS

The major goal of evaluation and treatment of ventricular arrhythmias is to minimize the risk of sudden cardiac death. An additional but secondary goal is to eliminate symptoms. When drugs are given to eliminate or reduce a patient's symptoms, the type, severity, and frequency of manifestation must be balanced against the side effects and potential toxicity of the agent. The clinician is justified in treating benign ventricular arrhythmias only in the rare patient who has severe symptoms, such as intolerable palpitations. Many patients with mitral valve prolapse have ventricular arrhythmias that are asymptomatic or minimally symptomatic and do not require therapy. Accelerated idioventricular rhythm, a type of automatic ventricular arrhythmia characterized by the discharge of a ventricular focus at a rate of 60 to 100 beats per minute, commonly occurs in the settings of acute myocardial ischemia, drug toxicity, particularly digitalis toxicity, or myocarditis. Patients are usually asymptomatic, and the arrhythmia does not usually degenerate into more malignant arrhythmias. Therefore this arrhythmia generally does not merit therapy. Although VT was once considered an arrhythmia that unconditionally mandated therapy, under many circumstances there is no need to institute antiarrhythmic agents.

In patients with "lethal" ventricular arrhythmias, such as prior out-of-hospital cardiac arrest from sustained VT or ventricular fibrillation (VF), prevention of subsequent major arrhythmic events is a major concern. Many studies have shown that there is a recurrence rate of 20% to 30% per year in these patients unless they are appropriately evaluated and treated. Prospective studies have demonstrated that the suppression of spontaneous arrhythmias in a highly structured protocol by use of ambulatory monitoring and exercise treadmill testing or the suppression of arrhythmias induced in the electrophysiology laboratory can significantly reduce the risk of sudden cardiac death.[4-6] However, there are no conclusive data that suppression of spontaneous "potentially lethal" ventricular arrhythmia improves survival in any patient population. As indicated in the box at the top of p. 31, all antiarrhythmic agents have risks, including the potential to cause an arrhythmia, to aggravate heart failure, to cause conduction defects, or to produce other noncardiac toxicity. Quantitative information about the frequency of the arrhythmia is essential and can be obtained by ambulatory monitoring and during exercise testing.

The decision to institute antiarrhythmic agents in a particular patient with ventricular arrhythmias can be made most rationally with additional data that establish the presence or absence of heart disease. Objective assessment of left ventricular function, obtained by an echocardiogram or a gated blood pool scan, is critically important. In selected patients at risk for coronary artery disease, exercise testing is

---

## Antiarrhythmic agents for ventricular arrhythmias

BENEFIT

Sudden death
Elimination of symptoms

RISKS

Arrhythmias
Aggravation of heart failure
Conduction defects
Organ toxicity (hepatotoxicity, agranulocytosis, thrombyocytopenia,
fever, systemic lupus erythematosus syndrome, and other toxicities)

---

reasonable before a final treatment decision is made. In the evaluation of a patient with an arrhythmia, quantitative data by Holter monitoring should be obtained to assess, in particular, any correlation of symptoms with the arrhythmia. The risk of the arrhythmias should be defined by establishment of the presence, type, and severity of the underlying heart disease by examination, electrocardiogram, and echocardiogram or a gated blood pool scan. Initiating factors, such as hypokalemia, hypomagnesemia, disturbances of pH, drug toxicity, or endocrine abnormalities, should be ruled out. Ischemia or left ventricular failure can contribute directly to worsening of acute ventricular arrhythmias and should be considered.

Electrocardiographic evidence of a prolonged Q-T interval should be excluded. In its presence, simple corrective measures such as treatment of hypokalemia or hypomagnesemia, treatment of bradycardia, and the removal of offending agents may be all that is required to rectify the arrhythmia. The clinician should be aware of multiple drugs that can result in Q-T prolongation (see the box below) and a type of polymorphic ventricular tachycardia known as *torsade de pointes.*

---

## Drugs implicated in prolonging the QT interval

*Antiarrhythmic agents:* quinidine, procainamide, disopyramide, amiodarone, sotalol, bepridil

*Psychotropic agents:* phenothiazines, tricyclic antidepressants

*Antimicrobial agents:* amantadine, chloroquine, pentamidine, erythromycin

*Liquid protein diets*

*Others:* Terfanadine

---

Based on this information, ventricular arrhythmias can be classified, as noted above, into the category of "benign," "potentially lethal," or "lethal." The quantitative arrhythmias data and objective information on the presence or absence of any structural heart disease allow the clinician to evaluate the risk versus the benefit of antiarrhythmic therapy. Benign ventricular arrhythmias present no risk of a future major arrhythmic event or sudden death; therefore, the only justification for treatment is intolerable symptoms, such as dizziness or palpitations.

As noted earlier, few data support the hypothesis that suppression of spontaneous high-grade ventricular arrhythmias affects survival in patients with potentially lethal arrhythmias. Moreover, evidence from the important Cardiac Arrhythmia Suppression Trial (CAST) study showed that the successful suppression of spontaneous ectopy after a myocardial infarction is associated with a significant increase in morbidity and mortality with the two antiarrhythmic agents encainide and flecainide.[7] As a result of the CAST study, treatment in this patient population currently is recommended only for clinically important symptoms. Although trials are currently underway evaluating the potential benefit of amiodarone use in this patient population, therapy with this potent antiarrhythmic is not justified in the postmyocardial infarction (MI) patient.

Patients with potentially lethal cardiac arrhythmias who have survived a recent myocardial infarction are problematic. The major mortality risk occurs during the first 6 months after an infarct with an equal distribution of sudden and nonsudden deaths. Based solely on the presence or absence of uniform or complex ventricular premature beats before discharge, one can stratify the risk of sudden coronary death in the 5 years after myocardial infarction. Additionally, nonsustained ventricular tachycardia detected on a Holter monitor shortly after the infarct doubles the mortality in the first year after myocardial infarction. The mortality of patients with ventricular tachycardia after myocardial infarction rises to as high as 38% at 3 years, whereas without ventricular tachycardia, it is one half that rate. Beta-blockers in the post-MI patient population have been shown to reduce mortality and the reinfarction rate and remain essential therapy in patients without clinical heart failure, bradycardia, or other contraindications.

The signal-averaged ECG (SAECG) also can be used as a noninvasive tool to further risk stratifying patients with ventricular tachyarrhythmias. Through a process of summation and amplification, SAECG allows for the detection of late potentials extending beyond the QRS complex. These potentials are from sites of slow conduction and serve as a marker of risk for development of sustained ventricular tachycardia. Although its value lies in its high negative predictive value, the combined use of Holter monitoring with frequent ectopy, low ejection fraction, and late potential after a myocardial infarction are associated with a more than 50% arrhythmic event rate in the first year after an MI.

Currently, noninvasive testing, including ambulatory monitoring, assessment of left ventricular function, and ischemia and the SAECG can identify a subset of patients at high risk of sudden death after a myocardial infarction. Unfortunately, however, multiple trials of antiarrhythmic agents in this patient population have failed to demonstrate benefit and, in several analyses, have been associated with an excess mortality when used for suppression of spontaneous arrhythmias. Whether therapy guided by programmed ventricular stimulation in the electrophysiology laboratory is warranted is currently under investigation through an ongoing trial (the Multicenter Automatic Defibrillator Implantation Trial) evaluating the role of drug therapy guided by electrophysiologic (EP) testing versus an implantable cardioverter defibrillator. An additional ongoing trial (the Multicenter Unsustained Tachycardia Trial) is randomizing high-risk patients with inducible VT in the electrophysiology laboratory to drug therapy or no treatment.

By definition, patients with "lethal" ventricular arrhythmias have a high risk of sudden death. Many of these patients have been resuscitated from out-of-hospital cardiac arrest or have had episodes of sustained ventricular tachycardia with hemodynamic collapse. Therapy of these patients includes initial stabilization of their rhythm with antiarrhythmic agents and treatment of any complication resulting from their arrhythmias. Generally these patients need cardiac catheterization to define their coronary anatomy and left ventricular function: frequently, therapy for ischemia and congestive heart failure is needed.

Over the last decade, numerous studies have shown that the incidence of a sudden cardiac death is reduced when antiarrhythmic agents prevent the induction of a ventricular arrhythmia in the electrophysiology laboratory in patients with lethal ventricular arrhythmias. In the electrophysiology laboratory, ventricular arrhythmias first are provoked after all drugs with antiarrhythmic effects have been discontinued for 5 half-lives (usually 2 to 4 days). Serial drug testing is then performed to identify an antiarrhythmic regimen that prevents induction of arrhythmias. The incidence of subsequent arrhythmias is considerably lowered when effective therapy is found by use of such electrophysiologic testing.

Although retrospective analysis of antiarrhythmic drug therapy guided by electrophysiologic testing or Holter monitoring had strongly suggested a better overall predictive accuracy of the former technique, one recent prospective comparative trial assessing electrophysiologic study versus electrocardiographic monitoring (ESVEM) for selection of antiarrhythmic drug therapy showed no difference in the ability of the techniques to prevent arrhythmia recurrence and sudden death.[6] The highly selected patient population in this study, the unconventional definitions of drug efficacy in the electrophysiologic limb, and the absence of a control group make it impossible to assess the true benefits or risks of antiarrhythmic drug therapy guided by either Holter monitoring or electrophysiologic testing. Furthermore, the sudden death rate of 7% at 1 year does not compare favorably with the 1% to 2% rate with the implantable cardioverter defibrillator.

One type of lethal ventricular arrhythmia that is best evaluated noninvasively is *torsade de pointes* because it is not reproducible in the electrophysiology laboratory. This term, which literally means 'twisted of the points', describes a rapid, polymorphic alternation of the electrical axis that occurs in the setting of a long Q-T interval.

Because the arrhythmia usually causes symptoms and can deteriorate to ventricular fibrillation, it always merits treatment. The arrhythmia is initiated by a ventricular premature beat that typically occurs as a late-cycle VPB. Prolonged Q-T interval is a prerequisite for the arrhythmia. The repolarization abnormality resulting in the long Q-T interval can be either congenital or acquired.

When the long Q-T syndrome occurs in the setting of congenital nerve deafness, it is known as the Jervell and Lange-Nielsen syndrome. When the long Q-T syndrome is an isolated congenital abnormality, it is known as the Romano-Ward syndrome. Recurrent episodes of torsade de pointes frequently are brought on by sudden sympathetic discharge, as in a fear or startle reaction. Whereas beta-blockers would promote torsade de pointes of the acquired form, they are usually effective in suppressing these arrhythmias in the congenital form of the prolonged Q-T syndrome. A sympathetic imbalance, with the left stellate ganglion being overactive relative to the right, predisposes to this arrhythmia by causing a heterogeneous repolarization of the myocardium. Permanent pacemaker therapy with beta-blocker therapy, surgical ablation of the left stellate ganglion or the implantable cardioverted defibrillator can be used in those individuals who do not respond to beta-adrenergic receptor blockade alone.

The acquired form is the more common and is secondary to drug treatment, particularly antiarrhythmic agents. The box at the bottom of p. 31 includes a list of drugs implicated in acquired Q-T prolongation. Type IA antiarrhythmic agent toxicity is a common cause of acquired long Q-T syndrome. Both hypokalemia and hypomagnesemia predispose to the condition. Q-T lengthening can occur in association with central nervous problems, such as subarachnoid hemorrhage, head trauma, and cerebral tumors. With acquired long Q-T syndrome, the life-threatening arrhythmias tend to develop in association with bradycardia. Acutely, the basis of therapy lies in identifying and removing the offending agent and rectifying electrolyte (hypokalemia and hypomagnesemia) imbalance. Treatment to increase the heart rate with isoproterenol or with a temporary pacemaker eliminates the runs of torsade de pointes. Chronically, avoidance of the offending agent or, if necessary, treatment of the bradycardia with a permanent pacemaker generally eliminates this life-threatening arrhythmia.

# DRUG THERAPY

Once the decision is made to institute antiarrhythmic agents the clinician must be familiar with the electrophysiologic and adverse effects of available drugs. Long-term pharmacologic therapy is difficult because of the unfavorable side-effect profile of antiarrhythmic agents. With the recent approval by the Food and Drug Administration (FDA) of tocainide, mexiletine, flecainide, propafenone, moricizine, sotalol, and amiodarone, there has been a dramatic expansion of the drugs available for treatment of ventricular arrhythmias.

Use of the classification scheme of Vaughn Williams for antiarrhythmic agents (Table 3–2) allows for a more systematic approach to therapeutic decisions in the treatment of ventricular arrhythmias. The class I agents are the membrane-active agents with local anesthetic action. Drugs with antisympathetic activity such as beta-adrenergic receptor blocking agents, are the class II drugs and include propranolol and acebutolol for treatment of ventricular arrhythmias. The class III agents include bretylium, sotalol, and amiodarone, which prolong the action potential duration by prolonging the repolarization process, thereby resulting in lengthening of the Q-T interval. Finally, the class IV drugs are the calcium-channel blocking agents, such as verapamil, and play no role in the treatment of ventricular arrhythmias. A summary of the pharmacologic properties of currently available antiarrhythmic agents for the treatment of ventricular arrhythmias is presented in Table 3–3.

Among the drugs that have been released recently in the last decade are two class III drugs that have been of particular interest to the clinician. Amiodarone, a class III antiarrhythmic agent, is a benzofuran derivative with potent antiarrhythmic effects. These effects include alpha- and beta-adrenergic inhibition, beta-blockade, and calcium-channel blockade in addition to its predominant potassium-channel blockade. This drug prolongs the effective refractory period in all cardiac tissues, including atrium, AV node, His-Purkinje system, ventricle, and bypass tracts in patients with ventricular preexcitation. It has a relatively minor negative inotropic effect.

The pharmacokinetics of amiodarone are complex and poorly understood. This drug has a very low clearance rate; one mode of its elimination is hepatic metabolism to desethylamiodarone with excretion through the biliary tract. It has a low bioavailability and an extremely large volume of distribution, is highly lipid soluble, and has a long elimination half-life of 26 to 107 days. A standard maintenance dose of

**Table 3-2.** *Classification of antiarrhythmic drugs*

| Class | Effect | Drugs |
|---|---|---|
| I | Local anesthetic action | Moricizine |
| IA | | Quinidine, procainamide, disopyramide |
| IB | | Lidocaine, mexiletine, tocainide |
| IC | | Flecainide, encainide, propafenone |
| II | Beta-adrenergic blockade | Propranolol, acebutolol, timolol, nadolol, pindolol, labetolol, atenolol, esmolol |
| III | Prolong repolarization | Bretylium, amiodarone, sotalol |
| IV | Calcium-channel blockade | Verapamil, diltiazem, nifedipine, nicardipine, bepradil |

**Table 3-3.** *Clinical pharmacology of antiarrhythmic agents for ventricular arrhythmias*

| Class | Agent | Total daily dose (mg) | Dosing interval (hours) | Oral bioavailability % of oral dose | Elimination half-life (hours) | "Therapeutic" serum level range (μg/mL) | Intravenous maximum loading dose | Infusion (mg/min) | Major side effects |
|---|---|---|---|---|---|---|---|---|---|
| IA | Quinidine | 600-1200 | 6-8 | 60-80 | 5-9 | 2-6 | — | — | GI, fever thrombocytopenia |
| | Procainamide | 2000-4000 | 4-6 | 70-85 | 3-5 | 3-8 | 1000 mg | 1-4 | Lupus-like syndrome, agranulocytosis |
| | Disopyramide | 400-900 | 6-8 | 85 | 6-9 | 2-5 | — | — | CHF, anticholinergic effects |

| Class | Drug | | | | | | | | Side effects |
|---|---|---|---|---|---|---|---|---|---|
| IB | Lidocaine | — | — | — | 1-2 | 1-5 | 200 mg | 1-4 | CNS, confusion, paresthesia, seizures |
| | Mexiletine | 300-900 | 6-8 | 90-100 | 10-15 | 1-2 | — | — | CNS, GI |
| | Tocainide | 1200-1800 | 6-8 | 100 | 10-15 | 3.5-10 | — | — | CNS, GI |
| IC | Flecainide | 100-400 | 12 | >90 | 12-20 | 0.2-1.0 | — | — | CHF, proarrhythmia |
| | Propafenone | 450-900 | 8 | >90 | 8-10 | — | — | — | CHF, bradycardia |
| III | Bretylium | — | — | — | — | — | 5-10 mg/kg | 2 | Hypotension |
| | Amiodarone | 200-400 | 24 | 50 | 26-107 days | 1-2.5 | — | — | All major organ systems |
| | Sotalol | 160-640 | 12 | 90 | 10-20 | 1-4 | — | — | Bradycardia, torsade de pointes, CHF |
| I | Moricizine | 600-900 | 8 | 90 | 8-6 | — | — | — | Proarrhythmia, dizziness |

*CHF*, Congestive heart failure; *CNS*, central nervous system; *GI*, gastrointestinal.

the drug is 200 to 400 mg daily after a loading period of 1 to 2 weeks with 1200 mg daily. The serum level should be kept between 1.0 to 2.5 $\mu$g/mL.

Amiodarone is effective in the suppression of spontaneous and inducible ventricular tachycardia. When VT recurs in patients receiving amiodarone, it is frequently slow (<150 bpm) and hemodynamically well tolerated. In the evaluation of patients who survived out-of-hospital cardiac arrest, the empiric use of amiodarone, compared to the use of conventional antiarrhythmic agents, significantly reduced cardiac death, arrhythmic death, and defibrillator discharges with syncope. Because of the complexity of its administration and the frequency and nature of its complication profile, amiodarone currently is indicated only for life-threatening ventricular arrhythmias.

Side effects are common with long-term use of amiodarone. Milder side effects include skin reactions with photosensitivity, or deposition of the drug in the skin that causes a peculiar slate-gray pigmentation. Gastrointestinal side effects include nausea and constipation. Corneal microdeposits develop in virtually all patients but rarely affect visual acuity. However, patients frequently complain of halos and difficulty with night vision. Neurologic toxicity includes peripheral neuropathy, tremors, ataxia, headaches, and proximal muscle weakness. The drug has a high iodine content, 37% by weight, and as a result hyperthyroidism or hypothyroidism develops in 3% to 5% of patients.

The more serious side effects of amiodarone include pulmonary alveolitis, which occurs in up to 15% of patients. Death has been reported in 5% to 10% of patients suffering from amiodarone pulmonary toxicity. Frequently, this toxicity manifests with subtle complaints of dyspnea or nonproductive cough. The chest roentgenogram shows diffuse interstitial or alveolar infiltrates. Routine screening of pulmonary function tests is the most sensitive indicator of amiodarone pulmonary toxicity. A reduction in diffusion capacity for carbon monoxide of 15% compared to a predrug study indicates probable amiodarone pulmonary toxicity. The presence of two out of three of the following has been recommended to be suggestive of amiodarone pulmonary toxicity: new symptoms, new chest roentgenogram findings, 15% or greater reduction in $DL_{CO}$ (carbon monoxide diffusion in the lungs), or total lung capacity in the absence of worsening heart failure or pulmonary infection. Amiodarone increases the serum digoxin level and can unpredictably potentiate the anticoagulant effects of warfarin. Although an extremely effective drug in the suppression of spontaneous arrhythmias, amiodarone use should be limited to patients with "lethal" ventricular arrhythmias, which are not controlled by alternative antiarrhythmic agents.

Sotalol recently has been approved for use in the United States. Sotalol, a beta-blocker with unique antiarrhythmic properties, is used as a racemic mixture. Although the D isomer has minimal beta-blocking effect, both the D and L isomers have a potassium-channel blocking effect. Sotalol is excreted unchanged by the kidneys; thus the dose should be adjusted in renal insufficiency. The starting dose is 80 mg twice a day; higher doses are necessary to achieve antiarrhythmic effect.

This effect manifests as a prolongation of the Q-T interval corrected for heart rate. These patients thus are susceptible to polymorphic ventricular tachycardia (torsade des pointes). In the ESVEM trial 35% of patients with ventricular tachyarhythmias randomly assigned to sotalol had electrophysiologic studies proving the drug efficacious compared to 16% for the other six drugs ($p < 0.001$). Sotalol caused a significant decline in cardiac and arrhythmic death and was better tolerated than the other drugs. As any beta-blocker, sotalol can worsen heart failure.

# GUIDELINES FOR ANTIARRHYTHMIC DRUG USE

If symptomatic, benign ventricular arrhythmias such as premature ventricular contractions or nonsustained ventricular tachycardia require therapy, the guiding principle should be to initiate treatment with agents that are associated with the least harm before one uses them with other drugs. In this patient population, such drugs as beta-blockers, the class IB agents, class IC agents, and moricizine have an extremely low risk of causing an arrhythmia.[7] The class IA agents and sotalol should be administered only when the patient is hospitalized to detect any early Q-T prolongation or torsade de pointes. In patients with prognostically significant, potentially lethal arrhythmias, specific antiarrhythmic therapy is not warranted unless the patient is symptomatic. If the patient has had a prior myocardial infarction, beta-blockers should be used unless contraindicated. In patients with symptomatic ventricular premature contractions or nonsustained VT in the setting of structural heart disease, the same principles for antiarrhythmic drug use should be applied as those for patients with benign ventricular arrhythmias. Based on its considerable toxicity, amiodarone is not an appropriate drug for suppression of symptomatic benign or potentially lethal ventricular arrhythmias.

In patients with prior episodes of sustained ventricular tachycardia, or ventricular fibrillation, multiple antiarrhythmic drugs have been associated with reduction in mortality when guided by Holter monitoring or electrophysiologic testing. Based on the ESVEM trial results, many experts believe that sotalol may have a survival benefit in the absence of contraindications. The class IA agents should be used alone or in combination with a class IB agent. In patients with prior sustained VT or VF, the class IC antiarrhythmic drugs, flecainide or propafenone, have a high risk of producing an arrhythmia; this observation also applies to moricizine. Accordingly, their use in patients with episodes of prior sustained VT or VF should be limited. Amiodarone is an option that should be considered if alternative antiarrhythmic drugs are unsuccessful or contraindicated. In patients with prior episodes of sustained VT or VF, however, drug therapy guided by electrophysiologic testing and Holter monitoring has not reduced the likelihood of sudden cardiac death as much as nonpharmacologic therapies such as the implantable cardioverter defibrillator (ICD). Accordingly, most arrhythmia experts consider the ICD as the preferred therapy in patients with prior episodes of sustained VT or VF.

## NONPHARMACOLOGIC APPROACHES TO VENTRICULAR ARRHYTHMIAS

For patients with prior episodes of sustained VT or VF, in the past pharmacologic therapy directed by programmed ventricular stimulation or Holter monitoring was accepted as the initial approach to management with surgical, ablative, or "device" therapy reserved for patients who did not respond to antiarrhythmic agents. A minority of patients with previous episodes of sustained ventricular tachycardia or fibrillation respond to drug therapy guided by electrophysiologic testing end points. Drug therapy is palliative, dependent on patient compliance, and frequently accompanied by side effects. Additionally, there is growing skepticism regarding the ability of such drugs to reduce arrhythmia recurrence and sudden death in patients with greatly reduced ejection fraction. Based on these considerations and the refinements in the last several years in mapping and guided surgery, ablative techniques, and ICD therapy, nonpharmacologic approaches now have emerged as accepted and in many patients the preferred treatment options.[8]

In selected patients with discrete anterior or anterior-apical aneurysms and coronary artery disease, mapping guided-subendocardial resection now has an operative mortality of approximately 5% without induced or spontaneous ventricular tachycardia in over 90% of patients. Although coronary artery bypass surgery improves symptoms, decreases the frequency of myocardial infarction, and decreases total mortality and sudden death in patients with left-main or three-vessel disease, sustained monomorphic ventricular tachycardia does not respond to revascularization alone. Although catheter ablation has revolutionized the treatment of supraventricular arrhythmias, providing a cure in over 95% of patients, its role in the treatment of ventricular tachycardia currently remains limited. In patients with coronary artery disease, congestive cardiomyopathies, or other forms of structural heart disease, the cure rate of ventricular tachycardia is approximately 30% with current catheter-based techniques, to the extent that it has been used in a limited fashion. However, certain types of ventricular tachycardia, such as those originating from the right ventricular outflow tract, idiopathic left ventricular tachycardia with a right bundle and superior axis originating from the region of the left posterior fascicle and ventricular tachycardia due to bundle-branch re-entry, have very high success rates with catheter ablation techniques.

ICD therapy has evolved from the first clinical implant in 1980 to a widely used and highly refined technology for the treatment of sustained VT or VF. The initial devices were able to recognize ventricular fibrillation and deliver a high-energy shock. Currently, clinically available devices also recognize ventricular tachycardia and have the ability to deliver tiered therapy with antitachycardia pacing, cardioversion, defibrillation, and bradycardia pacing as well as memory to store electrocardiographic data regarding detected arrhythmias. With nonthoracotomy lead systems and smaller devices allowing pectoralis implant, the operative mortality with device implantation is now less than 1%. Furthermore, there has been a consistent reduction in the sudden death rate to less than 1.5% per year with the implantable cardioverter defibrillator. A multicenter trial to assess whether ICDs use results in a lower mortality than that from pharmacologic therapy with sotalol and amiodarone in patients who have been resuscitated from sudden cardiac death caused by ventricular fibrillation or are otherwise at very high risk of death from ventricular tachycardia (AVID Trial) currently is enrolling patients. This study should determine whether implantation of an ICD or antiarrhythmic drug therapy results in longer survival.

# SUMMARY

The benefits of therapy with any antiarrhythmic agent include reduction in mortality or improvement or elimination of clinically important symptoms related to the arrhythmia. As yet, no antiarrhythmic drug has shown conclusive improvement in patient survival when used to suppress VPBs or nonsustained ventricular tachycardia in any setting. However, therapy is warranted in patients who have clinically important symptoms related to these arrhythmias. Currently in progress are clinical trials that will further define the relative risk and benefits of pharmacologic and nonpharmacologic therapy in patients with potentially lethal and lethal arrhythmias. Additionally, trials are in progress in patients with malignant ventricular arrhythmias examining the benefits, risks, and costs of pharmacologic therapy compared to the implanted cardioverter defibrillator. Future research on the basic mechanisms of ventricular arrhythmias and the influence of drugs on these arrhythmias should provide useful insights for improvements in treatment.

## References

1. Bigger JT: Definition of benign versus malignant ventricular arrhythmias: targets for treatment, *Am J Cardiol* 52(6):47-55, 1983.
2. Morganroth J: Premature ventricular complexes: diagnosis and indications for therapy, *J Am Coll Cardiol* 252:673-676, 1984.
3. Wellens HJJ, Bar FWH, Lie KI: The value of the electrocardiogram in the differential diagnosis of a tachycardia with a widened QRS complex, *Am J Med* 64:27-33, 1978.
4. Graboys TB, Lown B, Podrid PJ, DeSilva R: Long term survival of patients with malignant ventricular arrhythmia treated with antiarrhythmic drugs, *Am J Cardiol* 50:437-443, 1982.
5. Cameron J, Isner J, Salem D, Estes NAM: Cardiac electrophysiologic testing: its role in the selection of antiarrhythmic drug regimens for supraventricular and ventricular arrhythmias, *Pharmacotherapy* 5(2):95-108, 1985.
6. Mason JW for the Electrophysiologic Study Versus Electrocardiographic Monitoring Investigators: A comparison of electrophysiologic testing with Holter monitoring to predict antiarrhythmic-drug efficacy for ventricular tachyarrhythmias, *N Engl J Med* 329:445-451, 1993.

7. Reiffel JA, Estes NAM III, Waldo AL, et al: A consensus report on antiarrhythmic drug use, *Clin Cardiol* 17:103-116, 1994.

8. Estes NAM: Strategies for management of malignant ventricular arrhythmias: role of pharmacology, surgery, ablation and the implantable cardioverter defibrillator. In Estes NAM, Manolis AS, Wang PJ, editors: *The implantable cardioverter defibrillator: a comprehensive textbook,* New York, 1994, Marcel Dekker.

# Chapter 4

# *The Systolic Murmur*

Jeffrey M. Isner

Auscultation of a previously undescribed systolic murmur in an adult being seen by an internist for the first time or being evaluated for a noncardiac surgical procedure is one of the most common bases for cardiac consultation. The history, physical examination, and a variety of noninvasive diagnostic tests may be used to good advantage in most cases to avoid invasive evaluation of such a murmur. On the other hand, in occasional patients, the necessity for performing invasive evaluation is unequivocal. Therapeutic responses to the finding of a new systolic murmur are dependent on the results of the diagnostic workup.

## DIAGNOSIS

### History

Certain elements of the patient's personal medical history are essential to proper evaluation of the systolic murmur and include the age of the murmur, the age and sex of the patient, the presence or absence of syncope, chest pain, or dyspnea, and the family history. The first element is establishing whether the murmur is old or new. If the patient has been previously healthy and has not been followed regularly by a physician, no information may be available in this regard. A childhood history of a heart murmur is notoriously unreliable; a positive history often reflects a so-called innocent murmur, unrelated to organic heart disease; a negative history may be the result of limited examinations or limited information transmitted from the pediatrician to the mother to the patient. Two sources of routine examination that merit inquiry are examination for life insurance and examination on entry into or discharge from the armed forces. In these cases, a positive history is generally more reliable than a negative history.

If the history is known to be reliable, the absence of a previous history of a murmur virtually excludes the possibility that the systolic murmur is being generated across the right ventricular outflow tract or pulmonic valve. In the adult patient in whom the murmur is caused by left ventricular outflow tract obstruction, a history of a previous murmur is consistent with both a congenitally bicuspid aortic valve and a hypertrophic cardiomyopathy. In cases in which the systolic murmur is believed to be related to the mitral apparatus, a positive history most commonly indicates a preexisting floppy mitral valve, whereas a negative history indicates the likelihood of papillary muscle dysfunction or spontaneous rupture of mitral valve chordae tendineae.

The patient's sex and age are often overlooked in assessment of the basis for a systolic murmur. In general, valvular aortic stenosis is much more common in men than in women. Mitral regurgitation caused by mitral valve prolapse appears to be more common in women than in men. In the adult between 21 and 45 years of age, principle differential diagnostic considerations include a congenitally bicuspid aortic valve, mitral valve prolapse, and hypertrophic cardiomyopathy. In patients over 45 years of age, the principle considerations become aortic stenosis attributable to a calcified, congenitally normal, tricuspid aortic valve; mitral regurgitation caused by papillary muscle dysfunction; and mitral regurgitation caused by a calcified mitral anulus.

A history of syncope is likewise contributory because it generally indicates that the source of the systolic murmur is the left ventricular outflow tract. Syncope represents one of the classic manifestations of critical aortic stenosis and, as such, represents an ominous finding that is generally considered to be an indication for prompt, definitive therapy. On the other hand, when syncope complicates hypertrophic cardiomyopathy, it is not uncommon for the patient to complain of multiple syncopal episodes; in this setting syncope does not have the same ominous prognostic significance as in patients with critical aortic stenosis. Syncope is an unusual feature of a systolic murmur associated with the mitral valve apparatus unless it is attributable to associated conduction disturbances or tachyarrhythmias.

Complaints of anginal chest discomfort are most often associated with a systolic murmur generated in the left ventricular outflow tract. Chest discomfort that may be indistinguishable from angina is common in both critical aortic stenosis and hypertrophic cardiomyopathy. When anginal chest discomfort is associated with a systolic murmur that represents mitral regurgitation, the angina generally indicates that the systolic murmur is secondary to the basis for angina; a typical example is the patient with papillary muscle dysfunction attributable to ischemic heart disease. Angina is much less common in cases of primary mitral valve dysfunction, though patients with substantial mitral regurgitation may often complain of an anginal-equivalent pain resulting from severe pulmonary vascular congestion.

A complaint of dyspnea on exertion is less helpful in discriminating the source of a systolic murmur. Dyspnea on exertion is typically the first symptom that results from aortic stenosis but may occur in patients with hypertrophic cardiomyopathy and mitral regurgitation as well, because of pulmonary vascular congestion.

Although the patient's personal history may offer clues to the basis for the systolic murmur, the patient's family history is helpful in essentially only one situation, hypertrophic cardiomyopathy. In more than 50% of the cases, hypertrophic cardiomyopathy is a familial disease; accordingly a family history of premature sudden unexpected death, syncope, or heart murmur may constitute useful clues toward this diagnosis.

## Physical examination

Although the physical examination may leave undecided the magnitude of physiologic dysfunction represented by a systolic murmur, it may nevertheless be adequate to identify the source of the murmur.

Examination of the carotid pulses is extremely helpful: the classic *parvus et tardus,* bilaterally symmetrical carotid upstroke is typical of critical aortic stenosis. In the elderly patient, the contour of the pulse is more useful than auscultation of the pulse, inasmuch as the latter may be more unduly influenced by local carotid vascular disease. A "spike-and-dome" contour to the carotid pulse is the classic physical finding of hypertrophic cardiomyopathy. Mitral regurgitation classically produces a bounding pulse with a fast descent. In a younger patient, particularly if carotid disease is excluded, the finding of a bruit in association with an abnormal carotid examination is a clue that the systolic murmur is caused by the left ventricular outflow tract obstruction.

Examination of the jugular venous pulse is more useful in the evaluation of systolic murmurs generated on the right side of the heart than on the left side of the heart. The finding of large v waves in the jugular venous pulse is typical of tricuspid regurgitation. The finding of a well-defined, double-impulse (a-wave and v-wave) jugular venous contour is more typical of pulmonary outflow tract obstruction.

Palpation of the precordium is an often neglected examination that is crucial to the evaluation of the systolic murmur. Palpation of a systolic thrill (best performed using the portion of the palm at the base of the digits, with the patient lying in either the left lateral decubitus position or sitting upright) may indicate that the murmur is caused by the left ventricular outflow tract obstruction when the thrill is palpated along the upper sternal border. In contrast, when the thrill is palpated at the left ventricular apex, the murmur is more likely caused by mitral regurgitation. The exception to this is the patient with a recent myocardial infarction in whom a systolic thrill caused by a ruptured ventricular septum may be palpable at any site between the lower left sternal border and the left ventricular apex, though the lower left sternal border is the classic location of this murmur. The finding of a so-called triple ripple, that is, three distinct precordial palpatory impulses, is typical of hypertrophic cardiomyopathy. A well-localized, protracted precordial impulse generally represents left ventricular outflow tract obstruction; a diffuse, fleeting precordial impulse is more typical of a volume-overload lesion such as mitral regurgitation.

Although the auscultatory features of $S_1$ are generally not helpful, detection of two clear components to the $S_2$ may be extremely helpful: absence of an aortic component of the second heart sound indicates the presence of valvular aortic stenosis. Prolonged splitting of the second heart sound may be caused by pulmonic stenosis. The finding of gallop sounds are nonspecific, though the finding of gallop sounds that augment with inspiration may indicate that the associated systolic murmur is right sided.

Discrete sounds between $S_1$ and $S_2$ may be specific for the anatomic basis of the systolic murmur. An ejection sound is typical of a non-calcified, congenitally bicuspid aortic valve. The finding of a systolic click, particularly when it occurs during the latter two thirds of systole, is typical of a mitral valve prolapse. In the rare adult who escapes detection of a congenital right-sided murmur during childhood, an ejection click may be associated with valvular pulmonic stenosis.

Careful attention to the auscultatory features of the systolic murmur is critical in determining its origin and importance. A holosystolic blowing murmur almost always is caused by mitral regurgitation and is heard best at the left ventricular apex, radiating well to the left anterior axillary line. A harsh diamond-shaped murmur is generally caused by valvular aortic stenosis; it is important to note that in the elderly patient the murmur of valvular aortic stenosis may be heard better at the left ventricular apex than along the left upper sternal border. The murmurs of hypertrophic cardiomyopathy, mitral valve prolapse, and papillary muscle dysfunction are highly variable in configuration, intensity, and quality. As a result, the performance of several maneuvers is mandatory in the evaluation of the undefined systolic murmur. The most useful of these maneuvers, provided that the patient is physically able to cooperate, is the standing-squatting maneuver. An increase in the intensity of the murmur going from the squatting to the standing position is typical of patients with hypertrophic cardiomyopathy and mitral valve prolapse. A similar response to the Valsalva maneuver occurs in these two entities; however, the Valsalva maneuver is less reliable than standing-squatting for two reasons. First, it is difficult for many patients to perform the maneuver correctly, particularly if they are told to "bear down as if you are having a bowel movement." It is generally more useful to ask the patient either to purse his lips around his index finger and "blow on your finger as if you are blowing up a balloon," or to ask him to "press your belly against my hand." Second, if the outflow tract obstruction caused by hypertrophic cardiomyopathy is particularly severe, the Valsalva maneuver may result in total obstruction to the left ventricular outflow, causing a paradoxical diminution in the intensity of the murmur.

One "maneuver" that does not require any active participation on behalf of the patient is evaluation of the systolic murmur in response to a premature beat, or a short cycle followed by a long cycle in patients with atrial fibrillation. The murmur of valvular aortic stenosis typically increases during the long cycle, whereas the murmur of mitral regurgitation typically remains unchanged.

Whether the systolic murmur is accompanied by a diastolic murmur provides an important clue to the site at which the systolic murmur is being generated and to the morphology of the responsible valve. The diastolic "blowing" murmur of aortic insufficiency, best heard at the lower left sternal border, is common with either rheumatic aortic stenosis or valvular aortic stenosis attributable to a congenitally bicuspid aortic valve. On the other hand, aortic insufficiency present in more than trace amounts is rare in patients with a calcified, congenitally normal, tricuspid aortic valve. The presence of a diastolic murmur is rare in patients with dynamic subaortic left ventricular outflow tract obstruction, though common in patients in whom left ventricular outflow tract obstruction is attributable to a subvalvular discrete membrane. The finding of an opening snap and a diastolic low-frequency rumbling murmur at the left ventricular apex indicates that the systolic murmur of mitral regurgitation may be rheumatic in origin. Diastolic rumbles in the absence of an opening snap may be caused by torrential mitral regurgitation or severe mitral valve annular calcification.

## Electrocardiography

Until recently the electrocardiogram was more important in the evaluation of the systolic murmur than it is now with the currently available noninvasive imaging techniques. The absence of any electrocardiographic abnormalities is consistent with a nonorganic basis for the systolic murmur, such as anemia, an alternative high-output state, or innocuous valvular calcification. The most useful positive finding is left ventricular hypertrophy, which favors a diagnosis of left ventricular outflow tract obstruction. It is important to note that finding in elderly individuals because of changes in chest-wall configuration or voltage criteria, such as ST-T wave changes. Although the finding of left atrial enlargement is generally a clue to the presence of mitral valve disease, left atrial enlargement may occur in patients with left ventricular outflow tract obstruction caused by a hypertrophied noncompliant left ventricle. Electrocardiographic evidence of myocardial infarction indicates that papillary muscle dysfunction attributable to ischemic heart disease may be the basis for the systolic murmur. Finally, in any patient with systolic murmur and a "bizarre" electrocardiogram, the patient should be considered to have hypertrophic cardiomyopathy until proved otherwise.

Echocardiography. Cardiac ultrasonography has proved invaluable in the evaluation of the systolic murmur. Characterization of hypertrophic cardiomyopathy, for example, has paralleled the development of increasingly sophisticated ultrasound capabilities. The principal findings of an asymmetrically hypertrophied ventricular septum and systolic anterior motion of the mitral valve are the classic sine qua non findings for hypertrophic cardiomyopathy on M-mode echocardiography. Evaluation of such patients by two-dimensional echocardiography has indicated that the site of asymmetric hypertrophy may be occasionally located outside the M-mode beam; thus two-dimensional echocardiographic examination is recommended for thorough evaluation of this entity. Moreover, left ventricular outflow tract obstruction has been documented in a small number of patients with symmetric ventricular hypertrophy, and so even the finding of asymmetry may not be required to establish this diagnosis.

Likewise, the clinical description of the "floppy mitral valve" or "mitral valve prolapse" syndrome was fueled by the advent of M-mode echocardiography. An echocardiogram that is diagnostic of mitral valve prolapse, whether by M-mode or two-dimensional examination, is obviously helpful in establishing that mitral valve as the source of systolic murmur. On the other hand, it must be noted that echocardiographic patterns of mitral valve prolapse are highly variable and are extremely subject to viewer interpretation. Therefore the isolated finding of atypical mitral valve prolapse by cardiac ultrasonography, particularly if unaccompanied by typical clinical auscultatory findings, must be regarded with caution.

Evaluation of aortic stenosis perhaps is most valuable when the aortic valve is clearly seen, when the opening can be recognized to be totally normal, and when there is no increased echo intensity of the aortic valve to indicate fibrosis or calcification; in such a case, the diagnosis of hemodynamically significant aortic stenosis can be confidently excluded. On the other hand, when the aortic valve leaflets are heavily calcified, when no opening can be recognized, and when no discernible movement can be observed, a diagnosis of calcific aortic stenosis can be established with certainty. In intermediate cases, the echocardiogram may be useful in establishing that the aortic valve is the likely source of the systolic murmur but may not be adequate for defining the presence or absence of a hemodynamic deficit.

The recent addition of Doppler echocardiography to the ultrasound examination promises to be helpful in grading more accurately the severity of the deficit associated with the systolic murmur. Preliminary use of this modality has indicated a relatively close correspondence between gradients measured at the time of cardiac catheterization and gradients estimated on the basis of Doppler-derived algorithms. The use of color-coded Doppler scanning recently has been suggested as a promising means of quantifying the extent of mitral regurgitation, but further confirmatory studies are required to establish the accuracy of this technique.

**Radioisotope ventriculography.** Radioisotope ventriculography perhaps is most useful in the evaluation of mitral regurgitation. In such patients, the finding of a left ventricular stroke volume that is more than twice the right ventricular stroke volume indicates that the systolic murmur likely is attributable to mitral regurgitation, provided that a ventricular septal defect has been excluded. The finding of segmental wall-motion abnormalities, whether by radioisotope ventriculography or by two-dimensional echocardiography, indicates that papillary muscle dysfunction related to ischemic heart disease may be the basis for the systolic murmur.

**Fluoroscopy.** The importance of fluoroscopy in detecting aortic valve calcification is frequently overlooked. Hemodynamically significant aortic stenosis in patients over 55 years of age is rare in the absence of detectable valvular calcium. The converse, however, is not true: valvular calcification may exist and may cause a murmur to be heard without resulting in hemodynamic deficit.

## Invasive evaluation
A decision regarding the necessity for additional invasive examination is made after a synthesis of data gathered from the history, physical examination, and noninvasive tests.

Of the possible causes for a systolic murmur, the one that most often mandates invasive examination is valvular aortic stenosis. When two-dimensional echocardiography or cardiac fluoroscopy, or both, demonstrate a normal aortic valve, the need for invasive evaluation is obviated. If one of these evaluations is abnormal, however, determination of the hemodynamic severity of aortic stenosis becomes increasingly difficult as the appearance of the valve, determined noninvasively, becomes progressively more abnormal. Virtually every noninvasive evaluation that has been proposed at one time or another to be capable of discriminating hemodynamically significant from insignificant aortic stenosis has ultimately failed. The additional fact that so often dictates invasive evaluation for the question of aortic stenosis is the well-documented propensity for this lesion to cause sudden unexpected death. The 10-year follow-up study of patients with asymptomatic aortic stenosis in whom the calculated valve area is less than 0.5 cm$^2$ is poor enough that surgery is considered mandatory for all such patients. Thus the imperfect nature of noninvasive tests designed to evaluate aortic stenosis, combined with the frequently fatal nature of this lesion, most often leads to cardiac catheterization.

In contrast, the noninvasive diagnosis of hypertrophic cardiomyopathy in a patient who has not been previously treated for that condition does not require further invasive evaluation. Likewise, in most patients in whom mitral regurgitation is the basis for the systolic murmur, further invasive evaluation is unnecessary, provided that the patient is asymptomatic or only mildly symptomatic and that ventricular function is still intact (left ventricular ejection fraction greater than 55%). A possible exception to this rule is mitral regurgitation caused by papillary muscle dysfunction; in this case, the decision to proceed to invasive evaluation is based principally on considerations related to ischemic heart disease. For systolic murmurs originating on the right side of the heart, invasive evaluation is mandated only if the patient is symptomatic enough to be considered a candidate for operative intervention.

## TREATMENT

Treatment of the various lesions responsible for a systolic murmur differs greatly, depending on the anatomic basis for the murmur. In the case of a patient with mitral valve prolapse, for example, the only "treatment" required is antibiotic prophylaxis for bacterial endocarditis. Although recommendations have varied to some extent as to which patients with mitral valve prolapse require prophylaxis, my opinion is that all patients with this diagnosis should receive prophylaxis, provided that there is no demonstrated allergy to the particular antibiotic to be used. The bases for this recommendation are as follows:

1. Patients with isolated systolic clicks, in the absence of a murmur, have been documented to develop endocarditis.
2. The auscultatory findings in this syndrome, even in a given patient, are so variable that it is common for a patient to have a

murmur heard on one occasion and then on another occasion to demonstrate only a click.

3. If the echocardiographic pattern is absolutely diagnostic of mitral valve prolapse, it is possible that an associated murmur may be heard on some occasions but not on others; thus this group of patients should not be excluded from prophylaxis.

4. In patients with isolated clicks, the murmur may at times be provoked by various maneuvers, whereas at other times, in part because of poor patient cooperation, it may not be possible for it to be provoked; the presence or absence of a provokable murmur is thus an inadequate criterion on which to base the decision for prophylaxis.

5. The risk-to-benefit ratio of prophylaxis versus endocarditis justifies liberal use of prophylaxis in this syndrome.

At the other extreme is the treatment of the patient with hemodynamically significant aortic stenosis. Because of the well-documented propensity of this lesion to cause sudden unexpected death, surgical intervention is recommended for any symptomatic patient with hemodynamically significant aortic stenosis. Although controversy exists regarding the advisability of surgical versus medical therapy in asymptomatic patients, the scant data that exist in this regard indicate that in the younger patient surgical intervention may be advised. In the elderly patient, particularly the "oldest old," the natural history of hemodynamically significant aortic stenosis is unknown. Therefore in this age group, particularly when other confounding medical illness exists, the decision to recommend surgery may not be straightforward.

For the patient with hypertrophic cardiomyopathy, the first line of treatment is medical therapy with beta-adrenergic receptor blockade or calcium-channel blockers. Available evidence indicates that beta-blockers may be interchangeable for the treatment of this disorder. Among the calcium-channel blockers, verapamil has been used most extensively in the treatment of this disorder; nifedipine has been used successfully but less widely. Few data exist regarding the treatment of hypertrophic cardiomyopathy with diltiazem. Finally, Norpace (disopyramide phosphate preparations) has been used successfully in selected patients. The decision to recommend surgical intervention for the patient with hypertrophic cardiomyopathy can be made, with rare exception, only after failure of the patient to respond to medical therapy.

In the patient with mitral regurgitation caused by primary valve dysfunction, no surgical intervention is required, provided that the patient is asymptomatic or mildly symptomatic with intact ventricular function. In the patient with class III or class IV congestive heart failure symptoms who has failed to respond to conventional medical treatment and in whom ventricular function remains intact, surgical therapy is advised. The difficult decision concerns patients who, according to symptoms alone or in combination with the results of medical therapy, do not require surgical intervention but in whom there is evidence of progressive deterioration of left ventricular function. The decision to operate on these patients is strictly a matter of attempting to intervene at a time when further deterioration of left ventricular function may be prevented. Unfortunately, experience has been less than perfect with both noninvasive and invasive tests designed to allow one to predict the progression of left ventricular dysfunction. Thus a decision to operate on such patients must rest on the practitioner's preferred means of predicting the integrity of left ventricular function.

As mentioned previously, the decision for surgical intervention in the patient in whom a systolic murmur is caused by papillary muscle dysfunction rests principally on considerations related to ischemic heart disease. In particular, however, it should be noted that ejection-phase indices or other tests of left ventricular function do not have the same meaning in the patient with mitral regurgitation caused by ischemic heart disease that they may have in patients with primary mitral valve dysfunction. Specifically, the patient with impaired left ventricular function and secondary mitral regurgitation is more likely to improve after surgery as the result of revascularization combined with mitral valve replacement or left ventricular aneurysmectomy.

Finally, surgery is rarely required in the adult patient with a systolic murmur caused by pulmonary outflow tract obstruction. The same is true for isolated tricuspid regurgitation. One significant exception to the latter statement, however, is the patient with isolated tricuspid regurgitation caused by infective endocarditis, in whom simple excision without valve replacement is generally successful.

## References

1. Johnson LW, Grossman W, Dalen JE, Dexter L: Pulmonic stenosis in the adult: long-term follow-up results, *N Engl J Med* 287:1159-1163, 1972.
2. Roberts WC, Perloff JK: Mitral valvular disease: a clinicopathologic survey of the condition causing the mitral valve to function abnormally, *Ann Intern Med* 77:939-956, 1972.
3. Frank S, Johnson A, Ross J Jr: Natural history of valvular aortic stenosis, *Br Heart J* 35:41-45, 1973.
4. Maron BJ, Isner JM, McKenna WJ: Bethesda Conference #26: Recommendations for determining eligibility for competition in athletes with cardiovascular abnormalities. Task Force 3: hypertrophic cardiomyopathy, myocarditis and other myopericardial diseases, and mitral valve prolapse, *J Am Coll Cardiol* 24:845-899, 1994.
5. Isner JM: Aortic valve stenosis. In Al Zaibag MA, Duran CMG, editors: *Valvular heart disease,* New York, 1995, Marcel Dekker, Inc.
6. Verheul HA, van den Brink RBA, Bouma BJ, et al: Analysis of risk factors for excess mortality after aortic valve replacement, *J Am Coll Cardiol* 26:1280-1286, 1995.
7. Spirito P, Chiarella F, Carratino L, et al: Clinical course and prognosis of hypertrophic cardiomyopathy in an outpatient population, *N Engl J Med* 320:749-755, 1989.

# Chapter 5

# Anticoagulation in Cardiac Disorders

Jeffrey M. Isner

Interests frequently are called upon for an opinion regarding the use of anticoagulation in the treatment of certain forms of heart disease. In most cases the opinion rendered is just that—an "opinion." Uncertainty exists because of a paucity of data relating the *risks* of anticoagulation in an individual patient with a particular cardiac disorder and the *benefits* of anticoagulation. Such risk-to-benefit analyses are further confounded by the fact that the level of anticoagulation that represents the optimum compromise between efficacy and toxicity (bleeding) remains a matter of controversy. The conventional teaching states that the prothrombin time should be maintained at 1.5 to 2.5 times control. More recent data indicate that much lower levels of anticoagulation (1.2 to 1.5 times normal) may be effective and less likely to provoke bleeding, at least for treatment of recurrent venous thromboembolism. Furthermore, though for several cardiovascular disorders, there exists a consensus regarding the need, or the lack of need, for anticoagulation, for most situations in which the internist is consulted data are inadequate to allow definite recommendations. This caveat must be kept in mind when one is seeing patients with the conditions. I will focus on the situations in which the issue of anticoagulation is most often raised.

## RHEUMATIC MITRAL VALVE DISEASE

The subset of patients with documented mitral stenosis and atrial fibrillation and no contraindications to anticoagulant therapy represents the group of patients in whom there is least debate regarding the necessity for chronic anticoagulation. This consensus in favor of therapy exists even in the absence of a history of systemic emboli. I would recommend that all patients in this subgroup be prophylactically anticoagulated because of the high risk of peripheral embolic phenomena. Previous investigators have concluded that a patient with rheumatic valve disease has at least 1 chance in 5 of having a clinically detectable systemic embolus during the course of his or her disease. The incidence of such systemic emboli increases by a factor of 7 when mitral valve disease is complicated by atrial fibrillation. In the setting of mitral stenosis associated with atrial fibrillation, a correlation between systemic emboli and certain associated findings—such as atrial size, sex, mitral calcification, or age—is insufficiently weak to rely upon. Consequently, anticoagulation for all patients with mitral stenosis and atrial fibrillation, is needed at least up to "80" years of age.

Treatment of mitral stenosis in patients with atrial fibrillation—whether by operative commissurotomy, percutaneous valvuloplasty, or prosthetic valve replacement—does not eliminate the need for chronic anticoagulation. Some degree of mitral stenosis persists after all these procedures, including prosthetic valve replacement. The potential for systemic embolization thus persists, and as a consequence anticoagulation must be continued. Remember that the use of tissue valve prostheses in patients with mitral stenosis and atrial fibrillation does not obviate the need for chronic anticoagulation. The only utility of using a tissue valve is in case a patient subsequently develops an absolute contraindication to continued anticoagulation. Discontinuation of anticoagulation with warfarin is theoretically more acceptable in a patient with a tissue valve than in a patient with a mechanical valve; in this setting the efficacy of antiplatelet therapy as a substitute for warfarin therapy remains unproved.

The decision to anticoagulate patients with mitral stenosis who have not had a systemic embolus and who are in normal sinus rhythm is difficult. Some investigators have recommended that left atrial diameter greater than 55 mm in these patients serves as a good guideline instituting anticoagulant therapy. Other physicians have strongly recommended that these patients be prophylactically treated with anticoagulant therapy (regardless of left atrial size) because either atrial fibrillation or systemic embolization may represent the presenting manifestation of mitral stenosis. In individuals with no contraindications to anticoagulation, I believe therapy probably is indicated, particularly in patients who can be expected to adhere scrupulously to the plan of management.

Finally, the fact that the rheumatic mitral valve disease manifests as mild mitral stenosis with predominant mitral regurgitation does not, in my opinion, change the indications for chronic anticoagulation. Although previous studies had indicated that emboli may be more common in mitral stenosis than mitral regurgitation with a rheumatic cause, the fact that at least, mild, mitral stenosis complicates most cases of rheumatic mitral valve disease argues for anticoagulant therapy even in the patient with predominant mitral insufficiency.

# ATRIAL FIBRILLATION UNASSOCIATED WITH VALVULAR HEART DISEASE

Patients in whom atrial fibrillation is unaccompanied by valvular heart disease constitute a more controversial group of patients with regard to anticoagulant therapy than those in whom mitral stenosis coexists. There is no question that the risk of peripheral embolic events is increased in patients with chronic atrial fibrillation, as opposed to individuals with normal sinus rhythm. What remains unclear is the magnitude of this risk and its relation to the poorly defined risk of bleeding from warfarin in such patients. Some evidence indicates that the likelihood of peripheral embolic events in patients with atrial fibrillation is increased by the association of organic heart disease, such as left ventricular dilatation or hypertrophy. Certainly in patients with atrial fibrillation and a history of a previous embolic event, I would recommend chronic anticoagulation. I also recommend such therapy for patients in whom two-dimensional echocardiography or other noninvasive tests disclose evidence of atrial thrombus. Unfortunately, two-dimensional echocardiography is not optimally sensitive nor specific for the detection of such clots. Consequently, in the absence of a history of peripheral embolic events or noninvasive evidence of left atrial thrombus, I currently do not recommend anticoagulant therapy for "isolated" atrial fibrillation unassociated with organic heart disease. When chronic atrial fibrillation is complicated by coexistent organic heart disease, assessment of the relative risk of bleeding from warfarin must dictate the decision whether to anticoagulate such patients.

*Paroxysmal* atrial fibrillation previously had been suggested to constitute a more compelling basis for chronic anticoagulation than *chronic* atrial fibrillation. The rationale for this conclusion was based on the assumption that thrombus was likely to develop in the left atrial appendage during periods of atrial fibrillation and that such thrombus then could be dislodged when the patient spontaneously reverted to normal sinus rhythm with the onset of a coordinated left atrial contraction. We have reviewed a large series of patients with paroxysmal atrial fibrillation at our institution. We have found that in the absence of associated organic heart disease there is an exceptionally low incidence of peripheral embolic events and that this incidence of peripheral emboli does not exceed even the lowest estimates of complications from anticoagulation. Therefore I do not recommend chronic anticoagulant therapy to patients with paroxysmal atrial fibrillation unassociated with organic heart disease. Because we have observed systemic emboli in patients with paroxysmal atrial fibrillation in the *presence* of organic heart disease, however, I do recommend anticoagulant therapy for such patients.

# CARDIOMYOPATHY

Some studies have indicated that the incidence of ventricular and atrial thrombus in patients with dilated cardiomyopathy may be sufficiently high, when examined at necropsy, to constitute a sound basis for chronic anticoagulation. Clinical studies have shown a variable risk of peripheral embolic events in patients with dilated cardiomyopathy. Thus it is our policy to recommend chronic anticoagulation to such patients, provided that the basis for their dilated cardiomyopathy is not chronic ethanol use. Such therapy obviously is also contraindicated when a dilated cardiomyopathy is associated with secondary hepatic insufficiency.

In patients with hypertrophic cardiomyopathy, the basis for cerebrovascular accidents remains incompletely defined. Some investigations have suggested that such strokes are related to peripheral embolic events with a cardiac origin. Other studies have suggested, however, that the incidence of left atrial thrombus at autopsy is vanishingly rare and that cerebrovascular accidents are more likely to be caused by paroxysmal arrhythmias, intermittent outflow tract obstruction, or extracranial vascular disease. Left atrial size has been suggested as a useful guide in predicting the likelihood of cerebrovascular accidents if one argues that when the left atrial size exceeds 55 mm in diameter (by echocardiography), anticoagulation is warranted. I recommend anticoagulation to patients with hypertrophic cardiomyopathy and associated atrial fibrillation. At least some of these patients have mitral annular calcium deposits that may be associated with a transvalvular gradient in the absence of rheumatic mitral valve disease. Even without associated mitral annular calcium deposits, the considerable decrease in left ventricular compliance characteristic of such patients might be expected to produce variable degrees of left atrial stasis in association with atrial fibrillation: Such a combination of factors might constitute a basis for chronic anticoagulation. When hypertrophic cardiomyopathy is not accompanied by atrial fibrillation, I do not recommend chronic anticoagulation, unless there is a well-documented history of a focal cerebrovascular accident.

In general, the diagnosis of a restrictive cardiomyopathy does not constitute an indication for chronic anticoagulation. The exception to this rule is the patient with the hypereosinophilia syndrome in whom there is a higher likelihood of left atrial thrombus formation and in whom chronic anticoagulation may actually diminish the chronic deposition of ventricular cavity thrombus.

## DILEMMAS

Pregnancy in a patient with a preexisting indication for chronic anticoagulation constitutes a moderately difficult clinical problem. A more difficult dilemma exists with regard to a patient in whom infective endocarditis has been complicated by a cerebrovascular accident believed to be caused by a septic embolism. In both of these situations, hard data on which to base a firm clinical recommendation are not available. I believe that the best recommendations for these two situations are those given by the ACCP-NHLBI National Conference on Antithrombotic Therapy.

With regard to pregnancy, the conference stated the following: "It is recommended that pregnant patients . . . should be treated with adjusted-dose subcutaneous heparin (12 hourly subcutaneous heparin with a PTT 1.5-2 times control 6 hours after injection) from the time pregnancy is diagnosed until delivery. This recommendation is based on a study demonstrating a very high incidence of cerebral embolism when antiplatelet agents alone were used and a high frequency of embryopathy and fetal death in mothers treated with warfarin."

With regard to infective endocarditis, the recommendations of the same conference were as follows:

1. It is strongly recommended that antithrombotic therapy is not indicated in patients with uncomplicated infective endocarditis involving a native valve or a bioprosthetic valve in patients with normal sinus rhythm. This . . . recommendation is based on the increased incidence of hemorrhage in these patients and the lack of demonstrated efficacy of antithrombotic therapy in this setting.
2. It is recommended that long-term warfarin therapy be continued in patients with endocarditis involving a prosthetic valve unless there are specific contraindications. This . . . recommendation is based on the high frequency of systemic embolism in these patients. However, it is to be noted that the risk of intracranial hemorrhage in this circumstance is substantial.
3. The indications for anticoagulant therapy when systemic embolism occurs during the course of infective endocarditis involving a native or bioprosthetic heart valve are uncertain. The therapeutic decision should consider comorbid factors, including atrial fibrillation, evidence of left atrial thrombus, evidence and size of valvular vegetations, and the distribution and severity of embolism.

Recommendations regarding the use of anticoagulation obviously must be individualized. The INR (International Normalized Ratio) should be used to measure the intensity of anticoagulation in all patients receiving warfarin.

## References

Consensus Report of the ACCP-NHLBI National Conference on Antithrombotic Therapy, *Chest* 89:1S-99S, 1986.

The European Atrial Fibrillation Trial Study Group: Optimal oral anticoagulant therapy in patients with nonrheumatic atrial fibrillation and recent cerebral ischemia, *N Engl J Med* 333:5-10, 1995.

Cannegeiter, SC, Rosendaal FR, Wintzen AR, et al: Optimal oral anticoagulant therapy in patients with mechanical heart valves, *N Engl J Med* 333:11-17, 1995.

Becker RC, Ansell J: Antithrombotic therapy: an abbreviated reference for clinicians, *Arch Intern Med* 155:149-161, 1995.

Antiplatelet Trialists' Collaboration: Collaborative overview of randomised trials of antiplatelet therapy, I: prevention of death, myocardial infarction, and stroke by prolonged antiplatelet therapy in various categories of patients, *Br Med J* 308:81-106, 1994.

# Chapter 6

# *Management of Congestive Heart Failure*

Carey D. Kimmelstiel
Marvin A. Konstam

Heart failure is generally defined in terms of the effects of myocardial or valvular dysfunction on end-organ perfusion or venous hydrostatic pressure. Heart failure is present if systemic blood flow is inadequate to satisfy the aerobic metabolic needs of end organs, either at rest or during usual stress such as exercise. Alternatively, heart failure is present if pulmonary venous (left-sided heart failure) or systemic venous (right-sided heart failure) pressure rises to abnormal levels. Hydrostatic forces may then induce pulmonary edema (left-sided heart failure) or peripheral and systemic organ edema (right-sided heart failure).

Therapy for heart failure must be aimed at both the underlying cardiac functional disorder and the systemic manifestations of heart failure. Some modes of therapy are directed toward a given manifestation of heart failure, regardless of cause. For example, diuretics are used to reduce elevated venous pressure, regardless of cause. Other therapies are directed toward the cardiac functional disorder and may benefit all the manifestations of that disorder. An example is inotropic therapy, which may reduce all the consequences of myocardial systolic dysfunction. Still other forms of therapy act at multiple sites and therefore may benefit a given manifestation of heart failure but may be more effective in the presence of some functional disorders than in others. For example, calcium-channel antagonists, through peripheral arterial dilatation, will reduce systolic load and thus may augment systemic perfusion regardless of the functional disorder. Because calcium antagonists both accelerate relaxation and reduce contractility, these drugs are more effective in the presence of myocardial diastolic dysfunction and less effective, or possibly detrimental, when systolic dysfunction predominates.

In addition to being a debilitating illness, heart failure carries a poor prognosis, with 50% mortality within 6 months to 3 years, depending on the primary diagnosis and the severity of hemodynamic and clinical derangement. Despite the poor prognosis, therapy previously had been directed primarily to relief of symptoms, with little expectation that survival could be prolonged. This approach has changed, as treatment modalities such as angiotensin converting enzyme (ACE) inhibition have been shown to alter the natural history of disease.

This chapter is divided into two sections. In the first section, we discuss the physiologic factors that influence cardiac performance, categorize the disorders for each of these factors that lead to heart failure, and discuss therapeutic approaches in these specific myocardial functional disorders. In the second section, we discuss general treatment strategies and modalities, with attention to (1) the changing indications for treatment, (2) an approach to treatment, and (3) a review of available modes of therapy, with emphasis on matching treatment both to cardiac functional disorders and to peripheral manifestations.

# FACTORS INFLUENCING CARDIAC PERFORMANCE: THEIR CATEGORIZATION AND TREATMENT

## Preload

Preload, defined as the extent of myocardial fiber stretch immediately preceding contraction, is gauged experimentally as the length of an isolated muscle strip, or clinically as ventricular end-diastolic dimension, end-diastolic volume, or end-diastolic pressure. A commonly employed clinical index of left ventricular preload, mean pulmonary artery wedge pressure, generally reflects pulmonary venous pressure and, in the absence of mitral stenosis, parallels changes in left ventricular end-diastolic pressure. The pulmonary artery wedge pressure is not only an indicator of left ventricular preload, but also a gauge to judge the effectiveness of therapy directed against pulmonary interstitial and alveolar edema. Similarly, right atrial or central venous pressure, which may be judged clinically as jugular venous pressure, is both an indicator of right ventricular preload and a gauge for therapy directed toward the manifestations of right-sided heart failure.

The relation between ventricular preload and systolic performance is described by the Starling relation, which, in its clinical format, plots stroke volume, stroke work, or cardiac output against one of the indicators of preload. At relatively low levels of preload, systolic performance rises with preload until a relative plateau is reached. With additional increases in preload, ventricular systolic performance increases only modestly and may even decline. Further increases in preload, as with intravascular volume loading, will tend to worsen pulmonary edema and systemic venous congestion without substantial gain in forward output. In managing heart failure, it is often appropriate to maintain intravenous volume at a level that places preload near the start of this plateau. Further reduction in preload, as with diuretics or venodilators, may reduce the manifestations of elevated pulmonary or central venous pressure but also may reduce forward cardiac output.

In patients with reduced peripheral perfusion caused by myocardial infarction in the absence of antecedent cardiac disease, preload is optimized when pulmonary artery wedge pressure is in the range of 15 to 18 mm Hg. Further increases may result in pulmonary edema, whereas decreases may reduce cardiac output. When clinical evidence of low cardiac output is absent, there is no reason to maintain pulmonary artery wedge pressure at this level, which exceeds the normal range of 5 to 12 mm Hg. On the other hand, in patients with chronic elevation in ventricular filling pressure or with noncompliant ventricles (such as severe left ventricular hypertrophy), the "optimal" pulmonary artery wedge pressure may exceed 18 mm Hg. Under such circumstances either greater ventricular filling pressure is needed to achieve the same myocardial fiber stretch (because of diminished compliance) or the slope of the Starling curve is altered such that increases in pulmonary artery wedge pressure above 18 mm Hg may be accompanied by further increases in cardiac output. Furthermore, when pulmonary venous pressure is chronically elevated, mechanisms develop to diminish pulmonary interstitial or alveolar edema at any given pulmonary venous pressure. These mechanisms include an increase in pulmonary lymphatic flow and thickening of the alveolar-capillary membrane. For these reasons in management of heart failure the target ventricular filling pressures must be geared to the needs of the individual patient.

**Conditions of primary ventricular volume overload and their treatment.** Heart failure may be primarily the result of increased preload or ventricular volume overload. The most common causes of left ventricular volume overload are mitral regurgitation, aortic regurgitation, and ventricular septal defect with left-to-right shunt. Right ventricular volume overload most commonly results from tricuspid regurgitation (though tricuspid regurgitation is most often functional, secondary to pressure overload), atrial-level left-to-right shunt, or, less commonly, pulmonic regurgitation. In all these circumstances, the involved ventricle receives a diastolic volume that exceeds forward stroke volume, causing increased preload. Thus conditions of ventricular volume overload may directly cause manifestations of left- or right-sided heart failure because of excessive pulmonary or systemic venous pressure, respectively. Furthermore, chronic ventricular volume overload may cause progressive depression of myocardial contractility, thereby producing or worsening heart failure.

In these conditions of volume overload, therapy should be directed primarily toward reducing the excessive load. Under these circumstances, the most rational medical regimen includes diuretics, venodilators, or systemic arterial dilators.[1] Both diuretics and venodilators directly reduce ventricular preload, whereas arterial dilators augment systolic ejection performance, thereby secondarily reducing preload. Arterial dilators, by reducing aortic pressure and impedence to forward flow, are particularly effective in reducing diastolic load and augmenting cardiac output in settings of aortic regurgitation and ventricular-level left-to-right shunt. In the setting of mitral regurgitation, regurgitant flow is more closely related to systolic mitral orifice size than to left ventricular systolic pressure. Therefore therapy is best implemented by direct reduction in preload by use of diuretics and venodilators with resulting reduction in systolic mitral orifice size.

In aortic regurgitation, nifedipine has been shown to reduce left ventricular wall stress and volumes after 1 year of therapy.[2] Long-term nifedipine treatment of asymptomatic patients with chronic severe aortic regurgitation and normal left ventricular systolic function has been shown to delay the need for valve replacement when compared with digoxin treatment.[3] Symptoms of congestive heart failure indicate left ventricular systolic dysfunction, and therefore indicate the need for aortic valve replacement, even if symptoms are manageable with medical therapy. Delaying valve replacement may lead to irreversible loss of ventricular contractile function. In the absence of symptoms, noninvasive assessment of left ventricular systolic performance is employed to identify subclinical contractile dysfunction, thereby aiding in the timing of valve replacement. In patients with mitral regurgitation, since the left ventricle is ejecting directly into the left atrium and pulmonary veins, symptoms of heart failure may develop in the absence of substantial ventricular contractile dysfunction. Therefore, mitral valve replacement need be performed for mitral regurgitation only if symptoms persist despite medical therapy or if early left ventricular systolic dysfunction is evident by radionuclide ventriculography, echocardiography, or contrast ventriculography. More severe degrees of left ventricular systolic dysfunction (ejection fraction less than 40%) are associated with poorer prognosis after aortic or mitral valve replacement for regurgitant lesions.

## Afterload

In isolated myocardial tissue preparations, afterload may be defined as the degree of systolic tension developed during contraction. Clinically, afterload is defined as ventricular systolic stress; systolic stress is related directly to intracavitary pressure and radius and inversely to ventricular myocardial thickness. In most clinical circumstances acute changes in left and right ventricular afterload may be approximated by changes in systemic arterial and pulmonary arterial end-systolic pressure, respectively, as measured at the dicrotic notch. Acute changes in left ventricular afterload roughly parallel but frequently exceed acute changes in systolic blood pressure.

Increases in afterload reduce the effectiveness of ventricular systolic contraction. In isolated muscle preparations, the interaction between afterload and contractile function may be described by the relation between velocity of fiber shortening and systolic tension. With increasing levels of systolic load, myocardial-fiber shortening slows progressively. In patients, this interaction may be described by the relation of ventricular pressure on wall stress versus ventricular volume or dimension at end systole. As end-systolic pressure is reduced, a linear decrease in end-systolic volume is achieved. Herein lies the basis for afterload-reduction therapy in patients with heart failure and inadequate systemic perfusion.[4-7] Arteriolar dilatation causes reduction in systemic vascular resistance, thereby decreasing ventricular systolic pressure and myocardial stress, in turn, reducing end-systolic volume, and augmenting stroke volume and cardiac output.

Decreases in systemic perfusion pressure limit the extent to which afterload reduction may be employed in treating heart failure. When direct or indirect systemic arteriolar dilators are administered, care must be taken to maintain blood pressure in an acceptable range. Furthermore, in the clinical setting, it is unusual to reduce afterload without altering preload. Although combining these two effects may be desirable in managing the various manifestations of heart failure, concomitant preload reduction may diminish the degree to which afterload reduction augments cardiac output.

**Conditions of primary ventricular pressure overload and their treatment.** An abnormal increase in afterload may be the cause of left ventricular failure in patients with aortic stenosis, hypertrophic cardiomyopathy with left ventricular outflow obstruction, and severe systemic hypertension. Similarly an abnormal increase in afterload is the cause of right ventricular failure in patients with left-sided heart failure, mitral valve disease, pulmonary emboli, obstructive lung disease, and primary pulmonary hypertension and with stenosis of pulmonary arteries, pulmonic valve, or right ventricular infundibulum. In patients with left-sided heart failure of other causes, such as ischemic cardiomyopathy, afterload may be inappropriately high, because of stimulation of the sympathetic nervous system and renin-angiotensin axis, and may contribute to a vicious cycle of increasing heart failure.

Patients with severe systemic hypertension may develop manifestations of heart failure related to acute increases in systolic load in the absence of significant myocardial contractile impairment. Alternatively, patients with chronic severe hypertension may develop chronic heart failure secondary to myocardial hypertrophy, with resultant reduction in systolic performance, or, more commonly, diastolic performance. Treatment is best directed toward reduction in blood pressure through direct or indirect arteriolar dilators.

In patients with aortic stenosis, ventricular systolic performance is generally adequate if systolic wall stress has been normalized by an increase in myocardial thickness. In such cases, heart failure may still occur as a consequence of myocardial diastolic dysfunction (see below). In the absence of adequate myocardial thickening, afterload will be excessive, resulting in heart failure caused by reduced systolic performance. Although symptoms of heart failure may be improved by a variety of pharmacologic agents in aortic stenosis, such interventions are fraught with risk. For example, drugs that reduce preload, such as diuretics or nitrates, may diminish symptoms of pulmonary venous hypertension but carry the risk of greatly reducing stroke volume and cardiac output, which are highly preload dependent in the hypertrophied left ventricle of aortic stenosis. In addition, prognosis is poor in patients with aortic stenosis once symptoms of heart failure, syncope, or angina occur. Therefore the treatment of choice is correction of the primary abnormality, through aortic valve replacement or aortic valvuloplasty in symptomatic patients who are not surgical candidates. Once symptoms have appeared, surgery should *not* be delayed by a trial of medical therapy.

In hypertrophic cardiomyopathy with subaortic stenosis, heart failure may result from dynamic obstruction of the left ventricular outflow tract or from abnormal myocardial relaxation and compliance. Treatment should be initiated with a calcium-channel antagonist or a beta-adrenergic receptor blocker, or both.[8] Although these drugs are relatively contraindicated in patients with heart failure related to ventricular systolic dysfunction, systolic function is usually normal or hyperdynamic in patients with hypertrophic myopathy. Both beta-blockers and calcium-channel blockers may diminish dynamic outflow obstruction through reduction in myocardial contractility. Both classes of drugs also may improve ventricular filling through reduction in heart rate. Calcium-channel blockers have the additional action of augmenting relaxation (see below), which has been shown to be impaired in patients with hypertrophic myopathy. Both agents may reduce the incidence of supraventricular arrhythmias, which are often poorly tolerated in the preload-dependent hypertrophic ventricle. Additionally, beta-blockers may reduce the incidence of ventricular arrhythmias, which are frequently responsible for sudden death in patients with hypertrophic myopathy. However, neither calcium-channel blockers nor beta-blockers have been demonstrated to improve survival in this disease. Inotropic drugs are contraindicated, since these may augment the degree of outflow obstruction. Although venodilators and diuretics may directly reduce pulmonary venous hypertension, they must be employed with caution for two reasons: (1) reduction in left-ventricular end-diastolic volume may exacerbate outflow obstruction; (2) the hypertrophied ventricle is highly dependent on adequate preload to maintain forward flow. Cautious use of arteriolar dilators may have benefit, particularly if there is superimposed systemic hypertension. In patients who are significantly symptomatic despite medical treatment, benefit has been achieved from dual-chamber pacing or surgery directed at relieving the outflow obstruction through septal myotomy or myectomy, or both.

## Contractility

Contractility (or inotropic state) is defined as the effectiveness of myocardial contractile performance, independent of preload and afterload. In an isolated myocardial preparation under isometric conditions, inotropic state is gauged by the maximum tension developed or by the rate of tension development at a given end-diastolic fiber length. In a contracting preparation, the inotropic state may be gauged as velocity of shortening for a given end-diastolic length and a given systolic tension. In an intact ventricle, the inotropic state may be judged before ejection or during ejection. Before ejection (during isovolumic systole), contractility may be estimated by the peak rate of ventricular pressure rise ($dP/dt_{max}$) at a given level of preload. During ejection, contractility may be estimated when one examines the relation of the velocity of contraction versus maximum contractile tension at a given level of preload. With increased contractility, velocity of shortening is increased for any given level of systolic load. During ejection, contractility also may be judged by the relation of ventricular end-systolic pressure or wall stress versus end-systolic dimension or volume. With increased contractility, the volume to which the ventricle contracts (end-systolic volume) is reduced for any given level of systolic load (end-systolic pressure or wall stress). Increases in inotropic state also are accompanied by increases in the slope of the ventricular end-systolic pressure (or wall stress)-to-volume (or dimension) relation. In the assessment of contractility, this relation has the advantage of being independent of preload.

**Conditions where myocardial contractility is reduced and their treatment.** Decreased ventricular contractile function may result either from reduction in the mass of functional myocardium, as with ischemic heart disease, or with global reduction in myocardial contractility, as in dilated cardiomyopathy. These two conditions are the most common causes of heart failure in adults. In addition, the hypertrophied myocardium associated with chronically abnormal ventricular loads may manifest altered contractile properties. Reduction in myocardial contractility frequently contributes to the development of heart failure in patients with chronic volume overload (such as aortic or mitral insufficiency) and occasionally in patients with chronic pressure overload (such as aortic stenosis or long-standing hypertension).

Primary contractile abnormalities frequently are associated with secondarily altered ventricular loading conditions. Preload is increased because of an inability of the failing heart to eject its diastolic load. This effect serves to maintain forward output by the Starling mechanism. Afterload often is relatively high as a consequence of inappropriate "compensatory" mechanisms, which serve to maintain blood pressure at the expense of cardiac output. These mechanisms include vasoconstriction through activation of the sympathetic nervous system and of the renin-angiotensin system.

Therapy in patients with heart failure caused by reduced contractile performance has been directed toward reduction in preload and in afterload as well as to augmentation of contractility. Generally therapy is initially designed to reduce preload through sodium restriction, diuretics, and venodilators. These agents are particularly effective against manifestations of increased pulmonary and systemic venous pressure. Reduction in afterload, through use of direct arteriolar dilators, alpha-adrenergic receptor blockers, beta-adrenergic receptor agonists, or angiotensin-converting enzyme inhibitors, is particularly directed toward augmenting forward output. Inotropic agents may benefit manifestations of both "forward" and "backward" failure, though these agents are useful only in the short-term management of patients with decompensated heart failure (see below). Drugs that augment contractility of the failing heart, such as beta-adrenergic agents, often have several concomitant effects. These may include direct chronotropic effects and direct vascular effects, that is, vasoconstriction or vasodilatation. These effects may be desirable or undesirable, depending on the clinical circumstance. Additionally, since contractility is one of the major determinants of myocardial oxygen demand (others being wall stress and heart rate), beneficial effects of inotropic augmentation may be countered by an increase in myocardial oxygen requirement. When active myocardial ischemia reduces contractile performance, attempts should be made to reverse ischemia by medical or surgical means (see below).

## Relaxation, Compliance, and Ventricular Filling
The diastolic behavior of the myocardium may be divided into the active process of relaxation, during which calcium is actively transported from

the sarcolemma, and passive stretch (compliance) during ventricular filling. Relaxation properties are judged by examination of the rate of ventricular pressure decay during isovolumic relaxation. Compliance is judged by the relation of ventricular pressure and volume during filling. Alterations of either relaxation or compliance may produce manifestations of heart failure, since either may increase ventricular end-diastolic pressure, and therefore increase pulmonary or systemic venous pressure. Alternatively, decreased compliance (increased slope of the ventricular diastolic pressure-volume relation) may reduce forward flow, since a given level of end-diastolic pressure will be associated with lesser end-diastolic volume or fiber stretch. Cardiac output may therefore suffer because of reduced preload.

In addition to abnormalities of myocardial compliance or relaxation, ventricular filling may be mechanically impaired because of pericardial constriction, infiltrative processes that restrict filling (restrictive cardiomyopathy), or lesions that directly limit venous or atrial emptying into the right or left ventricle. Examples of the latter include mitral or tricuspid stenosis, atrial myxoma obstructing the atrioventricular valve, and pulmonary venous occlusive disease.

**Conditions of altered diastolic function or ventricular filling and their treatment.** Clinically relevant reductions in ventricular compliance or relaxation may occur as a result of acute myocardial ischemia, in which case, therapy is best directed toward medical or surgical relief of ischemia. Alternatively abnormalities of diastolic performance result from severe ventricular hypertrophy. The latter may be physiologic as a consequence of systemic hypertension, aortic stenosis (inducing left ventricular hypertrophy), pulmonary hypertension, or pulmonic stenosis (inducing right ventricular hypertrophy). Ventricular hypertrophy also may be nonphysiologic in the case of hypertrophic cardiomyopathy. In addition to relieving the stimulus to hypertrophy (see above), therapy may be instituted to directly improve myocardial relaxation. Calcium-channel antagonists improve relaxation in the setting of hypertrophic cardiomyopathy and may have a similar action in hypertensive hypertrophic cardiac disease. In patients with aortic stenosis, calcium-channel antagonists should generally be avoided, since any benefit afforded by improving relaxation is likely to be offset by the negative inotropic and vasodilatory actions of these agents.

Patients with restrictive cardiomyopathy may present with manifestations of pulmonary and systemic venous hypertension, though the latter generally predominates. Therapy consists primarily of sodium restriction and diuretic administration, with dosage limited by manifestations of low cardiac output. This condition must be distinguished from pericardial constriction, in which the treatment of choice is pericardial stripping.

Therapy for patients with mitral stenosis consists of sodium restriction, diuretics, and reduction in heart rate to maximize ventricular filling time. The latter may be achieved with digitalis (in the presence of atrial fibrillation), beta-blockers, or calcium-channel antagonists. When these measures fail to achieve adequate symptomatic benefit, correction by surgery or balloon mitral valvuloplasty should be undertaken.

# GENERAL TREATMENT STRATEGIES AND MODALITIES

## Indications for Treatment

In patients with left ventricular systolic dysfunction, therapy had been directed until recently primarily toward relief of symptoms. No data had proved that any medical treatment affected the progression of ventricular dysfunction or altered the natural history of disease. For this reason, a rationale had not existed justifing therapy in asymptomatic patients with depression of left ventricular systolic function caused by dilated cardiomyopathy or prior myocardial infarction. However, trials have emerged in the last decade indicating that long-term afterload reduction may prolong survival in such patients. In patients with symptomatic heart failure, the combination of hydralazine and nitrates improves survival slightly compared with placebo.[9] In symptomatic patients with left ventricular systolic dysfunction, angiotensin-converting enzyme inhibition with enalapril has likewise been found to prolong survival.[10,11] In addition, completed trials have documented that angiotensin-converting enzyme inhibition decreases the incidence of symptomatic heart failure and need for hospitalization in patients with asymptomatic left ventricular dysfunction.[12] Angiotensin-converting enzyme inhibitors have been documented to prevent progressive left ventricular dilatation and systolic dysfunction in patients with symptomatic and asymptomatic left ventricular dysfunction.[13,14] These findings, as well as others that substantiate the symptomatic benefit derived from certain vasodilator agents, have caused many clinicians to employ vasodilator agents, particularly angiotensin-converting enzyme inhibitors, earlier in the course of managing heart failure.

## Approaches to Therapy

The management of patients with congestive heart failure is rapidly evolving. A search for one of the remediable causes mentioned above always is indicated. The advent of powerful noninvasive diagnostic tools, particularly echocardiography, has considerably improved the ease and accuracy with which such remediable disorders may be recognized. These techniques also have permitted more precise categorization of functional myocardial disorders (such as systolic dysfunction, altered compliance, restrictive disorder), thereby facilitating the tailoring of therapy to the underlying pathophysiologic condition. Patients with heart failure must be divided based on left ventricular ejection fraction. Based on existing data, the therapy of patients with compromised left ventricular systolic performance is better defined than is the therapy of patients with heart failure who have normal or augmented left ventricular systolic function.

**Acute therapy.** When heart failure is accompanied by significant hypotension or inadequate systemic perfusion (such as altered mentation or reduced renal function), therapy must be carefully guided by monitoring pulmonary arterial wedge pressure, cardiac output, and blood pressure. Under these circumstances, measures must first be taken to maintain adequate blood pressure. If overt pulmonary edema is absent and pulmonary arterial wedge pressure is low enough to be safely raised, initial therapy should consist in isotonic saline administration to augment ventricular preload. Guidelines for optimizing pulmonary arterial wedge pressure are described in the section on *preload* above. If hypotension cannot be safely corrected with intravascular volume expansion, pressors should be administered. In heart failure, dopamine is the pressor of choice because of its pharmacologic actions described below. Where hypotension is accompanied by pulmonary edema, dopamine and a loop diuretic should be administered concomitantly. In patients with significant hypotension, drugs with predominant vasodilator action are contraindicated.

If pulmonary edema is present without hypotension or manifestations of low cardiac output, treatment may be instituted with loop diuretics alone. If diuresis cannot be readily achieved or inadequate cardiac output becomes evident, vasodilators with or without inotropic agents should be added. Vasodilators, such as intravenous nitroprusside or nitroglycerin, may be employed only if blood pressure is adequate. Under these circumstances, however, they may dramatically reduce ventricular filling pressures while augmenting cardiac output. Similar results may be achieved by administration of a nonpressor inotrope-vasodilator such as dobutamine or amrinone. Various combinations of inotropic and vasodilator agents may be employed where adequate improvement is not otherwise achieved.

When heart failure occurs in the setting of acute myocardial infarction, several additional considerations must be stressed. First, drugs with inotropic and particularly chronotropic action should be used less readily, since these agents may increase myocardial oxygen consumption, thereby potentially worsening ischemia and increasing infarct size. Second, as long as blood pressure is adequate, nitrates should be used readily, since these agents have been found in some studies to reduce infarct size and possibly subsequent left ventricular remodeling after infarction. Third, if ischemic symptoms are still manifest during the first 12 hours after onset of symptoms, consideration should be given to halting the progression of the infarction through thrombolysis or urgent coronary angioplasty, or both. If ischemia is noted in the presence of frank shock, emergent coronary angioplasty is preferable to chemical thrombolysis. Finally, specific remediable causes of heart failure and cardiogenic shock, that is, papillary muscle dysfunction or rupture, or acute ventricular septal defect should be considered and investigated rapidly.

Where medical measures are inadequate to remedy acute severe heart failure, intra-aortic balloon counterpulsation should be considered. This maneuver reduces ventricular preload and augments cardiac output through reduction in systemic arterial impedence. Intra-aortic balloon placement is most rational when a definable acute event is responsible for the abrupt deterioration, and correction or recovery reasonably may be expected. In acute myocardial infarction or severe ischemia, balloon counterpulsation serves the additional function of reducing ischemia, in part by augmenting diastolic coronary perfusion pressure. Counterpulsation is specifically indicated in the settings of severe acute mitral regurgitation or acute ventricular septal defect, where considerable benefit may be derived from reduction in aortic impedence. Counterpulsation is contraindicated in the presence of significant aortic regurgitation because of increases in aortic diastolic pressure.

**Chronic therapy.** Until recently, standard medical treatment in chronic heart failure began with the onset of symptoms and was initiated with restriction of physical activity, sodium restriction, and digitalis administration. If symptoms persisted, diuretics were added in increasing doses. More recently, data have indicated that vasodilator therapy, particularly with angiotensin-converting enzyme inhibitors, effect objective symptomatic improvement and alter the natural history of disease (Table 6-1). These findings have caused vasodilator therapy to be employed earlier in the course of heart failure. A variety of orally active inotropic agents have been studied, but, although these agents can produce long-lived hemodynamic improvement, chronic therapy failed to document improvement in symptoms or exercise tolerance. Moreover several trials employing these agents have documented excess mortality; consequently they are no longer employed for the long-term treatment of patients with heart failure. Several trials have underscored the importance of digitalis therapy in reducing heart failure symptoms[15] though whether digitalis has any effect on mortality is unknown. Some investigators have advocated a place for beta-adrenergic receptor blockade as a means for improving the natural history of disease in selected patients with severe ventricular systolic dysfunction. Several trials have documented improvement in symptoms, hemodynamics, and left ventricular ejection fraction in response to beta-blockade in heart-failure patients, and recent data indicate a survival benefit in at least some patient subgroups.

## Sodium restriction and diuretics

These measures are traditionally the first lines of intervention after the advent of symptoms of heart failure, and are primarily effective against symptoms of pulmonary venous hypertension: exertional dyspnea and orthopnea; and elevated systemic venous pressure: edema and ascites. As discussed above, diuresis may augment or reduce systemic perfusion, depending on the relationship between preload and cardiac output in the individual patient. Diuresis is most likely to be accompanied by an increase, or at least the maintainance, of cardiac output in the presence of functional mitral or tricuspid regurgitation, which may be diminished by reduction in ventricular volumes. In addition, when edema or ascites are present, considerable diuresis often may be achieved without significant reduction in forward output, since fluid may be mobilized from extravascular spaces without substantial reduction in intravascular volume. Although inducing diuresis, the patient must be monitored for manifestations of reduced systemic perfusion, particularly for worsening renal function, potassium depletion, and hyponatremia; the last may be avoided by free water restriction.

**Table 6-1.** *Drug therapy in chronic congestive heart failure*

| Drug class | Actions | Indications | Examples |
|---|---|---|---|
| Diuretics | Preload reduction by diuresis | Systemic and pulmonary venous congestion | Hydrochlorothiazide, 25-100 mg daily Lasix, 20-400 mg daily |
| ACE inhibitors | Inhibition of angiotensin II production Vasodilatation | Pulmonary congestion or low output; improves survival in symptomatic LV dysfunction; prevents LV dilatation in symptomatic and asymptomatic LV dysfunction | Captopril, 6.25-50 mg tid Enalapril, 2.5-10 mg bid Quinapril, 5-20 mg bid Lisinopril, 5-20 mg qd |
| Nitrates | Direct systemic venous and arterial vasodilatation Epicardial coronary artery vasodilatation | Pulmonary congestion, particularly associated with cardiac ischemia Shown to prolong survival in combination with hydralazine | Isosorbide dinitrate, 10-40 mg tid |
| Other vasodilators | Systemic arterial vasodilatation | Chronic low-output states Increased patient survival (hydralazine and nitrates) | 10-100 mg tid (Hydralazine) |
| Digitalis | Direct increase in cardiac inotropy | Chronic low output or pulmonary congestion Reduction of heart rate in atrial fibrillation | Digoxin, 0.125-0.375 mg qd |

*ACE,* Angiotensin-converting enzyme; *bid,* twice daily; *LV,* left ventricular; *qd,* once daily; *qid,* four times daily; *tid,* three times daily.

## Vasodilators

Vasodilator agents may be classified as predominantly arteriolar, such as hydralazine, predominantly venous, such as nitrates, and mixed arteriolar-venous, such as prazosin. Vasodilators also may be classified according to the mechanism of action: direct vascular smooth muscle relaxation (including calcium-channel antagonism), angiotensin-converting enzyme inhibition, or alpha-adrenergic receptor blockade. In addition, the beta-adrenergic agents and phosphodiesterase inhibitors, described below in the section on inotropic agents, also function as vasodilators.

In theory, predominant venodilators, such as nitrates, are most effective at reducing symptoms of systemic venous and pulmonary venous pressure, whereas predominant arteriolar dilators, such as hydralazine, are most effective at augmenting cardiac output. In practice, considerable overlap exists among the clinical benefits of these various drug classes. This overlap is partly attributable to the multiple sites of drug action; for example, nitrates reduce systemic vascular resistance as well as increasing systemic venous capacitance. In addition, drugs that directly reduce systemic vascular resistance secondarily reduce ventricular preload by augmenting ventricular systolic emptying. The need to maintain adequate systemic arterial pressure is always a factor limiting vasodilator drug dosage. Vasodilator therapy tends to effect the greatest hemodynamic and symptomatic benefit in patients with relatively large left ventricular end-diastolic volumes and in patients with valvular regurgitation, including those with functional mitral regurgitation.[16] Earlier institution of therapy in patients with less severely dilated left ventricles yields less evidence of acute benefit but limits the progression of left ventricular dilatation and systolic dysfunction.[12,14]

Angiotensin-converting enzyme inhibitors. In patients with heart failure, plasma renin levels tend to be elevated, resulting in increased systemic vascular resistance secondary to angiotensin effect. This response augments systemic arterial pressure at the expense of forward flow. The angiotensin-converting enzyme (ACE) inhibitors captopril and enalapril inhibit the conversion of angiotensin I to the active angiotensin II and, in patients with heart failure, reduce ventricular filling pressure and augment cardiac output. Although angiotensin-converting enzyme inhibitor administration may augment renal perfusion, prerenal azotemia may also emerge or worsen with initiation of therapy. This effect has been described especially in the presence of renal vascular disease but may occur in its absence. Prerenal azotemia may result from reduced glomerular filtration pressure related to a decrease in postglomerular, efferent vascular tone. For this reason and because of the potential for inducing symptomatic hypotension, administration of angiotensin-converting enzyme inhibitors always should be initiated with small doses, which may be increased as tolerated. Hyponatremia in patients with heart failure tends to be a marker for increased plasma renin levels, a finding that has several implications for therapy with angiotensin-converting enzyme inhibitors. Such patients may be more dependent on angiotensin levels for maintaining systemic arterial pressure and may be more prone to develop hypotension upon institution of therapy. However, if the drug is administered cautiously in gradually increasing doses, thereby avoiding hypotension, greater hemodynamic and symptomatic benefit may be expected. Institution of combined therapy with loop diuretics and an angiotensin-converting enzyme inhibitor has been reported to correct hyponatremia in patients with heart failure. This combination of agents may lead to elevation in serum creatinine levels most commonly in intravascularly volume-depleted patients. This does not mandate permanent discontinuation of converting enzyme inhibition, rather retrial at a lower diuretic dose.

ACE inhibitors have been most clearly demonstrated to chronically augment exercise capacity during placebo-controlled trials in patients with heart failure secondary to reduced left ventricular systolic function. The improvement in exercise capacity is not directly linked with the observed acute hemodynamic benefits and may require chronic drug administration to take effect. Angiotensin-converting enzyme inhibition effects improved survival in patients with severely symptomatic left ventricular systolic dysfunction. Similar therapy in patients with less severely dilated left ventricles limits the progression of left ventricular dilatation and systolic dysfunction.

**Nitrates.** Nitrates, as direct vasodilators that have greater effect on venous capacitance than on systemic arteriolar resistance, are particularly effective in reducing symptoms of systemic venous and pulmonary venous hypertension. However, they tend to reduce blood pressure and increase cardiac output as well, and chronic placebo-controlled trials have documented slightly improved exercise capacity induced by nitrate administration in patients with symptomatic left ventricular systolic dysfunction. Nitrate therapy has the additional benefit of reducing the frequency and severity of active myocardial ischemia in patients in whom ischemia contributes to symptoms of heart failure. Nitrates reduce myocardial ischemia through at least two mechanisms: by reducing myocardial oxygen demand and by reducing epicardial coronary arterial tone. The latter effect may be particularly important in patients in whom increased coronary tone augments the resistance to coronary flow imposed by fixed vascular occlusive disease. Nitrate therapy should not be administered continuously, either intravenously in the management of acute heart failure or topically in the management of chronic heart failure. Drug tolerance occurs under these circumstances and may be avoided by intermittent therapy.

**Calcium-channel antagonists.** Calcium-channel antagonists are agents that have several sites of action that contribute to their therapeutic effect in patients with heart failure. As systemic and pulmonary arteriolar dilators, they may reduce left and right ventricular systolic stress, thereby augmenting cardiac output and reducing pulmonary and systemic venous pressures. As dilators of both small and large coronary arteries, they may reduce any contribution of myocardial ischemia to altered ventricular systolic and diastolic performance. They may directly improve myocardial relaxation, thereby further reducing ventricular filling pressures. This effect is likely to be particularly beneficial in circumstances where altered relaxation is a primary pathophysiologic mechanism for development of heart failure, as in patients with hypertrophic cardiomyopathy. Calcium-channel antagonists variably reduce heart rate, an effect that will have particular benefit where myocardial compliance is reduced, as in patients with hypertrophic cardiomyopathy, or where ventricular filling is directly impeded, as in mitral stenosis. Reduced heart rate also will diminish myocardial ischemia by reducing myocardial oxygen demand. Of presently available agents, verapamil has the greatest negative chronotropic effect, and nifedipine the least, with diltiazam intermediate.

A potentially deleterious action of the calcium-channel antagonists is their variable negative inotropic action. In patients in whom heart failure results from depressed ventricular systolic performance, the risk of further reducing systolic function must be individually weighed against the potential beneficial effects described above. In such patients, therapy must be instituted cautiously. Indeed there are some data documenting heart failure exacerbation induced by calcium-channel blockade.[17] In addition, one large trial testing the effect of diltiazem in the postinfarction setting documented a reduction in mortality in patients without left ventricular systolic dysfunction but a disturbing increase in mortality in patients with impaired left ventricular systolic function.[18] Preliminary data with newer long-acting dihydropyridine calcium antagonists have suggested efficacy in heart failure, predominantly in those with a nonischemic cause; however, more data are needed.

The negative inotropic effect of the calcium-channel antagonists may be beneficial in patients with dynamic obstructive hypertrophic cardiomyopathy, in whom reduced contractility may be accompanied by reduction in the degree of dynamic aortic outflow obstruction. Of the presently available agents, verapamil has the greatest clinically relevant negative inotropic effect, diltiazem probably the least, with nifedipine probably being intermediate.

Similarly, calcium blockers have a theoretical role in patients with heart failure with normal left ventricular systolic function where they may exert a salutary effect on altered left ventricular relaxation. No consistent data from clinical trials have documented sustained improvement in response to calcium antagonism in patients with predominant diastolic dysfunction. Consequently, employing calcium blockers in such patients may be attempted with an eye toward symptomatic improvement in individual patients on a trial-and-error basis.

## Inotropic agents

A variety of drugs possessing positive inotropic action have been employed both acutely and chronically for the management of congestive heart failure caused by depressed left ventricular systolic function. Most of these agents enhance cardiac contractility by augmentation of intracellular myocardial cAMP. Orally active beta-adrenergic receptor agonists proved to be ineffective in clinical trials, primarily because of tolerance to the initial hemodynamic improvement. Clinical trials testing the efficacy of phosphodiesterase inhibitors in heart failure documented sustained hemodynamic improvement; however, clinical improvement was in general lacking. Indeed, excess mortality in patients receiving chronic phosphodiesterase inhibition has been demonstrated.[19]

Controversy surrounds the use of inotropic drug therapy in several respects. First, to what extent does chronic administration of inotropic drug therapy establish and maintain hemodynamic and clinical benefit? It may be argued that the failed ventricle is intrinsically exposed to near-maximal inotropic stimulation because of elevated levels of circulating catecholamines, and the degree to which long-term clinical benefit may be derived from additional inotropic stimulation may be questioned. Short-term hemodynamic benefit has been well documented, and trials are under way to investigate the chronic clinical efficacy of several newer orally active drugs with inotropic action. The second controversy surrounds the degree to which acute and chronic hemodynamic and symptomatic benefit of any inotropic agent results from augmented contractility, from concomitant vasodilator action possessed by many of these agents, or from still other mechanisms. Finally, since contractility is a determinant of myocardial oxygen requirement, inotropic drug therapy may increase this requirement, resulting in increased ischemic and arrhythmic events. Most studies up to now have failed to indicate consistent increases in myocardial oxygen consumption after administration of inotropically active drugs in patients with ventricular systolic failure. These findings are presumed to be related to reduction in systolic stress, which may offset any increase in myocardial contractility in the determination of oxygen demand. Nevertheless, the potential for increased myocardial oxygen requirement in individual patients must be considered whenever drugs possessing inotropic effect are administered.

Inotropic agents exert greatest direct benefit on symptoms of low cardiac output but also are likely to reduce ventricular filling pressures by augmenting systolic emptying or by exerting concomitant direct or indirect vasodilator effect. Inotropic augmentation has no role in the management of heart failure because of altered diastolic performance and is specifically contraindicated in patients with obstructive hypertrophic cardiomyopathy, where enhanced contractility may result in increased dynamic left ventricular outflow obstruction.

**Digitalis.** The digitalis glycosides were the first effective pharmacologic agents available for treating congestive heart failure, with clinical effects described by William Withering in the eighteenth century. The inotropic action of this class of drugs is related to its inhibition of myocardial sodium-potassium ATPase and may result from slight increases in intracellular sodium, leading to augmented sodium-calcium exchange. Digitalis has long been employed as an early intervention after development of symptoms of reduced cardiac output or pulmonary or systemic venous hypertension attributable to ventricular systolic dysfunction. The validity of this approach recently has been questioned by some investigators, and some placebo-controlled trials have failed to demonstrate effectiveness of digoxin in reducing the clinical manifestations of heart failure. Recent trials that withdrew digitalis from patients with moderate heart failure led to accelerated symptoms and worsened left ventricular systolic function.[20]

With the growing body of evidence demonstrating the clinical benefit of certain vasodilator agents, and the narrow toxic-therapeutic margin of digoxin, the use of digoxin early in the course of symptomatic heart failure may be questioned. Rather, it may be argued that therapy should be initiated with diuretics or vasodilators, or both, and an inotropic agent, such as digoxin, should be added only if symptoms persist.

In addition to its inotropic effect, digitalis is an important agent in the control of supraventricular arrhythmias and in the regulation of ventricular response to atrial fibrillation. In contrast with digitalis, other classes of agents with similar effects on atrioventricular conduction, namely, beta-adrenergic receptor blockers and calcium-channel antagonists, exert hypotensive and negative inotropic effects. Digoxin is therefore central in the management of patients in whom heart failure is complicated or exacerbated by supraventricular arrhythmias. Most clinicians continue to employ this drug for treating heart failure, but this issue remains controversial.[21]

**Beta-adrenergic receptor agents.** Beta-adrenergic agents exert their cellular effects after binding to cytoplasmic receptors of either the beta-1 class, with a preponderance in myocardium, or the beta-2 class, with a preponderance in vascular and bronchial smooth muscle. Cardiac beta-1 stimulation causes augmented inotropy and chronotropy, whereas smooth-muscle beta-2 stimulation causes vasodilatation and bronchodilatation. These effects are mediated by increased intracellular concentrations of cyclic AMP, resulting from augmented adenylate cyclase activity. Although various pharmacologic agents are said to be relatively beta-1 or beta-2 selective, in clinical practice this selectivity is relatively unimportant, and most beta-1 adrenergic agents exert chronotropic, inotropic, vasodilator, and bronchodilator actions. These actions, particularly the last three, have potential benefit in the acute management of severe congestive heart failure.

Dopamine and dobutamine are intravenously administered drugs, with beta-adrenergic receptor activity, that have a role in the management of patients with acute exacerbations of congestive heart failure, particularly when reduced cardiac output is a prominent feature.[22] In low-to-moderate doses, dopamine exerts beta-adrenergic as well as dopaminergic action. The former results in inotropic, chronotropic, and systemic vasodilator actions, whereas the latter results in renal vasodilatation, causing preferential increases in renal blood flow. In higher doses, dopamine exerts greater alpha-adrenergic action, resulting in systemic vasoconstriction, an effect that is undesirable in heart failure management unless blood pressure cannot otherwise be maintained. Used in moderate doses, dopamine tends to increase blood pressure while augmenting cardiac output and renal blood flow, with variable reduction in ventricular filling pressures. Its chronotropic action tends to be less evident in the presence of heart failure, where this action tends to be balanced by partial withdrawal of intrinsic catecholamines as cardiac output is improved.

Dobutamine possesses less alpha-adrenergic action and less dopaminergic action than dopamine. Because it is more exclusively beta-adrenergic, it effects greater degrees of systemic vasodilatation. Not a pressor agent, it should not be employed primarily in the setting of systemic hypotension. In patients with severe acute heart failure, it may be extremely effective at both augmenting cardiac output and reducing ventricular filling pressures. Some evidence exists to suggest that several days of dobutamine infusion achieves a more protracted improvement in hemodynamics and clinical status in patients with severe heart failure.[23]

Continued administration of a beta-adrenergic agent inevitably leads to tachyphylaxis because of a reduction in beta-adrenergic receptor density. Drug tolerance limits the usefulness of orally active beta-adrenergic agents in the management of chronic heart failure. Pulse therapy with either orally active agents or intravenous agents may serve some role in selected patients with intractible symptoms, but this possibility has not been adequately investigated.

**Phosphodiesterase inhibitors.** A series of nondigitalis, nonadrenergic, orally active agents such as amrinone, milrinone, and enoximone with inotropic effect has been investigated for both acute and chronic therapy in heart failure. The mechanism of their inotropic action may be related to their phosphodiesterase inhibitory effect, resulting in increased intracellular concentrations of cyclic AMP and augmented transmembrane calcium transport.[24] They exert bronchodilator and systemic and pulmonary vasodilator effect as well as inotropic action, and some investigators have contended that hemodynamic benefit is more closely related to vasodilator than to inotropic action. However, clinical inotropic action has been demonstrated by increases in isovolumic phase indices of contractility and by the fact that ventricular systolic performance is increased beyond that which may be explained by the degree of afterload reduction that occurs.[25]

Acute administration of intravenous amrinone in patients with severe left ventricular systolic dysfunction predictably augments cardiac output and variably reduces ventricular filling pressures. Blood pressure tends to be reduced slightly. Although this class of agents possesses chronotropic action, the heart rate remains unchanged or increases only slightly in patients with heart failure, presumably because of concomitant withdrawal of endogenous circulating catecholamines. At least one study has indicated that amrinone augments renal perfusion, though data on this matter are conflicting. Intravenous amrinone is an effective agent in managing patients with acute exacerbations of heart failure with reduced cardiac output and in maintaining acceptable hemodynamics during and after surgical procedures in patients with left ventricular systolic dysfunction.[26]

Unlike the beta-adrenergic agents, the phosphodiesterase-inhibitory inotropic agents have not been found to result in tachyphylaxis. Clinical outcome, however, has been disappointing. Currently, use of the phosphodiesterase inhibitors amrinone and milrinone is limited to intravenous administration for the short-term management of heart-failure patients who do not adequately respond to digoxin, diuretics, and vasodilators. Investigations are presently being conducted with newer agents such as vesnarinone, which has mechanistically distinct inotropic and electrophysiologic properties compared with other phosphodiesterase inhibitors. One recent trial documented a profound reduction in mortality in response to low-dose therapy with this agent in a population with greatly compromised left ventricular systolic function with excess mortality seen in patients exposed to higher vesnarinone doses.[27] Where this agent fits in our heart-failure therapeutic armamentarium awaits completion of an ongoing clinical trial.

## Beta-blockade

Patients with symptomatic heart failure are characterized by increases in circulating endogenous catecholamines, presumably in response to depressed systemic perfusion. Administration of beta-adrenergic receptor blocking agents to patients with heart failure caused by ventricular systolic dysfunction is hazardous, since endogenous catecholamines may be responsible for maintaining adequate blood pressure and cardiac output. For this reason these agents have long been considered contraindicated in this setting. In patients in whom heart failure is related to active myocardial ischemia, a cautious trial of beta-blockade is occasionally indicated. In addition, it has been speculated that chronic catecholamine stimulation may in part be responsible for progressive myocardial dysfunction, and blockade of this stimulation may therefore limit the progression of disease. Several clinical trials of beta-blocking agents have been carried out in patients with severe left ventricular systolic dysfunction, with varied results. Several trials have documented improvement in functional class and in the combined end point of death or need for heart transplantation. One recent trial documented a mortality reduction in patients with nonischemic cardiomyopathy treated with the beta-blocker bisoprolol.[28] This issue requires further study because this finding was noted only after subgroup analysis was performed in a trial in which there was no stratification based on the cause of heart failure. Newer beta-adrenergic receptor blocking agents with combined vasodilating properties have shown promise in recent clinical trials. Recently carvedilol has been documented to induce clinical and hemodynamic improvement in patients with advanced heart failure treated with diuretics, digitalis, and angiotensin-converting enzyme inhibitors.[29]

In patients with hypertrophic cardiomyopathy, beta-blocking agents augment ventricular filling through reduction in heart rate and decrease dynamic outflow obstruction through reduction in contractility. Likewise, in mitral stenosis, heart rate reduction by beta-blockade is effective in improving ventricular filling and reducing left atrial pressure, particularly in the presence of atrial fibrillation.

## Surgical approaches

Valvular disease. The aggressiveness with which a surgical approach should be taken in patients with congestive heart failure secondary to valvular disease depends on the lesion that is primarily responsible for symptoms. In both aortic stenosis and aortic regurgitation, valve replacement or repair should be undertaken at the onset of symptoms.

In the case of aortic stenosis, the advent of symptoms signifies a poor prognosis in the absence of surgical correction. Reduced left ventricular systolic function in the face of hemodynamically relevant aortic stenosis should not deter surgical intervention, since ventricular performance is likely to improve with relief of abnormal afterload. In patients with aortic regurgitation, symptoms of heart failure indicate at least moderate left ventricular systolic depression and represent a signal that further delay in surgical repair may lead to irreversible ventricular dysfunction. Aortic valve replacement in patients with chronic aortic regurgitation has been documented to increase ejection fraction and reduce left ventricular dilatation on both short-term and long-term follow-up study. A somewhat more conservative approach may be taken in the presence of mitral valve disease. In mitral regurgitation, a surgical approach need be taken only if symptoms cannot be readily controlled medically or if left ventricular function has begun to deteriorate. Mitral valve replacement with preservation of the papillary muscles and chordae tendineae leads to better preservation of left ventricular function postoperatively than surgery not preserving these structures.[30] As in aortic regurgitation, long-term prognosis is poor in patients who undergo mitral valve replacement for mitral regurgitation after development of severe left ventricular systolic dysfunction. In congestive heart failure caused by mitral stenosis, surgery is indicated primarily for relief of symptoms.

**Ischemic heart disease.** A subset of patients with heart failure related to ischemic heart disease has active myocardial ischemia, in addition to healed myocardial infarction, as the cause of left ventricular systolic dysfunction. Such patients may manifest improvement in systolic function, with relief of heart failure, after revascularization by either coronary bypass surgery or angioplasty. Identification of such patients represents a challenge. Evidence of active ischemia clinically or by thallium imaging should trigger consideration of coronary revascularization. Selected patients with heart failure benefit from resection of a left ventricular aneurysm, which is generally performed with coronary bypass surgery. In patients with severe heart failure after acute myocardial infarction, consideration should be given to the diagnoses of papillary muscle infarction (with or without rupture) or ventricular septal defect, which should be emergently surgically corrected.

**Cardiac transplantation.** In the last several years, cardiac transplantation has progressed from an experimental procedure to one of proved clinical benefit to selected patients with severe congestive heart failure. The two advances that have most improved survival after transplantation are (1) the use of endomyocardial biopsy to diagnose rejection and guide therapy and (2) the development and use of cyclosporin A as a component of the immunosuppressive regimen. At present, 1-year and 5-year survival after heart transplantation is approximately 80% and 60%, respectively. When compared with the 50% 6-month survival in patients with New York Heart Association functional class IV caused by congestive heart failure, it is evident that cardiac transplantation offers greater hope for improved survival in such patients than any other presently available form of therapy. Unfortunately, lack of donor availability considerably limits the application of this therapeutic modality. Approximately 2100 cardiac transplants were performed in the United States in 1991, whereas it is estimated that approximately 15 times that number of patients could have benefited from transplantation.[31] At present, consideration of transplantation is indicated in patients with less than 1-year expected survival in the absence of other significant disease processes.

## References

1. Chatterjee K, Parmley WW, Swan HJC, et al: Beneficial effects of vasodilator agents in severe mitral regurgitation due to dysfunction of subvalvular apparatus, *Circulation* 48:684-690, 1973.
2. Scognamiglio R, Fasoli G, Ponchia A, Dalla Volta S: Long-term nifedipine unloading therapy in asymptomatic patients with chronic severe aortic regurgitation, *J Am Coll Cardiol* 16:424-429, 1990.
3. Scognamiglio R, Rahimtoola SH, Fasoli G, et al: Nifedipine in asymptomatic patients with severe aortic regurgitation and normal left ventricular function, *N Engl J Med* 331:689-694, 1994.
4. Cohn JN: Physiologic basis of vasodilator therapy for heart failure, *Am J Med* 71:135-139, 1981.
5. Captopril Multicenter Research Group: A placebo-controlled trial of captopril in refractory chronic congestive heart failure, *J Am Coll Cardiol* 2:755-763, 1983.
6. Kramer BL, Masie BM, Topic N: Controlled trial of captopril in chronic heart failure: a rest and exercise hemodynamic study, *Circulation* 67:807-816, 1983.
7. Konstam MA, Weiland DS, Conlon TP, et al: Hemodynamic correlates of left ventricular versus right ventricular radionuclide volumetric responses to vasodilator therapy in congestive heart failure secondary to ischemic or dilated cardiomyopathy, *Am J Cardiol* 53:1131-1137, 1987.
8. Bonow RO, Ostrow HG, Rosing DR, et al: Verapamil effects of left ventricular systolic and diastolic function in patients with hypertrophic cardiomyopathy: pressure-volume analysis with a non-imaging scintillation probe, *Circulation* 25:1062-1073, 1983.
9. Cohn JN, Archibald DG, Phil M, et al: Effect of vasodilator therapy on mortality in chronic congestive heart failure, *N Engl J Med* 314:1547-1552, 1986.
10. The CONSENSUS Trial Study Group: Effects of enalapril on mortality in severe congestive heart failure: results of the Cooperative North Scandinavian Enalapril Survival Study (CONSENSUS), *N Engl J Med* 316:1429-1435, 1987.
11. The SOLVD Investigators: Effect of enalapril on survival in patients with reduced left ventricular ejection fractions and congestive heart failure, *N Engl J Med* 325:293-302, 1991.
12. The SOLVD Investigators: Effect of enalapril on mortality and the development of heart failure in asymptomatic patients with reduced left ventricular ejection fractions, *N Engl J Med* 327:685-691, 1992.
13. Konstam MA, Rousseau MF, Kronenberg MW, et al: Effects of the angiotensin converting enzyme inhibitor enalapril on the long-term progression of

left ventricular dysfunction in patients with heart failure, *Circulation* 86:431-438, 1992.

14. Konstam MA, Kronenberg MW, Rousseau MF, et al: Effects of the angiotensin converting enzyme inhibitor enalapril on the long-term progression of left ventricular dilatation in patients with asymptomatic systolic dysfunction, *Circulation* 88(part 1):2277-2283, 1993.

15. Packer M, Gheorghiade M, Young JB, et al: Withdrawal of digoxin from patients with chronic heart failure treated with angiotensin converting-enzyme inhibitors, *N Engl J Med* 329:1-7, 1993.

16. Weiland DS, Konstam MA, Salem DN, et al: Contribution of reduced mitral regurgitant volume to vasodilator effect in severe left ventricular failure, *Am J Cardiol* 58:1046-1050, 1986.

17. Elkayam U, Amin J, Mehra A, et al: A prospective, randomized, double-blind crossover study to compare the efficacy and safety of chronic nifedipine therapy with that of isosorbide dinitrate and their combination in the treatment of chronic congestive heart failure, *Circulation* 82:1954-1961, 1990.

18. The Multicenter Diltiazem Postinfarction Trial Research Group: The effect of diltiazem on mortality and reinfarction after myocardial infarction, *N Engl J Med* 319:385-392, 1988.

19. Packer M, Carver JR, Rodeheffer RJ, et al: Effect of oral milrinone on mortality in severe chronic heart failure, *N Engl J Med* 325:1468-1475, 1991.

20. Uretsky BF, Young JB, Shahidi E, et al: Randomized study assessing the effect of digoxin withdrawal in patients with mild to moderate chronic congestive heart failure: results of the PROVED trial, *J Am Coll Cardiol* 22:955-962, 1993.

21. Kimmelstiel C, Benotti JR: How effective is digitalis in the treatment of congestive heart failure? *Am Heart J* 116:1063-1070, 1988.

22. Leier CV, Heban PT, Huss P, et al: Comparative systemic and regional hemodynamic effects of dopamine and dobutamine in patients with cardiomyopathic heart failure, *Circulation* 58:466-475, 1978.

23. Sonnenblick EH, Frishman WH, LeJemtel TH: Dobutamine: a new synthetic cardioactive sympathetic amine, *N Engl J Med* 300:17-22, 1979.

24. LeJemtel TH, Keung E, Sonnenblick EH, et al: Amrinone: a new non-glycoside, non-adrenergic cardiotonic agent effective in the treatment of intractable myocardial failure in man, *Circulation* 59:1098-1104, 1979.

25. Konstam MA, Cohen SR, Weiland DS, et al: Relative contribution of inotropic and vasodilator effects to amrinone-induced hemodynamic improvement in congestive heart failure, *Am J Cardiol* 57:242-248, 1986.

26. Wilmshurst PT, Thompson DS, Jenkins BS, et al: Haemodynamic effects of intravenous amrinone in patients with impaired left ventricular function, *Br Heart J* 49:77-82, 1983.

27. Feldman AM, Bristow MR, Parmley WW, et al: Effects of vesnarinone on morbidity and mortality in patients with heart failure, *N Engl J Med* 329:149-155, 1993.

28. CIBIS Investigators and Committees: A randomized trial of β-blockade in heart failure. The Cardiac Insufficiency Bisoprolol Study (CIBIS), *Circulation* 90:1765-1773, 1994.

29. Krum H, Sackner-Bernstein JD, Goldsmith RL, et al: Double-blind, placebo-controlled study of the long-term efficacy of carvedilol in patients with severe chronic heart failure, *Circulation* 92:1499-1506, 1995.

30. Komeda M, David TE, Rao V, et al: Late hemodynamic effects of the preserved papillary muscles during mitral valve replacement, *Circulation* 90(part 2):II-190–II-194, 1994.

31. O'Connell JB, Gunnar R, Evans RW, et al: Task Force 1: Organization of heart transplantation in the U.S., *J Am Coll Cardiol* 22:8-14, 1993.

## Chapter 7

# Management of Atrial Fibrillation

Paul J. Wang
N.A. Mark Estes III

The evaluation of atrial fibrillation therapy has evolved considerably over the last several years. The scientific basis for warfarin and aspirin use in atrial fibrillation has been strengthened by prospective controlled trials that quantitate the risks and benefits of this therapy. Therapeutic options for controlling ventricular responses include digitalis, beta-adrenergic receptor blockers, calcium-channel blockers, and nonpharmacologic measures such as modification or ablation of the atrioventricular node. The efficacy and safety of antiarrhythmic regimens to restore and maintain normal sinus rhythm have been clarified. Controlled trials defining and comparing the relative risk and efficacy of rate control with anticoagulation versus antiarrhythmic agents to restore sinus rhythm are not yet available. Management strategies for anticoagulation, antiarrhythmics, and rate control to a large extent are left to the individual clinician's judgment. Future studies likely will refine current management strategies and provide better guidelines for rate control, restoration and maintenance of sinus rhythm, and anticoagulation in atrial fibrillation.

## DIAGNOSIS

Atrial fibrillation is by definition an atrial arrhythmia characterized by rapid irregular disorganized atrial activity with a rate greater than 300 beats per minute. Electrocardiographically, there are no discrete P waves and atrial activity manifests as irregular waveforms that continuously change in shape, duration, amplitude, and direction. The ventricular rate is usually irregular, reflecting variable conduction of atrial impulses through the atrioventricular (AV) node. Atrial fibrillation may be distinguished from atrial flutter and atrial tachycardias by the absence of discrete atrial activity and the irregular nature of the atrial impulses. Examining multiple ECG leads to confirm the absence of discrete atrial activity may aid in the diagnosis of atrial fibrillation. Vagal maneuvers may also be used to reveal irregular atrial activity during transient slowing of conduction to the ventricle. Since the mechanism of atrial fibrillation is believed to be multiple circulating wavelets of electrical activity following varying paths in the atria without critical involvement of the AV node, vagal maneuvers will not terminate atrial fibrillation. In addition atrial fibrillation is not terminated by pacing techniques.

Although there is no uniform definition, transient self-terminating episodes of atrial fibrillation lasting less than 24 hours are generally classified as paroxysmal atrial fibrillation. By definition, chronic atrial fibrillation represents sustained atrial fibrillation that, in the absence of therapy, does not revert to normal sinus rhythm.

## EVALUATION OF THE PATIENT WITH ATRIAL FIBRILLATION

The occurrence of atrial fibrillation demands prompt, full evaluation. A complete history and physical examination should be performed in order to identify conditions that may be associated with atrial fibrillation (see box below). Laboratory tests should include serum electrolytes and thyroid function tests to identify overt or latent hyperthyroidism, which often causes atrial fibrillation. A 12-lead electrocardiogram may identify abnormalities such as prior myocardial infarction or left ventricular hypertrophy. An assessment of cardiac function using an echocardiogram may be valuable in identifying left ventricular dysfunction, left

---

### Cardiovascular and Noncardiovascular Causes of Atrial Fibrillation

| CARDIOVASCULAR CAUSES | NONCARDIOVASCULAR CAUSES |
|---|---|
| Left ventricular hypertrophy | Hypothyroidism |
| Valvular heart disease | Diabetes |
| General heart disease | Chronic obstructive pulmonary disease |
| Coronary artery disease | Pneumonia |
| Cardiomyopathy | Alcohol |
| Pericardial disease | Carbon monoxide |
| Infiltrative heart disease | Acute toxic/metabolic abnormalities |
| Cardiac surgery | Electrolyte imbalances |
| Congestive heart failure | Exertion-induced |
| Pericarditis | Anxiety-induced |
| Myocarditis | Pheochromocytoma |
| Age-induced atrial fibrotic changes | Increased parasympathetic activity |
| Intracardiac tumors or thrombi | Idiopathic |
| Pulmonary hypertension | |
| Pulmonary embolism | |

atrial enlargement valvular abnormalities, and left ventricular hypertrophy not evident from physical examination. Patients with atrial fibrillation without evidence of any predisposing cardiac or metabolic condition are considered to have "lone" atrial fibrillation. Patients with lone atrial fibrillation have a low risk of stroke, especially if they are younger than 60 years of age. Atrial fibrillation is not commonly associated with an acute myocardial infarction. Thus, in the absence of symptoms, signs, or electrocardiographic evidence of myocardial ischemia, it is usually unnecessary to obtain serial cardiac enzymes or exercise testing.

## PREDICTORS OF ATRIAL FIBRILLATION

The incidence of atrial fibrillation rapidly increases with age, with a dramatic rise at 70 years or above. Structural heart disease greatly increases the risk of atrial fibrillation. The presence of mitral valve disease, mitral regurgitation, or mitral stenosis, is associated with a sharp increase in the incidence of atrial fibrillation. Congestive heart failure, hypertension, and diabetes also are risk factors for the development of atrial fibrillation. Disorders that result in chronic elevation of left atrial pressures, such as hypertensive heart disease, hypertrophic cardiomyopathy, dilated cardiomyopathy, and myocardial infarction, also are associated with an increased incidence of atrial fibrillation. Thus, increased left atrial size by echocardiography reflecting chronic elevation of left atrial pressure correlates with the risk of atrial fibrillation. The incidence of atrial fibrillation greatly increases as the left atrial size becomes greater than 4 cm in diameter, as measured on the echocardiogram.

## HEMODYNAMICS OF ATRIAL FIBRILLATION

The multiple electrical wavefronts in atrial fibrillation prevent coordinated mechanical contraction of the atria. The absence of atrial contraction at end diastole will decrease ventricular filling and cardiac output. Patients with impaired diastolic function are particularly susceptible to this decrease in cardiac output with the loss of atrial contraction. During atrial fibrillation, the degree of ventricular filling varies with the changing R-R intervals and diastolic filling periods. Thus, based on the Frank-Starling relationship of volume and cardiac output, each beat, having a different filling volume, will have a different stroke volume. During atrial fibrillation with a rapid ventricular response, the filling time may be insufficient, leading to poor cardiac output.

The mechanical inactivity in atrial fibrillation may predispose to thrombi, leading to thromboembolic events, and may persist even after conversion of atrial fibrillation. The longer the patient has been in atrial fibrillation, the longer the patient's atrial function will remain impaired, often for days to weeks. Thus anticoagulation remains important after cardioversion and is recommended for 4 weeks.

# ACUTE TREATMENT OF ATRIAL FIBRILLATION

Three major therapeutic issues must be addressed by the clinician in treating a patient with atrial fibrillation. These include heart rate control, restoration of sinus rhythm, and antithrombotic therapy. Control of ventricular rate is a primary goal of the treatment of acute atrial fibrillation. Rate control of acute fibrillation is usually achieved by the administration of intravenous agents that slow AV nodal conduction (Table 7-1). Intravenous calcium-channel antagonists and beta-adrenergic receptor antagonists may be used to decrease the ventricular response to less than 90 to 100 beats per minute. Diltiazem may be administered as an initial bolus injection of 0.25 mg/kg over 2 minutes and if needed a second bolus of 0.35 mg/kg 15 minutes later intravenously with a continuous infusion of 5 to 15 mg/hour. Intravenous infusions of esmolol consisting of an initial loading dose of 500 $\mu$g/kg/min over 1 minute

**Table 7-1.**  *Means to slow atrioventricular nodal conduction*

|  | Therapy | |
| Goal of therapy | Acute | Chronic |
| --- | --- | --- |
| Rate control | Beta-adrenergic blocking agents IV<br>Calcium-channel antagonist IV<br>Digoxin IV | Beta-adrenergic blocking agents oral<br>Calcium-channel antagonist oral<br>Digoxin oral<br>AV nodal ablation or modification |
| Restoration of normal sinus rhythm | Procainamide IV<br>Cardioversion | Class IA<br>Class IC<br>Class III<br>Surgical procedures |
| Prevention of thromboembolic complications | Heparin IV if atrial fibrillation duration >48 hours<br>Warfarin for 3 weeks before and 4 weeks after cardioversion | Warfarin<br>Aspirin |

*IV,* Intravenous(ly).

followed by a 4-minute maintenance infusion of 50 $\mu$g/kg/min, which may be titrated to achieve rate control of the acute fibrillation. These two agents have the advantage of allowing titration of infusion rate to achieve the desired slowing of ventricular response. Verapamil usually is administered as a bolus injection intravenously; continuous infusion is uncommonly used. Propranolol or metoprolol can be used for rate control of acute fibrillation. Digoxin may be used intravenously, but its onset of action is delayed for up to 30 minutes, and it frequently fails to control the ventricular rate adequately. Digoxin has no effect on conversion of atrial fibrillation to normal sinus rhythm. If the patient with atrial fibrillation has evidence of hemodynamic instability with hypotension, congestive heart failure, or angina, immediate electrical cardioversion is indicated.

Agents such as procainamide also may be used intravenously to attempt to convert atrial fibrillation acutely. Caution should be used because of the hypotensive effects of intravenous procainamide and the possibility of conversion of atrial fibrillation to atrial flutter frequently with a more rapid ventricular response. Intravenous procainamide is the drug of choice in patients with a wide complex irregular tachycardia considered most likely to be atrial fibrillation with Wolff-Parkinson-White syndrome. In patients with Wolff-Parkinson-White syndrome and atrial fibrillation, agents such as calcium-channel antagonists, beta-adrenergic receptor antagonists, and digoxin, which slow AV nodal conduction, should be avoided, since they will accelerate the ventricular response as the impulses are conducted to the ventricle through the more rapidly conducting bypass tract.

Patients presenting with atrial fibrillation of unknown duration usually are treated with control of the ventricular rate and are not immediately converted to the sinus rhythm. Instead, cardioversion is performed after acute anticoagulation with heparin and anticoagulation with warfarin for at least 3 weeks. If the patient is known to have atrial fibrillation of a less-than-48-hour duration, cardioversion may be performed without antecedent anticoagulation, unless there are significant risk factors for thromboembolism.

## CHRONIC TREATMENT OF ATRIAL FIBRILLATION

The goals of the chronic treatment of atrial fibrillation include the prevention of thromboembolic complications of atrial fibrillation and improving the hemodynamic effects and symptoms of atrial fibrillation (see Table 7-1). Maintenance of sinus rhythm and anticoagulation are two methods to reduce the risk of thromboembolic complications. Control of the ventricular response and maintenance of sinus rhythm are two strategies to improve the hemodynamic consequences of atrial fibrillation.

## RATE CONTROL

Calcium-channel antagonists, beta-adrenergic receptor antagonists, and digoxin may be used for the chronic control of the ventricular rate.

The calcium-channel antagonists verapamil and diltiazem may be used to regulate the ventricular rate chronically. The calcium-channel antagonists nifedipine and nicardipine have relatively little effect on AV nodal function. Beta-adrenergic receptor antagonists also are effective for rate control. The ventricular rate in atrial fibrillation is variable and highly dependent on sympathetic tone. Exercise commonly results in rapid ventricular rates in patients taking digoxin despite controlled rates at rest. Verapamil and beta-receptor antagonists may be superior to digoxin in modulating this exercise-related increase in ventricular rate.

In patients with atrial fibrillation and difficult-to-control ventricular rates, radiofrequency energy can be used to ablate the AV junction permanently by means of a catheter-based transvenous procedure. This procedure results in complete AV block and thus requires permanent pacemaker implantation. These procedures, 95% to 100% successful, are associated with a risk of life-threatening complications of less than 1%. Agents such as calcium-channel antagonists, beta-adrenergic receptor antagonists, and digoxin are discontinued after successful radiofrequency AV junction ablation. Studies have shown improvement in some patients' left ventricular function after this procedure. Additionally improved exercise tolerance and quality of life have been demonstrated after AV junction ablation.

More recently, radiofrequency energy has been used to modify AV nodal function to impair AV nodal function without total destruction of AV node. Because there remains some risk of complete AV nodal block during attempted modification of AV nodal function, the technique should be reserved for patients who are suitable candidates for complete AV junction ablation. Additional data on the short-term and long-term results of this procedure are needed before the technique is applied more widely. Ablation of the bypass tract in patients with Wolff-Parkinson-White syndrome who have atrial fibrillation is successful in greater than 95% of cases and also may eliminate atrial fibrillation.

## ANTICOAGULATION

Because of the lack of coordinated atrial contraction during atrial fibrillation, there is a significant incidence of thromboembolic complications in patients with atrial fibrillation. There are several clinical factors that increase the risk of thromboembolic complications including rheumatic heart disease, age, hypertension, congestive heart failure, and prior thromboembolic events.

The risk of thromboembolic events in patients with rheumatic heart disease and atrial fibrillation is significantly increased, mandating anticoagulation. The risk of thromboembolic events in the absence of rheumatic heart disease has been the focus of numerous recent studies. In patients less than 65 years of age without hypertension, diabetes mellitus, congestive heart failure, or evidence of structural heart disease, atrial fibrillation is associated with a very low incidence of thromboembolic events. Some recent studies have examined the efficacy of anticoagulation in patients with atrial fibrillation in preventing thromboembolic events. Studies such as Stroke Prevention in Atrial Fibrillation

(SPAF) and Boston Area Trial of Atrial Fibrillation (BAATAF) have demonstrated that the rate of thromboembolic events is significantly lower in patients treated with warfarin compared with patients treated with placebo. SPAF also demonstrated that aspirin treatment results in a lower incidence of thromboembolism compared to placebo.

In the clinical study SPAF II, aspirin was compared to warfarin therapy. A trend toward a decreased incidence of thromboembolism in the patients treated with warfarin compared with aspirin was found. However, this difference was not statistically significant. In addition, the increased incidence of hemorrhagic stroke in the warfarin-treated patients counterbalanced the trend toward a lower incidence of thromboembolic events. The presence of hypertension, congestive heart failure, diabetes mellitus, left atrial enlargement, and age greater than 75 are associated with an increased incidence of thromboembolic events. Anticoagulation for patients with atrial fibrillation and these risk factors is particularly important.

Anticoagulation is generally performed for 3 or more weeks before cardioversion and should be continued for at least 4 weeks after cardioversion. After this period of time it is important to document electrocardiographically that the patient remains in sinus rhythm before discontinuation of anticoagulation. Recently the identification of atrial thrombi using transesophageal echocardiography (TEE) has been proposed as an alternative to this strategy. In several studies, TEE has been performed in patients presenting with atrial fibrillation of either prolonged or unknown duration. In patients without evidence of atrial thrombi by TEE, cardioversion has been performed without antecedent anticoagulation and is followed by anticoagulation for at least 4 weeks. Although preliminary studies have demonstrated a very low incidence of thromboembolism, clinical trials, which currently are being performed, are needed before this strategy may be applied widely. Anticoagulation for 4 weeks is needed because the mechanical contraction of the atrium does not resume for several days, and patients remain at risk for stroke without anticoagulation.

For patients known to have atrial fibrillation of a less-than-48-hour duration, cardioversion may be performed without anticoagulation for the preceding 3 weeks. In patients with chronic atrial fibrillation who are treated with rate control alone without cardioversion, anticoagulation is usually continued indefinitely with a target international normalized ratio (INR) of 2.0 to 3.0. Based on the results of clinical experience and trials of antithrombotic agents, warfarin therapy sufficient to maintain a target INR of 3.0 should be prescribed for any patient with a prior stroke, transient ischemic attack, or other embolic event. Warfarin also is indicated in patients with clinical heart failure or subclinical left ventricular systolic dysfunction and in those with thyrotoxicosis-related atrial fibrillation because of the higher risk of embolic events. Warfarin therapy also should be strongly considered in patients with a history of hypertension in conjunction with vigorous attempts to control blood pressure. All patients with rheumatic mitral valvular disease or prosthetic valves should receive warfarin. For patients younger than 60 years without any risk factors for thromboembolism no clear increased risk of stroke has been demonstrated to exist; aspirin therapy (325 mg daily) may be considered in such patients. Aspirin also may be considered for patients younger than 75 years without diabetes, hypertension, heart failure, or prior stroke or embolic events. Patients greater than 75 years of age may benefit more from warfarin for embolic stroke reduction but have an increased risk of intracranial bleeding. Either aspirin or warfarin may be prescribed based on consideration in the individual patient of risk factors for stroke or bleeding.

# MAINTENANCE AND CONVERSION OF SINUS RHYTHM

Antiarrhythmic drugs may be used to convert atrial fibrillation to sinus rhythm. Drugs used chronically to convert atrial fibrillation and maintain sinus rhythm include quinidine, procainamide, disopyramide, flecainide, propafenone, sotalol, and amiodarone. Drug therapy alone may convert atrial fibrillation in approximately one third to one half of patients. In the remaining patients, electrical cardioversion is required. Synchronized electrical cardioversion using 50 to 300 J is typically conducted using deep sedation or anesthesia for patient comfort.

In some patients, particularly those in whom atrial fibrillation has a specific trigger such as surgery or other metabolic stress, antiarrhythmic drugs may not be needed after cardioversion. In the remaining patients, antiarrhythmic drug therapy is given chronically. The ability of a single drug to maintain sinus rhythm after cardioversion is approximately 50% at 1 year. When atrial fibrillation recurs, the patient may be converted again, alternative drug therapy may be employed, or antiarrhythmic drug therapy may be discontinued. In individual patients, one antiarrhythmic drug may be more effective than other agents, but overall most agents have similar success rates in long-term follow-up study.

Antiarrhythmic drugs may also be useful in decreasing the frequency of paroxysmal atrial fibrillation. In such patients, recurrence of atrial fibrillation is common, and drug therapy is mainly effective in decreasing the duration, severity, and freqency of paroxysms of atrial fibrillation. Thus, drug therapy is not regarded as a failure even if it results in recurrent episodes but ones that are better tolerated.

Recent data indicate that in some patients so-called antiarrhythmic drug therapy even may be associated with an increased risk of arrhythmic events and death. In a metanalysis performed by Coplen and associates there was an excess mortality in patients treated with quinidine compared to patients given placebo. However, total mortality and not sudden cardiac mortality was statistically different in these two groups. In a retrospective analysis of the SPAF trial, cardiac events in patients treated with antiarrhythmic drugs were increased compared to those not treated with antiarrhythmic drugs despite the adjustment for other patient characteristics.

When the benefits of normal sinus rhythm are judged to outweigh the risk of therapy (Fig. 7-1), antiarrhythmic therapy frequently is justified to decrease the high incidence of reversion to atrial fibrillation

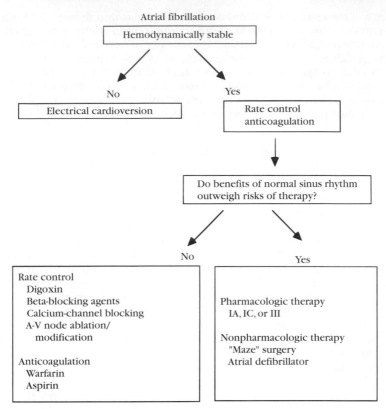

Figure 7–1. *Strategies for the treatment of chronic atrial fibrillation.*

after cardioversion. Multiple drugs have been shown to have efficacy in maintaining sinus rhythm, but all have cardiac and noncardiac side effects that should be considered by the clinician. Polymorphic ventricular tachycardia (torsade de pointes) associated with QT-prolongation is a widely recognized arrhythmia associated with antiarrhythmic drug therapy of atrial fibrillation. This arrhythmia is associated with type IA antiarrhythmic agents such as quinidine, procainamide, and disopyramide, with an estimated risk of 1.5% within the first 48 hours of starting therapy. Bradycardia, hypokalemia, excessive drug-induced QT prolongation have been associated with development of this arrhythmia. The common practice of initiation of these drugs on an outpatient basis or discharging the patients from the hospital shortly after electrical cardioversion has the obvious hazard of missing a significant portion of the cases of torsade de pointes occurring within the first 48 hours of therapy. Sotalol also is associated with torsade in a concentration-dependent fashion. The incidence is approximately 1% in patients receiving 160 to 240 mg daily but increases to 5% to 7% in patients receiving 480 to 640 mg daily for atrial fibrillation. Although the type IC agents have been implicated in increased frequency of sudden death and total mortality in patients after myocardial infarction, they are generally safe and well tolerated in patients with atrial fibrillation in the absence of any structural heart disease or ventricular arrhythmias. Amiodarone is a potent and highly effective antiarrhythmic drug for maintenance of sinus rhythm in low doses (less than 300 mg daily). Used for maintenance of sinus rhythm, amiodarone causes less toxicity than when the drug is used for ventricular arrhythmias. The use of amiodarone should be reserved for patients who have failed to benefit from alternative antiarrhythmic drugs and in whom maintenance of sinus rhythm is essential.

# NONPHARMACOLOGIC THERAPY

Radiofrequency ablation of the AV junction has been described as a method of establishing rate control as described above. A surgical procedure (called "maze" surgery) designed to prevent atrial fibrillation has been demonstrated to restore mechanical atrial contraction and transport by creating multiple blind alleys that prevent the wavefronts of depolarization that are responsible for atrial fibrillation. In addition, there are preliminary data indicating that it may be feasible to cure atrial fibrillation using a radio-frequency energy catheter-based procedure that creates linear lesions in the atria.

The atrial defibrillator, an implantable device using transvenous leads that can automatically convert atrial fibrillation, may emerge as a clinical option in the future. Data currently support the hypothesis that permanent dual-chamber pacemakers may result in a lower incidence of atrial fibrillation compared to single-chamber pacemakers. In patients with paroxysmal atrial fibrillation, dual-chamber pacemakers with the ability to avoid tracking the atrial activity also may be used effectively.

# STRATEGIES FOR THE TREATMENT OF ATRIAL FIBRILLATION

Several factors determine the best strategy for the treatment of atrial fibrillation in the individual patient. These factors include a relative contraindication to anticoagulation, rate of atrial fibrillation and difficulty controlling the rate, symptoms in patients with atrial fibrillation, underlying heart disease, and risk for thromboembolic events.

Two basic strategies exist for the patient presenting with chronic atrial fibrillation: (1) rate control possibly with anticoagulation and (2) conversion and maintenance of sinus rhythm using antiarrhythmic drugs (see Fig. 7-1). The primary advantage of the rate control strategy is the avoidance of adverse effects of antiarrhythmic drugs including a possibly increased mortality in some subgroups. The primary advantages of conversion with antiarrhythmic drugs are the potential improvement in hemodynamics and symptoms and possible elimination of the need for anticoagulation. At the present time, there are no large clinical trials that compare the efficacy and cost effectiveness of these two strategies.

For the patient with a relative contraindication to anticoagulation but with risk factors for thromboembolism, antiarrhythmic drug therapy may result in maintenance of sinus rhythm, obviating the need for anticoagulation. For patients in whom rate control in atrial fibrillation is very difficult, AV junction ablation will permit complete control of the rate but may require continued anticoagulation if indicated. For many patients, one may consider both the strategy of rate control and the strategy of maintenance of sinus rhythm with antiarrhythmic drugs. If a patient continues to be highly symptomatic despite adequate rate control, maintaining sinus rhythm may be the best strategy. For the patient who is asymptomatic after rate control is present with or without drug therapy, anticoagulation may be an alternative to cardioversion and maintenance of sinus rhythm. Renewed concern about the possible risks of antiarrhythmic drug therapy has made rate control a more attractive strategy.

## CONCLUSION

The treatment of atrial fibrillation is based on the principles of adequate rate control, anticoagulation, and maintenance of sinus rhythm. Individual factors determine the risk of thromboembolic events and the decision to anticoagulate. In addition, these factors affect the decision to convert atrial fibrillation and maintain sinus rhythm with antiarrhythmic drugs. AV junction ablation will play a particularly important role in controlling ventricular rate without pharmacologic therapy.

Over the last several years, multiple clinical trials have provided useful information on treatment options for atrial fibrillation. The risks and benefits of long-term anticoagulation with warfarin and aspirin have been evaluated and have clarified guidelines for warfarin therapy in patients with atrial fibrillation. The potential risks of antiarrhythmic agents for maintenance of sinus rhythm have become better appreciated, and prospective randomized trials are planned to compare the two strategies of maintenance of sinus rhythm with pharmacologic therapy, and rate control and anticoagulation. The role of transesophageal echocardiography in the management of atrial fibrillation is currently limited to exclusion of atrial thrombus in patients in whom immediate cardioversion is indicated or anticoagulation is contraindicated. Several options for pharmacologically refractory, symptomatic patients with atrial fibrillation have become available. These include treatment with amiodarone, ablation of the AV node, and newer surgical procedures. The current management strategies, which are formulated based on incomplete knowledge of the true risks and benefit of various therapeutic strategies, likely will be modified as the results of trials currently in progress become available in the future.

*Bibliography*

Coplen SE, Antman EM, Berlin JA, et al: Efficacy and safety of quinidine therapy for maintenance of sinus rhythm after cardioversion: a meta-analysis of randomized control trials, *Circulation* 82:1106-1116, 1990.

Cox JL, Boineau JP, Schuessler RB, et al: Successful surgical treatment of atrial fibrillation: review and clinical update, *JAMA* 266:1976-1980, 1991.

The European Atrial Fibrillation Trial Study Group: Optimal oral anticoagulation therapy in patients with nonrheumatic atrial fibrillation and recent cerebral ischemia, *N Engl J Med* 333:5-10, 1995.

Falk RH, Podrid PJ: Atrial fibrillation: mechanisms and management, New York, 1992, Raven Press.

Manning WJ, Silverman DI, Gordon SPF, et al: Cardioversion from atrial fibrillation without prolonged anticoagulation with use of transesophageal echocardiography to exclude the presence of atrial thrombi, *N Engl J Med* 328:750-755, 1993.

Manning WJ, Silverman DI, Keighley CS, et al: Transesophageal echocardiographically facilitated early cardioversion from atrial fibrillation using short-term anticoagulation: final results of a prospective 4.5-year study, *J Am Coll Cardiol* 26:1354-1361, 1995.

Morady F, Calkins H, Langberg JJ, et al: A prospective randomized comparison of direct current and radiofrequency ablation of the atrioventricular junction, *J Am Coll Cardiol* 21:102-109, 1993.

The National Heart, Lung, and Blood Institute Working Group on Atrial Fibrillation: Atrial fibrillation: current understanding and research imperatives, *J Am Coll Cardiol* 22:1830-1834, 1993.

Prystowsky EN, Benson DW, Fuster V, et al: Management of patients with atrial fibrillation: A statement for healthcare professionals from the subcommittee on electrocardiography and electrophysiology, American Heart Association, *Circulation* 93:1262-1277, 1996.

Stroke Prevention in Atrial Fibrillation Study: Final results, *Circulation* 84:527-539, 1991.

Stroke Prevention in Atrial Fibrillation Investigators: Warfarin versus aspirin for prevention of thromboembolism in atrial fibrillation: Stroke Prevention in Atrial Fibrillation II Study, *Lancet* 343:687-691, 1994.

Williamson BD, Man KC, Daoud E, et al: Radiofrequency catheter modification of atrioventricular conduction to control the ventricular rate during atrial fibrillation, *N Engl J Med* 331:910-917, 1994.

# Infectious Disease

## Chapter 8

## *Fever and the Hospitalized Patient*

Nelson M. Gantz

Fever is a common clinical problem and in one report occurred in 29% of hospitalized patients.[1] Fever may be classified as community-acquired fever if it is present or incubating on admission. Fever that occurs after hospitalization is called *nosocomial fever*. This chapter focuses on an approach to the patient with nosocomial fever on the medical service and the problem of postoperative fever. Discussions of the patient with fever of unknown origin or fever in the specialized host such as the patient with leukemia are presented elsewhere in this book.

## NOSOCOMIAL FEVER ON THE MEDICAL SERVICE

Multiple causes for fever, including infectious and noninfectious processes, exist in the patient on the medical service. Often the source of fever is obvious such as pain and erythema at an intravenous catheter site, which are suggestive of a diagnosis of phlebitis. At other times, the cause of the fever is at first not apparent. A detailed history with attention to the procedures, instrumentations, and drugs initiated since admission may provide a clue to the source of the fever. For example, a new cough and dyspnea in a patient with an underlying altered mental status are suggestive of an aspiration pneumonia. The physical examination may support the diagnosis of pneumonia by detecting the presence of localized crackles on auscultation of the lungs. A careful examination may note a decubitus ulcer or tender prostate gland that will help identify the source of the fever. Clues obtained from a detailed history and physical examination should provide the clinician with the appropriate tests to obtain to determine the cause of the fever. For example, the diagnosis of pseudomembranous colitis is suggested in a febrile patient receiving antibiotics who develops diarrhea. A "routine fever work-up" consisting of complete blood count, blood cultures, sputum culture, urine culture, and a chest roentgenogram is wasteful and not indicated. Instead, the studies ordered should be based on the likely sources of fever from the history and physical examination. For example, a febrile patient lacking pulmonary symptoms and signs is unlikely to have pneumonia, and a sputum culture and a chest roentgenogram will not contribute to finding the cause of the fever. In a febrile patient with an indwelling urinary catheter and an intravenous catheter, the results of blood cultures (two sets), urinalysis, and urine culture may reveal the diagnosis.

The box below lists the causes of nosocomial fever. The majority of diagnoses are infectious.[2] In one study, pneumonia and urinary tract

---

## Causes of Nosocomial Febrile Illnesses

### INFECTIOUS

Pneumonia
Urinary tract infection
Vascular catheter infection
Primary bacteremia (without a source)
*Clostridium difficile* colitis
Sinusitis
Cholangitis
Other

### NONINFECTIOUS

Drug reaction
Aspiration
Pulmonary embolus
Underlying illness
Myocardial infarction
Other

infections accounted for 35% of the causes. Approximately 33% of the diagnoses are attributable to noninfectious causes such as a drug reaction, tissue necrosis caused by a myocardial infarction or stroke, or the underlying illness such as a malignancy.[2]

**Pneumonia.** Pneumonia, a frequent cause of nosocomial fever in patients on the medical service, usually results from aspiration. Patients at high risk include those using a ventilator, the elderly, those with an altered mental status, and those having difficulty with their oropharyngeal secretions. The diagnosis is often difficult because congestive heart failure, atelectasis, pulmonary embolism with infarction, and adult respiratory distress syndrome may mimic pneumonia. Nosocomial pneumonia is usually caused by gram-negative bacilli and less often by *Staphylococcus aureus*. Pneumonia that occurs during the first 3 days of hospitalization may be caused by *Streptococcus pneumoniae* or *Haemophilus influenzae*. It is important to know the epidemiology of the indigenous pathogens in an individual hospital and in a special unit of that hospital. The etiologic diagnosis is often difficult because sputum may not be readily available. Cultures of pleural fluid or blood cultures may help confirm the diagnosis. Cultures of endotracheal aspirates or material obtained from a protected-specimen brush catheter or bronchoalveolar lavage may reveal the etiologic diagnosis. Therapy of nosocomial pneumonia is usually empiric, based on the patient's underlying illness, previous culture data, information on the nosocomial pathogens and their antimicrobial sensitivities, and results of sputum Gram stains and cultures.[3]

**Urinary tract infection.** Urinary tract infections (UTIs), the most frequent nosocomial infection in patients on the medical service, account for 40% of the infections.[4] The majority (80%) of the infections still are related to the use of a urethral catheter; genitourinary procedures are associated with another 10% of the infections. The duration of urethral catheterization is the factor that correlates best with the rate of infection. Approximately 5% to 10% of catheterized patients develop bacteriuria for each day the urethral catheter is in place. Rates of infection are greater for women than for men. Aerobic gram-negative rods account for the majority of infections. About 30% of patients with catheter-related bacteriuria develop symptoms, and only symptomatic patients need to be treated, with these exceptions: neutropenic patients with an obstructed genitourinary (GU) tract, pregnant patients, and organ-transplant recipients.

**Vascular catheter infections.** Intravascular catheters may be associated with fever caused by phlebitis, local infection, or catheter-related bacteremia. Phlebitis is a problem with peripheral rather than central lines and is a physicochemical phenomenon. Phlebitis is not usually caused by bacteria. A local cellulitis at the catheter insertion site and the more serious problem of suppurative phlebitis with pus filling the vein are recognized catheter-related complications. Catheter-related bacteremia or fungemia is another cause of nosocomial fever and occurs with central rather than peripheral lines. Clinical signs of infection at the catheter site are usually absent, and such absence makes the diagnosis more difficult. Coagulase-negative staphylococci are the most common pathogens, but *Staphylococcus aureus,* gram-negative rods, and *Candida* species may be associated with a bloodstream infection. The diagnosis is based on obtaining two sets of blood cultures and performing a semiquantitative culture of the catheter tip by rolling a segment of the catheter on an agar plate; a positive catheter-tip culture contains more than 15 colony-forming units of an organism.[5]

**Primary bacteremia.** Nosocomial bloodstream infections without a focus of infection are classified as primary bacteremias. Secondary bloodstream infections refer to bacteremias or fungemias with the same organism at another body site. Bloodstream infections secondary to an intravenous or arterial line are classified as a primary bacteremia unless signs of local infection at the catheter site are present. Two sets of blood cultures are usually adequate for detection of a nosocomial bacteremia.

**Cholangitis.** Cholangitis refers to infection involving the hepatic and common bile ducts. Obstruction by gallstones is a key factor in the pathogenesis of this disease. Liver function tests are usually elevated, and ultrasonography is helpful in evaluating the patient. Another cause of cryptic fever is acute acalculous cholecystitis. Diagnosis usually is suggested by the clinical picture such as history of trauma and the results of an abdominal computerized tomographic scan or ultrasonography.

The box on p. 94 lists some examples of noninfectious causes of nosocomial fever such as drug reactions. Almost any medication may cause fever, which is classically low grade but may be spiking. Drug fever may be secondary to new medications or drugs a patient has taken for years. A skin rash and eosinophilia may or may not be present. Drugs that are commonly involved include phenytoin sodium, procainamide, quinidine sulfate, and the sulfonamides. Drug fever usually occurs after 7 to 10 days of therapy and usually resolves within 48 to 72 hours of discontinuance of the drug.

Aspiration and atelectasis are other frequent causes of nosocomial fever. Pulmonary emboli always should be considered as a cause of unexplained nosocomial fever. A new myocardial infarction or cerebrovascular accident may cause nosocomial fever. Finally, fever secondary to the patient's underlying illness such as a lymphoma may be the cause of the nosocomial fever, but this is a diagnosis of exclusion.

# POSTOPERATIVE FEVER

Fever occurs frequently after surgery. The origin of the fever may be occult, or it may be obvious, as when a surgical wound dehisces and pus is extruded. The fever may have an infectious or a noninfectious cause. Atelectasis, the most frequent cause of postoperative fever, does not have an infectious basis. Any major surgical procedure can produce a fever for approximately 1 to 3 days after the operation. The fever is usually low grade (99° to 100° F; 37.2° to 37.8° C) and self-limited with no cause determined. However, a localized or a systemic infectious disease is always a consideration, especially when the patient's postoperative temperature exceeds 101° F (38.6° C) in magnitude, when the elevation persists for 72 hours, or when the temperature becomes elevated after an initial afebrile interval. If antitiotic therapy has been continued after surgery, the fever may be low grade, and the only clue may be the presence of leukocytosis with an increase in immature granulocytes ("left shift"). In the evaluation of a febrile postoperative patient, it is important to note the type of surgery, the anesthetic used, the transfusions administered, and the medication record, as well as to perform a meticulous physical examination to obtain clues to the source of fever.

Certain causes of postoperative fever, such as atelectasis or wound or urinary tract infection, are associated with a variety of surgical procedures. Other causes, such as mediastinitis or a prosthetic graft infection after the insertion of a heart valve, are specific for a particular type of operation. Occasionally, the fever represents an infectious disease problem unrelated to the surgical procedure, such as acute cholecystitis after a hernia repair.

**Fever during the first 24 postoperative hours.** In the evaluation of a patient with postoperative fever, it is important to note the temporal relation of the fever to the operation. Causes of fever during the procedure or within the first 24 hours include malignant hyperthermia, transfusion reactions, atelectasis, aspiration pneumonia, wound infection, drug reactions, or endocrine disorders such as acute adrenal insufficiency, thyroid storm, or pheochromocytoma. Malignant hyperthermia is a rare but life-threatening cause in which high fever (105° to 106° F; 40.6° to 41.6° C) and severe metabolic acidosis occur immediately after the introduction of the anesthesia.[6] The disease occurs in approximately one of every 40,000 adults having surgery. A family history of fatal reactions, such as anaphylactic shock associated with anesthesia, may be the only clue present. The disease is inherited as an autosomal dominant trait. Anesthetic agents that commonly trigger the reaction include halothane, enflurane, isoflurane, and succinylcholine. The susceptibility to malignant hyperthermia can be determined by obtaining a muscle biopsy and performing an in vitro contracture test on the muscle specimen. All patients with a family history of suspected malignant hyperthermia should undergo diagnostic muscle testing. Utilization of serum creatine kinase (CK) levels as a screening test for this disease should be abandoned, since false-positive and false-negative results occur frequently.[6]

Fever occurs commonly with blood transfusions. Although these reactions are usually self-limited, they may represent red blood cell or granulocyte incompatibility or contamination of the blood with microorganisms. Atelectasis is the most frequent cause identified for fever during the first 24 hours postoperatively. The aspiration of a foreign body, such as a denture, should be excluded. Although wound infections are usually not detected until after several days, those caused by group A streptococci or by clostridia may present during the first 24 hours after surgery.

**Fever that occurs 24 to 72 hours postoperatively.** The possible causes of fever that begins after the initial 24 to 48 postoperative hours are numerous. The most frequent causes, however, are infection at an intravenous or an arterial line site, infection of the wound, infection of the urinary tract, deep venous thrombosis, or a pulmonary problem.[5] "Third-day surgical fever" denotes fever that occurs on the third postoperative day as a result of an infection at the intravenous site.[7] Such fevers are not limited to the third day and may result from contaminated intravenous fluid as well as from infection at the catheter-insertion site. Inflammation may be absent from the intravenous site, thereby making the diagnosis more difficult. Arterial, pulmonary artery, and central venous pressure catheters are important sources of nosocomial bacteremias in patients hospitalized in intensive care units. This source of bacteremia can be decreased by removal of central lines when they are no longer medically indicated. Therapy consists of removal of the catheters, culture of the tips, and collection of several blood cultures. Never obtain a single set of blood cultures! Instead, draw two sets, using both aerobic and anaerobic bottles, before starting antibiotics.

**Wound sepsis.** Most wound infections are seen 4 to 10 days after an operation. Increased warmth, redness, pain, and tenderness, along with purulent drainage, may be detected. A Gram stain and culture of the discharge should identify the causative agent. Adequate drainage and antibiotics are usually required. Toxic shock syndrome (TSS) can develop as a complication of a surgical wound infection.[8] The syndrome usually develops within 2 days of surgery with a range of 1 to 7 days after the operation. The local signs of surgical wound infection may be unimpressive. *Staphylococcus aureus* is isolated from the wound culture. The diagnosis should be considered in a postoperative patient with fever, diffuse erythoderma that resembles a sunburn-like rash, watery diarrhea, and hypotension. Other findings that may be present include pyuria, an elevated CK level, abnormal liver function tests, a reduced serum calcium level, and a decreased platelet count. Treatment of TSS consists in fluid replacement, use of pressor agents, drainage of the local wound, and antistaphylococcal antibiotics.

**Urinary tract infection.** A urinary tract infection should be suspected in any patient with an indwelling catheter or who has had any urinary tract instrumention.[4] Although infrequent, the source of the fever may be in the prostate; thus a rectal examination should be done.

**Pulmonary problems.** Fever that develops 5 to 7 days or more after an operation should always raise the possibility of deep venous thrombosis, which can present with fever as its only clinical manifestation. The lungs are the other common site of infection. Atelectasis, aspiration, bacterial pneumonia, or pulmonary embolism are the most likely possibilities.[9, 10] Atelectasis with or without pleural effusion may be a clue to an intra-abdominal abscess beneath the diaphragm.

**Nosocomial sinusitis.** Nosocomial acute maxillary sinusitis is a frequently overlooked cause of fever in a postoperative patient with a nasogastric tube, nasotracheal tube, or other foreign body that causes mechanical obstruction of the sinus ostia.[11,12] A history of extensive facial or cranial fracture is often present. Purulent nasal discharge may provide a clue, but its absence does not exclude the diagnosis. Purulent discharge was present in only 25% of patients with sinusitis in one report.[11] Many of the patients are obtunded and unable to complain of facial pain. A leukocytosis is usually present, and roentgenograms of the maxillary sinuses or a computerized tomographic scan of the sinuses confirms the diagnosis. Unlike community-acquired acute maxillary sinusitis in otherwise healthy adults where the causative organisms are usually *Streptococcus pneumoniae* or *Haemophilus influenzae,* nosocomial sinusitis is most commonly caused by gram-negative aerobic bacilli, such as *Escherichia coli, Klebsiella* species, *Enterobacter* species, or *Pseudomonas aeruginosa.* Polymicrobic infections occur in 40% of patients.[11] Since it is difficult to predict the causative organisms in patients with nosocomial sinusitis, antibiotic therapy should be guided by the Gram stain and culture results of material obtained by sinus aspiration. Definitive therapy consists of removal of the nasal tube responsible for obstructing the sinus ostium and administration of appropriate antibiotics based on the results of the Gram stain and culture.

**Pseudomembranous colitis.** Fever, abdominal tenderness, and profuse watery diarrhea that occurs after surgery should raise the possibility that the patient has pseudomembranous colitis[13] caused by the gram-negative anaerobe *Clostridium difficile.* The disorder is more common and severe in the elderly patient who has undergone abdominal surgery and received antibiotics. The syndrome is highly variable, and some patients have fever and abdominal tenderness without diarrhea.[13] Fecal leukocytes are detected in about half of the patients. Symptoms occur as early as a few days after the start of an antibiotic to as long as 6 weeks after antibiotics have been discontinued. The diagnosis can be established by the visualization of pseudomembranes by proctosigmoidoscopy and by the detection of *C. difficile* cytotoxin in the stool. The extent of elevation of the cytotoxin titer does not correlate well with the disease severity, nor should it be used to follow response to therapy. Almost every antibiotic has been implicated as a cause of *C. difficile* colitis, except for vancomycin. Therapy consists in fluid and electrolyte replacement and oral administration of vancomycin or metronidazole. When postoperative patients have an ileus, metronidazole should be given intravenously as well as vancomycin given by enema and nasogastric tube. The offending antibiotic should be discontinued, though no firm data exist regarding the efficacy of this measure.

**Other causes of delayed postoperative fever.** Additional causes of fever with an onset at least 24 hours after an operation include the complications associated with anesthesia (such as halothane hepatitis), hepatitis C, cytomegalovirus (CMV), Epstein-Barr virus, protozoa transmitted through transfused blood such as *Babesia microti* (*babesiosis*) or *Plasmodium* species (malaria), sterile or infected hematomas, drug fever, and infections unrelated to the operation (such as acute cholecystitis). Halothane and methoxyflurane may cause postoperative fever, though this is infrequent. The features observed in a patient with halothane hepatitis are fever during the second postoperative week, malaise, anorexia, right upper quadrant pain, an increase in serum aspirate aminotransferase (AST) levels, and occasionally a rash or jaundice. Multiple exposures to halothane may be associated with a shorter postoperative incubation period. Risk factors associated with halothane hepatitis include middle age, previous closely spaced administrations of halothane, obesity, female sex, and genetic predisposition.[14] Chemical and bacterial meningitis are other reported causes of fever that may occur with spinal anesthesia. Transmission of CMV is not restricted to patients after open-heart surgery; CMV can develop after any blood transfusion. Fever that develops 2 to 4 weeks after an operation and accompanied by atypical lymphocytes is a clue to a mononucleosis syndrome caused by CMV or by Epstein-Barr virus.

The spectrum of disease associated with *B. microti* infection ranges from an asymptomatic disorder to an illness characterized by fever, myalgias, fatigue, and hemolytic anemia. Microscopic examination of Giemsa-stained blood smear reveals the intraerythrocytic protozoon. Patients who are seriously ill should receive treatment with clindamycin and quinine sulfate.

Hepatitis C is the major cause of transfusion hepatitis, but fever is usually absent. Drug fever is an important noninfectious cause of persistent postoperative fever, especially in patients taking antibiotics, quinidine, phenytoin, methyldopa, procainamide, allopurinol, or sleeping medications. Drug fever may be caused by any drug, however, and the associated rash and eosinophilia may be absent. Finally, there is always the possibility of an infection unrelated to an operation, such as cholecystitis, hospital-acquired influenza, or Legionnaire's disease.

Acute cholecystitis can occur after operative procedures unrelated to the biliary tract. This infection often develops in patients with no prior history of biliary tract disease. Symptoms include right upper quadrant pain, nausea, vomiting, and fever. At times, fever is the only feature. Right upper quadrant tenderness is a helpful finding. The inability to detect biliary stones by radiologic techniques does not exclude the diagnosis of acute cholecystitis, since the patient may have acalculous cholecystitis. Postoperative cholecystitis often results in gangrene, perforation, or empyema of the gallbladder. Other complications include intrahepatic abscesses, cholangitis, and intra-abdominal abscesses. Organisms recovered most often from patients with postoperative cholecystitis include *Escherichia coli, Klebsiella* species, enterococci, *Bacteroides fragilis,* and *Pseudomonas aeruginosa.*[15] Difficulties in establishing the diagnosis and in initiating appropriate therapy are reflected in high mortalities ranging from 10% to 50%. The mortality in patients with acalculous cholecystitis is usually twice that of patients who have calculi and acute cholecystitis.[15] Once the disease is recognized, early operative intervention and appropriate antibiotics are indicated.

Disseminated candidiasis is a consideration in patients who have had operations of the gastrointestinal tract.[16] Risk factors that predispose patients to systemic candidiasis include exposure to multiple broad-spectrum antibiotics, impaired host defenses caused by the patient's underlying illness, corticosteroids, parenteral catheters, and total parenteral nutrition. Fever, leukocytosis, and hypotension in a patient who has had abdominal surgery and who has received broad-spectrum antibiotics should raise the suspicion of disseminated candidiasis. Diagnosis depends on isolation of the yeast from the blood or detection of the typical focal chorioretinal lesions. Blood culture results are frequently negative, and serologic tests have not been helpful in establishing the diagnosis.

As previously mentioned, in addition to the complications that occur with various surgical procedures, the cause of the fever may be closely related to the particular kind of operation performed. An intra-abdominal, subphrenic, hepatic abscess or pancreatitis may develop after abdominal surgery. A foreign body, such as a surgical sponge retained after abdominal surgery, may be responsible for postoperative fever. A pelvic operation may be complicated by septic pelvic thrombo-phlebitis, pelvic abscess, or cellulitis. Diagnostic considerations after cardiovascular surgery are sternal osteomyelitis, endocarditis, medias-tinitis, venous graft-site infections, or the postcardiotomy syndrome. Similarly, in neurosurgical, orthopedic, and other specialist-performed operations, the causes of fever may be unique to the procedure. The cause of fever may become apparent only after an analysis of the fever onset and its relation to surgery in general or to the particular operation, the patient's complaints, and the physical and laboratory findings. As I have tried to stress, in the evaluation of a patient with nosocomial fever, it is important to perform a careful history and physical examina-tion and to obtain focused laboratory tests based on the likely source of the fever, rather than to order a routine battery of tests as part of a "fever work-up."[17-19]

## References

1. McGowan JE, Rose RC, Jacobs NF, et al: Fever in hospitalized patients, *Am J Med* 82:580, 1987.

2. Filice GA, Weiler MD, Hughes RA, Gerding DN: Nosocomial febrile illnesses in patients on an internal medicine service, *Arch Intern Med* 149:319, 1989.

3. Hospital Infection Control Practices Advisory Committee: Guideline for prevention of nosocomial pneumonia. Part I: Issues on prevention of noso-comial pneumonia. Part II: Recommendations for prevention of nosocomial pneumonia, *Am J Infect Control* 22:247-292, 1994.

4. Garibaldi RA: Hospital-acquired urinary tract infections. In Wenzel RP, editor: *Prevention and control of nosocomial infections,* ed 2, Balitmore, 1993, Williams & Wilkins.

5. Widmer AF: IV-related infections. In Wenzel RP, editor: *Prevention and control of nosocomial infections,* ed 2, Baltimore, 1993, Williams & Wilkins.

6. Heiman-Patterson TD: Neuroleptic malignant syndrome and malignant hy-perthermia, *Med Clinics North Am* 77:477, 1993.

7. Altemeier WA, McDonough JJ, Fuller WD: Third day surgical fever, *Arch Surg* 103:158-166, 1971.

8. Garbe PL, Arka RJ, Reingold AL, et al: *Staphylococcus aureus* isolates from patients with nonmenstrual toxic shock syndrome, *JAMA* 253:2538-2542, 1985.

9. Bartlett JG, Gorbach SL, Finegold SM: The bacteriology of aspiration pneu-monia, *Am J Med* 56:202-207, 1974.

10. Wynne JW, Modell JH: Respiratory aspiration of stomach contents, *Ann Intern Med* 87:466-474, 1977.
11. Caplan ES, Hoyt NJ: Nosocomial sinusitis, *JAMA* 247:639-641, 1982.
12. Kulber DA, Santora TA, Shabot MM, et al: Early diagnosis and treatment of sinusitis in the critically ill trauma patient, *Am Surg* 57:775, 1991.
13. Bartlett JG: *Clostridium difficile:* clinical consideration, *Rev Infect Dis* 12(suppl 2):S243, 1990.
14. Farrell G, Prendergast D, Murray M: Halothane hepatitis, *N Engl J Med* 313:1310-1314, 1985.
15. Devine RM, Farnell MB, Mucha P Jr: Acute cholecystitis as a complication in surgical patients, *Arch Surg* 199:1389-1393, 1984.
16. Burchard KW: Fungal sepsis, *Infect Dis Clin North Am* 6:677-692, 1992.
17. Cunha BA, Shea KW: Fever in the intensive case unit, *Insert Dis Clinic North Am* 10:185-209, 1996.
18. Stone HH: Infection in postoperative patients, *Am J Med* 81:39-44, 1986.
19. Arbo MJ, Fine MJ, Hanusa BH, et al: Fever of nosocomial origin: etiology, risk factors, and outcomes, *Am J Med* 95:505, 1993.

# Chapter 9

# *Assessing Fever in the HIV-Infected Patient*

Richard A. Gleckman

Fever frequently develops in HIV-infected patients, regardless of their degree of immunocompromise. This chapter offers the clinician a diagnostic strategy for the assessment of the HIV-infected patient who experiences fever. The foundation of the diagnostic assessment consists in a comprehensive medical history and physical examination, specific laboratory and radiographic studies, and the knowledge of a recent CD4 lymphocyte count (a surrogate marker for evaluating the degree of immunodeficiency).[1] The box at the top of p. 104 provides some general concepts that apply to the diagnostic considerations for the febrile HIV-infected patient.

When the clinician assesses fever in the HIV-infected patient, consideration should be given to those infections that are associated with specific life-styles. Homosexual and bisexual men are predisposed to *Salmonella* bacteremia. When intravenous drug users present with a febrile disorder, attention should be directed at a common infection (a viral or bacterial respiratory infection, bacterial pyelonephritis, pelvic inflammatory disease), an infection for which parenteral drug users are uniquely predisposed (see box at the bottom of p. 104), a noninfectious disorder (alcoholic hepatitis), and the possibility of one of the opportunistic infections or neoplasms that develop in the HIV-infected patient.[2] The decision to perform a detailed investigation to determine the cause of the patient's febrile state will depend on the patient's consent to be subjected to diagnostic studies and the "clinical stage" of the patient's disease. The clinician should provide comfort measures or hospice care exclusively when the patient experiences end-stage AIDS (advanced HIV-related dementia, uncontrolled opportunistic infections, or disseminated malignancies).

## DRUG-INDUCED FEVER

HIV-infected patients experience a high incidence of adverse reactions to drugs. Drug-induced fever has been attributed to antimicrobials (trimethoprim-sulfamethoxazole [TMP/SMX], clindamycin, dapsone),

---

### General Concepts
· · · · · · · · · · · · · · · · · · · · · · · · · · · · · · · · · · · · · · · · · · · · · · · · · · · · · · · · · · · · · · · · · · · · · · · ·

Infection is the most common cause of fever.

Resist temptation to attribute fever to the HIV infection itself in the patient with AIDS.

Fever can be exclusive manifestation of *Pneumocytis carinii* infection.

Compliant administration of prophylactic trimethoprim-sulfamethoxazole virtually excludes *Pneumocystis carinii* pneumonia and *Salmonella* bacteremia.

Fever can be caused by multiple simultaneous infections.

Prolonged unexplained (FUO) fever is usually caused by disseminated *Mycobacterium avium* complex, tubercule bacillus, *Pneumocystis carinii,* or non-Hodgkin's lymphoma.

---

antivirals (zidovudine, ganciclovir, interferon-alpha), antimycobacterials (isoniazid, rifampin), hematopoietic growth factors (erythropoietin, G-CSF), and antineoplastic agents (bleomycin, methotrexate).[3] When HIV-infected patients develop fever and there is no readily identifiable alternative explanation, the clinician should have little hesitation to recommend discontinuation of these medications.

## PRIMARY INFECTION

Fever is the most common manifestation of symptomatic primary infection caused by HIV. Fever is usually accompanied by additional findings, including malaise, sweats, weight loss, arthralgia, myalgia, photophobia, anorexia, retrosternal pain, odynophagia, headache, nausea, vomiting, diarrhea, pharyngitis, lymphadenopathy, skin rash, lesions of the oral cavity (ulcers, enanthemas, candidiasis), and, on occasion, splenomegaly and uclers of the penis and anus.[4] Symptomatic primary infection resolves spontaneously, usually within 2 to 3 weeks.

---

### Intravenous Drug User
· · · · · · · · · · · · · · · · · · · · · · · · · · · · · · · · · · · · · · · · · · · · · · · · · · · · · · · · · · · · · · · · · · · · · · · ·

Bacterial pneumonia

Tuberculosis (pulmonary or extrapulmonary)

Soft-tissue infections (cellulitis, abscess, necrotizing fasciitis)

Bacteremia/fungemia/septic thrombophlebitis

Endocarditis with or without meningitis, brain abscess, mycotic aneurysm, splenic or renal abscess

Septic arthritis or osteomyelitis

---

# CDC SYMPTOMATIC B

The disorder previously referred to as the persistent generalized lymph-adenopathy syndrome, or AIDS-related complex (ARC), has now been modified by the new CDC classification as *symptomatic B.* These individuals manifest the following: generalized lymphadenopathy of 3 months or greater, often accompanied by fever, fatigue, night sweats, weight loss, diarrhea, and splenomegaly. Once their CD4+ cell count drops below 200 cells/mm$^3$, or 14% of the total lymphocyte number, these HIV-infected persons are classified as having AIDS.

When patients classified as CDC B develop a febrile disease, the primary care physician should consider the following infectious disorders; traditional bacterial infections (including bronchitis, sinusitis, pneumonitis, bacteremia, pelvic inflammatory disease, pyelonephritis, cellulitis), viral respiratory infections, secondary syphilis, those infections associated with specific life-styles, and tuberculosis (pulmonary, extrapulmonary, or combined). On occasion, *Pneumocystis carinii* pneumonia develops in HIV-infected patients with CD4+ counts that exceed 200.

The approach to the HIV-infected febrile patient with a recent CD4+ cell count greater than 200 cells/mm$^3$ includes a thorough history and meticulous physical examination, complete blood count, chest roentgenogram, urinalysis, cultures of the blood, liver function tests (as an indicator for alcoholic, drug-induced, or viral hepatitis), serologic test for syphilis, serum amylase, and a tuberculin skin test (if a previous test was negative or if the patient has an unknown status to a purified protein derivative skin test) applied with other skin tests to ensure cutaneous reactivity. Further assessment of the patient is determined by the findings of the initial encounter, as determined by the results of the history and physical and laboratory studies. Patients who appear seriously ill, have a white blood cell count less than 500 mm$^3$, or are actively administering drugs intravenously are candidates for hospitalization and empiric antibiotic therapy. Additional indications for hospitalizing intravenous drug users include their unreliability to return for further assessment and the inability of the clinician to exclude the diagnosis of endocarditis during the initial patient encounter.

For patients who do not qualify for hospitalization the primary care physician should discontinue all medications that are not considered absolutely essential, discourage the use of antipyretics (when the cause of the fever remains unknown), and provide the patient with a means to contact the physician (or designee) 24 hours a day. If unexplained fever persists (the initial studies are nonrevealing, and there are no focal signs or symptoms such as cough, shortness of breath, headache, confusion, abdominal pain, or diarrhea), the primary care physician should confirm that all medications have been discontinued, inquire whether the patient has recently taken (by mouth or intravenously) an antibiotic, and arrange to have sinus roentgenograms performed. If the HIV-infected patient is an intravenous drug addict, persistent fever can signal the presence of osteomyelitis and "occult" tuberculosis.

HIV-infected patients who are intravenous drug users, immigrants from countries where tuberculosis is endemic (particularly Mexico, the Philippines, Vietnam, South Korea, China, Haiti), and individuals who are in contact with people who are disseminating *Mycobacterium tuberculosis* are predisposed to develop tuberculosis. HIV-infected patients with tuberculosis more often demonstrate extrapulmonary disease.[5] There is often a delay in considering a diagnosis of tuberculosis because the signs and symptoms are nonspecific, skin testing is insensitive, and the chest roentgenogram is neither sensitive nor specific.

## AIDS

Febrile HIV-infected patients with CD4+ counts less than 200 cells/ $mm^3$ merit an evaluation that searches for the disorders previously mentioned as well as those opportunistic infections caused by *Pneumocystis carinii, Histoplasma capsulatum, cryptococcus neoformans, Toxoplasma gondii,* mycobacteria causing disseminated disease (Mycobacterium avium–intracellulare [MAC], *M. genavense, M. chelonei*), *Bartonella henselae,* and occult neoplasm (particularly non-Hodgkin's lymphoma).[6,7]

A variable number of HIV-infected patients with symptomatic *Pneumocystis carinii* pneumonia will have a chest roentgenogram that fails to reveal an infiltrate.[7] A normal gallium scan in conjunction with a normal chest roentgenogram would virtually exclude *Pneumocystis carinii* pneumonia (PCP) as an explanation for the patient's persistent febrile state because gallium-scanning approaches 95% sensitivity for PCP.

Computerized tomography has an established role in the investigation of the HIV-infected, febrile patient with symptoms attributable to central nervous system disease and the patient being evaluated for evidence of ethmoid and sphenoid sinusitis. This technique also has considerable capability of indicating specific occult abdominal diseases that can produce fever, including MAC disease, tuberculosis, cytomegalovirus colitis, hepatic abscesses, hepatic masses, infectious cholangitis, and visceral non-Hodgkin's lymphoma.[8]

In contrast to tuberculosis, MAC disease develops exclusively in patients with an advanced stage of immunosuppression, and it often manifests as persistent occult fever. The clinical features associated with disseminated MAC disease (anorexia, weight loss, fever, night sweats, weakness, and diarrhea) simulate numerous alternative disorders in the AIDS patient.[9] Recognition of disseminated MAC disease has been accorded enhanced importance because medication is now available to reduce constitutional symptoms and prolong life. The diagnosis of MAC can usually be established by the isolation of the organism from blood, using both agar and radiometric methods. Unfortunately the procedure requires weeks. Demonstration of the organisms can be accelerated by microscopic examination of a bone marrow or liver biopsy specimen.[10]

In the HIV-infected patient histoplasmosis is a disseminated disease that is characterized by persistent fever and weight loss, often unassociated with respiratory symptoms.[11] The disease develops in patients who reside in endemic areas (such as the Ohio and Mississippi River valleys and Indianapolis), have previously lived in endemic areas (Puerto Rico, Colombia, Dominican Republic), or have hobbies that bring them into contact with foci contaminated with *Histoplasma capsulatum* (caves, farms, bird-roost sites). Diagnostic studies include serologic tests for antigen and antibody, demonstration of the organism in body fluids and tissues, and recovery of the organism from blood (lysis-centrifugation technique), bone marrow, cerebrospinal fluid, and bronchoalveolar lavage fluid.

Fever accompanied by night sweats, fatigue, and weight loss can herald systemic non-Hodgkin's lymphoma. Systemic lymphomas, in contrast to the primary central nervous system lymphomas, can develop in HIV-infected patients with CD4+ counts more than 200 cells/mm$^3$.[12] Two features characterize the systemic lymphomas: widespread extranodal dissemination on presentation (involving bone marrow, liver, meninges, and gastrointestinal tract) and appearance at unusual sites (such as testes, parotid gland, gingiva, appendix). The extranodal sites of systemic lymphomas are inaccessible to traditional physical examination. Abnormalities that would heighten the clinician's suspicion that systemic non-Hodgkin's lymphoma exists would include the following: asymmetric or rapidly progressive lymphadenopathy; hepatomegaly; splenomegaly; unexplained gastrointestinal symptoms/signs; obstructive biliary disease; radiographic detection of hilar adenopathy or an abdominal mass; and laboratory identification of an elevated serum alkaline phosphatase, a greatly abnormal serum LDH, or a sudden decrease in all blood cell lines.

It is important to recognize systemic non-Hodgkin's lymphomas because chemotherapy can produce symptomatic relief and, on occasion, for patients who are not greatly immunocompromised (CD4+ counts >200), enhance survival. The prognosis has generally been unfavorable, however, because patients often have extensive disease at presentation as well as detrimental risk factors (low Karnofsky performance status, marrow involvement, advanced immune incompetence), do not tolerate very intensive cancer regimens, and are predisposed to developing the "wasting syndrome," as well as life-threatening opportunistic infections.

# ADDITIONAL REMARKS

Some life-endangering opportunistic infections, both viral (cytomegalovirus, JC papovavirus) and parasitic (cryptosporidiosis, microsporidiosis, central nervous system toxoplasmosis), rarely cause fever in the HIV-infected patient.[13] Febrile HIV-infected patients who are seeking relief from the discomfort attributed to their fever can be encouraged to use aspirin or acetaminophen if the source of the fever has been established. The initial observation that acetaminophen enhanced the potential of zidovudine to cause neutropenia has not been subsequently confirmed.

## References

1. Turner BJ, Hecht FM, Ismail RB: CD4$^+$ T-lymphocyte measures in the treatment of individuals infected with human immunodeficiency virus type 1, *Arch Intern Med* 154:1561-1573, 1994.
2. Cherubin CE, Sapira JD: The medical complications of drug addiction and the medical assessment of the intravenous drug user: 25 years later, *Ann Intern Med* 119:1017-1028, 1993.
3. Jacobson MA, McGrath MS, Joseph P, et al: Zidovudine-induced fever, *J Acquir Immune Defic Syndr* 2:382-388, 1989.
4. Kinloch-deLoes S, Saussure PD, Saurat JH, et al: Symptomatic primary infection due to human immunodeficiency virus type 1: review of 31 cases, *Clin Infect Dis* 17:59-65, 1993.
5. Barnes PF, Block AB, Davidson PT, et al: Tuberculosis in patients with human immunodeficiency virus infection, *N Engl J Med* 324:1644-1650, 1991.
6. Sepkowitz KA, Telzak EE, Carrow M, et al: Fever among outpatients with advanced human immunodeficiency virus infection, *Arch Intern Med* 153:1909-1912, 1993.
7. Gleckman R, Czachor JS: Assessment of fever in HIV-infected patients, *Postgrad Med* 99:78, 1996.
8. Wyatt SH, Fishman EK: The acute abdomen in individuals with AIDS, *Radiol Clin North Am* 32:1023-1043, 1994.
9. Benson CA, Ellner JJ: *Mycobacterium avium* complex infection and AIDS: advances in theory and practice, *Clin Infect Dis* 17:7-20, 1993.
10. Bishburg E, Eng RHK, Smith SM, et al: Yield of bone marrow culture in the diagnosis of infectious diseases in patients with acquired immunodeficiency syndrome, *J Clin Microbiol* 24:312, 1986.
11. Wheat LJ, Stringfield PAC, Baker RL, et al: Disseminated histoplasmosis in the acquired immune deficiency syndrone: clinical findings, diagnosis and treatment, and review of the literature, *Medicine* 69:361-374, 1990.
12. Levine AM, Halley JS, Pike MC, et al: Human immunodeficiency virus–related lymphoma, *Cancer* 68:2466-2472, 1991.
13. Zurlo JJ, O'Neill D, Polis MA, et al: Lack of clinical utility of cytomegalovirus blood and urine cultures in patients with HIV infection, *Ann Intern Med* 118:12, 1993.

# Chapter 10

## Complicated Urinary Tract Infections: Therapeutic Concepts

Richard A. Gleckman

Traditionally, the term "complicated" has been applied to those urinary tract infections that occur in patients with structural or functional abnormalities impeding urine flow.[1] The term has also been extended to those urinary tract infections experienced by elderly patients as well as specific patients with altered host defenses (particularly the diabetic, the renal transplant recipient, the persistently granulocytopenic patient, and the patient receiving prednisone to manage a collagen vascular disorder.)[2]

Of interest is the observation that urinary tract infections have not represented a prominent theme for nonhomosexual HIV-infected individuals devoid of urinary catheters. Unfortunately the natural history of complicated infections for patients with abnormal urinary tracts and for patients with altered host defenses has not been adequately explored, and there is a dearth of well-designed, well-performed studies to serve as a resource to provide definitive therapeutic guidelines.

Compared to the uncomplicated infection, complicated infections are often recalcitrant to drug treatment, resulting in unresolved or recurrent (relapse) infection, and they represent a greater threat for the development of renal insufficiency. All patients with complicated urinary tract infections do not require antimicrobial therapy.[3,4] Drug treatment is not offered to some patients for the following reasons: the natural course of the untreated infection does not appear to represent a threat to life or cause serious morbidity; drug therapy is often unsuccessful and on occasion results in disease caused by a drug-resistant uropathogen, and drugs not only add to the costs of health care but also have the potential to contribute untoward events.

Treatment is certainly indicated for those patients who experience systemic abnormalities (rigors, sweats, fever, anorexia, nausea, vomiting), pain, or irritative voiding symptoms (frequency, urgency, dysuria, nocturia) attributed to the infection. A consensus has emerged that elderly asymptomatic individuals are not candidates for drug therapy. For many of these people asymptomatic bacteriuria is a transient event, and currently there is no method to identify those individuals who are at risk of developing symptomatic pyelonephritis. In addition, unless there is urinary tract obstruction, asymptomatic bacteriuria does not cause renal insufficiency, and, just as important, therapy frequently fails to achieve prolonged sterility of the urinary tract. The evidence indicates that asymptomatic bacteriuria may not allow one to predict death for geriatric patients, and antimicrobial therapy fails to reduce mortality for these infected elderly patients.[5] When the potential exists for serious illness, therapy would be appropriate for an asymptomatic patient. Examples include the patient with an infection stone, the patient with chronic bacterial prostatitis, and the patient with a renal transplant. Select compromised hosts, including the steroid recipient, the leukopenic cancer patient, and the diabetic, are at serious risk from the complications of asymptomatic bacteriuria. Diabetics are predisposed to the development of several unique life-endangering urinary tract infections, such as emphysematous pyelonephritis, pyelonephritis complicating papillary necrosis, and perinephric abscess. Whether these compromised hosts, harboring asymptomatic bacteriuria, are candidates for antimicrobial therapy is unknown.

It is important to stress that drug therapy is only one component of the management of the patient with a complicated urinary tract infection. Often radiologic and surgical intervention are essential. Abscesses must be drained, and impediments to urine flow must be corrected. Recent advances in endoscopic surgery and lithotripsy have added an important dimension in the therapy of complicated urinary tract infections.

## SYMPTOMATIC (COMPLICATED) PYELONEPHRITIS

Symptomatic, complicated (by obstruction, xanthogranuloma, or perinephric abscess) pyelonephritis is often heralded by the following features: continuous fever and pain despite antimicrobial therapy; bacteriuria that persists after drug treatment has commenced; and the development of septic shock with or without adult respiratory distress syndrome (ARDS). Symptomatic patients with complicated pyelonephritis are candidates for early drainage of perinephric abscesses, partial nephrectomy for xanthogranuloma, and relief of obstruction.[6] For the patient with symptomatic complicated pyelonephritis it would appear appropriate to prescribe an antibiotic when the disease is first considered and to continue drug administration for at least 10 to 14 days after the obstruction is relieved or the perinephric abscess is drained.

## CHRONIC BACTERIAL PROSTATITIS

Chronic bacterial prostatitis is characterized by recurrent urinary tract infection (relapse) caused most commonly by *Escherichia coli, Klebsiella* species, *Proteus mirabilis, Pseudomonas aeruginosa,* and *En-*

*terococcus faecalis.* Months of therapy have not resulted in impressive cure rates. Impaired drug penetration and infected prostatic calculi contribute to the difficulty in achieving cure.[7] The current recommendation is for prolonged treatment with trimethoprim-sulfamethoxazole or a fluoroquinolone. For select patients radical transurethral prostatectomy can be considered.

## RENAL TRANSPLANT RECIPIENT

When urinary tract infections are detected within 3 months of the transplant, they are most often a pyelonephritis rather than a cystitis, and when treated with the conventional 10 to 14 days of drug, they are frequently associated with relapse. Limited data indicate that these infections respond to a 6-week course of treatment.[8] When urinary tract infections occur more than 3 months after transplantation, a 2-week course of therapy is appropriate. If there is a concern that the disease is pyelonephritis or the patient experiences a relapse after therapy, the duration of drug treatment is 6 weeks.

## INFECTION STONE

Selective individuals, such as patients who have persistent or intermittent long-term catheterization to manage a neurogenic bladder, develop infection stones. The stones, consisting of calcium phosphate (apatite) and magnesium ammonium phosphate (struvite), are a threat to life because they are associated with silent obstruction with diminished renal function, xanthogranulomatous pyelonephritis, pyelonephritis, pyonephrosis, renal abscess, perirenal abscess, bacteremia, septic shock, and ARDS.[14] Infection stones contain urease-producing bacteria, particularly *Proteus mirabilis* and less commonly *Klebsiella pneumoniae* and *Pseudomonas aeruginosa*, in their interstices, and the organisms are protected from host defenses and antibiotics. Such protection explains why infection stones are prone to cause recurrent infections.[10]

Patients who experience acute symptomatic urosepsis are candidates for emergent relief of obstruction, intravenous administration of an antibiotic, and drainage of perinephric abscess or xanthogranulomatous pyelonephritis. Asymptomatic patients should be considered for stone dissolution with extracorporeal shock-wave lithotripsy, percutaneous nephrolithotomy, or a combination of these procedures. The urease inhibitor, acetohydroxamic acid, has not proved to be an effective agent to dissolve infection stones, and the compound has caused significant toxic reactions.[11]

## LONG-TERM CATHETERIZATION

Patients requiring long-term catheterization experience persistent polymicrobial infection recalcitrant to antimicrobial therapy. Attempts to rid the urine of organisms in an asymptomatic chronically catheter-ized patient are not recommended. Antimicrobial treatment fails to reduce the incidence of bacteriuria, the duration of bacteriuric epi-sodes, or the frequency of catheter obstruction. In addition, antimicro-bial treatment promotes the emergence of drug-resistant organisms. Antimicrobials should be reserved for patients who experience symp-tomatic urosepsis. These latter patients are candidates for a 10-day course of antimicrobial treatment, though the optimum treatment dura-tion is unknown.[12]

# CANDIDURIA

Candiduria is most often experienced by diabetics, intravenous drug abusers, recent recipients of an antibiotic, and patients with Foley catheters. Candiduria can be inconsequential (colonization), represent one manifestation of a focal urinary tract infection (urethritis, cystitis, pyelonephritis, fungal bezoar), or reflect disseminated (hematogenous) disease. Patients who demonstrate persistent candiduria and have not been subjected to instrumentation of the urinary tract merit assessment for diabetes mellitus, renal insufficiency, and an anatomic urinary abnor-mality.[13] Patients with candiduria and suspected bezoar, pyelonephritis with or without renal abscess, perinephric abscess, and papillary necro-sis, and those with disseminated disease (suggested by abnormalities of the optic fundi, skin lesions, the presence of vascular access sites, and evidence of multiple organ dysfunction with or without fungemia) should receive systemic antifungal therapy (in the form of parenteral amphotericin B or fluconazole), relief of obstruction, drainage of ab-scesses, and management of concomitant disorders. The safety, efficacy, ease of administration, and favorable pharmacokinetics make flucona-zole an appealing treatment. It should not be prescribed, however, when the candiduria is caused by non-*C. albicans Candida* species. Numerous treatments are available for the patient with symptomatic candidal cystitis. These include discontinuation of the antibiotic the patient is receiving and offering a single intravenous dose of amphoteri-cin B, orally administered flucytosine, orally administered fluconazole, or bladder irrigation with amphotericin B. There are no comparative controlled studies. Many patients with asymptomatic candiduria will experience spontaneous resolution. It has been suggested that the neutropenic host and the renal-transplant recipient are candidates for therapy. No studies have identified the optimum treatment duration of either focal or disseminated urinary tract infection caused by *Can-dida* species.

# DRUGS

The newer quinolones (norfloxacin, ciprofloxacin, ofloxacin, and enox-acin) rival trimethoprim-sulfamethoxazole (TMP-SMX) as the preferred medical management of patients with complicated urinary tract infections. The quinolones are available in oral form, have a spectrum of activity that includes most gram-negative aerobic bacilli that cause urinary tract infection, require infrequent dosing, have an established role for safety and efficacy, and are appropriate therapy for penicillin-allergic patients. The quinolones have demonstrated therapeutic efficacy for the management of complicated infections caused by bacteria resistant to TMP-SMX and aminoglycosides, and they have also ushered in a new era of oral treatment of *Pseudomonas aeruginosa*-related urinary tract infections.[14]

There are some concerns with regard to prescribing the new quinolones, however. These are expensive compounds that are not appropriate for pregnant women and require dose reduction when administered to patients with renal failure. The quinolones are not appropriate therapy for patients with infection caused by *Enterococcus* species and have the potential to produce hypersensitivity reactions as well as Achilles tendinitis or rupture. In addition, there are potential drug-drug interactions with ddi, antacids, sucralfate, multivitamins with zinc, iron sulfate, and theophylline. Limiting the enthusiasm for the new quinolones is the observation that some patients receiving a quinolone to treat a *Pseudomonas aeruginosa*-related urinary infection develop a relapse caused by a drug-resistant organism and that many recipients of these compounds develop superinfection with *Enterococcus* species or *Candida* species.[15]

## References

1. Preheim LC: Complicated urinary tract infections, *Am J Med* 79(suppl 2A):62, 1985.
2. Korzeniowski OM: Urinary infection in the impaired host, *Med Clin North Am* 75:391, 1991.
3. Gleckman R: Complicated urinary tract infections, *Int J Antimicrob Agents* 4.125, 1994.
4. Abrutyn E, Berlin J, Mossey J, et al: Does treatment of asymptomatic bacteriuria in older ambulatory women reduce subsequent symptoms of urinary tract infection? *JAGS* 44:293, 1996.
5. Abrutyn E, Mossey J, Berlin JA, et al: Does asymptomatic bacteriuria predict mortality and does antimicrobial treatment reduce mortality in elderly ambulatory women? *Ann Intern Med* 120:827, 1994.
6. Eastham J, Ashlering T, Skinner E: Xanthogranulomatous pyelonephritis: clinical findings and surgical considerations, *Urology* 43:296, 1994.
7. Meares EM Jr: Prostatitis, *Med Clin North Am* 75:405, 1991.
8. Rubin RH, Fang LST, Cosimi AB, et al: Usefulness of the antibody-coated assay in the management of urinary tract infection in the renal transplant patient, *Transplantation* 27:18, 1979.
9. Shortliffe LMD, Spigelman SS: Infection stones: evaluation and management, *Urol Clin North Am* 13:717, 1986.
10. Fowler JE Jr: Bacteriology of branched renal calculi and accompanying urinary tract infection, *J Urol* 131:213, 1984.
11. Griffith DP, Khonsari F, Skurnick JH, et al: A randomized trial of acetohydroxamic acid for the treatment and prevention of infection-induced urinary stones in spinal cord injury patients, *J Urol* 140:318, 1988.

12. Gleckman R, Blagg D, Hibert D, et al: Catheter-related urosepsis in the elderly, *J Am Geriatr Soc* 30:255, 1982.
13. Fisher JF, Newman CL, Sobel JD: Yeast in the urine: solutions for a budding problem, *Clin Infect Dis* 20:183, 1995.
14. Preheim LC, Cuevas JA, Roccaforte JS, et al: Oral ciprofloxacin in the treatment of elderly patients with complicated urinary tract infections due to trimethoprim/sulfamethoxazole-resistant bacteria, *Am J Med* 82(suppl 4A):303, 1987.
15. Ryan JL, Berenson CS, Greco TP, et al: Oral ciprofloxacin in resistant urinary tract infections, *Am J Med* 82(suppl 4A):303, 1987.

# Chapter 11
# *Nosocomial Pneumonia*

Nelson M. Gantz

Pneumonia is the second most frequent nosocomial infection in adults and a frequent problem for the internist. By definition, nosocomial pneumonia refers to an infection that is not present or incubating on admission to the hospital. Nosocomial pneumonia usually occurs at least 72 hours after admission and is associated with considerable morbidity and with a mortality of 20% to 50%.[2] Nosocomial pneumonia also prolongs the duration of hospitalization by about 6 days.[3]

## EPIDEMIOLOGY

Nosocomial pneumonia accounts for 15% of hospital-acquired infections, second in frequency to infections of the urinary tract in patients on the medical service. Overall rates of pneumonia are about 6 to 10 infections per 1000 patient discharges. Infection rates in patients in an ICU are at least 5 times the rate for patients in a non-ICU setting.[4] Risk factors that predispose patients for nosocomial bacterial pneumonia include age greater than 70 years, endotracheal intubation with or without mechanical ventilation, aspiration, prior antibiotic therapy, obesity, thoracoabdominal surgery, immunosuppression, underlying lung disease, and impaired consciousness.[5] The risk of pneumonia is 38-fold higher in patients who undergo thoracoabdominal surgery compared with control patients.[6]

## PATHOGENESIS

Nosocomial pneumonia occurs by three mechanisms: aspiration, inhalation, and hematogenous seeding from a distant focus of infection. Aspiration of oropharyngeal or stomach contents, the most important factor, occurs in about 70% of patients with diminished consciousness.[5] Colonization of the oropharynx with gram-negative bacilli is a key factor in the pathogenesis of pneumonia. Risk factors associated with oropharyngeal colonization with gram-negative bacilli include the presence of an endotracheal tube or tracheostomy, underlying lung disease, coma, hypotension, acidosis, azotemia, and use of antibiotics.[7]

115

The rate of colonization increases greatly in moribund patients compared with those who are not critically ill. Shortly after admission, an ICU patient will become colonized with gram-negative bacilli. An elevated gastric pH has also been shown to increase the colonization of the gastric flora particularly with gram-negative bacilli.[8] The issue of the relationship between the use of antacids, histamine (H$_2$)-blockers, or sucralfate to prevent gastrointestinal bleeding and the frequency of pneumonia continues to stir controversy. Antacids and H$_2$-blockers raise gastric pH, whereas sucralfate does not alter gastric pH. Sucralfate is effective by maintaining low counts of bacteria in the stomach by its ability to keep the gastric pH values low (pH <4). All the drugs appear to be effective in preventing gastric bleeding. In one report using metanalysis, sucralfate was associated with a reduced frequency of pneumonia compared with H$_2$-blockers or antacids. In another report using metanalysis, no significant difference between antacids, H$_2$-blockers, or sucralfate and the frequency of nosocomial pneumonia was identified.[10] In a recent study, there was a trend toward a lower incidence of nosocomial pneumonia in patients receiving sucralfate compared with antacids or ranitidine.[11] Interestingly the rate of pneumonia at least 4 days after mechanical ventilation was significantly lower in patients receiving sucralfate compared with pH-altering drugs. However, using mortality as an end point, there was no difference between sucralfate, antacids, or H$_2$-blockers.[11] Thus, for stress ulcer prophylaxis for patients in the ICU setting, the rate of nosocomial pneumonia is probably lower when sucralfate is used in selected patients.

Although aspiration of gastric contents appears to be important in the pathogenesis of pneumonia, another source of organisms appears to be the pooled secretions above the endotracheal tube in intubated patients.[12] In a group of patients receiving continuous suction of this area to remove secretions, the rate of pneumonia was 18% compared with a rate of 33% in the control group, which did not have the secretions aspirated.[12] Continuous aspiration of these subglottic secretions in intubated patients resulted in a decrease in pneumonia caused by gram-positive organisms and *Haemophilus influenzae* but not gram-negative bacilli. The explanation for this difference is unclear.

There are multiple sources for the flora that cause oropharyngeal colonization. In addition to the endogenous sources such as the gastric fluid and pooled secretions above the endotracheal tube, exogenous sources of colonizing flora include contaminated respiratory therapy equipment or the hands of hospital personnel caring for the patient. In the past, outbreaks of gram-negative pneumonia have occurred secondary to inhalation of aerosols of organisms from contaminated respiratory therapy equipment or anesthesia breathing machines.[13] At times, bacterial pneumonia can result from the hematogenous seeding of the lungs from another site of infection as in a patient with right-sided endocarditis with septic pulmonary emboli. Another potential source of organisms is from the gut lumen by a process called *translocation;* organisms cross the intestinal wall and seed the lungs. Translocation is postulated to occur in granulocytopenic hosts, but further data are needed to support this mechanism of pathogenesis. Figure 11-1 outlines the mechanisms by which organisms can invade the lungs and cause pneumonia.

## ETIOLOGY

In reviewing the studies listing the distribution of organisms causing nosocomial pneumonia, the discrepancies in pathogen frequencies are attributable to (1) different patient populations, (2) prior antimicrobial therapy, (3) diagnostic methods utilized, (4) season, and (5) indigenous flora of the hospital. Most studies show that the cause is polymicrobial with gram-negative bacilli predominating in about 10% to 50% of cases.[14,15] *Pseudomonas aeruginosa* is the most frequent isolate in some series, whereas in others, *Escherichia coli* or *Klebsiella species* occur most often.[14,16,17] *Staphylococcus aureus* and *Haemophilus influenzae* are also frequent pathogens. *Streptococcus pneumoniae* and *Haemophilus influenzae* tend to cause infection within 2 to 4 days after intubation.[1] The importance of anaerobes in causing nosocomial pneumonia is unknown, since studies rarely obtained transtracheal aspirates. In one report, using the technique of transtracheal aspiration in nonintubated patients, anaerobes were isolated in 35% of patients.[14] Today, transtracheal aspiration is rarely used, and the role for anaerobes as a cause of nosocomial pneumonia is unknown. The frequency of pneumonia caused by *Legionella* species or *Aspergillus* species, organisms that are inhaled, is dependent on the institution in which the data are collected.

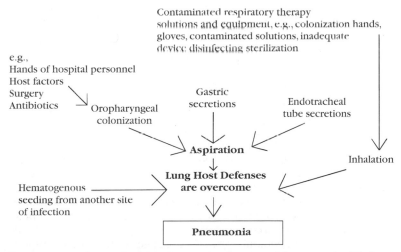

**Figure 11-1.** *Factors in the pathogenesis of nosocomial pneumonia. (Modified from Tablan OC, Anderson LJ, Arden NH, et al: Guidelines for prevention of nosocomial pneumonia. Am J Infect Control 22:247–292, 1994.)*

# DIAGNOSIS

The diagnosis of nosocomial pneumonia is difficult. The clinical criteria using fever, increase in respiratory symptoms, and a new infiltrate on chest roentgenogram are associated with both false-positive and false-negative values. Expectorated sputum or material obtained by endotracheal suctioning is associated with false-positive (colonization) or false-negative results. In patients with pneumococcal pneumonia, sputum is positive for *Streptococcus pneumoniae* in only 50% of patients. Similarly, prior antibiotic therapy can result in the sputum showing gram-negative bacilli such as *Serratia* species, which reflect colonization. Blood of pleural fluid cultures should be obtained, but the yield is low (<10% positives). Because of these problems, studies have used other methods to diagnose pneumonia, such as doing bronchoscopy and obtaining quantitative cultures. These bronchoscopic methods involve obtaining cultures of lung material by a protected specimen brush (PSB) or bronchoalveolar lavage (BAL).[4] These invasive techniques may be complicated by hypoxia, bleeding, or an arrhythmia, however. The sensitivity of these new techniques with bronchoscopy is between 70% to 100%, depending what is used as the standard. Most researchers consider a positive culture to have $\geq 10^3$ colony-forming units per milliliter (CFU/mL) of an organism to separate contamination or colonization from infection.[18] Other investigators favor using a cutoff of $10^6$ CFU/ml to decrease the frequency of false-positive results.[19] Studies support the efficacy of both PSB and BAL techniques in the diagnosis of pneumonia, and their results appear comparable. The value of these techniques for patients who have been receiving antibiotics is unclear. Use of an open-lung biopsy or transthoracic needle aspiration usually is reserved for the immunocompromised host. Despite these new techniques, often no specific organism is identified in many patients with nosocomial pneumonia.

# THERAPY

Therapy for nosocomial pneumonia remains empiric. Initial antibiotic selection is based on the status of the patient, compromised or normal host, prior use of antibiotics, results of preliminary laboratory data such as Gram stains, and antibiotic susceptibilities of known flora in the hospital or ICU. Most investigators favor a combination of antibiotics, but studies show the effectiveness of monotherapy.[4] Table 11-1 lists possible regimens to use, pending results of the studies. If *Legionella* species is suspected, erythromycin with or without rifampin must be given. If *Enterobacter* species or *Pseudomonas* species are identified, most investigators favor combination therapy. Once-a-day dosing of an aminoglycoside has certain advantages and requires study in patients with nosocomial pneumonia. Use of a drug such as ticarcillin or piperacillin and a beta-lactamase inhibitor extends the spectrum of the drug to include *Staphylococcus aureus* and anaerobes. However, ticarcillin with clavulanic acid and piperacillin with tazobactam are no better

**Table 11-1.** *Antimicrobial drugs for nosocomial pneumonia*

| Drug | Dose* | Comments |
|------|-------|----------|
| **THIRD-GENERATION CEPHALOSPORIN AND AMINOGLYCOSIDE** | | |
| ceftriaxone | 1-2 g IV q24h | Lacks anaerobic activity |
| or | | |
| ceftazidime | 2 g IV q8h | If *Pseudomonas* organisms are suspected |
| plus | | Poor anaerobic activity |
| gentamicin | 1.7 mg/kg IV q8h | |
| or | | Peak level 8 $\mu$g/mL (gent. and tobra.) |
| tobramycin | 1.7 mg/kg IV q8h | |
| or | | |
| amikacin | 7.5 mg/kg IV q12h | Peak level 25 $\mu$g/mL |
| **EXTENDED-SPECTRUM PENICILLIN AND AMINOGLYCOSIDE** | | |
| ticarcillin-clavulanic acid | 3.1 g IV q4-6h | |
| or | | |
| piperacillin-tazobactam | 3.375-4.5 g IV q6h | |
| plus | | |
| aminoglycoside | | |
| **PENEM AND AMINOGLYCOSIDE** | | |
| imipenem | 0.5 g IV q6h | Resistant *Pseudomonas* species may develop if imipenem is used alone |
| plus | | |
| aminoglycoside | | |
| **OTHER REGIMENS** | | |
| ciprofloxacin | 400 mg IV q8h | |
| plus | | |
| clindamycin | 600 mg IV q8h | |
| aztreonam | 2 g IV q8h | Decrease in nephrotoxity compared with aminoglycosides |
| plus | | |
| clindamycin | | |

*Need to reduce doses of ceftazidime, aminoglycosides, imipenem, extended-spectrum penicillins, quinolones, and aztreonam in renal failure.

than ticarcillin or piperacillin for *Pseudomonas* species. If methicillin-resistant *S. aureus* infection is suspected or identified, vancomycin should be used.

# PREVENTION

Several measures have been recommended to prevent nosocomial pneumonia.[20] Education of health care workers regarding infection control is highly advocated by the Centers for Disease Control and Prevention (CDC). It is important to determine the rates of nosocomial pneumonia expressed as infections per 100 ICU days or per 1000 ventilator days. Performance of routine surveillance cultures of the respiratory equipment or patients is not recommended. Use of high-level disinfection or sterilization of the respiratory equipment to interrupt the transmission of organisms is advocated. Postoperative patients should be encouraged to cough, take deep breaths, and ambulate as soon as possible after surgery. Patients receiving enteral feedings should have the head of the bed elevated 30 to 45 degrees to decrease the risk of aspiration. The issue of decreasing gastric colonization by using an agent (such as sucralfate) to prevent stress ulcers that does not raise the patient's gastric pH is unresolved.

Another approach that has been investigated to decrease the frequency of nosocomial pneumonia is the use of selective decontamination of the digestive tract (SDD). Most studies using SDD consist in administering anti-infective agents through the nasogastric tube and applying the drugs topically to the oropharynx as a paste. In some studies a 4-day course of parenteral antibiotic such as cefotaxime, a third-generation cephalosporin, is administered. Most reports using SDD show a decrease in colonization with gram-negative bacilli and *Candida* species. In some reports there has also been a decrease in the rate of nosocomial pneumonia. However, the overall mortality using SDD has not been reduced. One concern regarding the use of SDD is the development of colonization or infection with resistant organisms. At present, the data do not justify the routine use of SDD in the ICU setting.[21] Future studies may identify subsets of patients who could benefit from this approach. Another strategy to reduce gastric colonization is to acidify enteral feedings. Although this approach results in a decrease in the number of gastric organisms, the effect on the incidence of pneumonia is unknown.

# FUTURE DIRECTION

Several unresolved issues exist regarding nosocomial pneumonia. Therapy is often empiric, since bacteriologic confirmation of the cause is usually lacking. There is clearly a need for improved noninvasive diagnostic techniques. Better inhalation equipment would be beneficial to decrease this route as a source of organisms. Further studies are needed to define the importance of gastric colonization in the pathogenesis of pneumonia as well as the role of selective digestive decontamination in decreasing the incidence of pneumonia. The optimal therapy for nosocomial pneumonia is also unknown. Studies are needed to define the optimal type, duration, dose, and route (parenteral versus aerosolization) of antibiotics for therapy. Finally, research to examine the role of vaccines and immunoglobulins for prophylaxis as well as therapy would be beneficial.

## References

1. Tablan OC, Anderson LJ, Arden NH, et al: Guideline for prevention of nosocomial pneumonia, *Am J Infect Control* 22:247-292, 1994.
2. Pugliese G, Lichtenberg DA: Nosocomial bacterial pneumonia: an overview, *Am J Infect Control* 15:249-265, 1987.
3. Haley RW, Schaberg DR, Crossley KB, et al: Extra charges and prolongation of stay attributable to nosocomial infections: a prospective interhospital comparison, *Am J Med* 70:51 58, 1981.
4. Scheld WM, Mandell GL: Nosocomial pneumonia: pathogenesis and recent advances in diagnosis and therapy, *Rev Infect Dis* 13(suppl 9):S743-S751, 1991.
5. Celis R, Torres A, Gatell JM, et al: Nosocomial pneumonia: a multivariate analysis of risk and prognosis, *Chest* 93:318-324, 1988.
6. Hessen MT, Kaye D: Nosocomial pneumonia, *Crit Care Clin* 4:245-257, 1988.
7. Johanson WG, Pierce AK, Sanford JP, Thomas GD: Nosocomial respiratory infections with gram-negative bacilli: the significance of colonization of the respiratory tract, *Ann Intern Med* 77:701-706, 1972.
8. Driks MR, Craven DE, Celli BR, et al: Nosocomial pneumonia in intubated patients given sucralfate as compared with antacids or histamine type 2 blockers: the role of gastric colonization, *N Engl J Med* 317:1376-1382, 1987.
9. Tryba M: Sucralfate versus antacids or $H_2$-antagonists for stress ulcer prophylaxis: a meta-analysis on efficacy and pneumonia rate, *Crit Care Med* 19:942-949, 1991.
10. Cook DJ, Laine LA, Guyatt GH, Raffin TA: Nosocomial pneumonia and the role of gastric pH: a meta-analysis, *Chest* 100:7-13, 1991.
11. Prod'hom G, Leuenberger P, Koerfer J, et al: Nosocomial pneumonia in mechanically ventilated patients receiving antacid, ranitidine, or sucralfate as prophylaxis for stress ulcer, *Ann Intern Med* 120:653-662, 1994.
12. Valles J, et al: Continuous aspiration of subglottic secretions in preventing ventilator-associated pneumonia, *Ann Intern Med* 122:179-186, 1995.
13. Reinarz JA, Pierce AK, Mays BB, Sanford JP: The potential role of inhalation therapy equipment in nosocomial pulmonary infection, *J Clin Invest* 44:831-839, 1965.
14. Bartlett JG, O'Keefe P, Tally FP, et al: Bacteriology of hospital-acquired pneumonia, *Arch Intern Med* 146:868-871, 1986.
15. Fagon JY, Chastre J, Domart Y, et al: Nosocomial pneumonia in patients receiving continuous mechanical ventilation: Prospective analysis of 52 episodes with use of a protected specimen brush and quantitative culture techniques, *Am Rev Respir Dis* 139:877-884, 1989.
16. Schaberg DR, Culver DH, Gaynes RP: Major trends in the microbial etiology of nosocomial infection, *Am J Med* 91(suppl 3B):72S-75S, 1991.

17. Torres A, Aznar R, Gatell JM, et al: Incidence, risk, and prognosis factors of nosocomial pneumonia in mechanically ventilated patients, *Am Rev Respir Dis* 142:523-528, 1990.
18. Wimberley NW, Bass JB Jr, Boyd BW, et al: Use of a bronchoscopic protected catheter brush for the diagnosis of pulmonary infections, *Chest* 81:556-562, 1982.
19. Torres A, Martos A, de la Bellacasa JP, et al: Specificity of endotracheal aspiration, protected specimen brush, and bronchoalveolar lavage in mechanically ventilated patients, *Am Rev Respir Dis* 147:952-957, 1993.
20. Hamer DH, Barza M: Prevention of hospital-acquired pneumonia in critically ill patients, *Antimicrob Agents Chemother* 37:931-938, 1993.
21. Ferrer M, Torres A, Gonzalez J, de la Bellacasa JP, et al: Utility of selective digestive decontamination in mechanically ventilated patients, *Ann Intern Med* 120:389-395, 1994.
22. Lipchik RJ, Kuzo, RS: Nosocomial pneumonia (Review), *Radiol Clinics North Am* 34:47-58, 1996.

## Chapter 12

# *Fever of Unknown Origin in the Elderly*

Richard A. Gleckman

There are several reasons why the subject of fever of unknown origin (FUO) in the elderly merits attention. From 1960 to 1990 the number of Americans 65 years or older increased by 89%, and this segment of the population is expected to comprise 20% of the U.S. population by the year 2020. Diverse disorders, such as Still's disease, Crohn's disease, and factitious fever, that contribute to FUO in young adults fail to explain protracted fever in aged patients.[1,2] At a time when the clinician's ability to establish precise diagnoses is being enhanced by new technologic advances, voices are being raised to limit health resources, particularly for the elderly, as health care for older patients is perceived as too expensive or often futile. Most importantly, however, the lion's share of the entities (such as miliary tuberculosis, abdominal abscess, colonic neoplasm, temporal arteritis, and polyarteritis nodosa) that cause FUO in older adults are amenable to therapy.[2,3]

## DEFINITION

Traditionally FUO has been defined by a temperature of 101° F or higher for at least 3 weeks in duration and the failure to be explained despite a minimum of 7 days of in-hospital evaluation. Reflecting contemporary medical practice, the latter component of the definition has been altered to permit 3 days of hospitalization or exclusively outpatient assessment.[4] Timely use of abdominal ultrasound, computerized axial tomography, and echocardiography in the evaluation of the febrile geriatric patient has resulted in a change in the present range of disorders that contribute to FUO in older patients because these diagnostic studies have contributed significantly to the earlier detection of abdominal tumors and abscesses and, in conjunction with blood cultures, the recognition of endocarditis.

## HOSPITALIZATION

Elderly patients merit hospitalization for diagnostic assessment of FUO when there exists intractable pain, debilitating weakness, pronounced

123

confusion, or an inability for self-care. When nursing home residents experience FUO, there should be a heightened concern for occult tuberculosis, and, if the patient is immobile, the consultant should suspect deep venous thrombosis and consider pressure ulcer–induced contiguous deep soft-tissue abscess or osteomyelitis.

## INITIAL ASSESSMENT

Commonly, after the primary care physician has performed a medical history, physical examination, and tuberculin skin test and subjected the patient to a battery of laboratory investigations (including blood and urine cultures, routine urinalysis, complete blood cell count, liver chemistry tests, sedimentation rate, antinuclear antibody, rheumatoid factor, stools for occult blood, sputum for acid-fast stain or culture, urine cultures for the tubercle bacillus, serum electrophoresis) and radiographic studies (in the form of chest roentgenography, cardiac and abdominal ultrasonography, and abdominal computerized axial tomography), a consultation will be requested. As a general rule this initial assessment should reveal those patients with persistent fever caused by medication, subacute bacterial endocarditis, and abdominal or retroperitoneal neoplasms and abscesses.[5,6]

## APPROACHING THE CONSULTATION

A consultant can be intimidated by the impressive array of infectious, neoplastic, collagen vascular, and miscellaneous disorders that can cause FUO in older patients.[2,7] Equally overwhelming is the diversity of diagnostic studies that can be utilized.[8] The diagnostic strategy should, however, consist in a stepwise approach that is guided by information elicited from the patients' history, physical examination, and initial noninvasive tests (laboratory and radiographic).

When obtaining a comprehensive medical history, the consultant should inquire about the patient's illicit drug, transfusion, and sexual experiences. Elderly individuals who have received blood transfusions, engaged in intravenous drug abuse, or participated in heterosexual, bisexual, or homosexual relations with multiple or high-risk partners are candidates to develop human immunodeficiency virus (HIV) infection. It has been estimated that there are 1 million homosexual men over 65 years of age, and at-risk older adults are less likely to adopt AIDS prevention strategies. Prolonged unexplained fever in elderly HIV-infected patients requires a search for the traditional disorders that cause FUO in older patients as well as investigations to detect those infectious and neoplastic disorders (including disseminated caused by MAC, tuberculosis, histoplasmosis, toxoplasmosis, cryptococcosis, and non-Hodgkin's lymphoma) that have been identified in these immunocompromised hosts.

The consultant should analyze the fever pattern (a recurrent fever could be suggestive of Hodgkin's disease or colon cancer); investigate foreign travel (concern for malaria, TB, brucellosis, and hepatic amebiasis); and inquire about alcohol abuse (alcoholic hepatitis, hepatoma, TB), prior antibiotic ingestion (enhancing the possibility of culture-negative endocarditis, and perhaps the need for transesophageal echocardiography), and vague head (temporal arteritis), abdominal (polyarteritis nodosa, abscess, neoplasm), or back (osteomyelitis, neoplasm) pain.[6,9,10] The physical examination should be repeated to identify previously overlooked conjunctivitis (as a manifestation of systemic lupus erythematosus and polyarteritis nodosa), mononeuropathy multiplex (polyarteritis nodosa), lymphadenopathy (consistent with TB and lymphoma), or rectal neoplasm.

## INVASIVE STUDIES

If the consultant's assessment uncovers no helpful clues as to the cause of the patient's persistent fever, attention should be directed to the following entities: occult lymphoma or tuberculosis, cancer of the colon, temporal arteritis, and polyarteritis nodosa. The patient should be subjected to electrophysiological studies to confirm the presence of lower extremity nerve abnormalities (as a prelude to a biopsy to establish a diagnosis of polyarteritis nodosa) and colonoscopy to exclude colonic cancer.[5,11] If these studies are not diagnostic, consideration should be given to performing bilateral temporal artery biopsy, a procedure that can be safely performed in an outpatient setting. When, however, physical signs or biochemical studies indicate possible intra-abdominal disease, the preferred diagnostic approach is liver biopsy or laparoscopy. These invasive studies can establish the diagnosis of tuberculosis, lymphoma, hepatoma, and polyarteritis nodosa.[12,13] If the patient refuses these invasive tests or there is a contraindication to perform these tests, the consultant could recommend imaging with gallium-67 or indium-111–labeled white blood cells, but he or she must be aware of the fact that these studies often provide diagnostically noncontributory information.[14,15]

## EMPIRIC TREATMENT

When an elderly patient with persistent fever experiences evidence of accelerated deterioration and invasive studies are either refused or precluded, empiric therapy is essential. I would recommend commencing therapy for occult tuberculosis.[6] Most patients infected with drug-susceptible occult TB should become afebrile within 6 weeks. Unfortunately, however, resolution of fever after antituberculous therapy is not pathognomonic of tuberculosis because defervescence has been noted in patients harboring a lymphoma. Empiric treatment is not indicated if the patient's condition does not deteriorate.[16]

## References

1. Kazanjian PH: Fever of unknown origin: review of 86 patients treated in community hospitals, *Clin Infect Dis* 15:968, 1992.
2. Knockaert DC, Vanneste LJ, Bobbaers HJ: Fever of unknown origin in elderly patients, *J Am Geriatr Soc* 41:1187, 1993.
3. Esposito AL, Gleckman R: Fever of unknown origin in the elderly, *J Am Geriatr Soc* 26:498, 1978.
4. Durack DT, Street AC: Fever of unknown origin—reexamined and redefined. In Remington JS, Swartz MN, editor: *Current clinical topics in infectious diseases,* ed 11, Boston, 1991, Blackwell Scientific Publications.
5. Knockaert DC, Vanneste LJ, Vanneste SB, et al: Fever of unknown origin in the 1980s, *Arch Intern Med* 152:51, 1992.
6. Michel PL, Gleckman, RA: Fever of unknown origin: how the causes and workup differ in the elderly, *Consultant* 34:1665, 1994.
7. Knockaert DC: Fever of unknown origin, a literature survey, *Acta Clin Belg* 47:42, 1992.
8. Knockaert DC: Diagnostic strategy for fever of unknown origin in the ultrasonography and computed tomography era, *Acta Clin Belg* 47:100, 1992.
9. Knockaert DC, Vanneste LJ, Bobbaers HJ: Recurrent or episodic fever of unknown origin, *Medicine,* 72:184, 1993.
10. Smith KY, Bradley SF, Kauffman CA: Fever of unknown origin in the elderly: lymphoma presenting as vertebral compression fractures, *J Am Geriatr Soc* 42:88, 1994.
11. Wees SJ, Sunwoo JN, Oh SJ: Sural nerve biopsy in systemic necrotizing vasculitis, *Am J Med* 71:525, 1981.
12. Herruzo JAS, Benita V, Morillas JD: Laparoscopy in fever of unknown origin: a study of seventy cases, *Endoscopy* 13:207, 1981.
13. Herruzo JAS, Yague TM, Ruizdelgado C: Laparoscopic findings in polyarteritis nodosa, *Endoscopy* 13:9, 1981.
14. Davies SG, Garvie NW: The role of indium-labelled leukocyte imaging in pyrexia of unknown origin, *Br J Radiol* 63:850, 1990.
15. Knockaert DC, Mortelmaus LA, DeRoo MC, et al: Clinical value of gallium-67 scintigraphy in evaluation of fever of unknown origin, *Clin Infect Dis* 18:601, 1994.
16. Knockaert DC, Dujardin KS, Boffaers HJ: Long-term follow-up of patients with undiagnosed fever of unknown origin, *Arch Intern Med* 156:618, 1996.

# Chapter 13

# *Fever in the Leukopenic Cancer Patient*

Nelson M. Gantz

Neutropenia is the major risk factor for infection in patients with malignancy. One calculates the absolute neutrophil count by multiplying the total white blood cell count by the percentage of polymorphonuclear neutrophils plus band forms per cubic millimeter. The risk of infection increases when the absolute neutrophil count declines to less than a range of 500 to 750 neutrophils/mm.[1] The highest risk of infection occurs when the absolute neutrophil count is less than 100 cells/mm$^3$. Neutropenia occurs as a result of cytotoxic chemotherapy and the patient's underlying malignancy. The risk of infection not only correlates inversely with the level of neutropenia but also directly with the duration of neutropenia. Other factors that contribute to infection include the status of the humoral and cellular immune systems, which can be impaired by the patient's underlying illness or cytotoxic chemotherapy. Also, any factor that alters the normal defense barriers such as the presence of an indwelling intravenous catheter or oral mucositis predisposes patients to infections by providing a portal of entry for organisms.[2] Patients with malignancy often become colonized with resistant gram-negative bacilli and *Candida* species as a result of broad-spectrum antibiotic therapy and hospitalization. These endogenous organisms may cause disease as a result of cytotoxic chemotherapy or radiation therapy or enter the bloodstream at an indwelling intravenous catheter site.

## CAUSES OF FEVER

There are multiple causes for fever, both infectious and noninfectious, in patients with underlying malignancy and neutropenia. For the majority of patients, the cause of fever is never identified. Despite multiple blood cultures, only 20% to 30% of patients with fever and neutropenia will have a positive blood culture.[3] Noninfectious causes of fever include medications such as the chemotherapeutic drugs (such as bleomycin or ara-C), transfusion of blood products, deep venous thrombosis of the legs, phlebitis at an intravenous catheter site, pulmonary embolism, aspiration, atelectasis, or a hematoma. Fever as a result of the underlying malignancy may also occur. Malignancies that frequently cause fever include Hodgkin's disease, non-Hodgkin's lymphoma, leukemia, renal cell carcinoma, hepatoma, atrial myxoma, and metastatic disease to the liver. The diagnosis of fever caused by the underlying illness is one of exclusion. Common infections in the neutropenic patient include gingivostomatitis, pharyngitis, pneumonia, cellulitis, perirectal abscess, and phlebitis at the catheter site. Bloodstream infections also may occur because of disease-induced ulcerations of the gastrointestinal tract or related to a long-term intravascular device such as Hickman or Broviac catheters. Less frequently, fever can be attributed to sinusitis, urinary tract infection, pseudomembranous colitis, esophagitis, or meningitis. Rarely, fever may be caused by an infectious agent transmitted with a transfusion such as Epstein-Barr virus, or *Yersinia* organisms. More often fever is attributable to cytomegalovirus or hepatitis C acquired from a transfusion. Patients with leukemia may have fever caused by focal hepatic candidiasis.[4] Another infection that must be considered in a febrile neutropenic patient with abdominal pain is typhlitis, or inflammation of the cecum caused by gram-negative enteric organisms and anaerobes.

# EVALUATION

Evaluation of the febrile neutropenic patient begins with a detailed history and physical examination. The diagnosis of infection is more difficult in the febrile neutropenic host because of the subtleness of the symptoms and signs of infection.[5] For example, the patient with pharyngitis or cellulitis will have pain and erythema but lack exudates. Similarly, a patient with a perirectal abscess will complain of perineal pain and may have erythema but lack swelling, fluctuation, exudates, and regional adenopathy. Patients with pneumonia will have a nonproductive cough without crackles on examination and lack sputum production. Frank pus is rarely present because polymorphonuclear leukocytes are necessary for its production. An afebrile individual is unlikely to be infected, whereas fever indicates infection until it is excluded. Urinary tract infections often occur in the absence of irritative voiding symptoms such as dysuria and frequency.

The history can provide clues to the possible site of infection. A sore throat with fever and pharyngeal ulcerations can be a source for a bacteremia caused by *Pseudomonas aeruginosa* or a local herpes simplex virus infection. Dysphagia is suggestive of esophagitis caused most often by *Candida* species but may result from an infection with cytomegalovirus, herpes simplex virus, or rarely fungi such as aspergillus. Painful defecation should alert the clinician to the possibility of a perirectal infection. Fever, abdominal pain, and diarrhea may be a clue to the diagnosis of pseudomembranous colitis or typhlitis (inflammation of the cecum). In evaluating the febrile neutropenic patient, the physical examination must be meticulous and repeated often with special attention given to the oral cavity, pharynx, anorectal area, and skin lesions. For example, periodontal infection may be manifested by fever, gingival inflammation, and tenderness. Biopsy of skin lesions for Gram stain, histologic examination, and culture often provides invaluable diagnostic information. Cutaneous lesions with necrotic centers called ecthyma gangrenosum occur with *Pseudomonas* bacteremia but also with other pathogens such as *Candida, Mucor,* or other gram-negative bacilli.[6] Aspiration or biopsy of skin lesions is critical. Careful attention must be given to any indwelling catheters such as a Hickman catheter for examining the insertion site and tunnel. Redness and tenderness may be present, but generally no clinical evidence of infection is present.

In assessing the febrile granulocytopenic patient, it is important to obtain two or three sets of blood cultures, urinalysis and culture, and a chest roentgenogram. The yield of *Candida* species may be increased when blood cultures are processed by the lysis centrifugation technique. In the presence of granulocytopenia, urine, sputum, or any specimen from a suspected site of infection will not reveal polymorphonuclear leukocytes. In a patient with pneumonia, the chest roentgenogram will usually demonstrate an infiltrate though the findings may be minimal. If a central intravenous line is present, every lumen should be cultured separately in addition to obtaining peripheral blood cultures.[2] In patients with diarrhea, a stool specimen sent for *Clostridium difficile* toxin may establish the cause of the patient's symptoms. Use of routine surveillance cultures of the skin, nares, and stool is not indicated.

In recent years, there has been a change in the prominent pathogens causing infection in the granulocytopenic patient. Coagulase-negative staphylococci, which usually are susceptible only to vancomycin, have become a key pathogen in patients with indwelling intravenous catheters. Alpha-hemolytic streptococci may cause life threatening pulmonary disease in patients with leukemia.[7] The frequency of gram-negative infections especially attributable to *Pseudomonas aeruginosa* has decreased for no clear reason in recent years.[1] Anaerobes should be considered as possible pathogens in patients with gingivitis or perianal cellulitis. Two other anaerobic organisms, *Clostridium septicum* and *C. tertium,* may cause life-threatening septicemia. Of the viruses, one must always consider disease caused by the herpesviruses: herpes simplex virus, varicella-zoster virus, and cytomegalovirus. Fungi also have increased in frequency, with *Candida* species occurring most often.[2] Of the species of *Candida, C. albicans* predominates. Other yeasts that have increased have included *C. tropicalis, C. glabrata,* and *C. krusei,* the last of which is resistant to fluconazole. *Aspergillus* species occur second in frequency to *Candida* isolates. Some uncommon fungi such as *Fusarium, Trichosporon,* and *Saccharomyces* may also cause disease in the granulocytopenic patient. Another consideration in patients with persistent fever and abdominal pain is hepatosplenic candidiasis. The diagnosis of hepatosplenic candidiasis may be suggested by a CT scan of the abdomen and confirmed by liver biopsy.[8]

After appropriate cultures are obtained, the standard therapy for the febrile granulocytopenic patient consists in administering broad-spectrum antibiotics empirically.[9] Most febrile granulocytopenic patients are treated in the hospital setting. Recently, selected low-risk cancer patients with fever and granulocytopenia have been treated with antibiotics safely in the outpatient setting.[10] The advantages of outpatient antimicrobial therapy include lower cost, improved quality of life, and a decreased risk of acquiring nosocomial multidrug-resistant pathogens. Optimal antimicrobial therapy is unknown. Initial antimicrobial therapy is based on the knowledge of the likely infecting pathogens and their susceptibilities, allergies, renal and hepatic function, other drugs the patient is receiving, and cost. Therapy should be with use of bactericidal agents. Controversy continues to exist regarding the issue of combination therapy versus monotherapy.[11] Studies have demonstrated efficacy of broad-spectrum single agents with antipseudomonal activity with imipenem-cilastatin or ceftazidime. However, many experts continue to recommend a combination of drugs that include a beta-lactam drug such as ticarcillin, piperacillin, or ceftazidime with an aminoglycoside, such as gentamicin, tobramycin, or amikacin. Another approach is to avoid using an aminoglycoside and to select two beta-lactam drugs such as ceftazidime with piperacillin. The addition of vancomycin as a third drug for initial empiric therapy for its gram-positive activity has not been shown to improve survival. However, in patients with an indwelling intravenous catheter, vancomycin should be included in the initial antibiotic regimen for the possibility of the many *staphylococci* that are coagulase negative and *Staphylococcus aureus,* which is coagulase positive, but both types of which may be resistant to methicillin. Vancomycin also is effective against *Corynebacterium jeikeium,* an important pathogen in patients with indwelling intravenous catheters.

Selected initial antibiotic regimens are listed in Table 13-1 for patients with fever and granulocytopenia. In choosing the initial antibiotic regimen, one should consider the antibiotic susceptibilities of the indigenous flora in the community and the hospital, drug allergies, renal or hepatic dysfunction, and other drugs the patient is receiving. Drugs such as cisplatin, amphotericin B, cyclosporin A, and the aminoglycosides should be used together with great caution because of potential nephrotoxicity. Of the four schemes listed in Table 13-1, (1) aminoglycoside with an antipseudomonal beta-lactam, (2) two beta-lactam drugs, (3) a single drug, and (4) vancomycin plus aminoglycoside plus antipseudomonal beta-lactam, one of the combination therapies is preferred by most experts.[9] Advantages of combination therapy include potential synergistic effects against some gram-negative bacilli, a decrease in emergence of resistant strains during treatment, and a wider efficacy than that of just one drug. The major disadvantages are the increased risk of adverse effects, expense, and inconvenience. Once started on a course of therapy the patient must be monitored closely for a response. If vancomycin was not included in the initial regimen, the drug can be added if gram-positive bacteria are isolated in culture or if no response occurs after 3 days. No increase in mortality has been reported if there has been a delay in starting vancomycin therapy when cultures reveal gram-positive organisms.

**Table 13-1.** *Selected initial antibiotic regimens to use for the febrile granulocytopenic patient*

| Drug | Dose* |
|---|---|
| **AMINOGLYCOSIDE + ANTIPSEUDOMONAL BETA-LACTAM** | |
| Aminoglycoside | |
| gentamicin | 1.7 mg/kg q8h |
| or | |
| tobramycin | 1.7 mg/kg q8h |
| or | |
| amikacin | 7.5 mg/kg q12h |
| plus | |
| beta-lactam | |
| ticarcillin | 4 g q4-6h |
| or | |
| ticarcillin-clavulanic acid | 3.1 g q4-6h |
| or | |
| piperacillin | 4 g q4-6h |
| or | |
| piperacillin-tazobactam | 3.375 to 4.5 g q6h |
| or | |
| ceftazidime | 2 g q8h |
| or | |
| aztreonam | 2 g q8h |
| **COMBINATION OF TWO BETA-LACTAM DRUGS** | |
| ceftazidime | |
| plus, | |
| e.g., piperacillin | |
| **MONOTHERAPY** | |
| ceftazidime | 0.5 g IV q6h |
| or | |
| imipenem/cilastatin | |
| **VANCOMYCIN + AMINOGLYCOSIDE + BETA-LACTAM** | |
| vancomycin | 1 g q12h |
| plus, | |
| e.g., tobramycin | |
| plus, | |
| e.g., ceftazidime | |

Modified from Hughes WT, Armstrong D, Bodey GP, et al. Guidelines for the use of antimicrobial agents in neutropenic patients with unexplained fever, *J Infect Dis* 161:381-396, 1990.

*Dosage of drugs needs to be reduced in renal failure.

After initiation of antibiotic therapy, clinical response, results of cultures, and absolute granulocyte count dictate subsequent management. If clinical improvement occurs and cultures reveal a pathogen, antibiotic therapy should be dictated by culture and sensitivity results. However, it is important to continue broad-spectrum antibiotic therapy until the patient is no longer granulocytopenic (granulocyte count >500 cells/mm$^3$) to prevent a breakthrough of bacteremia.[12-13] Antibiotics should be continued until the infection has resolved, the patient is no longer granulocytopenic, and at least 7 days have passed. If no organism is isolated and clinical improvement occurs, antibiotics should be given for at least 7 days with monitoring of clinical response and degree of granulocytopenia. If the patient remains febrile after 3 to 4 days, a meticulous reassessment of the patient is critical. Causes of fever include noninfectious ones such as drug fever, inadequate drug levels, infection at a catheter site, hepatic candidiasis, splenic abscess, pseudomembranous colitis, or a viral infection attributable to herpes simplex virus or cytomegalovirus. Reassessment should include performing a careful physical examination, obtaining blood cultures, and diagnostic imaging of any organ suspected of harboring a localized infection. For example, a computerized scan of the abdomen may show an infection caused by a *Candida* or *Aspergillus* species. If after the reassessment, no cause is identified and fever persists, the three options include (1) continuance of the initial antibiotics, (2) a change of antibiotics, or (3) addition of amphotericin B with or without changing antibiotics. If the patient is febrile but doing well with no progression of disease, the initial antibiotics can be continued, especially if the granulocytopenia can be expected to improve shortly. Another option is changing to different antibiotics, especially if there is progression of the symptoms and signs of disease such as worsening mucous membrane lesions, increasing abdominal pain, or a new pulmonary infiltrate appearing on the chest roentgenogram. The third choice is to consider the addition of amphotericin B if the fever persists after 7 days and no cause is identified.[14] One report in 1980 showed that about 33% of patients with fever and granulocytopenia who failed to respond to 1 week of antibiotics had a fungal infection usually caused by a *Candida* or *Aspergillus* species.[15] With the addition of amphotericin B, the aminoglycoside should be discontinued to decrease the likelihood of nephrotoxicity. Further studies are needed to define the role of empiric fluconazole in this setting as an alternative to amphotericin B.[16] Fluconazole has been effective in patients with hepatosplenic candidiasis.[17] Empiric antiviral therapy is not indicated unless patients have proved or suspected viral infections, such as acyclovir for herpes simplex or herpes zoster, or use of ganciclovir for cytomegalovirus. Granulocyte transfusions are not indicated. Further studies are indicated for assessing the role of granulocyte and granulocyte-macrophage colony-stimulating factors in this setting. Granulocyte and granulocyte-macrophage colony-stimulating factors may reduce the duration and severity of the neutropenia in patients receiving chemotherapy.[18,19] The use of these growth factors has been associated with fewer infections but no decrease in overall mortality.

Indwelling intravenous catheters often are used in patients with malignancy. As foreign bodies, they may be associated with bacteremia or fungemia. Infection can occur at the exit site or along the subcutaneous tunnel of the catheters. Coagulase-negative *Staphylococci* are the most common pathogen, but *S. aureus*, gram-negative bacilli, *Bacillus* species, *Corynebacterium jeikeium*, and fungi such as *Candida* species, *Aspergillus* species, and *Malassezia furfur* may also cause catheter infections. Tunnel infections and disease caused by *Bacillus* species or fungi will not be cured without removal of the catheter along with appropriate anti-infective therapy.[2]

## References

1. Bodey GP, Buckley M, Sathe YS, Freireich EJ: Quantitative relationships between circulating leukocytes and infection in patients with acute leukemia, *Ann Intern Med* 64:328-340, 1966.
2. Pizzo PA: Management of fever in patients with cancer and treatment-induced neutropenia, *N Engl J Med* 328:1323-1332, 1993.
3. Pizzo PA: Evaluation of fever in the patient with cancer, *Eur J Cancer Clin Oncol* 25(suppl 2):S9-S16, 1989.
4. Thaler M et al: Hepatic candidiasis in cancer patients: the evolving picture of the syndrome, *Ann Intern Med* 108:88-100, 1988.
5. Sickles EA, Greene WH, Wiernik PH: Clinical presentation of infection in granulocytopenic patients, *Arch Intern Med* 135:715-719, 1975.
6. Wolfson JS, Sober AJ, Rubin H: Dermatologic manifestations of infections in immunocompromised patients, *Medicine* 64:115, 1985.
7. Dybedal I, Lamvik J: Respiratory insufficiency in acute leukemia following treatment with cytosine arabinoside and septicemia with streptococcus viridans, *Eur J Haematol* 42:405-406, 1989.
8. Lee JW, Pizzo PA. Management of the cancer patient with fever and prolonged neutropenia, *Hemat/Oncol Clinics North Am* 7:937-960, 1993.
9. Hughes WT, Armstrong D, Bodey GP, et al: Guidelines for the use of antimicrobial agents in neutropenic patients with unexplained fever, *J Infect Dis* 161:381-396, 1990.
10. Malik IA, Khan WA, Karim M, et al: Feasibility of outpatient management of fever in cancer patients with low-risk neutropenia: results of a prospective randomized trial, *Am J Med* 98:224-231, 1995.
11. Wade JC: Antibiotic therapy for the febrile granulocytopenic cancer patient: combination therapy vs. monotherapy, *Rev Infect Dis* 11(suppl 7):S1572-S1581, 1989.
12. Pizzo PA, Commers J, Cotton D, et al: Approaching the controversies in the antibacterial management of cancer patients, *Am J Med* 76:436-449, 1984.
13. Pizzo PA, Robichaud KJ, Gill FA, et al: Duration of empiric antibiotic therapy in granulocytopenic patients with cancer, *Am J Med* 67:194-200, 1979.
14. Walsh TJ, Lee J, Lecciones J, et al: Empiric therapy with amphotericin B in febrile granulocytopenic patients, *Rev Infect Dis* 13:496-503, 1991.
15. Pizzo PA, Robichaud KJ, Gill FA, Witebsky FG: Empiric antibiotic and antifungal therapy for cancer patients with prolonged fever and granulocytopenia, *Am J Med* 72:101-111, 1982.
16. Sugar AM: Empiric treatment of fungal infections in the neutropenic host: review of the literature and guidelines for use, *Arch Intern Med* 150:2258-2264, 1990.

17. Kauffman CA, Bradley SF, Ross SC, Weber DR: Hepatosplenic candidiasis: successful treatment with fluconazole, *Am J Med* 91:137-141, 1991.
18. Lieschke GJ, Burgess AW: Granulocyte colony–stimulating factor and granulocyte-macrophage colony–stimulating factor, *N Engl J Med* 327:28-35, 99-106, 1992.
19. Anaissie EJ, Vartivarian S, Bodey GP, et al: Randomized comparison between antibiotics alone and antibiotics plus granulocyte-macrophage colony-stimulating factor, *Am J Med* 100:17-23, 1996.

# Chapter 14

# *New Pathogens*

Richard A. Gleckman

This chapter describes three new infectious organisms that present a diagnostic challenge, occur in numerous areas of the country, and are capable of causing life-threatening disease. When the astute clinician considers these infections and institutes prompt therapy, much morbidity and mortality can be reduced.

## EHRLICHIOSIS

Since 1986 there has been the recognition of human ehrlichiosis in the United States. This disease, which has been reported in more than 23 states, particularly in southern Atlantic and south central states, is caused by a small gram-negative, obligate intracellular bacterium that parasitizes the cytoplasmic phagosomes of mononuclear cells of blood and bone marrow. Ehrlichiosis is caused by *Ehrlichia chaffeensis,* an organism that has been cultivated in tissue culture from the blood leukocytes of infected patients.

The disease is considered a tick-borne zoonosis with March to October seasonality. Patients may experience no symptoms, a self-limited nonspecific brief febrile disorder, significant systemic symptoms, or a fatal course characterized by hypotension, gastrointestinal hemorrhage, renal failure, disseminated intravascular coagulation, adult respiratory distress syndrome, or life-endangering suprainfection. After an incubation period of 4 to 33 days after tick exposure, patients develop nonspecific symptoms, predominantly fever, malaise, chills, and headache. Additional symptoms have included anorexia, meningeal irritation, lethargy, confusion, hallucinations, arthralgias, myalgias, nausea, vomiting, diarrhea, and abdominal pain. Usually, other than fever, patients have no consistent physical findings.[1] On occasion, there can be conjunctival erythema or hemorrhage, and some patients demonstrate a rash. The rash can appear as transient mottled or diffuse erythema, or as purpuric or petechial lesions. Ehrlichiosis has also presented as a severe, life-threatening disease that displays all the features of the toxic shock syndrome.[2]

During the first week of illness patients often manifest a decrease in leukocytes and platelets but elevated aspartate aminotransferase and alanine aminotransferase concentrations.[1] Cerebrospinal fluid abnormalities have an increased concentration of protein and lymphocytes, rarely neutrophilic pleocytosis. Incorrect diagnoses have included Rocky Mountain spotted fever, Lyme disease, leptospirosis, tularemia, meningococcemia, influenza, and "viral" syndrome.

The demonstration of cytoplasmic inclusions (morulae) in peripheral lymphocytes, bone marrow, or cerebrospinal mononuclear cells can provide the initial diagnostic clue, but this is a difficult and insensitive procedure. The definitive diagnosis is usually established by the demonstration of a fourfold rise in antibody, using the indirect immunofluorescence technique on a patient's serum, when both acute and convalescent phase sera are analyzed. There are false-negative test results, however, for HIV patients and normal hosts.[3] A polymerase chain-reaction test, applied to the patient's blood, can usually confirm the diagnosis in 48 hours. This test can also establish the diagnosis when there is a false-negative immunofluorescence serum antibody test.[1] Unfortunately, however, the polymerase chain-reaction test is not widely available, and it also has not been 100% sensitive.

The provisional diagnosis of ehrlichiosis is a clinical one, and the physician should intervene early by prescribing supportive treatment with either tetracycline qid or doxycycline bid.[1] Treatment diminishes the need for hospitalization and accelerates the rate of resolution of the clinical manifestations. Severity of illness has been correlated with delay in initiating antibiotic therapy. Patients usually defervesce within 3 days of the onset of doxycycline treatment. Rarely, disease can persist and progress despite antibiotic administration.

In 1994 reports from the upper midwest United States, namely, Wisconsin and Minnesota, indicated that there was an additional form of ehrlichiosis and that the disease is not caused by *Ehrlichia chaffeensis*. This new entity is human granulocytic ehrlichiosis, a disorder that resembles ehrlichiosis associated with *Ehrlichia chaffeensis,* but is caused by an organism related to the *Ehrlichia phagocytophila/ Ehrlichia equi* group, and the organisms are located in the cytoplasm of neutrophils, not mononuclear white blood cells. Human granulocytic ehrlichiosis also appears to be a tick-borne disease, and patients respond to doxycycline treatment. Currently the diagnosis is established by the demonstration of *Ehrlichia*-like inclusions only in the cytoplasm of circulating neutrophils.[4]

# BARTONELLA HENSELAE

Since its initial description in 1982, *Bartonella henselae* has been identified as a cause of bacteremia (without an obvious portal of entry); bacillary angiomatosis (cutaneous vascular lesions); bacillary peliosis hepatis (blood-filled hepatic cysts in patients with fever, weight loss, abdominal pain, or fullness); focal and disseminated disease that involves the bone, brain, liver, spleen, lymph node, bronchial mucosa, larynx, lung, bone marrow, and gastrointestinal tract; and cat-scratch disease in immunocompetent hosts, organ-transplant recipients, and, most commonly, patients with advanced HIV infection.[5-7] Presumably the disorder caused by this small, curved, gram-negative bacillus is acquired by a cat scratch or a bite from a kitten or cat flea.[8,9]

Bacillary angiomatosis manifests as solitary or multiple, dermal or subcutaneous dusky red papules or nodules that can involve contiguous bone and resemble Kaposi's sarcoma, pyogenic granuloma, and infections caused by fungi or mycobacteria.[10] Patients with extracutaneous disease experience fever, weight loss, anorexia, and vomiting, thereby resembling HIV-infected patients with disseminated fungal or mycobacterial infection.

The diagnosis is established by isolation of the organism from blood using the lysis-centrifugation procedure, culture of tissue, histologic features with Warthin-Starry staining of the bacterium, or electron microscopy or PCR performed on tissue. Serologic tests (indirect fluorescent-antibody and enzyme immunoassay for IgG antibodies) are available, but they should be interpreted with caution.

Patients with cat-scratch disease require no antibiotic therapy.[7] All patients with bacillary angiomatosis, bacteremia, bacillary peliosis of the liver and extracutaneous focal or disseminated infection, merit antibiotic treatment because of the morbidity and mortality associated with progressive disease. Erythromycin (as 500 mg qid) is prescribed for 8 weeks to HIV-infected patients with cutaneous disease. Patients who relapse are treated for at least 4 additional months. Alternative therapies include clarithromycin, azithromycin, and doxycycline. Antibiotic therapy can be associated with a Jarisch-Herxheimer reaction.[5] Patients with disease of the bone or disseminated disease are candidates for intravenous therapy initially, followed by numerous months of additional oral treatment. Relapses require lifelong maintenance treatment.

# HANTAVIRUS PULMONARY SYNDROME

First recognized in the United States in the spring of 1993 as a febrile illness occurring in previously healthy young adults living in the rural Southwest, the *Hantavirus* (Four Corners virus, Muerto Canyon virus, *sin nombre* virus) pulmonary syndrome has developed in more than 80 patients, representing 19 states. The disease, presumably caused by the inhalation of virus from the excreta of deer mice, has a prodromal phase manifesting as fever, myalgias, and headache, with or without nausea, vomiting, abdominal pain, and diarrhea.[11-13] Four or 5 days later patients experience a cardiovascular phase characterized by cough, dyspnea, tachypnea, and tachycardia. Laboratory abnormalities include leukocytosis with a left shift, atypical lymphocytes, thrombocytopenia, and elevated aspartate aminotransferase and alanine aminotransferase. Radiographic findings include interstitial edema, bibasilar or perihilar airspace disease, and pleural effusions. The initial chest roentgenogram can reveal normal findings.[12] A serologic test, IgM antibody, is available to establish the diagnosis because the illness resembles bacteremia, a rickettsial disorder, and an infectious pneumonia. The disease is associated with considerable mortality. Death is attributed to the adult respiratory distress syndrome and myocardial depression with irreversible hypotension.[12]

Treatment, consisting of respiratory support, fluid administration monitored by a flow-directed pulmonary artery catheter, infusion of an inotropic agent, and management of arrhythmias, is conducted in the intensive care unit. Intravenous ribavirin has been used as an antiviral compound, but this medication can produce hemolytic anemia, is contraindicated for pregnant patients, and has not been documented to be beneficial.[11] Person-to-person transmission of the disease has not been documented.

## References

1. Everett ED, Evans KA, Henry B, et al: Human ehrlichiosis in adults after tick exposure, *Ann Intern Med* 120:730, 1994.

2. Fichtenbaum CJ, Peterson LR, Weil GJ: Ehrlichiosis presenting as a life-threatening illness with features of the toxic shock syndrome, *Am J Med* 95:351, 1993.

3. Paddock CD, Suchard D, Grumbach KL, et al: Brief report: fatal seronegative ehrlichiosis in a patient with HIV infection, *N Engl J Med* 329:1164, 1993.

4. Bakken JS, Dumler S, Chen SM, et al: Human granulocytic ehrlichiosis in the upper midwest United States, *JAMA* 272:212, 1994.

5. Adal KA, Cockerell CJ, Petri JA Jr: Cat scratch disease, bacillary angiomatosis, and other infections due to *Rochalimaea, N Engl J Med* 330:1509, 1994.

6. Dolan MJ, Wong, MT, Regnery RL, et al: Syndrome of *Rochalimaea henselae* adenitis suggesting cat scratch disease, *Ann Intern Med* 118:331, 1993.

7. Schwartzman WA: Infections due to *Rochalimaea:* the expanding clinical spectrum, *Clin Infect Dis* 15:893, 1992.

8. Koehler JE, Glaser CA, Tappero JW: *Rochalimaea henselae* infection, *JAMA* 271:531, 1994.

9. Tappero JW, Boetani JM, Koehler JE, et al: The epidemiology of bacillary angiomatosis and bacillary peliosis, *JAMA* 269:770, 1993.

10. Koehler JE, Tappero JW: Bacillary angiomatosis and bacillary peliosis in patients infected with human immunodeficiency virus, *Clin Infect Dis* 17:612, 1993.

11. Butler JC, Peters CJ: Hantaviruses and hantavirus pulmonary syndrome, *Clin Infect Dis* 19:387, 1994.

12. Duchan JS, Koster FT, Peters CJ, et al: Hantavirus pulmonary syndrome: a clinical description of 17 patients with a newly recognized disease, *N Engl J Med* 330:949, 1994.

13. Levy H, Simpson SQ: Hantavirus pulmonary syndrome, *Am J Respir Crit Care Med* 149:1710, 1994.

14. Walker DH: Human ehrlichiosis: more trouble from ticks, *Hosp Practice* 31:47, 1996.

# Chapter 15

# *Infections in Diabetics*

Richard A. Gleckman
Pierre Abi Hanna

It has been estimated that there are approximately 10 million diabetics in the United States. Diabetic patients are considered compromised hosts because they are predisposed to some unique infections and, on occasion, demonstrate impaired host defenses (abnormality of polymorphonuclear leukocyte function, including impairment of adherence, chemotaxis, phagocytosis, and intracellular killing) that retard their ability to prevent or restrict infections.

Selective diabetics experience ischemia, trauma, and neuropathies, resulting in skin, soft tissue, and bone infection. The box on p. 140 depicts those bacterial and fungal infections that research has suggested diabetics are at greater risk to experience. In addition to those common infections that involve the skin, urinary tract, and lung, there are some infections relatively unique to diabetics: malignant external otitis, rhinocerebral mucormycosis, emphysematous cholecystitis, emphysematous pyelonephritis, and aggressive soft-tissue infections (necrotizing fasciitis, necrotizing cellulitis).[1] These infections as well as infections of the feet are the subject of this chapter. The consultant also appreciates the fact that ketoacidosis and the hyperosmolar state are often precipitated by infection.

## INVASIVE EXTERNAL OTITIS

Invasive external otitis, the invasive infection of the external auditory canal caused predominantly by *Pseudomonas aeruginosa,* occurs most often in elderly patients with long-standing diabetes mellitus. The infection begins in the external canal and often crosses the cartilaginous-osseous junction into the temporal bone and the mastoid process. The facial nerve becomes involved as it leaves through the stylomastoid foramen. The infection can advance along the base of the skull, cause other cranial nerve palsies, thrombosis of the sigmoid sinus, and death. Ear irrigation with nonsterile tapwater has been considered a predisposing factor. Poor glucose control is not a predisposing condition.[2]

Severe, persistent otalgia and otorrhea are the dominant presenting features. Facial nerve palsy occurs in one third to one half of the patients

## Diabetes as a Risk Factor

......................................................................

### BACTERIAL INFECTION

Urinary tract infection (women; nosocomial)
Emphysematous cystitis/pyelonephritis
Renal carbuncle/corticomedullary abscess
Papillary necrosis with pyelonephritis
Perinephric abscess

Foot infections

Endocarditis secondary to bacteremia originating from a soft-tissue *Staphylococcus aureus* infection

Group B streptococcal infections

Necrotizing fasciitis
Synergistic necrotizing cellulitis

Emphysematous cholecystitis
*Klebsiella* liver abscess

Endophthalmitis
Invasive external otitis

Lower lobe tuberculosis

### FUNGAL INFECTION

Candidal vulvovaginitis, Candiduria, pyelonephritis
Cutaneous, endobronchial, rhinocerebral mucormycosis

---

and portends a poor prognosis. The external auditory canal is inflamed and contains granulation tissue. Patients do not appear toxic, are usually afebrile, and fail to muster a leukocytosis. An elevated erythrocyte sedimentation role is almost always present, and one investigator suggested that it can be monitored, subsequent to therapy, as an indicator for recurrence.[2]

Plain films have not been helpful to define the process. Technetium and gallium scintigraphy are more sensitive than conventional x rays but lack specificity. Some investigators suggest that gallium citrate scanning can be used to assess radiographic resolution after successful antimicrobial therapy. CT scan to detect bone destruction and magnetic resonance imaging (MRI) to identify nervous system involvement remain the modalities of choice for defining the extent of the disease.

They are not useful to follow disease progression or healing. Differential diagnosis includes traditional external otitis and carcinoma.

A two-antibiotic combination therapy, with an aminoglycoside and an antipseudomonal penicillin, administered parenterally for 6 to 8 weeks, has been the standard treatment to manage invasive external otitis caused by *Pseudomonas aeruginosa,* particularly when there is evidence of cranial neuropathy, osteomyelitis, or spread to the contralateral base of the skull. Alternatively, imipenem, or a third-generation parenteral antipseudomonal cephalosporin, such as ceftazidime, can also be used. Limited data indicate that prolonged oral ciprofloxacin therapy, with or without rifampin, provides effective treatment. Surgery, consistency of local débridement and excision of accessible foci of infection, plays an ancillary role to antibiotic treatment. After the initial treatment, patients need to be evaluated for recurrent disease. Relapse is most commonly caused by persistent skull-base osteomyelitis, and it may not be apparent for a year after antibiotic treatment has ended.

# RHINOCEREBRAL MUCORMYCOSIS

Rhinocerebral mucormycosis (zygomycosis, phycomycosis), a rapidly spreading life-endangering fungal infection caused by *Mucor* species, is usually accompanied by ketoacidosis.[3] A similar syndrome has resulted from infection caused by other fungi and bacteria. The disease begins in nasal tissue or the palate, where the *Mucor* organisms initially invade, and extends to the paranasal sinuses, where it threatens the orbit and brain. The fungus that causes this potentially life-threatening infection has the unique predisposition to invade blood vessels, both arteries and veins, thereby producing thrombosis, infarction, and necrosis. There may be thrombosis of the internal jugular vein or sinuses of the brain.

Onset is usually but not invariably sudden, and the clinical presentation manifests as facial or ocular pain and on occasion a characteristic blood-tinged nasal discharge. Additional features include fever, lethargy, headache, proptosis, periorbital edema, visual blurring, increased lacrimation, tenderness over the maxillary sinus, and facial cellulitis. Physical exam can also reveal a darkened area of tissue necrosis in hard palate, nares, or face. The disease resembles orbital cellulitis and cavernous sinus thrombosis.

Roentgenograms of the maxillary sinus reveal mucosal thickening, with or without air fluid levels, and spotty destruction of the bony walls. CT scan and MRI are helpful to visualize the extent of the disease (bone, soft tissue, and intracranial complications). The diagnosis should be confirmed by biopsy specimens of infected tissues, which are submitted for both histologic examination and culture.

Treatment consists in control of the hyperglycemia and ketoacidosis, administration of amphotericin B as 1.5 mg/kg daily, and early surgical débridement of necrotic tissue, an activity that may need to be repeated.

Limited data indicate a possible role for adjunctive hyperbaric oxygen therapy.

# EMPHYSEMATOUS CHOLECYSTITIS

This unique form of note cholecystitis affects more men than women, and often there is no concomitant cholelithiasis. Presumably, ischemia is an important pathogenic component. The clinical manifestations are suggestive of acute cholecystitis. Gangrene and perforation of the gallbladder occur more frequently. Diagnosis is made when gas is seen in the gallbladder wall on plain films of the abdomen in the absence of abnormal communication with the gastrointestinal tract. Organisms responsible are predominantly clostridial species, but other organisms can be associated. Treatment consists in cholecystectomy and the infusion of antibiotics that inhibit the growth of clostridia and gram-negative aerobic bacilli.

# EMPHYSEMATOUS PYELONEPHRITIS

Emphysematous pyelonephritis is a necrotizing, gas-forming, potentially life-threatening bacterial infection usually caused by aerobic gram-negative bacilli, particularly *Escherichia coli*. These patients appear critically ill[4] and experience fever, vomiting, flank pain, and on occasion bacteremia. Rarely, diabetic intravenous drug abusers develop a more smoldering form of emphysematous pyelonephritis caused by *Candida* species. Diagnosis is made when gas is identified in the kidney or perirenal space. There may be concomitant obstructive uropathy. Nephrectomy is often required in addition to antibiotics.[4] Transcutaneous drainage should be attempted before nephrectomy, so that one may salvage the infected kidney.

# RENAL PAPILLARY NECROSIS WITH PYELONEPHRITIS

Renal papillary necrosis with pyelonephritis can appear as an acute fulminating disorder, or it can manifest as a subacute process. The diagnosis should be considered when the diabetic patient manifests florid pyelonephritis, hematuria, renal colic, or ketoacidosis, or does not respond well to antibiotic treatment or develops renal insufficiency. The intravenous pyelogram has a distinctive appearance, however, because of concomitant renal impairment, a retrograde pyelogram is the preferred study. Therapy of the seriously ill diabetic patient resembles that offered the patient with traditional bacterial pyelonephritis, that is, supportive measures, antibiotic infusion, regulation of concomitant ketoacidosis, and relief of obstruction.

# FOOT INFECTIONS

Foot infections are among the most common reasons for hospital admission in the diabetic patient. They range from local fungal infections of the nail to severe, necrotizing, life-threatening infections. More than 70% of all nontraumatic lower extremity amputations are performed on diabetic patients.

## Dermatophytosis

Fungal infection of the foot develops in 60% to 80% of diabetic patients. Most common causative organisms are *Trichophyton, Microsporum,* and *Epidermophyton.* Tinea pedis manifests with skin breakdown and maceration, primarily between the toes, and it should be treated because it can lead to a superimposed bacterial infection of the lower extremity.[5]

## Paronychia

Paronychia is an infection adjacent to the toenail usually attributable to nail dystrophy, ill-fitting shoes, or improper nail cutting.[5] It can be caused by a bacterial infection, usually, *Staphylococcus aureus* or to a fungal infection, usually *Candida* species.[6] The disorder is manifested as tenderness and inflammation of the nail folds. Therapy is directed to local care, incision and drainage when necessary, and to an antimicrobial agent as adjunctive therapy.

## Neuropathic ulcers

Neuropathy predisposes the diabetic to develop neuropathic ulcer, or *mal perforans,* which is commonly found on the sole (plantar ulcer), primarily at the site of bony prominence, such as metatarsal heads, and is usually circular, punched out, and associated with a callus. Claw deformity, which accompanies motor neuropathy, leads to unequal weight distribution, which exposes the foot to repetitive trauma and development of neutrophic ulcer.[7] Felted foam dressing is helpful in the management of a noninfected neuropathic ulceration. Heat, soaks, and whirlpools are not recommended.

**Prevention.** Local foot care and modification of the weight-bearing plantar surface are important in preventing infection. Patients should be educated not to walk barefoot and to inspect their feet daily, prevent trauma, and report to their physician any abnormality.

## Bacterial infection

Foot infections in the diabetic commonly originate at the nail plates or the interdigital web spaces. Puncture wounds or small foreign bodies can also be the cause of infection.[8] The most common risk factor, however, is the neuropathic ulcer. If left untreated, local infection can evolve into deeper soft-tissue infection, plantar space infection, osteomyelitis, suppurative tendinitis, gangrene, and bacteremia. Microbiologic features involve multiple organisms in the form of aerobes, facultative anaerobes, and strict anaerobes.

Deep-tissue cultures provide the most accurate microbiologic data. It is preferable to obtain a curettage of the ulcer base and needle aspiration after saline injection, rather than swabs of the ulcer or draining material. Evaluation should include a plain roentgenogram to help exclude the presence of foreign bodies, soft-tissue gas, or osteomyelitis.

Treatment of foot infections include foot elevation to decrease edema, control of the hyperglycemic state, broad-spectrum antibiotics, and local tissue débridement when indicated. Saline-moistened sterile gauze is applied over the wound and changed two or three times a day. Relieving the pressure at the site of the ulcer to permit healing can be accomplished by the use of felted foam inserts for small shallow ulcers and total-contact cast for more serious ulcers. All diabetics presenting with a foot infection should be evaluated for the presence of correctable vascular disease and concomitant osteomyelitis.[7,9]

## Deep space infection

Deep space infections of the feet frequently show little plantar or dorsal foot abnormality.[7] Cellulitis or abscess formation of the plantar spaces necessitates early and aggressive surgical therapy, including drainage and excision of the necrotic tissue, as well as broad-spectrum antimicrobial treatment.

## Osteomyelitis

Osteomyelitis is a common complication of a diabetic foot infection. The microbiologic characteristics are similar to those found in diabetic foot infections secondary to neuropathic ulcers. Osteomyelitis has often been demonstrated by bone biopsy in chronic, benign-appearing plantar ulcers. Lytic lesions require more than 30% bone loss to be demonstrated on plain roentgenograms, and this can take more than 14 days. Lack of sensitivity and specificity is a concern with all imaging devices used to detect osteomyelitis.[10] Adjacent soft-tissue infection and presence of diabetic osteopathy (Charcot joints) can give false-positive imaging results in this population of diabetic patients.[11-14]

A recent study showed that palpating bone at the base of an infected ulcer with a probe was consistent with underlying osteomyelitis. Failure to detect palpable bone does not, however, exclude osteomyelitis. This led the investigators to suggest combining the use of plain roentgenograms with probing of the bone. If both tests are negative, the patient should be initially treated as having soft-tissue infection. Plain x-ray films should be repeated after 2 weeks because an occult osteomyelitis should manifest at that time.[9,15] The standard for the diagnosis of osteomyelitis remains the recovery of a pathogen in culture from bone. The traditional therapeutic approach includes surgical débridement followed by prolonged antibiotic therapy. Limited data indicate benefit with long-term antibiotic therapy exclusively.[16,17]

## Choice of antibiotics

**Non-limb threatening lower extremity infections.** Most uncomplicated acute foot infections in diabetic patients, not recently treated with antibiotics, are caused by *Staphylococcus aureus*. A 2-week oral course of an antibiotic, such as clindamycin or cephalexin, would be considered appropriate. Cultures by curettage or aspiration should be done in all patients when possible. Treatment should be modified if and when valid culture results are available.[9,18]

**Limb-threatening infections.** Initially, intravenous antibiotic with broad-spectrum coverage should be used. Examples include imipenem-cilastatin, a beta-lactam/beta-lactamase-inhibitor combination (such as ticarcillin-clavulanate or piperacillin-tazobactam), or a combination of either clindamycin-ciprofloxacin or clindamycin-aztreonam. A recent study showed no significant difference between imipenem-cilastatin and ampicillin-sulbactam, despite the broader range of the former regimen.[19] It is desirable to avoid an aminoglycoside in this diabetic population because of concomitant renal disease, the risks of protracted aminoglycoside therapy, and the need to obtain sequential meaningful serum assays.

# NECROTIZING SOFT-TISSUE INFECTIONS

Necrotizing soft-tissue infections include a variety of disorders that produce progressive inflammation and necrosis of skin, subcutaneous tissues, fasciae, and occasionally muscles and can be accompanied by bacteremia. These infections occur most frequently in areas previously affected by trauma, surgery, or skin disorders. They usually involve the sacrum, perineum, and lower extremities and can be associated with the presence of gas in tissue, which is more consistently demonstrated by plain roentgenogram than by palpation.[5,20]

Necrotizing soft-tissue infection can be subdivided into two broad categories, superficial infection and deep infection. *Superficial infection*, defined as superficial to deep fasciae, includes nonclostridial anaerobic cellulitis and necrotizing fasciitis. Nonclostridial anaerobic cellulitis is characterized by mixed organisms, gradual or rapid onset, and usually absence of systemic toxicity. The relative mildness of the process helps to distinguish it from true gas gangrene. This disorder manifests as discoloration of skin, presence of gas, mild pain, dark pus, and foul odor.

Necrotizing fasciitis is a rapidly progressive, usually polymicrobial infection, accompanied by prominent systemic toxicity. Disease is usually characterized by rapid onset, areas of skin necrosis, and seropurulent drainage. Fournier's gangrene is classified as a necrotizing fasciitis.

*Deep infection* involves muscle tissue underneath the deep fascia. It includes synergistic nonclostridial anaerobic myonecrosis and clostridial gas gangrene. Synergistic nonclostridial anaerobic myonecrosis, known as *necrotizing cellulitis,* has the following features: overlying skin that appears normal (because muscle rather than skin is involved), rapid onset, severe pain, gas, skin necrosis (on occasion), and "dishwater" pus.

Clostridial gas gangrene, a clostridial myonecrosis, is a very unusual disorder among diabetics. This illness occurs within hours of an insult or surgery. A thin, watery discharge and large hemorrhagic bullae can appear on the skin near the wound. *Clostridium perfringens* causes the most severe and rapidly progressive form of these infections.

The definitive diagnosis of these infections is established by a combination of surgical intervention and precise microbiologic identification. Treatment of necrotizing soft-tissue infection consists in prompt and extensive surgery (débridement of all necrotic tissue) with parenteral antibiotics.[21] Potential initial treatment could be the use of imipenem-cilastatin. If the patient is allergic to penicillin or has a history of seizures, empiric therapy could be the infusion of clindamycin and aztreonam. Limited data indicate that hyperbaric oxygen therapy has an adjunctive role.

## References

1. Gleckman RA: Usual and unusual infections complicating diabetes mellitus, *Contemp Intern Med* 3:13-24, 1991.
2. Rubin J, Yu VL: Malignant external otitis: insights into pathogenesis, clinical manifestations, diagnosis, and therapy, *Am J Med* 85:391-398, 1988.
3. Adam RD, Hunter G, DiTomasso J, et al: Mucormycosis: emerging prominence of cutaneous infections, *Clin Infect Dis* 19:67-76, 1994.
4. Patel NP, Lavengood RW, Fernandes M, et al: Gas-forming infections in genitourinary tract, *Urology* 39(4):341-345, 1992.
5. Kemmerly SA: Dermatologic manifestations of infections in diabetics, *Infect Dis Clin North Am* 8(3):523-532, 1994.
6. Perez MI, Kohn SR: Cutaneous manifestations of diabetes mellitus, *J Am Acad Dermatol* 30:519-531, 1994.
7. Bridges RM, Deitch EA: Diabetic foot infections, pathophysiology and treatment, *Surg Clin North Am* 74:537-555, 1994.
8. Lavery LA, Harkless LB, Felder-Johnson K, et al: Bacterial pathogens in infected puncture wounds in adults with diabetes, *J Foot Ankle Surg* 33:91-97, 1994.
9. Caputo GM, Cavanagh PR, Ulbrecht JS, et al: Assessment and management of foot disease in patients with diabetes, *N Engl J Med* 331(13):854-860, 1994.
10. Eckman MH, Greenfield S, Mackey WC, et al: Foot infections in diabetic patients, *JAMA* 273(9):712-720, 1995.
11. Keenan AM, Tindel NL, Alavi A: Diagnosis of pedal osteomyelitis in diabetic patients using current scintigraphic techniques, *Arch Intern Med* 149: 2262-2266, 1989.
12. Newman LG, Waller J, Palestro CJ, et al: Unsuspected osteomyelitis in diabetic foot ulcers: diagnosis and monitoring by leukocyte scanning with indium [In 111] oxyquinoline, *JAMA* 266(9):1246-1251, 1991.
13. Tumeh SS, Tohmeh AG: Nuclear medicine techniques in septic arthritis and osteomyelitis, *Rheum Dis Clin North Am* 17(3):559-583, 1991.
14. Weinstein D, Wang A, Chambers R, et al: Evaluation of MRI in the diagnosis of osteomyelitis in diabetic foot infections, *Foot Ankle* 14(1):18-22, 1993.
15. Grayson ML, Gibbons GW, Habershaw GM, et al: Probing to bone in infected pedal ulcers, *JAMA* 273(9):721-723, 1995.
16. Bamberger DM, Daus GP, Gerding DN: Osteomyelitis in the feet of diabetic patients, *Am J Med* 83:653-660, 1987.
17. Peterson LR, Lissack LM, Canter K, et al: Therapy of lower extremity infections with ciprofloxacin in patients with diabetes mellitus, peripheral vascular disease, or both, *Am J Med* 86:801-808, 1989.

18. Lipsky BA, Pecoraro RE, Larson SA, et al: Outpatient management of uncomplicated lower-extremity infections in diabetic patients, *Arch Intern Med* 150:790-797, 1990.
19. Grayson ML, Gibbons GW, Balogh K, et al: Use of ampicillin/sulbactam versus imipenem/cilastatin in the treatment of limb-threatening foot infections in diabetic patients, *Clin Infect Dis* 18:683-693, 1994.
20. McHenry CR, Brandt CP, Piotrowski JJ, et al: Idiopathic necrotizing fasciitis: recognition, incidence, and outcome of therapy, *Am Surg* 60(7):490-494, 1994.
21. Lille ST, Sato TT, Engrav LH et al: Necrotizing soft tissue infections: obstacles in diagnosis, *J Am Coll Surg* 182:7, 1996.

## Chapter 16

# Medical and Surgical Indications for Systemic Antimicrobial Prophylaxis

Nelson M. Gantz

The use of antimicrobial agents given before the onset of disease to prevent infection constitutes prophylaxis. On the surgical service, antimicrobial prophylaxis can decrease the incidence of wound infections after certain operations. The benefit of prophylaxis must be weighed against the risk of adverse effects of the antibiotic, emergence of resistant organisms, and the possiblity of superinfection.[1] On the medical service, anti-infective agents can prevent certain infections such as malaria and rheumatic fever. Prophylactic antibiotics can prevent the acquisition of an exogenous organism that is not normally part of the individual's flora. An example is the use of amantadine to prevent influenza A. Another goal of prophylaxis is to prevent organisms normally present in one site from gaining access to a normally sterile body site. An example is the attempt to prevent recurrent urinary tract infections from flora normally present in the stool or vagina. Antimicrobial prophylaxis is most effective when an antibiotic is selected for a specific pathogen. For example, penicillin is active against group A beta-hemolytic streptococci, which are involved in the pathogenesis of rheumatic fever. Thus penicillin can be given to prevent streptococcal pharyngitis to avoid a possible sequela, rheumatic fever. For prophylaxis to be effective, the antimicrobial agent needs to be present at the site where the infection is likely to occur. Prophylaxis should be differentiated from the use of antibiotics for situations in which contamination has occurred as after an animal bite or with an open fracture. Antibiotic use in these settings is an example of therapy for an "early infection." Use of isoniazid for tuberculosis prophylaxis also constitutes therapy of an existing infection. Prophylaxis is most effective when the aim is to prevent infection caused by a single organism. In contrast, antibiotics are less effective when multiple organisms are involved such as the use of antibiotics for patients with chronic bronchitis to prevent an acute exacerbation.

# PRINCIPLES OF
# ANTIBIOTIC PROPHYLAXIS

Effective use of prophylactic antibiotics requires that adequate drug levels be present at the appropriate site at the time of the event posing the risk of transient bacteremia. To accomplish this goal, the antimicrobial should initially be given 1 to 2 hours before the procedure and continued for one dose after. An increase in the duration of treatment beyond one dose after the initial loading dose only raises the cost and increases the possibility of an adverse drug reaction.

The antibiotic selected for dental procedures and other procedures involving the airway should be directed against viridans streptococci. Genitourinary manipulations and gastrointestinal, gynecologic, and obstetric procedures require that the antibiotic prophylaxis be adequate for enterococci. Antibiotics should be directed against penicillinase-producing staphylococci in a predisposed person having incision and drainage of an abscess. A urine culture should be obtained before a genitourinary procedure so that any infection can be identified and treated before the instrumentation. Tables 16-1 to 16-3 list the regimens of antibiotic prophylaxis preceding dental and surgical procedures as well as those for incision and drainage of skin abscesses.

# ANTIMICROBIAL PROPHYLAXIS
# ON THE MEDICAL SERVICE

Table 16-4 lists examples of using antimicrobial prophylaxis to prevent infections in patients on the medical service.[2]

**Endocarditis prophylaxis.** The subject of endocarditis prophylaxis continues to stir controversy. Recommendations for prevention of endocarditis from the committee of the American Heart Association (AHA) are not based on controlled clinical studies.[3] No such studies have been published or are likely to be forthcoming. A few questions regarding prophylaxis remain unanswered: Can endocarditis be prevented by giving prophylactic antibiotics? What is the risk of endocarditis after procedures, such as dental extraction, associated with transient bacteremia? Which antibiotic regimens for prophylaxis are the best? Are parenteral antibiotics more effective than oral drugs? Which procedures merit the use of prophylactic antibiotics to prevent endocarditis? How should patients with mitral valve prolapse who are to undergo various diagnostic or therapeutic manipulations be managed? Should patients with arterial grafts or orthopedic devices (such as a prosthetic hip) receive prophylactic antibiotics for special clinical situations associated with a transient bacteremia? This is only a partial list of questions that the clinician faces daily when caring for patients at risk for endocarditis. Despite the widespread availability of antibiotics, the incidence of endocarditis has not declined in recent years.

Infective endocarditis has major morbidity and mortality, despite the availability of antimicrobial agents. Patients who have underlying valvular heart disease are at risk for the development of infective endo-

**Table 16-1.**  *Antibiotic prophylactic regimens (dental procedures)\**

| Drug | Initial dose | Route | Regimen |
|------|------|------|------|
| Amoxicillin | 3.0 g | po | 1 hour before, then 1.5 g 6 hours later |
| Ampicillin | 2.0 g | IV or IM | 30 min before, then ampicillin, 1.0 g IV or IM, or amoxicillin, 1.5 g po, 6 hours later |
| Ampicillin plus gentamicin[†] | 2.0 g 1.5 mg/kg (to a maximum of 80 mg) | IV or IM IV or IM | 30 min before, then amoxicillin 1.5 g po 6 hours later; or repeat parenteral drugs 8 hours later |
| Erythromycin ethylsuccinate[‡] *or* | 1600 mg | po | |
| | | | 2 hours before, then half the dose 6 h later |
| Erythromycin stearate[‡] | 1.0 g | po | |
| Clindamycin[‡] | 300 mg | po | 1 hour before, then 150 mg 6 hours later |
| Vancomycin[†‡] | 1.0 g | IV | Administer over 1 hour, and perform procedure immediately when finished |

*IM,* Intramuscularly; *IV,* intravenously; *po,* by mouth (*per os*).
*Parenteral regimens are recommended for patients with prosthetic or biosynthetic heart valves.
[†]May be preferred for patients in highest-risk groups though data to support this practice are not available.
[‡]If patient is allergic to penicillin or receiving continuous oral penicillin.
Modified from Dajani AS, Bisno AL, Chung KJ, et al: Prevention of bacterial endocarditis, *JAMA* 264:2919, 1990.

carditis when organisms invade the bloodstream. A key factor in the pathogenesis of infective endocarditis is the occurrence of a transient bacteremia.[4] The AHA recommends that patients with rheumatic, congenital, or other cardiovascular diseases, as well as those with a prosthetic heart valve, receive prophylactic antibiotics when they have a procedure associated with a transient bacteremia.[3]

Most cases of endocarditis are not preventable by the administration of prophylactic antibiotics. Only half of the patients who develop endocarditis have a recognized cardiac lesion for which prophylaxis would be a consideration. Furthermore, less than 25% of patients with endocarditis caused by viridans streptococci and about 40% of patients

**Table 16-2.** *Endocarditis prophylaxis\* for adults before genitourinary or gastrointestinal or gynecologic procedures*

| Drug | Initial dose | Route | Regimen |
|------|------|------|------|
| Ampicillin plus gentamicin | 2.0 g 1.5 mg/kg (to a maximum of 80 mg) | IV or IM | 30 min before, then repeat 8 hours later or amoxicillin 1.5 g 6 hours later |
| *or* | | | |
| Vancomycin plus gentamicin† | 1.0 g 1.5 mg/kg (to a maximum of 80 mg) | IV IV or IM | 1 hour before, then repeat 8 hours later |
| *or* | | | |
| Amoxicillin‡ | 3.0 g | po | 1 hour before, then 1.5 g 6 hours later |

*IM,* Intramuscularly; *IV,* intravenously; *po,* by mouth (*per os*).
\*Parenteral regimens are recommended for patients with prosthetic or biosynthetic heart valves.
†If allergic to penicillin.
‡Alternative for low-risk patient.
Modified from Dajani AS, Bisno AL, Chung KJ, et al: Prevention of bacterial endocarditis, *JAMA* 264:2919, 1990.

with endocarditis caused by entrococci have an identified portal of entry for which prophylaxis could be given. In addition, the usually recommended antibiotics are likely to be effective in only two thirds or so of cases of endocarditis. Therefore, it is estimated that only 8% to 10% of cases of endocarditis are potentially preventable.

**Transient bacteremia.** Transient bacteremias occur commonly.[4] They may occur spontaneously, as with chewing food or with defecation. They may result from many procedures that traumatize mucuous membranes with an indigenous microbial flora, as with a dental extraction or a urethral catheterization. Bacteremias that follow procedures resulting in mucosal trauma are asymptomatic, usually occur about 1 to 5 minutes after the procedures, and generally last less than 15 minutes. Blood cultures are usually sterile 30 minutes after the procedures. Transient bacteremias also occur with local infections, such as those that occur with incision and drainage of an abscess or with manipulation of the urinary tract in a patient with asymptomatic bacteriuria. The organisms associated with these bacteremias reflect either the normal flora at the manipulated site or the pathogen causing the local infection.

A history of a predisposing event can at times be elicited from patients with endocarditis. A preceding dental procedure has been

**Table 16-3.** *For incision and drainage of skin abscesses caused by coagulase-positive staphylococci\**

| Drug | Initial dose | Route | Regimen |
|------|------|-------|---------|
| Nafcillin or oxacillin | 2 g | IV | ½ to 1 hour before procedure, then 2 g IV q4h |
| Dicloxacillin | 500 mg | po | 1 hour before procedure, then 500 mg q6h |
| Cefazolin† | 1 g | IM | 1 hour before procedure and then 1 g IV or IM q8h |
| Vancomycin*† | 1 g | IV | Over 60 min; start infusion 1 hour before procedure, then 1 g q12h IV |

*IM*, Intramuscularly; *IV*, intravenously; *po*, by mouth (*per os*).
\*Route and duration of therapy depend on the severity of the infection and whether the predisposed person is at risk (as with a prosthetic heart valve). Results of Gram stains and cultures should also guide antibiotic selection.
†If patient is allergic to penicillin.
Modified from Dajani AS, Bisno AL, Chung KJ, et al: Prevention of bacterial endocarditis, *JAMA* 264:2919, 1990.

noted in 15% to 20% of patients with nonenterococcal streptococcal endocarditis. A preceding genitourinary tract procedure has been reported in 40% of patients with enterococcal endocarditis. A preceding infection of the skin or soft tissue has been noted in 35% of patients with staphylococcal endocarditis.[5]

The oropharynx is a frequent portal of entry for organisms into the bloodstream. Blood cultures are positive in 18% to 85% of patients after a dental extraction.[4] The frequency of bacteremia correlates with the severity of gingival infection and the extent of tissue trauma. The organisms isolated reflect the normal mouth flora. Viridans streptococci are isolated most frequently, but anaerobic streptococci, coagulase-negative staphylococci, diphtheroids, and fusobacteria are also seen. Strains of viradans streptococci account for 50% to 75% of cases of endocarditis and are usually penicillin sensitive. Prophylaxis should begin 1 to 2 hours before a procedure so that serum levels of the antibiotic are adequate at the time of anticipated bacteremia.

Other dental procedures that may result in a transient bacteremia include periodontal operations, such as gingivectomy, root canal surgery, and dental cleaning. Blood cultures are positive in up to 88% of patients, depending on the severity of gum disease.[4] The predominant organisms are the same as those found after dental extraction. Positive blood cultures are also seen after tooth brushing (0 to 26%), after the use of oral irrigation devices (7% to 50%), after the use of dental floss (20%), and after gum cleaning or eating hard candy (0 to 22%). Antibiotic prophylaxis obviously is impractical for prevention of transient bacteremias secondary to these common daily activities. The cumulative risk of transient bacteremia is far greater for the usual events of living, such as eating, brushing the teeth, or defecation, compared with the risk from an occasional surgical procedure.[6] Maintenance of good oral hygiene decreases the amount of gum disease, which is a key determinant of the frequency of transient bacteremia after any dental manipulation.

Other procedures involving the oropharynx and the respiratory tract may result in bacteremia; these include tonsillectomy, nasotracheal intubation, and rigid-tube bronchoscopy. Positive blood cultures, however, rarely occur in association with flexible fiberoptic bronchoscopy and lung biopsy; this finding contrasts with the 15% rate of bacteremia associated with the use of a rigid bronchoscope.[4]

Diagnostic procedures that involve the gastrointestinal tract are another source of transient bacteremias.[4,7] Positive blood cultures are found in 0 to 10% (4% overall) of patients having fiberoptic gastrointestinal endoscopy, in 0 to 9.5% (5% overall) of patients undergoing rigid sigmoidoscopy, in 3% to 14% of patients undergoing liver biopsy, in 11% of patients having a barium enema, and in 0 to 27% (5% overall) of patients undergoing colonoscopy.[7] The predominant organisms isolated with these procedures are enterococci, which are frequent causes of endocarditis, and gram-negative bacilli, organisms rarely involved in endocarditis.

Transient bacteremia and infective endocarditis can occur after urinary tract, obstetric, and gynecologic procedures.[4] The urinary tract is the portal of entry in 20% to 50% of patients with enterococcal endocarditis, whereas 20% of cases caused by this organism are related to obstetric and gynecologic procedures. A genitourinary tract source is implicated in about 15% of all patients with endocarditis. A transient bacteremia occurs in 8% of patients undergoing urethral catheterization, in 24% of patients undergoing urethral dilatation, in 17% of patients having cystoscopy, and in 12% to 31% of patients having transurethral prosthetic resection. The frequency of positive blood cultures increases severalfold in patients with infection at the instrumented site.[8] One example of such an infection is that of the urinary tract.

Transient bacteremia also occurs in 0 to 5% of patients after vaginal delivery, cesarean section, and dilation and curettage of the uterus and during insertion or removal of an intrauterine contraceptive device.[4] Manipulation of an infected focus, such as massage of an infected prostate or incision and drainage of an abscess, is associated with bacteremia and the risk of endocarditis. Transient bacteremia, however, is rare with cardiac catheterization and angiographic procedures. The box on p. 159 lists the procedures associated with transient bacteremia and the indications for antibiotic prophylaxis.

**Cardiac lesions predisposing to endocarditis.** Prevention of endocarditis requires a knowledge of the events likely to produce bacteremia, as well as the patients with predisposing cardiac lesions. Unfortunately, half the patients with endocarditis have no recognized underlying heart disease, thus making antibiotic prophylaxis impossible for this group.[5] Rheumatic valvular disease still remains the most common form of

**Table 16-4.** *Examples of antimicrobial prophylaxis in patients on the medical service*

| Disease | Organism | Anti-infective agent | Dose/route | Comments |
|---|---|---|---|---|
| Rheumatic fever | Group A beta-hemolytic streptococci | Benzathine penicillin | 1.2 million units IM once every 3 to 4 weeks | Continue for at least 5 years and patient is no longer at risk of exposure to streptococcal infections |
| | | Penicillin V | 250 mg po twice a day | |
| | | Sulfisoxazole | 1 g po daily | |
| Plague | *Yersinia pestis* | Tetracycline | 250 mg po four times a day for 7 days | |
| Meningitis | *Neisseria meningitidis* | Rifampin | 600 mg po twice a day for 2 days | |
| | | Ceftriaxone | 250 mg IM | |
| | | Ciprofloxacin | 500 mg po once | Not for persons less than 18 years of age |
| Recurrent cellulitis | Group A beta-hemolytic streptococci | Penicillin | 250 mg po twice a day | |
| | *Staphylococcus aureus* | Clindamycin | 300 mg po two times a day | |
| Tuberculosis | *Mycobacterium tuberculosis* INH sensitive | Isoniazid | 300 mg po once daily for 9 months | |

| Condition | Organism | Drug | Dose | Comments |
|---|---|---|---|---|
| | INH resistant | Rifampin plus pyrazinamide | 600 mg po once daily / 25 mg/kg po once daily for 9 months | No data on effectiveness |
| Pertussis | *Bordetella pertussis* | Erythromycin | 500 mg orally four times a day for 14 days | For all close contacts irrespective of vaccination status |
| | | Trimethoprim-sulfamethoxazole | 1 DS tablet twice a day for 14 days | Efficacy? |
| Fungal infections in acute leukemia | *Candida* species other than *Candida krusei* | Fluconazole | 400 mg orally once daily | Decrease in *Candida* colonization and superficial infections; no effect in preventing deep fungal infections or reducing mortality |
| Spontaneous bacterial peritonitis in cirrhosis | Gram-negative bacilli | Norfloxacin | 400 mg orally per day | Decrease in infection Controlled trial needed |
| Cytomegalovirus after liver transplantation | Cytomegalovirus | Ganciclovir | 5 mg/kg intravenously twice daily for 7 days | Decrease in CMV disease compared with oral acyclovir |

*(continued)*

**Table 16-4.** Examples of antimicrobial prophylaxis in patients on the medical service—cont'd

| Disease | Organism | Anti-infective agent | Dose/route | Comments |
|---------|----------|---------------------|------------|----------|
| Traveler's diarrhea | Enterotoxigenic *Escherichia coli, Campylobacter, Shigella, Salmonella,* parasites | Ciprofloxacin | 500 mg once daily | Antibiotic not usually recommended for prophylaxis |
| | | Bismuth subsalicylate | 2 tablets four times a day | Do not take for more than 3 weeks |
| Malaria | *Plasmodium* species | Mefloquine | 250 mg weekly; start 1 week before, during, and 4 weeks after return | For chloroquine-resistant strains See *Health Information for International Travel, 1994,* for further advice or call the CDC at 404-332-4559 |
| | | Doxycycline | 100 mg once daily; begin 1 day before travel, during, and 4 weeks after return | |
| | | Chloroquine | 500 mg of salt once weekly; begin 1 week before, during, and 4 weeks after return | |
| Influenza | Influenza A virus | Amantadine | 100 mg orally once daily for 4 to 8 weeks | Decrease dose in renal failure |
| | | Rimantadine | 100 mg orally once daily for 4 to 8 weeks | Decrease in CNS adverse effects compared with amantadine |

| Condition | Organism | Drug | Dose | Comments |
|---|---|---|---|---|
| Genital herpes simplex virus (HSV) in transplant recipients; in acute leukemia | Herpes simplex virus | Acyclovir | 400 mg orally twice daily; 250 mg/m² q8h for 1 month | Well tolerated for years; Duration of therapy is less if patient is discharged or HSV infection develops |
| Recurrent cystitis | Gram-negative enterics | Trimethoprim-sulfamethoxazole; Trimethoprim | ½ tablet at bedtime; 100 mg at bedtime or shortly after sexual intercourse | |
| Human bite wounds | Mouth anaerobes | Penicillin | 250 mg orally three times daily for 3 to 5 days | |
| Following splenectomy | Encapsulated bacteria, e.g., *Streptococcus pneumoniae* | Pneumococcal vaccine | 1 dose every 7 years | |
| *Pneumocystis* pneumonia | *Pneumocystis carinii* | Trimethoprim-sulfamethoxazole; Dapsone; Pentamidine | 1 DS orally once daily or 3 times a week; 50 mg orally twice daily; Aerosol 300 mg once a month by Respirgard II Nebulizer | Start with CD4 count <200/mm³ |
| Toxoplasmosis | *Toxoplasma gondii* | Trimethoprim-sulfamethoxazole | 1 DS orally daily or 3 times a week | IgG titer positive for Toxoplasma and CD4 < 100 cells/mm³. |

*(continued)*

**Table 16-4.** *Examples of antimicrobial prophylaxis in patients on the medical service—cont'd*

| Disease | Organism | Anti-infective agent | Dose/route | Comments |
|---------|----------|---------------------|-----------|----------|
| Disseminated mycobacteria | *Mycobacterium avium–intracellulare* complex | Rifabutin Clarithromycin Azithromycin | 300 mg orally daily 500 mg orally twice daily 250 mg orally once daily | Begin with CD4 < 75 cells/mm$^3$ |
| Histoplasmosis | *Histoplasma capsulatum* | Itraconazole | 200 mg orally once daily | Consider for selected patients with AIDS in endemic areas |
| Cytomegalovirus | Cytomegalovirus | Ganciclovir | 1 g orally tid | CD4 <100 cells/mm$^3$ |
| Recurrent oral or vaginal candidiasis | *Candida* species | Fluconazole | 100 mg orally daily | Limited data |

*AIDS,* Acquired immunodeficiency syndrome; *CDC,* Centers for Disease Control and Prevention, Atlanta, Ga.; *CMV,* cytomegalovirus; *CNS,* central nervous system; *DS,* double strength; *HSV,* herpes simplex virus; *IM,* intramuscularly; *INH,* isoniazid; *po,* by mouth (*per os*); *tid,* three times a day.

## Indications for Antibiotic Prophylaxis in Procedures Associated with Transient Bacteremia

ANTIBIOTIC PROPHYLAXIS RECOMMENDED FOR ALL PATIENTS WITH VALVULAR HEART DISEASE

### Dental procedures with gingival bleeding

Dental extraction
Dental cleaning
Periodontal surgery (such as gingivectomy)

### Procedures involving the airways

Tonsillectomy or adenoidectomy
Bronchoscopy with a rigid bronchoscope

### Genitourinary manipulations

Cystoscopy
Transurethral prostatic resection
Urethral dilatation

### Gastrointestinal tract

Cholecystectomy
Intestinal surgery

### Gynecologic and obstetric conditions

Dilatation and curettage of uterus
Vaginal hysterectomy
Vaginal delivery (complicated)
Cesarean section

### Manipulation of septic foci

Incision and drainage of abscesses

ANTIBIOTIC PROPHYLAXIS RECOMMENDED ONLY FOR PATIENTS AT HIGH RISK, THAT IS, PRESENCE OF PROSTHETIC OR BIOPROSTHETIC HEART VALVES

### All procedures listed previously

### Procedures involving the airway

Nasotracheal intubation
Fiberoptic bronchoscopy(?)

### Gastrointestinal procedures

Sigmoidoscopy
Barium enema

*continued*

*continued*

---

Colonoscopy
Liver biopsy
Upper gastrointestinal endoscopy with biopsy
Endoscopic retrograde cholangiopancreatography

### PROCEDURES FOR WHICH ANTIBIOTIC PROPHYLAXIS IS NOT INDICATED FOR PATIENTS WITH VALVULAR HEART DISEASE

***Procedures involving the airway***
Orotracheal intubation
Nasotracheal suctioning

***Gynecologic procedures***
Insertion or removal of intrauterine device
Vaginal delivery (uncomplicated)

***Other procedures***
Cardiac catheterization and angiographic procedures
Pacemaker insertion
Peritoneal dialysis

---

underlying cardiac disease in patients in whom endocarditis develops. The frequency has declined in recent years, however, because of the decreasing incidence of rheumatic fever. Patients with a bicuspid aortic valve are predisposed to endocarditis, as are patients with calcific or atherosclerotic changes in the aortic and mitral valve or anulus.

Patients with mitral valve prolapse, the click murmur syndrome, have been reported to be at increased risk of endocarditis. In a case-controlled study, the risk of endocarditis in patients with mitral valve prolapse was approximately eight times higher than that for the matched controls.[9] In a study of endocarditis prophylaxis failures, mitral valve prolapse was the most frequent cardiac abnormality identified and accounted for 33% of the cases of endocarditis.[10] Prophylaxis in all such patients would be difficult because of the high incidence of mitral valve prolapse; 5% to 6% of the American population is affected. I therefore recommend that antibiotic prophylaxis should be given only to those patients with associated mitral insufficiency documented by a holosystolic murmur and not to those patients who have only a systolic click.

Patients with a previous episode of endocarditis should receive prophylaxis for predisposing events. Patients with prosthetic or bio-prosthetic heart valves are also predisposed to endocarditis. Because infection of a prosthesis is often difficult to eradicate and carries a high mortality, antibiotic prophylaxis is recommended both for the usual predisposing events and for additional procedures that are associated with a transient bacteremia but with a lower risk of infection, such as sigmoidoscopy (see box on pp. 159 and 160).[4]

Although there are no controlled studies to establish the effectiveness of prophylactic antibiotics in patients with predisposing cardiac lesions, prophylaxis is generally recommended. The value of prophylaxis for procedures that may be associated with a transient bacteremia is unclear in patients with transvenous pacemakers, arteriovenous shunts for hemodialysis, and ventriculoatrial shunts. The risk in the last situation is probably low, and the majority of experts do not recommend prophylaxis in such cases. Only rough estimates are available for the incidence of endocarditis in susceptible persons after exposure to an event associated with transient bacteremia. The incidence is clearly low.

## SURGICAL PROPHYLAXIS

For more than 30 years, the use of antibiotics to prevent surgical infections has been the standard of therapy.[11] Controversial issues have centered around the procedures that merit prophylaxis, the choice of drug, the time to begin therapy, and the duration the agent should be administered. Some of these issues have been resolved by carefully performed controlled trials. Other questions remain unanswered, and at times, in practice, the antibiotic selected for prophylaxis is based on belief rather than on science.[12]

Surgical site infections, formerly called wound infections, represent the most frequent nosocomial infection in patients on the surgical service. The risk of infection varies with the type of surgical procedure. Operations can be classified as clean, clean-contaminated, contaminated, and dirty (Table 16-5). The rate of infection is lowest with a clean operation, less than 5%, and highest with a dirty procedure, with an infection rate of about 30%.[12] Rates of infection are intermediate with clean contaminated and contaminated procedures. A clean procedure such as a breast biopsy or hernia repair refers to an operation in which no entry into the respiratory, alimentary, or genitourinary tract occurs. In a clean operation, there is also no break in sterile technique. In a dirty procedure, there is fecal contamination of the wound with devitalized tissue and often the presence of foreign bodies. Some traumatic wounds can be classified as dirty cases. Since the infection rate is low in clean cases, antibiotics are not usually administered. The potential consequences of antibiotic usage such as cost, possible adverse drug effects, influence on the bacterial flora in terms of resistance, usually exceeds the benefit in clean procedures. The major exception occurs in clean cases in which a prosthetic device is inserted such as a heart valve, vascular graft, CFS or cerebrospinal fluid shunt or an artificial joint. In these situations, infection is difficult to eradicate without removal of the device, and prophylactic antibiotics are administered as a standard practice. In contaminated or dirty operations, organisms are present, and antibiotics are used as early therapy

**Table 16-5.** *Prevention of wound infection in surgical patients*

| Nature of operation | Likely pathogens | Recommended drugs | Adult dosage before surgery* |
|---|---|---|---|
| CLEAN | | | |
| Cardiac | | | |
| Prosthetic valve, coronary artery bypass, other open-heart surgery, pacemaker implant | *Staphylococcus epidermidis, S. aureus* | cefazolin *or* vancomycin[†] | 1-2 g IV 1 g IV |
| Vascular | | | |
| Arterial surgery involving the abdominal aorta, a prosthesis, or a groin incision | *S. aureus, S. epidermidis* | cefazolin *or* vancomycin[†] | 1-2 g IV 1 g IV |
| Lower-extremity amputation for ischemia | *S. aureus, S. epidermidis* | cefazolin *or* vancomycin[†] | 1 g IV 1 g IV |
| Neurosurgery | | | |
| Craniotomy | *S. aureus, S. epidermidis* | cefazolin *or* vancomycin[†] | 1 g IV 1 g IV |
| Orthopedic | | | |
| Total joint replacement, internal fixation of fractures | *S. aureus, S. epidermidis* | cefazolin *or* vancomycin[†] | 1-2 g IV 1 g IV |

## CLEAN-CONTAMINATED

| | | |
|---|---|---|
| **Head and neck** | | |
| Entering oral cavity or pharynx | *S. aureus*, streptococci, oral anaerobes | cefazolin *or* clindamycin | 1-2 g IV<br>600 mg IV |
| **Abdominal** | | |
| Gastroduodenal | Enteric gram-negative bacilli, gram-positive cocci | cefazolin<br>*High-risk procedures only:* e.g., for gastric bypass for obesity, percutaneous endoscopic gastrostomy, disorders with decreased gastric acidity or motility | 1-2 g IV |
| Biliary tract | Enteric gram-negative bacilli, enterococci, clostridia | *High risk only:* cefazolin | 1-2 g IV |
| Colorectal | Enteric gram-negative bacilli, anaerobes | *Oral:* neomycin + erythromycin base‡; cefoxitin *or* cefotetan | 1-2 g IV |
| Appendectomy | Enteric gram-negative bacilli, anaerobes | cefoxitin *or* cefotetan | 1-2 g IV |
| **Gynecologic** | | |
| Vaginal or abdominal hysterectomy | Enteric gram-negative bacteria, anaerobes, group B streptococci, enterococci | cefazolin | 1 g IV |
| Cesarean section | Same as for hysterectomy | *High risk only:* cefazolin | 1 g IV after cord clamping |
| Abortion | Same as for hysterectomy | *First trimester, high risk‖:* aqueous penicillin G *or* doxycycline<br>*Second trimester:* cefazolin | 1 million units IV<br>300 mg PO‖<br>1 g IV |

*(continued)*

**Table 16-5.** *Prevention of wound infection in surgical patients—cont'd*

| Nature of operation | Likely pathogens | Recommended drugs | Adult dosage before surgery* |
|---|---|---|---|
| **DIRTY (OR CONTAMINATED) SURGERY** | | | |
| Ruptured viscus¶ | Enteric gram-negative bacilli, anaerobes, enterococci | cefoxitin<br>*or* cefotetan<br>+ gentamicin<br>*or* clindamycin<br>+ gentamicin | 2 g IV q6h<br>1-2 g IV q12h<br>1.5 mg/kg IV q8h<br>600 mg IV q8h<br>1.5 mg/kg IV q8h |
| Traumatic wound¶# | *S. aureus*, group A streptococci, clostridia | cefazolin | 1-2 g IV q8h |

*Parenteral prophylactic antimicrobials can be given as a single intravenous dose just before the operation. For prolonged operations, additional intraoperative doses should be given q6-8h for the duration of the procedure.
†For hospitals in which methicillin-resistant *Staphylococcus aureus* and *S. epidermidis* frequently cause wound infection, or for patients allergic to penicillins or cephalosporins. Rapid IV administration may cause hypotension, which could be especially dangerous during induction of anesthesia. Even if the drug is given over 60 minutes, hypotension may occur; treatment with diphenhydramine (Benadryl and others) and further slowing of the infusion rate may be helpful. For procedures in which enteric gram-negative bacilli are likely pathogens, such as vascular surgery involving a groin incision, cefazolin should be included in the prophylaxis regimen.
‡After appropriate diet and catharsis, 1 gram of each at 1 PM, 2 PM, and 11 PM the day before an 8 AM operation.
§Patients with previous pelvic inflammatory disease in inflammatory disease, previous gonorrhea, or multiple sex partners.
∥Divided into 100 mg 1 hour before the abortion and 200 mg ½ hour after.
¶For "dirty" surgery, therapy should usually be continued for 5 to 10 days.
#For bite wounds, in which likely pathogens may also include oral anaerobes, such as *Eikenella corrodens* (human) and *Pasteurella multocida* (dog and cat), some consultants recommend use of amoxicillin-clavulanic acid or ampicillin-sulbactam.
Modified from Anonymous: *Med Letter* 37:79–82, 1995.

rather than as prophylaxis. In clean-contaminated cases such as an elective colon resection, it is impossible to avoid minor spillage of the normal bowel flora. Prophylactic antibiotics are given to decrease the number of organisms to a level so that normal host defenses can handle them.

**Timing of antibiotic administration.** In animal models, administering antibiotics before or shortly after the inoculation of a pathogenic organism reduced the size of the ensuing skin lesion compared with waiting 4 hours when the antibiotic had no effect. In a study, the wound infection rate was the lowest when the antibiotics were given preoperatively, which was defined as occurring up to 2 hours before the incision.[13] Infection rates were highest when the drug was given early, 2 to 24 hours before the operation, or postoperatively if the drug was given more than 3 hours after the incision. In this study, 30% of patients received the prophylactic antibiotics inappropriately, either early or postoperatively.[13] Thus the goals of antibiotic prophylaxis are to achieve inhibitory levels of drug present at the time of the incision and for the duration of the procedure. I therefore recommend starting the parenteral antibiotic about 1 hour before the incision.

**Duration of prophylaxis.** The optimal duration of prophylaxis is unknown.[14] Studies have failed to show a benefit of drug after the patient has left the operating room. For most procedures, antibiotics should be stopped within 24 hours of the operation. This is an area of controversy especially for cardiac surgeons who believe that longer durations are needed, despite lack of confirmatory data.[10]

**Choice of antibiotics.** Table 16–5 lists the recommended drugs and dosages for prophylaxis adopted from the 1995 *Medical Letter.*[15] Further randomized controlled trials are needed in certain areas such as neurosurgery to better define the optimal agent.[16,17]

## References

1. Kaiser AB. Antimicrobial prophylaxis in surgery, *N Engl J Med* 315:1129-1138, 1986.
2. VanScoy RE, Wilkowski CJ: Prophylactic use of antimicrobial agents in adult patients, Mayo Clin Proc 67:288-292, 1992.
3. Dajani AS, Bisno AL, Chung KJ, et al: Prevention of bacterial endocarditis, *JAMA* 264:2919, 1990.
4. Everett ED, Hirschmann JV: Transient bacteremia and endocarditis prophylaxis: a review, *Medicine* 56:61-76, 1977.
5. Kaye D: Prophylaxis against bacterial endocarditis: a dilemma in infective endocarditis. In Kaplan E, Taranta AV, editors: Infective endocarditis, *American Heart Association Monograph Series,* No. 52, Dallas, 1977, American Heart Association.
6. Guntheroth WG: How important are dental procedures as a cause of infective endocarditis? *Am J Cardiol* 54:797-801, 1984.
7. Shorvan PJ, Eykyn SJ, Cotton PB: Gastrointestinal instrumentation, bacteremia, and endocarditis, *Gut* 24:1078-1093, 1983.
8. Sullivan NM, Sutter VL, Mims MM, et al: Clinical aspects of bacteremia after manipulation of the genitourinary tract, *J Infect Dis* 127:49-55, 1973.

9. Clemens JD, Horowitz RI, Jaffe CC, et al: A controlled evaluation of the risk of bacterial endocarditis in persons with mitral-valve prolapse, *N Engl J Med* 307:776-781, 1982.

10. Ariano RE, Zhanel GG: Antimicrobial prophylaxis in coronary bypass surgery: a critical appraisal, *DICP (Drug Intell Clin Pharm)* 25:478-484, 1991.

11. Burke JF: The effective period of preventive antibiotic action in experimental incisions and dermal lesions, *Surgery* 50:161-168, 1961.

12. Hirschmann JV, Inui TS: Antimicrobial prophylaxis: a critique of recent trials, *Rev Infect Dis* 2:1-23, 1980.

13. Classen DC, Evans RS, Pestonik SL, et al: The timing of prophylactic administration of antibiotics and the risk of surgical wound infection, *N Engl J Med* 326:281-282, 1992.

14. Dellinger EP, Gross PA, Barrett TL, et al: Quality standard for antimicrobial prophylaxis in surgical procedures, *Control Hosp Epidemiol* 15:182-188, 1994.

15. Anonymous: *Med Letter* 37:79-82, 1995.

16. Committee on Antimicrobial Agents, Canadian Infectious Disease Society, Waddell TK, Rotstein OD: Antimicrobial prophylaxis in surgery, *Can Med Assoc J* 151:925-931, 1994.

17. Holloway KL, Smith KW, Wilberger JE, et al: Antibiotic prophylaxis during clean neurosurgery: A large, multicenter study using cefuroxime, *Clinical Therapeutics* 18:84-94, 1996.

# Part 3

# Gastrointestinal Disease

## Chapter 17

## Dysphagia

Karim A. Fawaz

Dysphagia is defined as difficulty in swallowing. In most instances the term *dysphagia* should be used whenever the patient describes a sensation of "sticking" of an ingested bolus of food or liquid. However, the term *dysphagia* is also used when the patient describes an inability to initiate swallowing or an inability to transfer food from the mouth to the esophagus. Dysphagia is different from odynophagia, which implies the presence of pain on swallowing, though the two conditions may coexist in certain disorders.

An accurate clinical history is extremely useful in categorizing the cause of dysphagia and in planning for diagnostic steps and therapy. There are two major categories of disorders that cause dysphagia, mechanical and neuromuscular. In general, difficulty in swallowing only solids is suggestive of a mechanical disorder, whereas difficulty in swallowing both solids and liquids is suggestive of a neuromuscular disorder. Rapidly progressive dysphagia is consistent with an expanding lesion causing progressive mechanical narrowing of the lumen, whereas episodic dysphagia associated with specific solid foods is suggestive of a fixed, nonprogressive narrowing.

Remember that there is no good correlation between the location that the patient identifies as, "The food sticks here," and the actual site of the disorder. A lesion in the esophagus may cause a sensation of sticking that corresponds to the site of the disorder or to anywhere proximally along the esophagus but never distal to the lesion.

There are many causes of dysphagia (see box on next page). In this discussion, the conditions that are commonly seen in consultation are discussed in more detail than the rarer causes of dysphagia. In my experience, benign peptic stricture of the esophagus, lower esophageal ring, and carcinoma account for approximately 90% of all cases of dysphagia.

# MECHANICAL CAUSES OF DYSPHAGIA

## Benign peptic stricture

Peptic stricture of the esophagus usually is the result of chronic reflux of gastric acid into the esophagus. The acid reflux causes the sensation of heartburn and the pathologic entity of esophagitis.[1] If untreated, the esophagitis becomes chronic and scarring sets in, thereby leading to the formation of a stricture. When a stricture forms, the patient may lose the symptom of heartburn and acquire a new symptom, namely, dysphagia. The dysphagia is usually to solid food only unless the lumen becomes so narrow that even liquids have trouble passing.

The diagnosis usually is made after one performs a barium swallow that shows a tapered narrowing of the lumen with smooth edges in the distal third of the esophagus. If the stricture is of long-standing duration, dilatation of the esophagus proximal to the stricture may be seen. Endoscopy and esophageal biopsy specimens should be performed if the history or barium swallow provides the slightest suspicion of malignancy. The best treatment is prevention of acid reflux (by vigorous treatment of esophagitis) before a stricture develops.

Once a stricture develops, several different therapeutic options are available, depending on the diameter of the stricture: (1) antireflux measures such as antacids, $H_2$-blockers, omeprazole, lansoprazole, elevation of the head of the bed, avoidance of alcohol and cigarettes, a low-fat diet, and avoidance of an increase in intra-abdominal pressure; (2) antireflux measures and dilatation of the esophagus with bougies or balloons; (3) surgical treatment; and (4) preoperative dilatation followed by surgery. In the medical treatment of severe esophagitis and stricture, omeprazole and lansoprazole are superior to any other agent.[2,3]

A note of caution is in order concerning patients with long-standing reflux. They are prone to the development of the so-called Barrett's esophagus, which is considered a premalignant condition.[4] The disease involves a metaplastic change in the chronically inflamed squamous epithelium of the esophagus, which leads to replacement of this epithelium by columnar cells. Most commonly, the stricture in Barrett's esophagus occurs in the middle third of the esophagus in contrast to the usual benign peptic stricture, which occurs in the lower third of the esophagus. The presence of a stricture in the upper or middle third

# Causes of Dysphagia

## MECHANICAL

### Intrinsic

Benign peptic stricture
Carcinoma
Lower esophageal ring (Schatzki's ring)
Candidal esophagitis
Esophageal web
Stricture secondary to endoscopic sclerotherapy
Benign tumor
Caustic injury
Zenker's diverticulum

### Extrinsic

Malignant tumors (direct extension or metastasis)
Retrosternal thyroid
Vascular compression

## NEUROMUSCULAR

### Smooth muscle disorders

Achalasia
Diffuse esophageal spasm
Scleroderma
Chagas's disease
Hypothyroidism

### Striated muscle disorders

Cricopharyngeal achalasia
Polymyositis
Myasthenia gravis
Myotonia dystrophica
Thyrotoxicosis

### Neural disorders

Brainstem lesion or stroke
Demyelinating disease
Degenerative disease

of the esophagus is a definite indication for endoscopy, cytology, and biopsy to rule out a malignancy. Unfortunately, neither medical nor surgical treatment of reflux has been shown to cause regression of Barrett's epithelium.

## Carcinoma

A history of rapidly progressive dysphagia points to the presence of carcinoma of the esophagus until proved otherwise. Associated symptoms include weight loss and anorexia. By far the most common histologic type of esophageal cancer is squamous cell carcinoma.

Squamous cell carcinoma of the esophagus occurs with almost equal frequency in the upper, middle, and lower thirds of the esophagus. The diagnosis is made by a barium swallow that reveals an intraluminal, irregular, ulcerated mass. Sometimes the radiographic picture is one of smooth narrowing, which is difficult to distinguish radiologically from a benign stricture. It is in such instances that the location of the stricture assumes great importance. Benign strictures occur in the lower third of the esophagus, whereas malignant strictures can occur anywhere along the esophagus. A stricture in the upper or middle third of the esophagus thus should be considered malignant until proved otherwise. Endoscopy, biopsy, and cytology are a must in this latter group.

A smaller group of patients (less than 10%) has adenocarcinoma of the esophagus. Adenocarcinoma is confined to the distal third of the esophagus except if it arises in Barrett's epithelium. It is often difficult to differentiate between primary esophageal adenocarcinoma and one arising from the fundus of the stomach and secondarily invading the lower esophagus. In both instances, dysphagia is the major symptom.

Unfortunately for patients with esophageal cancer, when they start complaining of dysphagia, the lesion is already large and has spread at least locally, thereby making prognosis dismal no matter what type of therapy is employed. In general, tumors in the lower third of the esophagus are best treated by surgical resection with or without preoperative irradiation, whereas tumors of the upper and middle third are treated by irradiation unless surgical resection is believed to be technically possible. The prognosis is poor for all patients, with less than a 5% 5-year survival rate.[5]

## Lower esophageal ring

The classic symptom of a lower esophageal ring is episodic dysphagia to solid food. The presence of daily dysphagia or progressive dysphagia over days is not suggestive of the presence of a lower esophageal ring. A typical history is one of dysphagia to meat, relieved by vomiting, followed by an asymptomatic period of weeks or months. A protracted history of symptoms of reflux esophagitis is uncommon and should alert the physician to the presence of a peptic stricture, rather than a lower esophageal ring. The diagnosis of a lower esophageal ring is cinched by a barium swallow that reveals a concentric mucosal ring, 2 to 4 mm in thickness, projecting into the lumen of the distal part of the esophagus.

The prevalence of the lower esophageal ring is reported to be between 6% and 14% as seen on routine barium swallow; however, only 0.5% of patients with a ring suffer from dysphagia.[6] Most patients with rings measuring 13 mm or less in diameter are symptomatic. Rings 13 to 17 mm in diameter may produce dysphagia, but patients with rings greater than 17 mm in diameter are usually asymptomatic. The treatment of a lower esophageal ring is rupture of the ring with dilators or balloons and is usually successful in most cases and affords relief for a prolonged period. Treatment may have to be repeated in months or years, and the result is equally good. Only on rare occasions is surgery required.

## Candidal esophagitis

Most patients with acute esophagitis caused by *Candida albicans* complain of dysphagia. This clinical picture is in contrast to patients with herpetic esophagitis who complain of odynophagia. The diagnosis should be suspected in diabetic patients, immunocompromised hosts (especially patients with AIDS), and patients receiving steroids. The presence of oral thrush makes the diagnosis of a *Candida* infection much more likely.

Chronic candidal esophagitis may occur in patients with chronic mucocutaneous candidiasis, a disease characterized by chronic involvement of the skin, nails, and oral cavity. In this condition, the major symptom of esophageal involvement is also dysphagia, whereas odynophagia is uncommon. The diagnosis may be suspected after a barium swallow that reveals esophagitis, ulceration, or intramural pseudodiverticulosis or stricture. The diagnosis is confirmed by endoscopy and demonstration of the organism by cytologic examination, culture of the brushing, or biopsy performed at endoscopy. Fluconazole (100 to 200 mg/day) and ketoconazole (200 to 400 mg/day) for 2 weeks are very effective, but the latter's absorption is dependent on the presence of acid, and so fluconazole is the treatment of choice.[7] In severe cases that do not respond to fluconazole, low-dose intravenously administered amphotericin B may be required.

## Esophageal web

Esophageal web, single or multiple, may occur anywhere along the esophagus. The most common type is a single web in the postcricoid region of the upper third of the esophagus, which, when associated with dysphagia, is referred to as the *Plummer-Vinson syndrome*. Esophageal web has a higher incidence in females and an association with iron-deficiency anemia, autoimmune disease, and postcricoid carcinoma. The most common presenting symptom is dysphagia to solids, which may be accompanied by regurgitation and aspiration. Diagnosis is made by barium swallow or by cineradiography. Treatment is by dilatation with mercury bougies.

## Stricture secondary to endoscopic sclerotherapy

Endoscopic sclerotherapy of esophageal varices is now commonly used for the treatment of bleeding esophageal varices. Complications of this procedure include esophageal ulcers and stricture formation. Patients who develop strictures complain of dysphagia to solids. The treatment is esophageal dilatation, and the results usually are excellent. Theoretically, one would expect bleeding to be a frequent complication of esophageal dilatation in such patients; fortunately this has not been the case.

# NEUROMUSCULAR CAUSES OF DYSPHAGIA

## Achalasia

Achalasia, a motor disorder of the esophagus, results from a sharp decrease in Auerbach's ganglion cells. Dysphagia to both solids and liquids is the most common presenting symptom in achalasia. Onset is usually between 20 and 40 years of age, though it has been reported in infancy and in the elderly. Regurgitation of food or liquid, particularly in the recumbent position, is the next most common symptom in achalasia; this may lead to repeated spells of coughing and, when severe and recurrent, to pneumonia. The combination of progressive dysphagia to solids and liquids coupled with regurgitation of material ingested hours or days earlier should alert the physician to a motor abnormality such as achalasia.

The radiologic picture of late achalasia is quite specific, though not absolutely diagnostic. A barium swallow usually reveals a dilated, aperistaltic esophagus that terminates with a very narrow segment referred to as a "beak." The diagnosis is confirmed by esophageal manometry that typically shows a hypertensive lower esophageal sphincter, absence of contractions in the esophagus, and incomplete relaxation of the lower esophageal sphincter on swallowing.

Occasionally a carcinoma of the cardia of the stomach with submucosal invasion of the distal esophagus may mimic achalasia radiographically and manometrically. Although endoscopy is not necessary to establish a diagnosis of achalasia, it is advisable in order to differentiate true achalasia from a high gastric ulcer.

Until recently, treatment of achalasia was either by pneumatic dilatation (rupture of the lower esophageal sphincter with aid of fluoroscopy or with direct endoscopic vision) or by Heller's myotomy. Both modes of therapy provide relief of symptoms in most patients.[8] Pharmacologic treatment of achalasia with nitrates and calcium-channel blockers may help in a small percentage of patients.[9] A reasonable approach to treatment is to start with pneumatic dilatation, to add pharmacologic therapy if the response is not satisfactory, and to reserve surgery for patients who fail multiple attempts with conservative measures. A new method of medical therapy under investigation is the intrasphincteric injection of *Botulinum* toxin.[10]

## Diffuse esophageal spasm

Diffuse esophageal spasm is a motor abnormality that usually presents after 40 years of age, but it does occur at an earlier age. The clinical presentation includes chest pain and dysphagia. The dysphagia does not necessarily accompany the chest pain, and the chest pain is not necessarily related to the act of swallowing. The dysphagia is to solids and liquids and is intermittent rather than progressive. Symptoms of dysphagia or chest pain, or both, may be triggered by very hot or very cold liquids.

A barium swallow may be normal at a time when the patient is asymptomatic, or it may show tertiary contractions that, when extreme, give the appearance of a corkscrew esophagus. Esophageal manometry in a typical patient shows simultaneous high-amplitude, prolonged waves called *tertiary contractions*. A group of patients with similar symptoms in whom barium swallow appearance is normal and in whom primary peristaltic waves recorded on esophageal manometry also appear normal has been reported. However, the contractions are of extremely high amplitude and are prolonged. This group of patients is considered a variant of diffuse esophageal spasm, and the condition is referred to as a *Nutcracker esophagus*.

The results of therapy in this disorder are less than desirable. Some patients may respond to pharmacologic agents such as nitrates and calcium-channel blockers. Others may respond to dilatations, and those with severe symptoms may have to undergo a long esophageal myotomy.[11]

Several investigators of esophageal motor dysfunction believe that achalasia and diffuse esophageal spasm are at opposite ends of the spectrum of one disease entity.

## Scleroderma

The clinical presentation of the motor defect in the esophagus of a patient with scleroderma is one of dysphagia and heartburn. The presence of Raynaud's phenomenon with these symptoms makes the diagnosis of scleroderma almost a certainty. Unlike achalasia, barium swallow is not diagnostic. It may show a dilated esophagus, a decrease in or absence of contractions in the lower two thirds of the esophagus, and gastroesophageal reflux. The diagnosis is confirmed by esophageal manometry that reveals a weak lower esophageal sphincter and absent peristalsis in the lower two thirds of the esophagus.[12]

The two causes underlying dysphagia in scleroderma are motor disorder and esophageal stricture secondary to chronic gastroesophageal reflux. There is no specific treatment for scleroderma. Treatment is directed toward preventing esophagitis and stricture formation by antireflux measures including antacids, $H_2$-blockers, omeprazole, and cisapride (promotility agent).

## Other neuromuscular disorders

Dysphagia may be associated with diseases of striated muscle such as polymyositis, myasthenia gravis, and myotonia dystrophica. Dysphagia is evoked by both solids and liquids. Neurologic disorders such as a brainstem lesion of stroke, multiple sclerosis, and Parkinson's disease may cause dysphagia. The dysphagia results from an inability to initiate a swallow or to transfer food from the mouth to the esophagus. Invariably, the dysphagia is accompanied by choking and aspiration because of trickling into the larynx, especially when liquids are swallowed. Cineradiography, rather than an ordinary barium swallow, is the examination of choice in the preceding conditions. Treatment is directed at the primary disease.

## References

1. Pope CE: Acid-reflux disorders, *N Engl J Med* 331:656-660, 1994.
2. Marks RD, Richter JE, Rizzo F, et al: Omeprazole versus $H_2$-receptor antagonists in treating patients with peptic strictures and esophagitis, *Gastroenterology* 106:907-915, 1994.
3. Castell DO, Richter JE, Rohmon M: Large trial compares lansoprazole to omeprazole, *Gastroenterology* 108:A67, 1995.
4. Cameron JA, Lomboy CT: Barrett's esophagus: age, prevalence, and extent of columnar epithelium, *Gastroenterology* 103:1241-1250, 1992.
5. Earlam R, Cunha-Melo JR: Esophageal squamous cell carcinoma: I. A critical review of surgery, *Br J Surg* 67:381-390, 1980.
6. Goyal RK, Glancy MB, Spiro HM: Lower esophageal ring, *N Engl J Med* 282:1298-1305, 1970.
7. López-Duplá M, Mora-Sanz P, Pintado-García V, et al: Clinical, endoscopic, immunologic, and therapeutic aspects of esophageal candidiasis in HIV-infected patients: a survey of 114 cases, *Am J Gastroenterol* 87:1771-1776, 1992.
8. Abid S, Champion G, Richter JE: Treatment of achalasia: the best of both worlds, *Am J Gastroenterol* 89:979-985, 1993.
9. Gelfoud M, Rozen P, Gilat T: Isosorbide dinitrate and nifedipine treatment of achalasia: a clinical, manometric and radionuclide evaluation. *Gastroenterology* 83:963-969, 1982.
10. Pasricha PJ, Ravich WJ, Hendrix TR: Treatment of achalasia with intrasphincteric injection of *Botulinum* toxin, *Ann Intern Med* 121:590-591, 1994.
11. Vantrappen G, Hellemans J: Treatment of achalasia and related motor disorders, *Gastroenterology* 79:144-154, 1980.
12. Clements PJ, Kadell B, Ippolite A, et al: Esophageal motility in progressive systemic sclerosis, *Dig Dis Sci* 24:639-644, 1979.

## Chapter 18

# *Chronic Abdominal Pain*

Sanjeev Arora
Karim A. Fawaz

Abdominal pain is an unpleasant subjective sensation produced by noxious stimuli from most intra-abdominal and some extra-abdominal organs. Noxious stimuli such as burning, cutting, or crushing produce severe pain when applied to the skin. The visceral organs, however, are insensitive to these stimuli. Visceral pain is produced by stimuli such as distension, ischemia, inflammation, or neoplastic infiltration. The rate of distension is important because slow distension as seen in malignant biliary obstruction is painless whereas rapid distension as seen in gallstone or renal colic is often extremely painful. Ischemia to intra-abdominal organs produces pain by slowing the rate of blood flow and therefore allowing the accumulation of tissue metabolites around the sensory nerves. Inflammation causes increased local production of hormones such as prostaglandin, bradykinin, and serotonin, which in turn can cause pain by stimulating the peripheral nerve endings. Neoplastic infiltration of peripheral sensory nerves as seen in carcinoma of the pancreas can produce severe and unrelenting abdominal pain.

For purposes of this discussion, we define chronic abdominal pain as discomfort that has lasted longer than 2 weeks or that has been intermittently recurring for a period greater than 2 weeks. We will therefore exclude causes of acute abdominal pain such as acute appendicitis, acute pancreatitis, or perforated viscus.

A detailed history and a careful physical examination are essential when consultation is done on a patient for chronic abdominal pain. Emphasis on the history can avoid many unnecessary and expensive diagnostic tests and can aid in early diagnosis by focusing the diagnostic work-up.

## HISTORY

**Site and nature of pain.** Most upper abdominal organs such as stomach, duodenum, gallbladder, common bile duct, and pancreas are innervated by nerves from dermatome T6 to T10.[1] These organs are innervated bilaterally and therefore cause pain at or near the midline anteriorly. Pain from a gastric ulcer is located in the midline or slightly to the left in the epigastric region, whereas pain from an ulcer in the duodenal bulb may be slightly to the right of midline. Pain originating from the jejunum and the ileum, as seen in Crohn's disease, is often located in the midline near the umbilical region. Colonic pain usually is poorly localized and present in the lower midabdomen. Gallbladder or common bile duct pain is present in the midepigastric region or in the right upper quadrant and may radiate to the back. Visceral pain from these organs often is associated with other autonomic symptoms such as nausea or sweating. Pancreatic pain is usually a dull ache and can radiate to the back. Table 18-1 summarizes various causes of chronic abdominal pain.

**Duration.** Pain that lasts for several years without weight loss or other complications is suggestive of irritable bowel syndrome. Persistent and worsening midabdominal pain that is present for several weeks or months with associated weight loss is suggestive of cancer of the pancreas.

**Relationship to meals: aggravating and relieving factors.** Relief of pain with ingestion of food is suggestive of peptic ulcer disease. It is difficult to differentiate gastric ulcer from duodenal ulcer based on historical data alone. Colicky abdominal pain brought on by meals may indicate gallbladder disease, obstructing inflammatory bowel disease (such as Crohn's disease), or pyloric channel ulcer producing gastric outlet obstruction. In an elderly individual with diffuse vascular disease, midabdominal pain beginning 20 to 30 minutes after meals in association with weight loss may be caused by chronic intestinal ischemia. Relief of pain with use of antacids is seen in peptic ulcer disease. One can often aggravate pancreatic pain by lying supine and relieve it partially by bending forward. Crampy lower abdominal pain with tenesmus that is relieved by a bowel movement indicates a colonic source of pain.

**Radiation of pain.** Radiation of abdominal pain to the back is seen with pancreatic disease, gallbladder disease, and disease of the common bile duct.

**Associated symptoms.** A history of weight loss associated with abdominal pain should alert the physician to serious disease. In the elderly, malignancy such as pancreatic, gastric, or colonic carcinoma has to be considered. In the young, inflammatory bowel disease may be the cause. The presence of hematochezia associated with abdominal pain can indicate colonic carcinoma or diverticulosis in the elderly. In the young, inflammatory bowel disease such as Crohn's disease may be responsible. Alternating diarrhea and constipation in a young patient with abdominal pain is suggestive of irritable bowel syndrome. In the middle-aged or elderly, however, the diagnosis of irritable bowel syndrome should not be entertained as a primary diagnosis unless investigations of the intestine have excluded neoplasms.

Vomiting associated with abdominal pain may indicate subacute intestinal obstruction, such as Crohn's disease, or gastric outlet obstruction, such as pyloric channel ulcer. Colicky pain caused by acute distension of the gallbladder, the common bile duct, or the renal pelvis and ureter can also produce vomiting attributable to autonomic stimuli.

**Table 18-1.** *Chronic abdominal pain*

| Clinical diagnosis | Site of pain | Description |
| --- | --- | --- |
| Peptic ulcer | Epigastric region: right of midline = duodenal ulcer; left of midline = gastric ulcer | Gnawing pain, burning pain, hunger pain, nocturnal pain, relief with food and antacids in duodenal ulcer |
| Biliary colic | Epigastric region, right upper quadrant radiating to back, interscapular region | Recurrent pain, rapid onset, severe intensity, duration of several hours, associated nausea and vomiting |
| Pancreatic carcinoma | Epigastric region, right or left of midline, bandlike pain around abdomen | Anorexia and weight loss, constant pain, increasing severity, radiation to back |
| Chronic pancreatitis | Epigastric region, left of midline | Persistent or episodic pain, radiates to back, history of alcoholism |
| Crohn's disease | Umbilical region, right lower quadrant | Colicky pain, postprandial vomiting, weight loss |
| Chronic intestinal ischemia | Umbilical area | Postprandial pain 20 to 30 minutes after meals, lasts 60 to 90 minutes, weight loss |
| Irritable bowel syndrome* | Umbilical region, left lower quadrant, or diffuse pain | Diarrhea or constipation, long-standing symptoms, no nocturnal pain, no weight loss, negative diagnostic tests |

* From Swarberick ET et al: *Lancet* 2:443–446, 1980.

The presence of abdominal pain with menstrual bleeding may represent menstrual cramps or intra-abdominal bleeding caused by endometriosis.

**Family and personal history.** The patient should be queried about a family history of peptic ulcer disease, gallstones, inflammatory bowel disease, and malignancy. A strong history of smoking in a patient with abdominal pain predisposes the patient to peptic ulcer disease and carcinoma of the pancreas. A history of alcoholism may indicate chronic pancreatitis as a cause for chronic abdominal pain.

## PHYSICAL EXAMINATION

A physical examination may yield useful clues to the diagnosis of chronic abdominal pain. The presence of icterus and a palpable gallbladder (Courvoisier's sign) may indicate carcinoma in the head of the pancreas. The presence of arthritis and erythema nodosum is suggestive of inflammatory bowel disease. Diminished peripheral pulses and abdominal bruits often are detected in patients who are later diagnosed to have chronic intestinal ischemia. A palpable abdominal mass obviously aids in the diagnosis. The presence of occult blood in the stool should lead to a search for inflammatory or malignant lesions of the gastrointestinal tract.

## DIAGNOSTIC TESTS AND PROCEDURES

When the history and physical examination are suggestive of peptic ulcer disease as the most likely etiologic factor for abdominal pain, it is reasonable to attempt a therapeutic trial with histamine ($H_2$)-blockers, such as cimetidine or ranitidine, before any further investigations are done. If the initial manifestations are atypical or of new onset in an elderly person, an upper gastrointestinal (GI) endoscopy is the procedure of choice. Although this approach is more expensive than a roentgenogram of the stomach and duodenum, it is much more sensitive and specific than upper GI roentgenograms for the diagnosis of ulcer disease.[2] In addition endoscopy allows a biopsy to be done in patients with gastric ulcers. The recent association of *Helicobacter pylori* with peptic ulcer disease and the low recurrence rate after appropriate treatment with antibiotics and acid-reducing agents have swayed many to prove the presence of an ulcer and the bacterium and treat accordingly rather than treat empirically with acid-reducing or acid-neutralizing agents with or without antibiotics, but the debate between these two strategies remains a lively one.[3]

When biliary tract disease is being investigated, an ultrasonogram of the abdomen is the procedure of choice to diagnose gallstones because of its high sensitivity and lack of any radiation hazard. Ultrasonography has virtually replaced the oral cholecystogram as the first procedure for diagnosis of gallstones; this test also detects obstruction of the biliary tree. A hepatobiliary scan or a liver and spleen scan is of little use in the investigation of chronic abdominal pain. If stones in the common bile duct are suspected, the procedure of choice is an endoscopic retrograde cholangiogram because ultrasound, the computerized tomographic (CT) scan, and the intravenous cholangiogram are not sensitive tests to allow one to diagnose common bile duct stones.

For neoplastic disease of the pancreas and retroperitoneum, a CT scan of the abdomen, though expensive, is the most sensitive preferred primary diagnostic test. Ultrasonography of the abdomen is also a good

**Table 18–2.** *Diagnostic procedures for chronic abdominal pain*

| Clinical suspicion | Condition | Diagnostic test or procedure |
| --- | --- | --- |
| Stomach and duodenum | Peptic ulcer | Therapeutic trial or upper Gastrointestinal endoscopy |
| | Obstruction, such as pyloric obstruction | Upper GI x-ray film with barium |
| Small intestine | Crohn's disease | Upper GI x-ray film and small bowel followthrough |
| | Obstruction Crohn's disease Tumors Adhesions | As above |
| Biliary tract | Gallbladder stone disease | Ultrasonography of right upper quadrant |
| | Common duct stone | ERCP |
| Pancreas and retroperitoneum* | Chronic pancreatitis | Flat-plate abdomen for calcification or ERCP, or both |
| | Carcinoma of pancreas | CT scan of abdomen or ERCP, or both |
| Colonic disease | Diverticulosis | Barium enema |
| | Neoplasms | Colonoscopy or flexible sigmoidoscopy and barium enema |
| | Inflammatory bowel disease | Colonoscopy |

* From Currie DJ: *Abdominal pain,* New York, 1979, Hemisphere. *CT,* Computerized tomography; *ERCP,* endoscopic retrograde cholangiopancreatography.

test; however, it is often unable to visualize the entire pancreas and may be limited because of technical problems. The use of ultrasound as a first test often necessitates a CT scan as a follow-up test and therefore voids its cost advantage and lack of radiation.

An endoscopic retrograde cholangiopancreatography (ERCP) or a needle biopsy of the pancreas may be necessary to confirm diagnostic impressions on a CT scan. Table 18-2 summarizes diagnostic procedures for chronic abdominal pain.

## References

1. Way LW: Abdominal pain. In Sleisenger MH, Fordtran JS, editors: Gastrointestinal disease: pathophysiology, diagnosis, management, ed 5, Philadelphia, 1993, Saunders.

2. Wilson DI: Evaluation of patients with upper abdominal pain, *Pract Gastroenterol* 8(5):6-17, 1984
3. Fendrick AM, Chernew ME, Hirth RA: Alternative management strategies for patients with suspected peptic ulcer diseases, *Ann Intern Med* 123:260-268, 1995.

# Chapter 19

# *Upper Gastrointestinal Bleeding*

Karim A. Fawaz

Upper gastrointestinal (UGI) bleeding is a common and serious medical emergency. Despite remarkable improvements in diagnostic techniques and accuracy in the determination of the bleeding site, UGI bleeding continues to carry a mortality of up to 8% to 10%. The mortality increases with age and with the presence of other serious diseases. The diagnosis and management of such patients require close cooperation among the internist, the surgeon, and the radiologist.

## GENERAL REMARKS

The approach to a patient who presents with UGI bleeding depends on the general condition of the patient. The sequence of steps in the diagnosis and management of a patient with massive bleeding and shock is different from the sequence followed in a patient with melena for a few days without orthostatic hypotension. Although the diagnostic steps may be the same, the former scenario requires an immediate and vigorous approach with an emphasis on resuscitative measures that include (1) intravenous access adequate for rapid infusion of saline and blood products, (2) withdrawal of blood for typing, crossmatching, and measurement of hemoglobin, hematocrit, platelets, prothrombin time, partial thromboplastin time, urea nitrogen, and creatinine. The primary goal of the physician in the treatment of such patients is the restoration of blood volume, regardless of the diagnosis. Initially either normal saline solution or Ringer's lactate solution may be used until blood is available. The modern emergency room should be able to provide blood to the patient within 60 to 75 minutes. The use of albumin and plasma expanders is not necessary unless bleeding is continuous and massive and packed cells are not available. Although replenishing the blood volume is the most important goal, care should be taken not to "overexpand" the blood volume in elderly patients and in those at risk of congestive heart failure. In such patients, it is advisable to monitor central venous pressure (CVP) and to gauge fluid replacement accordingly.

The cardiovascular response to volume loss correlates with the rapidity and severity of blood loss but is modified by age, medications, previous cardiovascular disease, and other associated diseases. A prompt examination of the pulse and blood pressure allows the physician to estimate the magnitude of blood loss roughly. In general, in an otherwise healthy person the following guidelines apply: (1) a systolic blood pressure below 100 mm Hg or a pulse above 100 beats per minute indicate a 20% volume loss, (2) an orthostatic increase in the pulse of 20 beats per minute or a decrease in the blood pressure of more than 10 mm Hg in response to a postural change indicates a 20% volume loss. These measurements should be repeated frequently while saline is being administered. Caution, however, should be exercised in performing postural signs in the elderly because such maneuvers may precipitate a cerebrovascular ischemic attack.

After a quick examination is performed to estimate blood loss and after vigorous saline and blood administration have restored the blood pressure and pulse to normal, a nasogastric (NG) tube should be introduced and the stomach contents aspirated. Aspiration of the stomach contents serves several purposes: (1) it identifies the site of bleeding, (2) it provides a more accurate index about the rate of blood loss, (3) it establishes whether bleeding continues or has stopped, and (4) it prevents aspiration, a known complication of UGI bleeding, especially in the elderly.

There are some controversies regarding the use of nasogastric tubes in UGI bleeding. Should a nasogastric tube be introduced in a patient who is suspected of having bleeding esophageal varices? Does gastric lavage help stop bleeding? If gastric lavage is to be done, what type of fluid should be used and at what temperature? Most gastroenterologists believe that the presence of esophageal varices is not a contraindication to a nasogastric tube since there is no evidence that the tube initiates or prolongs bleeding. Gastric lavage is performed as a force of habit, rather than on the basis of objective data. It is empirically believed that lavage with cold fluids helps to stop the bleeding, but no such data exist. Further, there is no evidence that saline is superior to tap water, nor is there evidence that cold fluid is superior to room temperature fluid. My approach is to perform gastric lavage with tap water initially to know whether the bleeding persists and, before diagnostic endoscopy, to have a clear view of the stomach.

Measurement of hemoglobin and hematocrit on admission and in 6 to 12 hours is essential to follow the progress of a bleeding patient. Initial values are often misleadingly high, however, because compensatory physiologic mechanisms to reestablish intravascular volume, such as the release of aldosterone and antidiuretic hormone, lag behind. The initial levels of hemoglobin and hematocrit do not fall because the blood lost has the same concentration of red blood cells as the blood remaining. The fall in these measurements with time is often the consequence of hemodilution secondary to administered saline or to ingested fluid.

The measurement of platelets, prothrombin time, and partial thromboplastin time is important to rule out a bleeding diathesis. The bleeding disorder could be primary or could be secondary to medications, liver disease, consumption coagulopathy, or autoimmune disease.

## HISTORY AND PHYSICAL EXAMINATION

After resuscitative measures are instituted and the patient is relatively stable, a detailed history should be taken and a physical examination performed. A history of drug intake, such as salicylates, nonsteroidal anti-inflammatory agents, anticoagulants, and antineoplastic drugs, should be taken. A history of previously known disease such as alcoholism, chronic liver disease, blood dyscrasias, neoplasm, and arthritis may help in narrowing the differential diagnosis. The following findings are of high diagnostic value:

1. Hematemesis indicates bleeding above the ligament of Treitz; however, patients with bleeding duodenal ulcers may present with melena only.
2. Hematemesis shortly after forceful vomiting should raise the possibility of a Mallory-Weiss tear.
3. A history of epigastric distress and pain for several days before bleeding is suggestive of peptic ulcer disease or gastritis.
4. Trauma, burns, or surgery hours to days before bleeding are suggestive of stress ulcerations as the cause of bleeding.
5. Previous surgical procedures, such as partial gastrectomy, raise the possibility of an anastomotic ulcer.
6. Dysphagia indicates possible esophageal lesions such as esophagitis, esophageal ulcer, or carcinoma.
7. The presence of signs of portal hypertension, such as splenomegaly, ascites, abdominal collateral circulation, and spider nevi, indicates the possibility of bleeding esophageal varices.
8. Examination of the skin, mucous membranes, and fingertips is important for the diagnosis of hereditary hemorrhagic telangiectasia, Peutz-Jeghers syndrome, and blue rubber bleb nevus. All of the preceding may present with bleeding.

## THE ROLE OF ENDOSCOPY IN UGI BLEEDING

UGI endoscopy has been proved to be the quickest and most accurate means of finding the source of UGI bleeding. In controlled trials the diagnostic yield of UGI endoscopy is 75% to 90%, whereas the yield for barium roentgenography is 20% to 50%.[1, 2] Since earlier and more accurate diagnosis is provided by endoscopy, one might expect a reduction in the mortality of UGI bleeding. Unfortunately, controlled studies have failed to show a difference in mortality between patients undergoing routine early endoscopy and those who do not.[3] Medications such as $H_2$-blockers, omeprazole, and antacids are not effective in the treatment of mucosal UGI bleeding. Endoscopic therapy with heater or bipolar probes and endoscopic sclerotherapy is effective in achieving hemostasis, but large studies are needed to find out if they reduce mortality.

The fact that endoscopy does not reduce mortality does not mean that the procedure should be abandoned. For instance, endoscopic sclerosis of varices is effective in treating bleeding esophageal varices. Endoscopy remains the first and usually the only diagnostic procedure that is performed. When should endoscopy be performed? Recent studies have shown that there is no significant difference between the yield of emergency endoscopy and that done within 24 to 48 hours, but beyond 48 hours the diagnostic yield declines significantly. Endoscopy should be performed on a more emergent basis when bleeding is suspected to be from esophageal varices because successful treatment hinges on the correct diagnosis.

Although there is agreement on the diagnostic value of endoscopy, there are situations when it is relatively contraindicated. An endoscopy performed on a patient with massive, active hematemesis may cause aspiration without allowing one to identify the source of bleeding (because of inadequate visualization). Endoscopy also is not indicated in an elderly patient with severe hypoxic pulmonary disease who has recently been diagnosed to have a duodenal ulcer unless it is done for therapeutic purposes. The risk of performing endoscopy in such situations often outweighs the benefit.

# RADIOLOGY

Three diagnostic roentgenologic techniques are useful in patients with gastrointestinal bleeding: radionuclide imaging, barium x-rays, and angiography. I follow the scheme illustrated in Fig. 19-1 for the evaluation of patients with UGI bleeding.

**Radionuclide imaging.** Radionuclide imaging as a technique is the least invasive and most useful in lower gastrointestinal bleeding. Its yield in UGI bleeding is low, and therefore radionuclide imaging is rarely used in UGI bleeding.

**Barium roentgenography.** Barium studies are inferior to endoscopy in UGI bleeding. In addition, the use of barium has some disadvantages. First, endoscopy or angiography performed soon after a barium study showing negative results is difficult because the barium compound coats the mucosa, and adequate visualization is precluded. Second, a barium study may show only one of two coexisting lesions, and that lesion may not be the bleeding site. In general, a barium study is indicated only when endoscopy is contraindicated and active bleeding has ceased. Enteroclysis, which is a rapid fluoroscopic study of the small intestines, is sometimes helpful in the diagnosis of lesions in the small bowel.

**Angiography.** The development of better endoscopic techniques and equipment has led to a sharp decline in the use of angiography in UGI bleeding. Studies have demonstrated that peripheral infusion of vasopressin (antidiuretic hormone, ADH, or somatostatin are as effec-

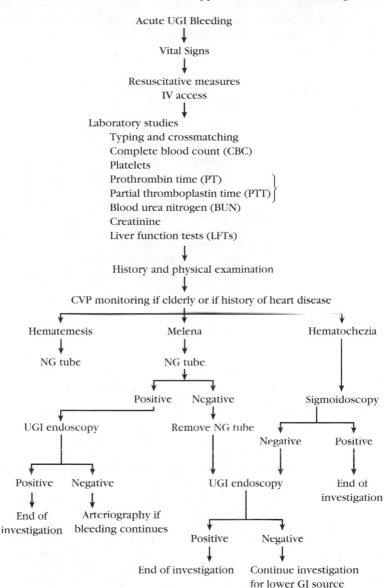

**Figure 19-1.** *Schema for the investigation of a patient with upper gastrointestinal bleeding.*

tive as selective arterial infusion of ADH in the treatment of bleeding varices and thus have further reduced the need for angiography. In general, I reserve angiography for situations where endoscopy is contraindicated or has failed to reveal the source of bleeding, yet active bleeding continues. In such cases the bleeding source may be identified, and therapeutic intervention such as embolization of an arterial bleeder may be attempted.

# INCIDENCE OF THE VARIOUS CAUSES OF UGI BLEEDING

The incidence of the various causes of UGI bleeding varies from one hospital to another and depends on the type of patients the hospital caters to and attracts. The box on p. 187 provides a list of the possible sources of UGI bleeding. In a review and analysis of 2014 patients with UGI bleeding, Domschke reported the following incidence of endoscopically diagnosed sources of bleeding:[4] gastric and stomal ulcers, 25.1%; duodenal ulcers, 24%; esophageal and gastric varices, 18.1%; Mallory-Weiss tear, 10%; esophagitis, 9.5%; gastric erosions, 9.1%; gastric neoplasm, 2.8%; Osler-Weber-Rendu disease and telangiectasia, 0.4%. These figures seem representative, but in my experience in an inner-city tertiary-care hospital, the incidence of bleeding from gastritis and gastric erosions is higher and that from Mallory-Weiss tear is lower.

In the following discussion, I concentrate on the diagnosis and management of the most common sources of bleeding.

## Ulcer disease
The presentation and management of ulcer disease at any site in the upper gastrointestinal tract are similar. Typical epigastric pain of ulcer disease may precede bleeding for days or weeks. When bleeding occurs, however, the pain usually disappears because blood is a good buffering agent. Bleeding gastric ulcers more commonly result in hematemesis and melena, whereas melena alone more commonly results from duodenal ulcers. A negative (for blood) nasogastric tube aspirate eliminates the presence of a bleeding gastric ulcer but not of a duodenal ulcer. In some instances, a competent pylorus prevents regurgitation of blood into the stomach; the nasogastric tube aspirate thus remains negative for blood. These patients obviously present with melena or hematochezia only. The diagnosis of a bleeding ulcer is best achieved by endoscopy. In addition to its accuracy, endoscopy provides valuable information regarding the likelihood of recurrent bleeding. The finding of what endoscopists refer to as a "visible vessel" is associated with a high incidence of recurrence of bleeding during the same hospitalization. Storey reported a 56% incidence of rebleeding in patients with a visible vessel compared to 8% in patients without a visible vessel.[5]

Regardless of the site, the treatment of bleeding ulcers is the same. We clinically refer to acid-reducing agents ($H^2$-blockers and omeprazole) and ulcer-coating agents (sucralfate) as treatment. However, there is considerable evidence that they play no role in stopping bleeding or in preventing its recurrence. *Helicobacter pylori* is present in over 90% of patients with duodenal ulcers and in the majority of patients with gastric ulcers who are not taking NSAIDs, and so treatment should

## Sources of UGI Bleeding

### MUCOSAL DISEASE

Duodenal ulcer and duodenitis
Gastric ulcer and gastritis
Stomal or anastomotic ulcer
Superficial stress ulcer or erosions
Dieulafoy's ulcer

### VASCULAR

Varices: esophageal, gastric, and upper intestinal
Portal gastropathy
Vascular malformation
Telangiectasia
Mesenteric ischcmia
Vasculitis
Postbypass aortoduodenal fistula

### MECHANICAL OR TRAUMATIC

Mallory-Weiss tear
Strangulated hiatus hernia
Hemobilia
External trauma

### NEOPLASIA

**Benign**

Polyps
Leiomyoma

**Malignant**

Carcinoma
Melanoma
Lymphoma
Leiomyosarcoma

**Miscellaneous**

Blood dyscrasia
Iatrogenic ovcranticoagulation
Uremia
Radiation enteritis
Intestinal lymphangiectasia
Parasitic infection, such as strongyloidiasis

be directed accordingly, but this has no effect on bleeding. Since pharmacologic treatment is ineffective, investigators have moved on to more invasive techniques to stop bleeding in an attempt to avoid surgery. These techniques use some form of electrocoagulation by means of endoscopy, such as heater and bipolar probe treatment or injection therapy using epinephrine or alcohol. Numerous studies have shown the effectiveness of the above compared to controls.[6,7]

Surgical intervention is the last resort in the treatment of bleeding ulcers. However, the surgical service should be consulted on admission. Close cooperation between the medical and surgical teams is imperative, especially if a visible vessel is seen on endoscopy. No general rule exists as to when to intervene surgically. Although one hopes to avoid surgery, the decision should not be delayed until the patient is moribund. In general, in an otherwise healthy person, I suggest surgery in such a patient whose blood requirement has exceeded 10 units in 24 hours and in the patient who rebleeds despite endoscopic therapy. About 10% of patients presenting with active bleeding require urgent surgery because of failure of endoscopic therapy.

## Gastritis and gastric erosions

Although epigastric pain may be a prominent symptom in ulcer disease before bleeding, pain is much less common in patients who have gastritis or gastric erosions. The offending agents or situations that usually are associated with this condition are alcohol, salicylates, nonsteroidal anti-inflammatory agents, stress, neurologic or neurosurgical insults, and possibly steroids. A careful history and immediate discontinuation of any potentially offending agent are mandatory. The diagnosis is made by endoscopy; barium roentgenograms usually miss these superficial lesions.

The pharmacologic treatment of gastritis and gastric erosions, as for ulcer disease, is not effective. Electrocoagulation holds less promise because the lesions are multiple and diffuse. Intravenous vasopressin has been used, but with mixed results. Care should be taken with vasopressin use in the elderly because of possible complications, such as coronary and cerebral vasoconstriction. Surgery should be avoided, if possible, especially when the erosions are in the fundus or are diffuse because the operative procedure increases in magnitude and in risk.

## Mallory–Weiss tear

The most common setting for a Mallory-Weiss tear is in the alcoholic who develops hematemesis after vomiting forcefully. However, neither alcoholism nor initial nonbloody vomitus is a requirement for its presence. In one study of 40 patients with this lesion, 17 (42%) had an associated hiatus hernia. Endoscopy is the diagnostic method of choice. The tears usually are seen in the gastric side of the gastroesophageal junction, especially if there is an associated hiatus hernia. The tear also may extend to the distal esophagus. Fortunately, more than 80% of patients stop bleeding spontaneously. Intravenous vasopressin has been shown to be effective in case reports and is worth trying in the minority of patients whose bleeding does not cease spontaneously. If pharmacologic treatment fails, endoscopic therapy with electrocoagulation or injection therapy is quite effective in stopping the bleeding.[6] Surgical treatment consists in oversewing the laceration, but it is rarely needed.

## Bleeding varices

Bleeding from varices is one of the most serious complications of portal hypertension. Esophageal varices are the most common site of bleeding; however, gastric varices and varices along the rest of the intestinal tract may bleed. Most patients suffer from cirrhosis, but extrahepatic causes, such as portal and splenic vein thrombosis, Budd-Chiari syndrome, are also possible. A history of chronic alcoholism and other chronic liver diseases, as well as signs of portal hypertension (such as splenomegaly, ascites, abdominal collateral veins, and spider nevi) should alert the physician to varices as the possible source of bleeding. However, it should not be assumed that every bleeding cirrhotic patient is actually bleeding from varices. Endoscopy has demonstrated that, even when esophageal or gastric varices are present, 50% of cirrhotic patients bleed from other causes, such as gastritis, portal gastropathy, duodenitis, a Mallory-Weiss tear, peptic ulcer, or esophagitis. Because of this observation (and the resulting difference in management) urgent endoscopy is indicated in patients with cirrhosis and UGI bleeding.

The initial treatment of bleeding varices is not different from any other type of UGI bleeding. However, because of the high incidence of coagulopathy associated with severe liver disease, the need for fresh frozen plasma and platelets is much more common. Several specific means of treatment of bleeding varices are available, such as balloon tamponade, intravenous vasopressin or somatostatin infusions,[8] percutaneous transhepatic embolization, endoscopic sclerotherapy or ligation,[9] transjugular intrahepatic portosystemic shunt (TIPS),[10] and emergency portal decompression surgery. None of these therapies except surgery provides a predictable and consistent lasting effect. However, emergency surgery carries a prohibitive mortality of 80%. Endoscopic sclerotherapy and ligation are the most widely used methods to control active bleeding worldwide. Endoscopic ligation is gaining ground on sclerotherapy because of its lower incidence of short-term and long-term complications.[11]

Generally I adhere to the following plan for treating acute variceal bleeding:

1. Continuous intravenous infusion of vasopressin starting at 0.4 U min/IV with upward titration to 0.6 if needed and simultaneous infusion of nitroglycerin, if the systolic blood pressure is above 100 mm Hg, in a dose that will maintain the systolic blood pressure at 100 mm Hg or above. Nitroglycerin is used to neutralize the systemic vasoconstrictive side effects of vasopressin. Alternatively, one can use a continuous infusion of somatostatin or octreotide (a sympathetic analog that is more potent and has a longer half-life) at a dose of 25 to 50 $\mu$g/min. Somatostatin and octreotide are preferred to vasopressin because of the

absence of systemic side effects such as hyponatremia, bradycardia, and systemic vasoconstriction.

2. If pharmacologic therapy does not control bleeding, endoscopic sclerotherapy or ligation should be performed. In general either procedure is successful in stopping the bleeding in most of the cases.

3. If bleeding continues despite endoscopic therapy, a Sengstaken-Blakemore tube should be introduced. The gastric balloon is inflated first, and if bleeding continues, the esophageal balloon should be inflated.

4. If bleeding is controlled by balloon tamponade for 24 to 36 hours, another attempt at sclerotherapy or ligation should be undertaken immediately after removal of the Sengstaken-Blackmore tube.

5. If the bleeding is not controlled or recurs despite the above procedures, a transjugular intrahepatic portosystemic shunt (TIPS) should be inserted, provided that the patient does not have severe hepatic encephalopathy, since encephalopathy is a known complication of this procedure.

6. An emergency surgical shunt for surgical decompression should be left as a last resort because of its high associated mortality (80%).

If bleeding is controlled without the need for a shunt procedure, endoscopic sclerotherapy or ligation should be repeated in 5 to 7 days and then every 2 to 4 weeks until obliteration of the varices is accomplished.

## References

1. Hoare AM: Comparative study between endoscopy and radiology in acute upper gastrointestinal haemorrhage, *Br Med J* 1:27-30, 1975.

2. McGinn FP, Guyer PM, Wilken BJ, et al: A prospective comparative trial between early endoscopy and radiology in acute upper gastrointestinal haemorrhage, *Gut* 16:707-713, 1975.

3. Peterson WL, Barnett CC, Smith HJ, et al: Routine early endoscopy in upper-gastrointestinal tract bleeding: a randomized controlled trial, *N Engl J Med* 304:925-929, 1981.

4. Domschke W, Lederer P, Lux G: The value of endoscopy in upper gastrointestinal bleeding: review and analysis of 2,014 cases, *Endoscopy* 15:126-131, 1983.

5. Storey DW, Bown SG, Swain CP, et al: Endoscopic prediction of recurrent bleeding in peptic ulcers, *N Engl J Med* 305(16):915-916, 1981.

6. Laine L: Multipolar electrocoagulation in the treatment of active gastrointestinal hemorrhage: a prospective controlled trial, *N Engl J Med* 316:1613-1617, 1987.

7. Laine L, Peterson W: Bleeding peptic ulcer, *N Engl J Med* 331:717-727, 1994.

8. Kravetz D, Bosch J, Teres J, et al: A controlled comparison of continuous somatostatin and vasopressin in the treatment of acute variceal hemorrhage, *Hepatology* 4:442, 1984

9. Hou MC, Lin HC, Kuo BIT, et al: Comparison of endoscopic variceal injection sclerotherapy and ligation for the treatment of esophageal variceal

hemorrhage: a prospective randomized trial, *Hepatology* 21:1517–1522, 1995.

10. Rossle M, Haag K, Ochs A, et al: The transjugular intrahepatic portosystemic stent-shunt procedure for variceal bleeding, *N Engl J Med* 330:165–171, 1994.

11. Laine L, Cook D: Endoscopic ligation compared to sclerotherapy for treatment of esophageal variceal bleeding, *Ann Intern Med* 123:280–287, 1995.

# Chapter 20

# *Recurrent Lower Gastrointestinal Bleeding*

Karim A. Fawaz

Lower gastrointestinal bleeding, a serious and life-threatening condition, can have a wide variety of causes (see box on p. 193). Many of these causes (such as inflammation, infection, and neoplasm) are relatively easy to diagnose by sigmoidoscopy, colonoscopy, barium roentgenography, stool cultures, and stool microscopy. These conditions are not discussed here. Rather, the focus of this chapter is on the difficult problem of *recurrent* lower gastrointestinal bleeding. A definitive diagnosis usually cannot be made either on initial presentation or during subsequent episodes of bleeding. Despite considerable improvement in our diagnostic tools, most gastroenterologists are haunted by a small cadre of patients with recurrent episodes of lower gastrointestinal bleeding of unknown cause. The fact that most of these patients are elderly[1] and do not tolerate major bleeds well makes the problem more serious and frustrating.

## RESUSCITATIVE MEASURES

The initial resuscitative measures for patients with lower gastrointestinal bleeding are the same as for patients with upper gastrointestinal (UGI) bleeding (see Chapter 19).

## DIAGNOSIS

The history is extremely helpful in the diagnosis of lower GI bleeding. For instance, a history of tenesmus, abdominal cramping, and diarrhea is suggestive of an inflammatory or infectious cause. A history of radiation therapy for cancer is suggestive of radiation enteritis. However, in patients with recurrent lower GI bleeding, likely causes are diverticulosis and vascular lesions,[2] and history is not helpful. No historical features distinguish these lesions.

I generally follow the schematic plan in Fig. 20-1 when investigating a patient with lower gastrointestinal bleeding. I will discuss only diverticulosis (including Meckel's) and vascular lesions (angiodysplasia).

## Causes of Lower Gastrointestinal Bleeding

DIVERTICULOSIS

VASCULAR

Angiodysplasia
Vascular malformation
Vascular ischemia
Hemorrhoids and fissures
Ileal and colonic varices
Vasculitis

INFLAMMATORY BOWEL DISEASE

Ulcerative colitis
Crohn's disease

INFECTION

Bacterial
Parasitic
Viral
Toxic

NEOPLASM

**Benign**

Polyps
Leiomyoma

**Malignant**

Carcinoma
Lymphoma
Melanoma
Leiomyosarcoma

RADIATION ENTERITIS

MISCELLANEOUS

Blood dyscrasias
Meckel's diverticulum
Solitary rectal ulcer

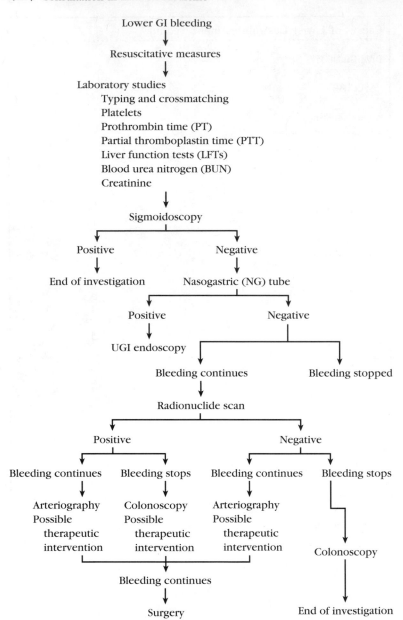

**Figure 20-1.** *Schema for the investigation of a patient with lower gastrointestinal bleeding.*

## Diverticulosis

Colonic diverticula are especially common in the older age group. Autopsy studies have shown an incidence of up to 50% in patients over 60 years of age. Diverticula are uncommon under 30 years of age. Left-sided diverticula are more common than right-sided ones by a ratio of 10 : 1. It is important to stress two points in relation to diverticular bleeding: (1) Diverticulitis may be associated with guaiac-positive stools but rarely presents with massive lower gastrointestinal bleeding. (2) Bleeding from right-sided diverticula is more common than from left-sided diverticula. This observation is in contrast to diverticulitis, which almost always is left-sided.

There is some difference of opinion on the diagnostic method of choice in the evaluation of diverticular bleeding, but all investigators agree that it is *not* a barium enema. A barium enema shows diverticula very nicely but does not identify the bleeding diverticulum. In addition, barium tends to be retained in diverticula, thereby making subsequent tests such as colonoscopy and arteriography difficult to interpret. A barium enema may be performed later in the hospital course to search for colonic lesions other than the identified site of bleeding.

In acute diverticular bleeding, colonoscopy also is of little value. During active bleeding, colonoscopy should not be performed because of inadequate visualization of the colon. Colonoscopy may be performed when bleeding stops, but blood, like barium, tends to be retained in diverticula, and identification of the specific bleeding diverticulum is difficult. Radionuclide scanning may help to diagnose the location of the bleeding site but not the cause of the bleeding.[3]

If conventional barium roentgenography, radionuclide scanning, and direct visualization by colonoscopy are of little use, what diagnostic tool should we use? I strongly believe that selective angiography is the diagnostic test of choice. In addition to its diagnostic superiority, angiography has a potential therapeutic role. Selective arterial infusion of vasopressin has been shown (by angiography) to stop diverticular bleeding.[4] If bleeding does not respond to vasopressin and remains massive, that is, greater than 10 units per 24 hours, surgery is indicated. Some investigators believe that selective surgery is indicated after the first massive diverticular bleed, even if the bleeding stops, because of the high incidence (25% to 50%) of rebleeding. I do not agree with this opinion.

If arteriography is so accurate, why do many patients with diverticular bleeds remain undiagnosed? The main reason is that, to make the diagnosis angiographically, the patient has to be actively bleeding at a rate that exceeds 0.4 mL/min. Many patients stop bleeding spontaneously before arteriography is carried out, and others bleed in an erratic fashion, thereby eluding diagnosis. Angiography must be done immediately in the patient admitted to the hospital with a third or more episode of recurrent lower GI bleeding.

## Angiodysplasia

Angiodysplasia,[5,6] an acquired localized vascular lesion, occurs mainly in the right side of the colon and the distal ileum and can be single or multiple. Histologically, the lesion consists of ectatic submucosal capillaries or veins. There is a strong correlation between angiodysplasia and aging and a weaker association between angiodysplasia and aortic stenosis.

The diagnosis of angiodysplasia can be made by angiography and colonoscopy. In the undiagnosed patient with recurrent lower GI bleeding, angiography is preferable for the reasons discussed in the section on diverticulosis. Again, barium enema is not helpful except to eliminate other lesions. Radionuclide scanning may localize the general site of bleeding and aid the angiographer to catheterize selectively the artery suspected of feeding the angiodysplasia.

The treatment of angiodysplasia is endoscopic or surgical. If the bleeding stops and the angiodysplasia can be identified by colonoscopy, cauterization with a heater probe, bipolar probe, or laser should be attempted. If bleeding does not stop, surgical intervention is indicated. If chronic bleeding persists or recurs after endoscopic or surgical treatment, a trial of treatment with estrogen and progesterone is indicated. This has been reported to be effective in some patients, particularly if they have renal failure. Angiodysplasia is a difficult entity to treat because it may be multiple with a different site of bleeding on different occasions and because it has a tendency to recur, even after surgical resection.

## References

1. Boyel SJ, Dilirase A, Brandt LJ, et al: Lower intestinal bleeding in the elderly, *Am J Surg* 137:57-64, 1979.
2. Reinus JF, Brandt LJ: Vascular ectasias and diverticulosis: common causes of lower intestinal bleeding, *Gastroenterol Clin North Am* 23:1-20, 1994.
3. Colacchio TA, Forde KA, Patros TJ, et al: Impact of modern diagnostic methods on the management of active rectal bleeding, *Am J Surg* 143:607-610, 1982.
4. Baum S, Rosch J, Dotter CT: Selective mesenteric arterial infusions in the management of massive diverticular hemorrhage, *N Engl J Med* 288:1269-1271, 1973.
5. Richter JM, Hedberg SE, Athanesoulis CA: Angiodysplasia: clinical presentation and colonoscopic diagnosis, *Dig Dis Sci* 29(6):481-485, 1984.
6. Foutch PG: Angiodysplasia of the gastrointestinal tract, *Am J Gastroenterol* 88:807-818, 1993.

# Chapter 21

# *Acute Diarrhea*

Karim A. Fawaz

Diarrhea may be defined in qualitative terms, in which case the consistency and frequency of stools are taken into consideration, or in quantitative terms, where stool volume or weight is measured. The qualitative definition may be misleading because it depends on subjective interpretation by the patient. With the quantitative definition one considers an individual stool volume of more than 200 mL as diarrhea. To ascertain the presence of true diarrhea is more of a problem in patients who complain of chronic rather than acute diarrhea. For the purposes of this discussion, acute diarrhea will be defined as a sudden change in stool consistency that results in liquid stool with a significant increase in stool volume.

## THE ROLE OF HISTORY

A detailed history and a complete physical examination are crucial in the differential diagnosis of the various causes of acute diarrhea listed in the box on p. 198.

Key questions asked should pertain to the following:

**Recent travel.** A history of recent travel to a foreign country is suggestive of an infectious cause for the diarrhea. *Escherichia coli* is the most common offender in traveler's diarrhea, but other bacterial agents, giardiasis and amebiasis, also should be considered.

**Intake of undercooked beef, chicken, and eggs.** Diarrhea after eating an undercooked hamburger should raise the possibility of *E. coli* infection. Diarrhea after eating undercooked chicken or raw eggs should raise the possibility of *Salmonella* gastroenteritis.

**Institutions.** Diarrhea in institutions such as day care centers or retarded care facilities where individual hygiene is difficult to maintain is associated with pathogens such as *Clostridium difficile, Shigella, Campylobacter,* and *Giardia* organisms.

**Medications.** Many drugs can cause diarrhea, and the following are some common examples: laxatives, magnesium-containing antacids, digoxin, quinidine, chemotherapeutic agents, and antibiotics, especially penicillin derivatives. The effect of the drug is usually immediate. On the other hand, antibiotic-associated colitis (pseudomembranous

## Causes of Acute Diarrhea

| INFECTIOUS CAUSES | NONINFECTIOUS CAUSES |
|---|---|
| **BACTERIAL CAUSES** | **INFLAMMATORY BOWEL DISEASE** |
| *Escherichia coli*<br>*Shigella*<br>*Salmonella*<br>*Staphylococcus*<br>*Campylobacter*<br>*Yersinia*<br>*Clostridium difficile* | Ulcerative colitis<br>Crohn's disease<br>Ischemic colitis<br>Lactase deficiency |
| **VIRAL CAUSES** | **DRUGS** |
| Norwalk virus<br>Rotavirus | Laxatives<br>Antacids<br>Antibiotics<br>Antimetabolites |
| **PARASITIC CAUSES** | |
| *Giardia*<br>Amebiasis<br>*Cryptosporidium*<br>Microsporidia-<br>Cyclospora | Acute radiation injury<br>Mechanical causes<br>Fecal impaction<br>Partial small bowel obstruction |

colitis) may occur while the patient is receiving an antibiotic such as ampicillin or clindamycin, but it also may present several days to weeks after cessation of therapy.

**Radiation treatment.** Acute diarrhea may occur secondary to mucosal sloughing from acute radiation injury. Acute radiation diarrhea occurs closely after treatment, unlike the diarrhea secondary to mesenteric vascular injury that may occur months later.

**Heart disease.** Patients with congestive heart failure, especially those on diuretic therapy, are prone to develop acute ischemic colitis with bloody diarrhea secondary to a "low-flow" state.

**Tenesmus.** The presence of this symptom usually indicates rectal involvement. It is a common symptom in inflammatory bowel disease and in infections involving the distal area of the colon.

**Bloody diarrhea.** The presence of bloody diarrhea indicates mucosal inflammation and should direct the physician's attention toward inflammatory bowel disease and organisms that cause inflammation or ulceration, such as *Shigella, Campylobacter, Salmonella,* amebas, and *Clostridium difficile.*

**Change in eating habits.** The question "Have you changed your eating habits?" is rarely asked by a physician seeing a patient with acute diarrhea. It is an important question to ask, however, because the answer may prevent a long and expensive diagnostic investigation. Postoperative patients are often prescribed a liquid diet rich in dairy products. Because some of these patients have a lactase deficiency that they are not aware of, diarrhea develops. I also have seen many patients who have been advised by old-timers or by friends that milk is good for their ulcer pain. Large amounts of milk are consumed, thus unmasking lactase deficiency and causing diarrhea.

**Rectal intercourse.** Diarrhea occurring after rectal intercourse should direct the physician's attention to infections such as gonorrhea, shigellosis, amebiasis, giardiasis, and *Chlamydia* and *Campylobacter* infections.

**Extraintestinal manifestations of inflammatory bowel disease.** Diarrhea associated with joint pain, iridoscleritis, or skin eruptions such as erythema nodosum and pyoderma gangrenosum is suggestive of the presence of inflammatory bowel disease.

Questions in these 11 simple areas help the physician to decide which diagnostic tests if any should be ordered and in what sequence. In many instances, however, the patient recovers by the time the diagnosis is made. Detailed investigation need not be done in patients with mild diarrhea until the diarrhea lasts for longer than 2 to 3 weeks.

# DIAGNOSTIC TESTS

Reaching the correct diagnosis in a patient with an acute diarrheal illness usually requires results from four tests: stool microscopy, stool culture, endoscopic visualization with or without biopsy, and x-ray studies. Not all patients need to undergo all these tests. Furthermore, if barium studies are planned, they should be performed last because barium interferes with the detection of ova and parasites for 2 to 3 weeks. In addition, patients with suspected acute severe colitis have a relative contraindication to a barium enema because of the danger of precipitation of toxic megacolon.

In the following discussion I will focus on the clinical presentation, diagnosis, and management of the more common causes of acute diarrhea in adults.

# BACTERIAL INFECTION

Bacterial infections,[1,2] the most common causes of acute diarrhea, are usually caused by contaminated food or water. Acute diarrhea that develops in association with travel to developing countries is referred to as "traveler's diarrhea" and is caused by bacterial infection in most cases.

**Escherichia coli diarrhea.** Most strains of *E. coli* are harmless. However, some strains are pathogenic, such as enteropathic *E. coli,* which are common causes of diarrhea in neonates and infants, and enterotoxigenic *E. coli,* which are responsible for diarrhea in 45% to 85% of cases of traveler's diarrhea.[3,4] The diarrhea, usually nonbloody, is associated with abdominal cramps. Systemic manifestations of fever and chills are not common. The incubation period is 2 to 3 days. The diagnosis of *E. coli* diarrhea is not easy to make, since it is a normal finding in stool cultures. A presumptive diagnosis may be made if the stool culture grows pure *E. coli;* otherwise special culture techniques are needed to differentiate pathogenic from nonpathogenic strains.

Specific treatment is not necessary in most instances because this illness is usually self-limiting, lasting only a few days. Adequate hydration should be maintained, and nonspecific antidiarrheal agents, such as lopamide or bismuth subsalicylate, may be used if the diarrhea is bothersome. When symptoms are severe and disabling, antibiotic therapy with trimethoprim-sulfamethoxazole (two double-strength tablets) for 3 to 5 days is effective.

Epidemic outbreaks as well as sporadic cases of hemorrhagic colitis associated with *E. coli* strain 0157:H7 have been reported.[5,6] This illness is much more severe than the usual *E. coli* diarrhea and is associated with systemic manifestations such as the hemolytic uremic syndrome and mucosal damage causing bloody diarrhea. There is no known effective therapy, and so management should be directed at rehydration and prevention.

**Shigellosis.**[1] Shigellosis, referred to as *bacillary dysentery,* is the cause of diarrhea in 15% to 22% of traveler's diarrhea. The incubation period may be as short as 24 hours. The clinical presentation includes abdominal cramping, fever, and diarrhea that often becomes bloody. Fecal leukocytes are present. The findings on sigmoidoscopy depend on the severity of the disease and are indistinguishable from those of idiopathic ulcerative colitis. The diagnosis is made by stool culture.

There is controversy on whether antibiotic treatment is indicated in mild cases of shigellosis. Most investigators agree that severe cases should be treated. The antibiotics of choice are ampicillin (2 g daily for 5 to 7 days) and trimethoprim-sulfamethoxazole (two double-stength tablets for 5 to 7 days). Nonspecific antidiarrheal drugs such as loperamide and diphenoxylate, which act by delaying intestinal motility, should be used with caution because they may prolong the illness by increasing the time of contact between the bacteria and the colon and may precipitate a toxic megacolon in severe cases.

**Salmonellosis.**[1] *Salmonella* may cause gastroenteritis, typhoid fever, and bacteremia. *Salmonella* gastroenteritis has an incubation period of 12 to 36 hours. *Salmonella* organisms, cultured in 4% to 5% of cases of traveler's diarrhea, is a common cause of epidemic forms of gastroenteritis. It is usually a self-limiting illness characterized by abdominal cramps and diarrhea that may become bloody. Systemic manifestations of fever, chills, and headache may be present. Leukocytosis is common, but blood cultures have negative results. Sigmoidoscopy may show colitis that cannot be distinguished from idiopathic ulcerative colitis. Diagnosis is established by stool culture. Specific treatment with antibiotics is not indicated; symptomatic treatment and adequate hydration are sufficient.

**Campylobacter enteritis.** *Campylobacter* enteritis recently has emerged as a common cause of acute diarrhea. Most clinical laboratories now look (and should look) for *Campylobacter* organisms in addition to *Salmonella* and *Shigella* organisms in routine stool cultures. The clinical picture is that of diarrhea, abdominal pain, and fever; bloody diarrhea occurs in 46% of the cases.[7] The stool cultures are positive for fecal leukocytes, and sigmoidoscopy again reveals a colitis indistinguishable from ulcerative colitis. The illness may last longer than *Salmonella* and *Shigella* infection but is similar in that it is self-limiting in most instances. The diagnosis is made by a positive stool culture. Again, antibiotic treatment is not necessary in most cases, but when the illness is severe or lasts for greater than 7 days, erythromycin (250 mg three times daily for 7 days) should be administered.

**Clostridium difficile colitis.**[1] Many antibiotics cause *C. difficile* colitis, but the most frequent offenders are ampicillin, clindamycin, and cephalosporins. The clinical presentation is the same as with the other bacterial diarrheas. The illness may commence during the course of antibiotic treatment and up to 3 months after cessation of therapy. Sigmoidoscopy may be normal or may resemble ulcerative colitis. The most characteristic finding is the presence of membranous plaques and hence the term *pseudomembranous colitis.* The diagnosis is made by a positive *C. difficile* stool toxin assay or a positive stool culture. Specific treatment is indicated in this illness; the agents of choice are metronidazole (500 mg three times daily for 7 days) and vancomycin (125 mg four times daily for 7 days).

# PARASITIC INFECTION[1]

**Giardiasis.** *Giardia* protozoons, a common cause of diarrhea, are responsible for 3% of traveler's diarrhea.[3,4] The most common symptom is diarrhea that is never bloody. Abdominal pain and malabsorption are more common in children. There is an association with dysgammaglobulinemia, especially in IgA deficiency. The diagnosis is made by stool microscopy, duodenal aspiration, or duodenal biopsy. A negative stool examination does not rule out giardiasis because up to 50% of cases with a positive duodenal aspirate have a negative stool microscopy. Sigmoidoscopy shows normal results. Specific treatment is indicated and consists in the use of metronidazole (250 mg three times daily for 7 days) or quinacrine (100 mg three times daily for 7 days).

**Amebiasis.** Amebiasis may be acute or chronic. Its clinical manifestations vary from an asymptomatic carrier state to severe colitis. The acute form of colitis is similar to ulcerative colitis and bacterial diarrhea discussed earlier. Sigmoidoscopy is helpful when typical discrete ulcers with undetermined edges are present, but this picture is not universally present. One may obtain trophozoites by scraping the base of the ulcers suspected. A serum test for amebic titer by indirect hemagglutination is an adjunct to diagnosis. Specific treatment is indicated and consists in the use of metronidazole (750 mg three times daily for 7 to 20 days). Diiodohydroxyquin (650 mg three times daily for 20 days) is the treatment for asymptomatic carriers in combination with metronidazole in severe cases.

**Cryptosporidiosis.** The pathogen *Cryptosporidium* was believed to affect immunocompromised hosts only, but it is now clear that this waterborne parasite is an important cause of acute diarrhea.[1] The diarrhea is frequently associated with abdominal cramps, nausea, vomiting, and weight loss. Chills and fever are usually absent. The diagnosis is made by identification of eggs on stool microscopy using an acid-fast stain or by direct immunofluorescence. No effective therapy is available.

# DIARRHEA IN PATIENTS WITH AIDS

Diarrhea is very common in patients with AIDS, occurring in 50% to 60% of patients with an identifiable infectious cause in 50% to 85% of the cases.[8] Patients who are immunocompromised are susceptible to the usual pathogens that affect immunocompetent patients, but in addition they are susceptible to other pathogens such as protozoans in the Microsporidia order, *Cytomegalovirus* (CMV), and Mycobacteria. The prevalence of microsporidiosis is reported to be 10% to 30% in patients with AIDS and diarrhea,[8] and symptoms include abdominal discomfort, weight loss secondary to malabsorption, but no fever.

# INFLAMMATORY BOWEL DISEASE

Patients with ulcerative colitis and Crohn's disease may present acutely or have a more insidious presentation. When the initial presentation is acute, it must be differentiated from infectious colitis. The clinical and sigmoidoscopic picture may be the same, but the presence of extraintestinal manifestations, such as arthralgia, arthritis, erythema nodosum, pyoderma gangrenosum, and associated liver disease, is suggestive of inflammatory bowel disease.

In ulcerative colitis only the colon is involved, and the rectum is always involved. The disease is diffuse and continuous without "skip" segments. In contrast, Crohn's disease may involve the small or large intestines. The rectum may be spared, and "skip" areas of normal mucosa may be present. The diagnosis is established by a process of elimination of specific causes of colitis. Colonic biopsies may be helpful but are not specific. Involvement of the small intestine favors the diagnosis of Crohn's disease. Treatment depends on the type, severity, and location of the disease. The drugs used are steroids, sulfasalazine, azathioprine, purinethol, and metronidazole.

## References

1. Guerrant RL, Bobak DA: Bacterial and protozoal gastroenteritis, *N Engl J Med* 325(5):327-340, 1991.

2. Guerrant RL, Shields DS, Thorson SM, et al: Evaluation and diagnosis of acute infectious diarrhea, *Am J Med* 78(suppl 6B):91, 1985.

3. DuPont HI, Reves RR, Galindo E, et al: Treatment of traveler's diarrhea with trimethoprim/sulfamethoxazole and with trimethoprim alone, *N Engl J Med* 307(14):841-844, 1982.

4. Johnson PC, DuPont HL, Ericsson CD: Travelers' diarrhea—common misconceptions, *Pract Gastroenterol* 9(3):14-18, 38-40, 1985.

5. Remis RS, MacDonald KL, Lee WR, et al: Sporadic cases of hemorrhagic colitis associated with *Escherichia coli* 0157:H7, *Ann Intern Med* 101:625-626, 1984.

6. Consensus Conference Statement: *Escherichia coli* 0157:H7 infections—an emerging national health crisis, *Gastroenterology* 108:1923-1934, 1995.

7. Blaser MJ, Wells JG, Feldman RH, et al: *Campylobacter* enteritis in the United States, *Ann Intern Med* 98:360-365, 1983.

8. Simon D, Brandt LJ: Diarrhea in patients with the acquired immunodeficiency syndrome, *Gastroenterology* 105:1238-1242, 1993.

# Chapter 22

# *Chronic Diarrhea*

Karim A. Fawaz

Chronic diarrhea is defined as recurrent diarrhea or diarrhea that lasts for more than 3 to 4 weeks. Under normal circumstances, 1 to 2 liters of fluid are ingested orally and 7 liters are secreted into the intestinal lumen by the stomach, liver, pancreas, and small intestines in a 24-hour period. Intestinal absorption is so efficient that 99% of the fluid ingested and secreted is reabsorbed. In a normal individual, stool weight is less than 200 g per 24 hours, with water accounting for about 75% of stool weight.

Diarrhea may be caused by any condition that disturbs the delicate balance between secretion and absorption and results in a decrease in net water absorption. In a patient with diarrhea, water rises to 90% of stool weight. Since water is the major factor in determining stool weight, diarrhea is defined quantitatively as the excretion of more than 200 g or 200 mL of stools per 24 hours. Exceptions to this quantitative definition are patients with distal colitis or proctitis and patients with the irritable bowel syndrome who may have an increased stool frequency but a normal stool weight. Pathophysiologically, diarrhea may be caused by any one of the following mechanisms: increased intraluminal osmotic load (osmotic diarrhea); decreased absorption (malabsorption); defective digestion (maldigestion); exudation of protein, blood, and fluid into the lumen (exudative diarrhea); excessive intestinal secretion of water and electrolytes (secretory diarrhea); and abnormal intestinal motility (motility-related diarrhea). An excellent review on the outpatient and inpatient evaluation of patients with chronic diarrhea recently has been written by Donowitz and associates.[1]

The box on pp. 205 and 206 lists the specific causes of chronic diarrhea in relation to the preceding pathophysiologic mechanisms. First, I review my approach to the initial and subsequent evaluation of a patient with chronic diarrhea and then discuss the more common causes of chronic diarrhea.

## Causes of Chronic Diarrhea
..........................................................................

### I. OSMOTIC DIARRHEA

Disaccharidase deficiency (such as lactase deficiency)
Laxatives

### II. MALABSORPTION

A. Small bowel disease
   Celiac sprue
   Whipple's disease
   Tropical sprue
   Giardiasis
   Extensive Crohn's disease
     or intestinal resection
   Collagenous sprue
   Amyloidosis

Radiation enteritis
Intestinal lymphangiectasia
Intestinal lymphoma
Eosinophilic gastroenteritis
Bacterial overgrowth
Chronic intestinal ischemia
Infections associated with
   immunodeficiency syn-
   dromes, including AIDS

B. Maldigestion
   Chronic pancreatitis
   Pancreatic cancer
   Bacterial overgrowth
   Bile acid deficiency
   Cystic fibrosis

### III. EXUDATIVE DIARRHEA

Ulcerative colitis
Crohn's disease
Colon cancer
Amebiasis
Tuberculosis

### IV. SECRETORY DIARRHEA

Cholera
Pancreatic cholera (pancreatic tumor that secretes vasoactive intestinal
  polypeptide, VIP)
Zollinger-Ellison syndrome
Carcinoid
Medullary carcinoma
Drugs (laxatives, theophylline)
Bile acids
Villous adenoma
Partial small bowel obstruction
Mucosal injury (celiac sprue, inflammatory bowel disease, ischemia)

*continued*

*continued*

| V. MOTILITY-RELATED DIARRHEA |
| --- |
| Hyperthyroidism<br>Carcinoid syndrome<br>Scleroderma<br>Diabetes<br>Irritable bowel syndrome |

# INITIAL WORK-UP OF CHRONIC DIARRHEA

**History.** In the evaluation of a patient with diarrhea, the history should direct the physician to the most appropriate tests and the sequence in which they are performed. After establishing that the diarrhea is truly chronic, the following historical features are helpful clues:

1. *Stool character and number.* A large volume of stools is suggestive of a secretory diarrhea or malabsorption. Greasy malodorous stools often are seen in patients with malabsorption. The presence of blood is suggestive of a neoplastic or inflammatory process. The presence of mucus and pus indicates inflammation. Diarrhea alternating with constipation or the passage of several small bowel movements within a short period of time in the morning only is most consistent with irritable bowel syndrome.
2. *Stool timing.* Nocturnal diarrhea almost always indicates the presence of an organic cause of the diarrhea rather than a functional cause.
3. *Associated intestinal symptoms.* The presence of tenesmus points to the presence of an inflammatory or neoplastic condition in the rectum. The presence of abdominal cramps that are relieved by a bowel movement is not specific and may occur in functional or organic diarrhea. Flushing or a reddish discoloration of the skin in a patient with chronic diarrhea is suggestive of carcinoid syndrome.
4. *Associated extraintestinal manifestations.* Diarrhea associated with arthralgia, arthritis, erythema nodosum, pyoderma gangrenosum, and iridoscleritis is suggestive of the presence of inflammatory bowel disease.
5. *Weight loss.* The presence of weight loss in association with chronic diarrhea points to the presence of malabsorption, neoplasia, or inflammatory bowel disease rather than irritable bowel or lactose intolerance.
6. *Dietary habits.* The association of diarrhea with eating dairy products should raise the suspicion of lactose intolerance.
7. *Previous abdominal surgery.* Gastric surgery with vagotomy may cause postvagotomy diarrhea. Gastrointestinal surgery may

result in diarrhea because of several problems, including bacterial overgrowth, short bowel syndrome, or bile salt malabsorption. Cholecystectomy may lead to postcholecystectomy diarrhea probably induced by bile acids.[2]

8. *Other associated diseases.* In diabetics, diarrhea, particularly nocturnal, is not uncommon when other manifestations of neuropathy are present. In patients with scleroderma, abnormal small bowel motility may lead to stasis and bacterial overgrowth resulting in diarrhea.

9. *Radiation therapy.* Pelvic and abdominal radiation damage can cause chronic diarrhea that can occur months to years after radiation treatment.

10. *Drugs.* Antibiotics and many other drugs may cause acute diarrhea. In addition, regular ingestion of drugs, such as laxatives, lactulose, bronchodilators, magnesium-containing antacids, colchicine, and guanidine, may cause chronic diarrhea.

11. *Sexual habits.* Male homosexuals are at significantly higher risk of developing chronic amebiasis, giardiasis, and opportunistic infections associated with AIDS.

12. *Travel history.* Most infectious diarrhea states associated with travel are acute; however, diseases such as amebiasis and giardiasis often lead to chronic diarrhea.

13. *Fever.* The presence of fever should raise the strong possibility of inflammatory bowel disease or lymphoma, since it is uncommon in all other causes of chronic diarrhea.

**Physical examination.** The physical examination usually is less helpful than the history in the work-up of chronic diarrhea, but occasionally it clinches the diagnosis. The presence of a right lower quadrant mass and perianal fistulous disease is almost diagnostic of Crohn's disease. Examination of the skin for pyoderma gangrenosum and erythema nodosum is helpful in the diagnosis of inflammatory bowel disease. Hyperpigmentation of the skin is suggestive of Whipple's disease or Addison's disease.

**Stool examination.** Every patient with chronic diarrhea should have an initial stool examination that includes testing for the presence of blood and white blood cells (WBCs), a Sudan stain for fat, and microscopy for ova and parasites. In contrast to acute diarrhea, the yield from sending stools for culture in patients with chronic diarrhea is extremely low, since most of the organisms that are grown on stool culture cause self-limited, brief illnesses. The exception to this statement is the immunocompromised patient, especially the patient with AIDS. The presence of blood in the stool is suggestive of an inflammatory or neoplastic condition, whereas the presence of WBCs is suggestive of an inflammatory condition. A Sudan III stain for fat is a good screening test for fat malabsorption. Stool microscopy for ova and parasites should be done two or three times, especially if the index of suspicion for a parasitic infection is high. Remember that stool microscopy for ova and parasites should be performed on fresh specimens *before* any barium x-ray studies are performed because barium may interfere with the yield and lead to false-negative results for at least 2 to 3 weeks after the barium x-ray test.

**Blood tests.** WBC and differential studies need to be done to look for an increase in neutrophils or in eosinophils. Obviously, if bloody diarrhea is present, the hematocrit and hemoglobin need to be checked frequently.

**Sigmoidoscopy.** A sigmoidoscopy should be part of the initial evaluation of every patient with chronic diarrhea unless the diagnosis of a parasitic infection is made by stool microscopy. Sigmoidoscopy should be performed without cleansing preparation so that the mucosa and any exudate that may be present on it are not distorted.

## SUBSEQUENT WORKUP OF CHRONIC DIARRHEA

The decision to continue the investigation and the sequence of tests that are ordered depend on the results of the initial investigation and the clinical suspicion of the physician. In a young patient whose initial workup is completely negative and in whom the clinical suspicion for irritable bowel syndrome is high, a therapeutic trial of dietary manipulation and symptomatic treatment is in order before embarking on a "megaworkup." Similarly if the clinical suspicion of lactose intolerance is high, a 2-week trial of a lactose-free diet is the next logical step to take. On the other hand, chronic diarrhea that occurs in a 60-year-old person without a previous history of diarrhea deserves full investigation despite a negative initial workup.

The following is a list of tests that may be indicated in the subsequent workup of chronic diarrhea. One or more of these tests may be indicated, depending on the clinical suspicion formulated from the initial workup:

1. *Routine blood work.* BUN, creatinine, electrolytes, albumin
2. *Special blood work.* Gastrin, cortisol, vasoactive intestinal peptide (VIP), thyroid function tests, immunoglobulins
3. *Roentgenography.* Upper gastrointestinal (UGI) series, barium enema, computerized tomography (CT) scan of the abdomen, endoscopic retrograde cholangiopancreatography (ERCP)
4. D-*Xylose.* Two-hour serum sample and 5-hour urine collection
5. *Small bowel aspirate. Giardia*
6. *Small bowel biopsy*
7. *Urine.* 5-Hydroxyindoleacetic acid (5-HIAA), vanillylmandelic acid (VMA)

The sequence of tests depends on the initial formulation. In the following section, I review the major causes of chronic diarrhea, my diagnostic approach, and my plan of management.

## LACTOSE INTOLERANCE

Lactose intolerance secondary to mucosal lactase deficiency, a common cause of diarrhea worldwide, is an acquired condition that manifests itself in early adulthood. In the United States 70% to 75% of blacks and 5% to 20% of whites suffer from this ailment.[3] Its prevalence in Asia and the Middle East is as high as 90%. Typically the patient with lactose intolerance complains of diarrhea associated with bloating, gaseous distension, and crampy abdominal pain. The diagnosis of lactase deficiency should be suspected in any patient who complains of the preceding symptoms after the ingestion of milk or dairy products, but not all patients recognize this association. Remember that patients may be able to tolerate varying amounts of lactose without any symptoms; the mucosal deficiency of lactase is a graded one and not an all-or-nothing phenomenon. There are several different tests to confirm the diagnosis. The most accurate, but most invasive and therefore least used, is a small bowel biopsy with quantitative measurement of mucosal lactase activity. Other less invasive tests include a lactose tolerance test and labeled breath tests that utilize carbon dioxide and hydrogen. I favor utilizing a therapeutic trial of a lactose-free diet for 1 to 2 weeks rather than any of these tests. I resort to the breath test only when the therapeutic trial is inconclusive.

The treatment of lactose intolerance is obviously a lactose-free diet. That does not mean, however, that a patient is condemned to a dairy-free diet forever. There are commercial milk products that are pre-treated with lactase and enzyme preparations, which can be added to milk products. It is also important to know that the ingestion of yogurt by such patients does *not* cause symptoms because, in the process of producing yogurt, bacterial lactase digests the lactose present in the milk.

## CELIAC SPRUE

Celiac sprue is also known as *gluten sensitive enteropathy*. It is the gluten, and particularly the gliadin moiety in gluten, that is toxic to the intestinal mucosa of patients who suffer from this condition. The result is flattening of the intestinal villa, thereby leading to malabsorption. The most common symptoms in celiac sprue are diarrhea, abdominal distension, and weight loss; abdominal pain is unusual. The causes of diarrhea in these patients are multiple and include decreased absorption of carbohydrate, protein, and fat and increased secretion of water and electrolytes. Also fat reaching the colon is broken down by bacteria to fatty acids, which in turn cause fluid secretion into the intestinal lumen.

The diagnosis of celiac sprue is based on the following findings: increased 72-hour stool fat (greater than 7 g per 24 hours); abnormal serum and urine D-xylose test (2-hour serum sample greater than 25 mg/dL and urine greater than 5 g per 5 hours of collection); abnormal laboratory findings such as iron and folate deficiencies, prolonged prothrombin time, and low calcium, and vitamin $B_{12}$ blood levels; and abnormal small bowel pattern with dilated proximal loops. Antibodies to gliadin and endomysium have been used with variable degrees of sensitivity and specificity, but it seems that the serum IgA antibody to endomysium is more specific and more sensitive for celiac sprue.[4] A flat mucosa with absence of villi on small bowel biopsy is the test I rely on most heavily. The treatment of celiac sprue is a gluten-free diet. Every patient suspected of having this condition must have a small bowel biopsy to confirm the diagnosis. The patient also should meet with a dietitian to receive proper instructions on a gluten-free diet. The treatment is simple in concept, but following a strict gluten-free diet is not easy because gluten is present in so many additives and preservatives in addition to natural food. The clinical response to treatment is relatively quick, but the histologic improvement lags months behind. A decrease in the antiendomysial antibody titer correlates with response to therapy too.

# CHRONIC PANCREATITIS

Pancreatic exocrine insufficiency, a frequent complication of chronic pancreatitis, causes malabsorption and hence diarrhea. The scenario is usually one of chronic abdominal pain with acute exacerbations for years before the development of diarrhea. Typically, more than 90% of the pancreas is destroyed before diarrhea sets in. The pathophysiologic mechanism is maldigestion of protein, carbohydrates, and fat secondary to insufficient enzyme production by the diseased pancreas. The diagnosis should be suspected when a patient presents with diarrhea after a long history of abdominal pain. Findings such as calcification of the pancreas on kidney, ureter, and bladder (KUB) studies and elevated 72-hour stool fat confirm the diagnosis. In some patients, calcification of the pancreas may not occur, and ERCP is required to establish a diagnosis. The bentiromide test[5] has gained acceptance over the last decade as a more specific and less cumbersome test than the 72-hour stool fat test. Bentiromide, a synthetic peptide, is cleaved by chymotrypsin in the small intestine resulting in the release of *para*-aminobenzoic acid (PABA), which in turn is absorbed and excreted in the urine. The test consists in giving 500 mg of bentiromide after an overnight fast and collecting urine for 6 hours. In normal people, greater than 50% of PABA is recovered in the urine. This test has a 5% false-positive and a 20% false-negative result.

# INFLAMMATORY BOWEL DISEASE

Chronic diarrhea is the most prominent symptom in ulcerative colitis and Crohn's disease.[6] The pathophysiologic mechanisms are multiple and include exudation of protein, blood, and mucus from inflammatory sites, malabsorption, and net fluid secretion. The diarrhea is frequently bloody and may contain pus. Nocturnal diarrhea is not unusual. Abdominal cramping is often an accompanying symptom. The diagnosis is made by sigmoidoscopy, colonoscopy, and barium roentgenography singly or in combination. Caution is necessary during the investigation of patients with inflammatory bowel disease, especially acute ulcerative colitis. A limited sigmoidoscopy without bowel preparation is sometimes the only indicated procedure in patients with severe bloody diarrhea and accompanying systemic manifestations and physical findings such as fever, tachycardia, hypotension, and a distended and tender abdomen. A barium enema or complete colonoscopy are contraindicated because of possible precipitation of a toxic megacolon, which is a life-threatening condition. The treatment options include sulfasalazine, steroids, azathioprine, and 6-mercaptopurine, depending on the type of disease and its severity.

## COLON CANCER

Symptoms in colonic cancer are not uniform; they vary according to the site of the lesion. A change in bowel habits manifested by constipation or alternating constipation and diarrhea are much more common in left-sided colonic lesions than in right-sided ones. Diarrhea occurs more frequently in distal colonic lesions. If gross blood or guaiac-positive stools accompany these symptoms, it becomes mandatory to rule out colonic cancer. The diagnosis of colonic cancer can be made by a sigmoidoscopy and a barium enema or colonoscopy.

## IRRITABLE BOWEL SYNDROME

Abdominal pain and constipation are more common than diarrhea in this common syndrome. However, diarrhea alternating with constipation or steady diarrhea occurs in a significant number of patients. The diarrhea is more frequent in the morning, especially after breakfast, and in the early evening. The bowel movments are usually multiple, small in volume, and "mucusy." Nocturnal diarrhea that wakes the patient up from sleep is extremely rare, and dehydration and weight loss do not occur. The condition usually occurs in early adulthood. The onset of similar symptoms for the first time in middle-aged and older persons is rare and should alert the physician to search for a more serious organic condition. The pathophysiologic mechanism is presumed to be a motility disturbance. However, studies have not been conclusive. The personal experience of many gastroenterologists, as well as epidemiologic studies, indicates that stress and emotional tensions may play a role in precipitating this condition.[7]

There is no diagnostic test that clinches the diagnosis, so the diagnosis is made by a consistent clinical picture and by exclusion of other conditions, such as villous adenoma and inflammatory bowel disease. The history of emotional stress in patients with an episodic bowel pattern is also helpful. The management of patients suffering from the irritable bowel syndrome is often difficult. It is of paramount importance to stress to the patient the benignity of this condition. Alterations in diet, anticholinergics, and antidiarrheal agents may be used, but controlled studies have failed to show a beneficial long-term effect for any particular regimen.

# CHRONIC DIARRHEA OF UNKNOWN CAUSE

A cause of chronic diarrhea is usually found in most patients.[1,8] However, every gastroenterologist is referred an occasional patient who remains undiagnosed despite an extensive workup, including routine blood tests, stool examinations, malabsorption workup, endoscopic procedures, x-ray studies, dietary manipulation, and therapeutic trials.

The list of causes in these unusual patients is long, but among the conditions that must be considered are laxative abuse, bile acid diarrhea, neuroendocrine tumors such as VIP-secreting pancreatic tumors, idiopathic secretory diarrhea, microscopic colitis, intestinal lymphoma, and irritable bowel syndrome. In a prospective study of 87 such patients,[8] the most common diagnoses in order of frequency were laxative abuse (30), irritable bowel (14), idiopathic secretory diarrhea (13), and bile acid diarrhea (9).

Certain additional tests are needed in this group of patients. I usually perform them in the following sequence:

1. Alkalinization of the stools (to test for laxatives containing phenolphthalein)
2. Serum hormone levels (VIP, calcitonin, gastrin)
3. 48-hour fasting (to determine that the diarrhea is secretory and not related to absorption)
4. Stool electrolyte levels and osmolarity
5. Colonoscopy and multiple biopsies (to diagnose microscopic colitis)
6. Levels of fecal excretion of $^{14}$C-cholyglycine (to diagnose bile acid diarrhea), or a therapeutic trial of cholestyramine, which binds bile acids

In summary, the work-up of a patient with chronic diarrhea requires a sound understanding of the pathophysiologic mechanisms underlying the different causes of diarrhea, an accurate history, and common sense in choosing the right tests in the right order. Haphazard testing or a course of "order everything on the checklist" is frustrating, time consuming, expensive, and unrewarding.

## References

1. Donowitz M, Kokke FT, Saidi R: Evaluation of patients with chronic diarrhea, N Engl J Med 332:725-729, 1995.
2. Hutcheon DF, Bayless TM, Gadacz TR: Post-cholecystectomy diarrhea, JAMA 241:823-824, 1979.
3. Bayless TM, Rothfeld B, Massa C, et al: Lactose and milk intolerance: clinical implications, N Engl J Med 292:1156-1203, 1975.
4. Volta U, Molinaro N, Fusconi M, et al: IgA antiendomysial antibody test, Dig Dis Sci 36:752-756, 1991.
5. Toskas PP: Bentiromide as a test of exocrine pancreatic function in adult patients with pancreatic insufficiency, Gastroenterology 85:565-569, 1983.

6. Young JL, Miner PB: The differential diagnosis of inflammatory bowel disease, *Practical Gastroenterol* 19:10-22, 1995.
7. Medeloff AI, Monk M, Siegel CI, et al: Illness experience and life stresses in patients with irritable colon and with ulcerative colitis, *N Engl J Med* 282:14-17, 1970.
8. Read NW, Krejis GJ, Read MG, et al: Chronic diarrhea of unknown origin, *Gastroenterology* 78:264-271, 1980.

# Chapter 23

## *Elevated Transaminases*

Karim A. Fawaz

Measurement of the serum levels of hepatic enzymes and aminotransferases (transaminases) provides sensitive assessments of liver cell injury. Elevation of alanine aminotransferase (ALT), formerly referred to as serum glutamic pyruvic transaminase (SGPT), is more specific for liver cell injury. Elevation of aspartate aminotransferase (AST), formerly referred to as serum glutamic oxaloacetic (SGOT), also may be seen in myocardial and skeletal muscle injury. I am frequently asked to interpret the significance of elevated aminotransferases in a variety of clinical settings. The ease or the difficulty of correctly interpreting the data depends on several factors, including the availability of previous measurements, the results of other liver function tests, the results of serologic tests for hepatitis A, B, and C, and the general medical condition of the patient. Many patients are referred for asymptomatic aminotransferase elevations, with negative serologic markers for hepatitis, and it is not always easy to decide on how extensive an investigation is warranted.[1]

Aminotransferases normally are present in the serum in concentrations of less than 30 to 40 units per liter. Although the rise in serum aminotransferases does not correlate well with severity of liver disease, the level of aminotransferase elevation does frequently correlate with the type of liver cell injury. In general, elevations of up to eight to ten times the upper limit of normal are seen in any type of acute or chronic liver disease. Values in the low thousands or above are seen exclusively in disorders associated with acute extensive hepatocellular necrosis, such as viral and drug hepatitis and acute cardiocirculatory collapse.

The variety of liver diseases that result in elevated serum aminotransferases is extensive. To focus the differential diagnosis, I divide the aminotransferase elevations into two sections, that is, below or above 500 units per liter. This is an arbitrary but convenient way of highlighting the type of liver disease that a physician should consider first. Considerable overlap does exist between the two groups, however.

# AMINOTRANSFERASES ABOVE 500 UNITS

Aminotransferase elevations above 500 units are seen almost exclusively in conditions that are associated with acute hepatocellular necrosis. Acute viral hepatitis, the most common cause of acute hepatocellular necrosis, accounts for more than 95% of cases. Other likely causes include drug hepatitis and acute cardiocirculatory failure.

## Acute viral hepatitis

Three main types of viral hepatitis—A, B, and C—account for more than 95% of all episodes of acute viral hepatitis. Hepatitis D (the delta virus) occurs only in the presence of acute or chronic hepatitis B. Hepatitis E is similar to hepatitis A, but is extremely rare in the United States. Acute hepatitis attributable to the Epstein-Barr virus and to cytomegalovirus account for the remaining episodes. The prodromal symptoms of all types of hepatitis are similar and manifest as anorexia, nausea, malaise, and fatigue. A serum sickness-like syndrome may be seen with hepatitis B. The physical examination usually reveals tender hepatomegaly. Splenomegaly and atypical lymphocytes are more common in Epstein-Barr virus and cytomegalovirus infections than in hepatitis A, B, or C. The aminotransferases are usually about 500 units, except in the extremely early stages of the illness, but can rise to as high as several thousand units. The AST-to-ALT ratio is of no value in the differentiation of one type of hepatitis from the other. Aminotransferases tend to be lowest when the disease is caused by cytomegalovirus, Epstein-Barr virus, and hepatitis C, higher when caused by hepatitis A, and highest when caused by hepatitis B. Serum bilirubin elevation depends on the severity of the disease. Alkaline phosphatase is usually only mildly elevated, but in a third of patients with Epstein-Barr virus infection, it is disproportionately elevated (with respect to the rise in bilirubin).

The diagnosis of a particular type of viral hepatitis is established by serologic tests. Type A hepatitis is diagnosed by the presence of an IgM antibody to hepatitis A (anti-HAV, IgM). The presence of an IgG antibody to hepatitis A (anti-HAV, IgG) indicates either past exposure to or present infection with hepatitis A. The diagnosis of hepatitis B is made by the presence of a hepatitis B surface antigen (HBsAg). The physician, however, should remember that an acute hepatitis of a different type may be superimposed on a carrier state of hepatitis B in patients with a high risk of developing multiple episodes of viral hepatitis, such as male homosexuals, intravenous drug addicts, hemophiliacs, and dialysis patients. To confirm the diagnosis of acute hepatitis B in such cases, the presence of an IgM core antibody (anti-HBc) is necessary. The diagnosis of hepatitis C is made by the presence of antibody (anti-HCV). Unlike that in hepatitis A, the antibody to hepatitis C does not always show its presence during clinical symptoms, and it may take several months for it to become positive. The diagnosis of hepatitis

D is made by the presence of an antibody (anti-HDV), but keep in mind that the delta virus is a defective virus and needs the hepatitis B virus to survive. Epstein-Barr virus and cytomegalovirus hepatitis are best diagnosed by the presence of a rising titer of the corresponding antibody.

## Drug hepatitis

Drugs may cause three types of reaction in the liver: (1) hepatocellular necrosis, (2) cholestasis, and (3) mixed hepatocellular and cholestatic picture.

Aminotransferase levels above 500 units, in the range of acute viral hepatitis, are commonly seen with drugs that cause hepatocellular necrosis; in this setting the alkaline phosphatase level is normal or only slightly elevated. The degree of hyperbilirubinemia depends on the severity of the hepatitis. Aminotransferase values that are one to 10 times normal are seen with drugs that cause a predominantly cholestatic picture; there is a concomitant moderate to pronounced elevation of the alkaline phosphatase and the bilirubin. Drugs that cause a mixed picture are associated with a wide range of aminotransferase values. Drugs that cause hepatocellular necrosis produce their damage by two mechanisms:

1. *Direct hepatotoxicity.* The direct form is a dose-dependent type of hepatotoxicity that affects all subjects who are exposed to the offending agent. Examples of such agents are acetaminophen, carbon tetrachloride, and poisonous mushrooms.
2. *Hypersensitivity or metabolic idiosyncrasy.* The liver injury caused by drugs that belong to the hypersensitivity group by definition is not dose dependent. Liver injury produced by a hypersensitivity to a drug usually manifests itself clinically within 1 to 4 weeks and is frequently accompanied by fever, rash, and eosinophilia. When rechallenged with the drug, subjects exhibit immediate aminotransferase elevations. Common examples of such drugs are sulfonamides and *para*-aminosalicyclic acid.

   On the other hand, some drugs cause injury by the slow accumulation of toxic metabolites. The duration of exposure may be weeks or months, and the response to a rechallenge may be delayed. Isoniazid is a prime example of a drug that causes drug hepatitis by this mechanism. Both mechanisms of idiosyncrasy are suspected with some drugs, such as halothane and phenytoin.

The list of drugs that can cause hepatitis is virtually endless. In the following discussion I review the more commonly used agents that may cause hepatitis with aminotransferase elevations of about 500 units.

### Acetaminophen

Acetaminophen is a safe analgesic when taken in the usual therapeutic doses. However, ingestion of an overdose is a common method of attempted suicide. Hepatic necrosis and pronounced aminotransferase elevations may be seen in subjects who ingest more than 6 g. Doses that exceed 15 g are reported in 80% of fatal cases. Signs of hepatic necrosis appear when the plasma acetaminophen level exceeds 300 mg/mL at 4 hours after ingestion.[2] A correct, early diagnosis is crucial because therapy with acetylcysteine (Mucomyst) within 12 hours of ingestion of an acetaminophen overdose can be lifesaving.

### Halothane

Halothane is a widely used and relatively safe anesthetic, but on rare occasions it can cause fatal hepatitis. Obese, elderly females seem to be more susceptible. Halothane and related compounds always should be considered in the differential diagnosis of postoperative aminotransferase elevations. The average time between exposure to halothane and the onset of aminotransferase elevations is 1 week for a first exposure and as short as 3 days for repeat exposures. Fever, anorexia, vomiting, and eosinophilia are the most common associated findings. There is no treatment.

### Isoniazid

Isoniazid (INH) itself is not hepatotoxic, but its metabolite hydrazine has been implicated in the production of liver necrosis. Hydrazine produces subclinical hepatic injury in 12% to 20% of recipients. However, the aminotransferases are usually less than six times normal and eventually return to normal in the majority of subjects despite continuation of the drug.[3] Hepatitis from this agent is more common in older patients and in Orientals. The time of the onset of liver disease is within 2 months of the start of drug therapy in 50% of cases but may be as late as 12 months after drug commencement. I recommend that patients receiving isoniazid have liver function tests at monthly intervals.

## Acute cardiocirculatory failure

Aminotransferase elevations in the acute viral hepatitis range (and even higher) may be seen in patients who suffer from acute heart failure or from circulatory collapse.[4] The distinguishing feature of this entity is the fact that the aminotransferases quickly return to normal if the patient's circulation is restored to normal. It is not unusual to have values as high as 10,000 units fall to 100 to 200 units in 3 to 4 days. Such rapid recovery is not encountered in any other type of liver disease.

# AMINOTRANSFERASES BELOW 500 UNITS

## Alcoholic hepatitis

The majority of patients with alcoholic liver disease have a typical pattern of serum aminotransferase elevation. In 95% of cases, the AST is higher than the ALT, and both usually are below 300 units. Even in patients with severe acute alcoholic hepatitis, which carries a mortality of 20%, the aminotransferases are rarely above 300 units. The lower serum ALT level reflects the decreased synthesis of ALT in the liver secondary to a deficiency of pyridoxal phosphate in alcoholic liver disease.[5] Pyridoxal phosphate is required for ALT synthesis in the liver more than for AST synthesis. The AST-to-ALT ratio is usually of little value in distinguishing the different types of liver disease. If the ALT is below 300 units, an AST-to-ALT ratio of more than two is suggestive of alcoholic liver disease and a ratio of more than three is highly suggestive of alcoholic liver disease.[6]

Long-term heavy alcohol intake causes fatty infiltration of the liver in all subjects, but only 10% to 15% of those subjects develop alcoholic hepatitis or cirrhosis. Fat accumulation in the liver may cause an enlarged liver but does not usually lead to abnormalities in liver function tests except for occasional mild aminotransferase elevations. Symptomatic alcoholic hepatitis is usually associated with bilirubin elevation in addition to aminotransferase elevations. Such patients usually complain of fatigue, anorexia, nausea, and fever and have tender hepatomegaly and leukocytosis. The prothrombin time may be elevated, and the serum albumin may be low. Alcoholic hepatitis is a potentially reversible condition if cirrhosis has not yet developed. Alcoholic cirrhosis is manifested by hepatomegaly, splenomegaly, palmar erythema, and spider nevi. Liver function tests are the same as in alcoholic hepatitis, but a lower serum albumin level is more common with cirrhosis.

The diagnosis of alcoholic liver disease may be suspected by the history and the typical AST-to-ALT ratio, but it is established by liver biopsy. The decision to do a liver biopsy should be made on an individual basis after one weighs the risks and benefits of the procedure. For example, the risk of bleeding after a liver biopsy outweighs the benefit in a patient with a history of chronic heavy alcohol intake and the presence of massive ascites, a low platelet count, and a prothrombin time 3 seconds or more above control (with an INR >1.5).

## Chronic hepatitis

Chronic hepatitis, defined as a chronic inflammatory disease of the liver that persists for at least 6 months, is almost always associated with mild to moderate aminotransferase elevations. The most common cause of chronic hepatitis is viral, but other causes include drug hepatitis and autoimmune hepatitis.

One has to rely on the history and the results of serologic tests to determine the cause of elevated aminotransferases in chronic hepatitis. An accurate history is of paramount importance. Key information includes the duration of symptoms, medications, sexual habits, transfusions, and intravenous drug use. The two most important serologic tests are those for hepatitis B and hepatitis C. The presence of an HBsAg usually clinches the diagnosis of chronic hepatitis B, except in rare circumstances when the patient is a chronic carrier of hepatitis B and has a superimposed hepatitis C or smooth muscle antibody in high titers or drug hepatitis. The presence of an anti-HCV usually denotes chronic hepatitis C, but you should be aware that there are false-positive results particularly in patients with autoimmune hepatitis and hypergammaglobulinemia. The presence of an antinuclear antibody is consistent with autoimmune hepatitis, but its absence does not rule out this condition.

### Chronic viral hepatitis

Type A hepatitis does not cause chronic hepatitis because it is never associated with the presence of a chronic carrier state. In contrast, both types B and C hepatitis are common causes of chronic hepatitis and account for more than 95% of all cases of chronic hepatitis. Between 5% to 10% of patients with acute hepatitis B become chronic carriers. The chronic carrier state occurs predominantly in males and is more common in male homosexuals. The incidence of chronic hepatitis after an acute episode of hepatitis C is 50% to 70%.[7] Chronic hepatitis D can occur in patients with hepatitis B and is most commonly seen in drug addicts.

The presence of considerable overlap makes it impossible to differentiate between chronic persistent hepatitis (benign form) and chronic active hepatitis (may progress to cirrhosis) on the basis of the degree of aminotransferase elevations. In general, however, aminotransferases are usually below 250 units in chronic persistent hepatitis. When these levels are above 250 units, chronic active hepatitis is more likely. Occasionally, aminotransferases above 500 units are encountered during exacerbation of chronic active hepatitis B. Patients with chronic persistent hepatitis do not show any abnormalities in other liver function tests. In contrast, patients with chronic active hepatitis may have low albumin levels or elevated bilirubin, globulin, and alkaline phosphatase levels and an elevated prothrombin time. The physical examination usually reveals an enlarged liver in both conditions. When splenomegaly is present, chronic active hepatitis is much more likely. Remember, however, that patients with either condition may have only elevated aminotransferase levels, and the diagnosis of either cannot be established, short of performing a liver biopsy.

### Autoimmune hepatitis

The autoimmune type of chronic hepatitis most commonly affects young women and was formerly referred to as "lupoid hepatitis" because of the frequent presence of a positive lupus erythematosus (LE) cell in the serum. The distinguishing feature of this type of chronic hepatitis is its frequent association with extrahepatic manifestations, such as arthralgia, arthritis, skin rash, fever, and amenorrhea. An elevated sedimentation rate, an increase in gamma globulin, and a positive antinuclear antibody (ANA) or smooth muscle antibody (SMA) in titers above 1 : 40 are frequent associated laboratory findings.[8] Serum aminotransferases are usually below 500 units but may become higher during an acute exacerbation. Other liver function tests initially may be normal, but with progression of the disease the albumin level decreases and the bilirubin level rises. The correct diagnosis is important because this entity is the only known form of chronic hepatitis that responds to treatment.[9] Treatment is with corticosteroids and azathioprine.

### Chronic drug hepatitis

In general, most drugs cause an acute hepatitis; however, several drugs have been shown to cause chronic hepatitis. The common offenders are alpha-methyldopa, oxyphenisatin, isoniazid, and nitrofurantoin.

## Cirrhosis

The degree of aminotransferase elevation in cirrhosis depends on the cause and the activity of the disease. Patients with cirrhosis secondary to alcohol, schistosomiasis, hemochromatosis, and alpha$_1$-antitrypsin deficiency tend to have a mild elevation of aminotransferases. Patients with cirrhosis secondary to chronic active hepatitis, Wilson's disease, sclerosing cholangitis, and primary biliary cirrhosis tend to have higher elevations. Because any of these diseases reach an end-stage form, the aminotransferases decrease and may even become within the normal range. Therefore a decline in aminotransferases should not always be interpreted as a good prognostic sign. The serum bilirubin and the liver function tests that reflect the synthetic ability of the liver, such as albumin and prothrombin time, are the more important and useful tests to follow in the patient with progressive cirrhosis. The diagnosis of cirrhosis is established by the performance of a liver biopsy, but it should be emphasized that the cause of the cirrhosis cannot always be determined by the biopsy.

## Bile duct obstruction

Bile duct obstruction secondary to gallstones, tumor, pancreatitis, and postoperative strictures may be accompanied by mild aminotransferase elevations. Occasionally, high values reaching 1000 units may be seen in the first 24 to 48 hours after an acute bile duct obstruction secondary to gallstones. However, these values usually drop to below 300 units soon thereafter. As the aminotransferases drop, the alkaline phosphatase and the bilirubin rise if the obstructing stone does not pass spontaneously. A right upper quadrant ultrasound is the first screening test if common bile duct obstruction is suspected.

## Congestive heart failure

Patients with congestive heart failure may have mild aminotransferase elevations accompanied by an elevated alkaline phosphatase two to three times normal and, in some instances, a mild bilirubin elevation. The presence of congested neck veins, tender hepatomegaly, and a hepatojugular reflux on physical examination should alert the physician to this condition as the cause of aminotransferase elevations. A liver biopsy specimen shows passive congestion around the central veins, but biopsy is only rarely indicated.

## Fatty infiltration of the liver

Fat accumulation in the liver (with hepatomegaly) secondary to alcohol, diabetes, obesity, hyperlipemia, and postintestinal bypass surgery may cause a rise in aminotransferases up to six to eight times normal. The diagnosis requires a liver biopsy. In patients with hyperlipemia, control of the serum lipids by diet or by medications, or both, is advised before a liver biopsy is performed. A return of the serum aminotransferases to the normal range with normalization of the serum lipids is the rule rather than the exception, and biopsy can be obviated. Nonalcoholic steatohepatitis is a condition that may progress to cirrhosis and its pathologic characteristics almost mimic alcoholic liver disease. The only way to diagnose this condition is by a liver biopsy, and recently this condition has been reported in people who are not even overweight.

## Other conditions

Other conditions that cause mild serum aminotransferase elevations are intravenous hyperalimentation, granulomatous hepatitis, primary or metastatic liver cancer, sarcoidosis, amyloidosis, hepatic vein thrombosis, pericholangitis associated with inflammatory bowel disease, primary sclerosing cholangitis, myocardial infarction, hemolysis, and myositis. In the last three conditions the AST elevation is significantly higher than that of ALT and should be differentiated from alcoholic liver disease (in which the AST is also higher than the ALT).

*References*

1. Goddard CJ, Warnes TW: Raised liver enzymes in asymptomatic patients: investigation and outcome, *Dig Dis Sci* 10:218-226, 1992.
2. Hamlyn AN: The spectrum of paracetamol (acetaminophen) overdose: clinical and epidemiological studies, *Postgrad Med J* 54:400-404, 1978.
3. Mitchell JR, Zimmerman HJ, Ishak KG, et al: Isoniazid liver injury: clinical spectrum, pathology, and probable pathogenesis, *Ann Intern Med* 84:181-192, 1976.
4. Johnson RD, O'Connor ML, Kerr RM: Extreme serum elevations of aspartate aminotransferases, *Am J Gastroenterol* 90:1244-1245, 1995.
5. Diehl AM, Potter J, Boitnott J, et al: Relationship between pyridoxal 5'-phosphate deficiency and aminotransferase levels in alcoholic hepatitis, *Gastroenterology* 86:632-636, 1984.
6. Matloff DS, Selinger MJ, Kaplan MM: Hepatic transaminase activity in alcoholic liver disease, *Gastroenterology* 78:1389-1392, 1980.
7. Alter HJ, Purcell RH, Shih JW, et al: Detection of antibody to hepatitis C virus in prospectively followed transfusion recipients with acute and chronic non-A, non-B hepatitis, *N Engl J Med* 321:1494-1500, 1989.
8. Johnson PJ, McFarlane IC: Meeting report, International Autoimmune Hepatitis Group, *Hepatology* 18:998-1005, 1993.
9. Maddrey WC, Combes B: Therapeutic concepts for the management of idiopathic autoimmune chronic hepatitis, *Sem Liver Dis* 11:248-256, 1991.

# Chapter 24

# *Clinical Approach to Jaundice*

Karim A. Fawaz

Bilirubin, a breakdown product of heme, is produced in the reticuloendothelial system. The sequence of the reaction is as follows:

$$Heme \xrightarrow{\text{Heme oxygenase}} Biliverdin$$

$$Biliverdin \xrightarrow{\text{Biliverdin reductase}} Bilirubin$$

Fat-soluble, not water-soluble, bilirubin has to be bound by albumin to be transported in blood to the liver where it is conjugated to glucuronic acid. The conjugated bilirubin, now water-soluble, is transported into the bile canaliculi by an energy-requiring process that seems to be the rate-limiting step in bilirubin metabolism.

The traditional van den Bergh assay for measuring bilirubin, still used in most laboratories, measures both the total bilirubin and the direct fraction; the indirect fraction is the difference between the total and direct levels. The direct and indirect fractions are approximate determinations of the conjugated and unconjugated bilirubin, respectively. Newer and more accurate methods of bilirubin measurement are replacing the van den Bergh method in some laboratories. One such method that is increasingly gaining acceptance is based on photographic film technology. Three fractions of bilirubin are reported by this method: unconjugated bilirubin, conjugated bilirubin, and delta bilirubin; the delta bilirubin is conjugated bilirubin bound to albumin.[1] The fractionation of bilirubin differentiates jaundice caused by hemolysis or by Gilbert's disease (indirect hyperbilirubinemia) from jaundice caused by hepatobiliary disease (direct hyperbilirubinemia). The challenge to the physician lies primarily in the differential diagnosis of direct hyperbilirubinemia. The central clinical question is: Is the elevated direct bilirubin secondary to liver disease or to bile duct obstruction; that is, is the jaundice medical or is it surgical?

The evaluation of the patient who presents with jaundice must be rigorous, thorough, and systematic. The initial impression is based on the history and physical examination. Liver function tests help to confirm or refute the initial clinical impression and to point to the next step. If common bile duct obstruction is suspected, noninvasive radiologic studies are required to confirm the suspicion. Invasive radiologic or endoscopic diagnostic procedures may be indicated, depending on the results of the workup to that point.[2] If hepatocellular disease is suspected, serologic tests should be ordered, and, depending on the clinical picture, liver biopsy may be required to make a definitive diagnosis.

# CLINICAL CLUES

## History

When one is taking a history, several features such as age, exposure, and type of presentation help formulate the initial impression. Viral hepatitis is more common in the younger age group, whereas malignant obstruction is more common over 60 years of age. Alcoholic liver disease is not common before 30 years of age but may occur at any time later. Choledocholithiasis is more common over 40 years of age. A history of exposure to friends or to family members with known viral hepatitis, a history of needle sticks, a history of exposure to dialysis patients, a history of intravenous drug use, and a history of blood transfusion should direct attention toward the strong possibility of viral hepatitis. A history of heavy alcohol intake is suggestive of alcoholic liver disease, but a history of a recent or a chronic drug intake makes drug-induced hepatitis a likely contender.

The type of onset of jaundice and the associated symptoms also is helpful in formulating the initial clinical impression. The sudden onset of jaundice, preceded or accompanied by constitutional symptoms of fatigue, loss of appetite, nausea, and vomiting, is typical for hepatitis. On the other hand, the gradual onset of jaundice without constitutional symptoms is typical of malignant obstruction and is sometimes recognized by relatives or friends, rather than the patient. The presence of fever, chills, and colicky abdominal pain associated with jaundice is suggestive of choledocholithiasis. High-grade fever and abdominal pain are not common in parenchymal liver disease, except for alcoholic hepatitis and infectious mononucleosis. Itching, more common in obstructive jaundice, can be the earliest symptom in primary biliary cirrhosis[3] and is common in other conditions causing intrahepatic cholestasis. Jaundice and an elevated alkaline phosphatase in a patient with inflammatory bowel disease should raise the suspicion of primary sclerosing cholangitis.[4,5] A history of dark urine indicates the presence of direct bilirubin in the urine. Patients with hemolysis and Gilbert's disease do not excrete dark urine because the elevated bilirubin is indirect and hence bound to albumin, which does not traverse the glomerular membrane. Postoperative jaundice, especially after long abdominal or cardiac surgery with large transfusion requirements, should alert the physician to the possibility of benign postoperative jaundice. Prolonged hypotension during surgery or associated with cardiac shock makes the diagnosis of ischemic liver damage the most likely cause of jaundice.

## Physical examination

The size of the liver is not an important differentiating sign between parenchymal and obstructive liver disease because hepatomegaly occurs in both conditions. A firm and nodular liver is seen in cirrhosis and in primary or metastatic cancer of the liver. Although an enlarged spleen is suggestive of the presence of portal hypertension (and hence the presence of chronic liver disease), splenomegaly also is present in infectious mononucleosis and in up to 20% of patients with acute hepatitis. The presence of ascites and stigmas of chronic liver disease, such as abdominal collaterals, spider nevi, and palmar erythema, are diagnostic of cirrhosis. A gallbladder not tender to palpation is suggestive of malignant obstruction of the common bile duct below the takeoff of the cystic duct. When the gallbladder is palpable and tender, empyema of the gallbladder secondary to cystic duct obstruction by a stone should be suspected.

## Hemogram

A sudden drop in hematocrit without evidence of bleeding is suggestive of a hemolytic process as the cause of jaundice; the majority of the bilirubin should be indirect. Leukocytosis with a left shift, commonly seen in choledocholithiasis and alcoholic hepatitis, is uncommon in viral hepatitis and malignant obstruction. The presence of pancytopenia should alert the clinician to the possibility of chronic liver disease, portal hypertension, and hypersplenism. Atypical lymphocytosis is seen in viral infections, particularly infectious mononucleosis. Finally, eosinophilia should raise the possibility of drug-induced hepatitis.

## Liver function tests

Although an individual liver function test abnormality may be characteristic of a certain type of hepatobiliary disease, it is essential that it be interpreted in the context of other liver function test abnormalities (Table 24-1), the time period from the onset of the illness, and the whole clinical setting. A perfect example is acute common bile duct obstruction secondary to a stone. In the first 24 to 48 hours the aminotransferases may be greatly elevated and in the range of hepatitis, whereas the bilirubin and alkaline phosphatase may be minimally elevated. With time, however, the aminotransferases drop quickly, whereas the bilirubin and alkaline phosphatase continue to rise.

**Bilirubin.** Elevation of the serum bilirubin level may occur in response to the following pathophysiologic mechanisms:

1. Overproduction of bilirubin, such as hemolysis
2. Impaired uptake or conjugation of bilirubin, such as Gilbert's syndrome
3. Impaired hepatic excretion of bilirubin, such as Dubin-Johnson syndrome, obstruction, or cholestasis

**Table 24-1.** *Liver function test abnormalities in various conditions*

| Condition | Bilirubin | Alkaline phosphatase | Aminotransferases |
|---|---|---|---|
| HEMOLYSIS | 2 to 6 × N* | N | N |
| **DEFECTS IN BILIRUBIN METABOLISM** | | | |
| Gilbert's syndrome | 2 to 6 × N | N | N |
| Dubin-Johnson syndrome | 2 to 6 × N | N | N |
| Rotor's syndrome | 2 to 6 × N | N | N |
| **HEPATOCELLULAR DISEASE** | | | |
| Viral hepatitis | N to 40 × N | N to 3 × N† | 10 to 100 × N (ALT > AST) |
| Drug-induced hepatitis | N to 40 × N | N to 3 × N | 5 to 100 × N (ALT > AST) |
| Alcoholic hepatitis | N to 40 × N | N to 3 × N | 2 to 8 × N (AST > ALT) |
| Chronic active hepatitis | N to 15 × N | N to 3 × N | 2 to 10 × N |
| Cirrhosis | N to 20 × N | N to 3 × N | N to 3 × N |
| **CHOLESTATIC LIVER DISEASE** | | | |
| Drug-induced hepatitis | N to 40 × N | 2 to 10 × N | N to 8 × N |
| Primary biliary cirrhosis | N to 40 × N | 3 to 20 × N | N to 5 × N |
| Sclerosing cholangitis | N to 40 × N | 3 to 10 × N | N to 10 × N |
| **EXTRAHEPATIC OBSTRUCTION** | | | |
| Common bile duct stone | N to 15 × N | 2 to 15 × N | N to 8 × N‡ |
| Malignant obstruction | N to 40 × N | 3 to 10 × N | N to 5 × N |
| **INFILTRATIVE DISEASE** | | | |
| Tumor | N to 5 × N | 2 to 15 × N | N to 8 × N (AST > ALT) |
| Sarcoidosis | N to 5 × N | 2 to 8 × N | N to 5 × N |

N, Normal.
* Indirect bilirubin.
† Higher in Epstein-Barr virus infection.
‡ Initially increased.

4. Regurgitation of unconjugated and conjugated bilirubin from damaged liver cells, such as in hepatitis

In general, the presence of an elevated bilirubin level without any other abnormality in liver function tests indicates the presence of hemolysis or a genetic abnormality in bilirubin metabolism. The exception to this rule is the occasional patient with inactive stable cirrhosis. Fractionation of the bilirubin narrows the differential diagnosis; indirect hyperbilirubinemia is suggestive *only* of hemolysis or Gilbert's syndrome, whereas direct hyperbilirubinemia is suggestive *only* of Dubin-Johnson syndrome or Rotor's syndrome. When hyperbilirubinemia is associated with other liver function test abnormalities, the degree of elevation is not helpful in the differential diagnosis.

**Alkaline phosphatase.** Extrahepatic obstruction and intrahepatic cholestasis stimulate the renewed production of the hepatic enzyme alkaline phosphatase. Thus the serum alkaline phosphatase is moderately to considerably elevated (three to 10 times normal) in such instances. On the other hand, acute or chronic hepatocellular disease is associated with only minor elevation of alkaline phosphatase, usually less than three times normal.

**Aminotransferases.** The aminotransferases—alanine aminotransferase (ALT); (formerly serum glutamic-pyruvic transaminase, SGPT) and aspartate aminotransferase (AST); (formerly serum glutamic-oxaloacetic transaminase, SGOT)—are usually much higher in acute hepatocellular diseases than with extrahepatic obstruction and intrahepatic cholestasis. The values are highest in acute viral hepatitis and drug-induced hepatitis; usually the ALT is higher or equal to the AST (10 to 100 times normal). There are some exceptions to this rule; the two most frequent exceptions are alcoholic liver disease and acute gallstone obstruction of the biliary tract.

Although acute alcoholic hepatitis is a hepatocellular disease, the aminotransferases are rarely above 300 units (less than eight times normal), and characteristically the AST is higher than the ALT. On the other hand, acute gallstone obstruction of the common bile duct may be associated with pronounced elevation of the aminotransferases, particularly in the first 48 hours (up to 25 times normal). However, they drop quickly to less than eight times normal. Hepatic enzymes, other than aminotransferases, often are measured in a battery of liver function tests. One example is lactate dehydrogenase, the highest levels of which are seen in hepatocellular carcinoma and liver metastases.

**Prothrombin time.** Prothrombin, produced by the liver, requires vitamin K for its production. The prothrombin time could be elevated in hepatocellular and obstructive liver disease because of different mechanisms. An elevated prothrombin time that does not correct with the intramuscular injection of vitamin K indicates severe liver disease because it reflects the inability of the diseased liver to produce prothrombin. On the other hand, if the prothrombin time returns to normal after the administration of vitamin K, the presence of vitamin K malabsorption is established. Vitamin K, being fat-soluble, may be malabsorbed in obstructive jaundice because of inadequate micelle formation owing to the lack of bile salts in the small intestine.

**Serum proteins.** Generally, serum protein determinations are not helpful in the differential diagnosis of acute jaundice. They may, however, be helpful in cirrhosis. In severe cirrhosis the serum albumin is usually low, whereas hypergammaglobulinemia is more characteristic of Laënnec's cirrhosis and of autoimmune chronic active hepatitis.

**Serologic studies.** When acute or chronic hepatitis is suspected as the cause of jaundice, serologic tests such as antibody to hepatitis A virus (anti-HIV), hepatitis B surface antigen (HBsAG), and antibody to hepatitis C (anti-HCV) are indicated. Antibody to delta hepatitis (anti-HDV) is indicated in patients with severe acute hepatitis B or exacerbation of known chronic hepatitis B. If primary biliary cirrhosis is suspected, antimitochondrial antibody (AMA) should be done. Other tests such as smooth muscle antibody (SMA) and antinuclear antibody (ANA) are indicated if autoimmune hepatitis is suspected.

### Radiologic noninvasive studies

The history, physical examination, and laboratory tests provide the data for the initial impression. If common bile duct obstruction is suspected, one of two noninvasive radiologic studies is indicated—ultrasonography (ECHO) or computerized tomography (CT) scanning. Both techniques give the needed information regarding the size of the bile duct. Ultrasonography is more readily available, quicker, and cheaper than the other. Its disadvantage is that overlying gas often hinders adequate visualization of the pancreas and retroperitoneal structures. The CT scan provides more information about the pancreas, retroperitoneum, and liver; its disadvantage lies in its high cost and lack of availability. I believe that the best screening test to rule out extrahepatic obstruction is ultrasonography.[6] The common bile duct is considered dilated if it measures more than 6 to 8 mm in diameter depending on whether there is a previous history of cholecystectomy or a history suggestive of passage of gallstones. False-negative results can occur with both techniques if the obstruction is intermittent or of short duration.

### Invasive endoscopic or radiologic studies

The decision to perform an invasive procedure to visualize the biliary system usually is made after one finds a dilated bile duct by ultrasonography or by CT scan. These procedures, however, may be indicated when the noninvasive radiologic tests are equivocal or when the clinical suspicion of biliary tract obstruction is high. The two invasive techniques that visualize the biliary tree are endoscopic retrograde cholangiopancreatography (ERCP) and percutaneous transhepatic cholangiography (PTC). These techniques have diagnostic as well as therapeutic capabilities.[7-9] Endoscopic sphincterotomy of the ampulla of Vater, stone extraction, and biliary stent placement for drainage may be accomplished by ERCP, whereas external and internal drainage may be accomplished by PTC. Several factors deserve consideration before one of these procedures is carried out:

1. Suspected cause of the obstruction
2. General condition of the patient
3. Availability of the test
4. Skill of the operator in diagnostic and therapeutic maneuvers
5. Long-term plan of treatment

For example, if a common bile duct stone is suspected, the procedure of choice is ERCP with endoscopic sphincterotomy and stone extraction, which has a success rate of 90% to 95%. If cancer of the pancreas or chronic pancreatitis causing common bile duct obstruction is suspected (and the patient is a good surgical candidate), ERCP is superior because it may visualize the pancreatic duct, help to confirm the diagnosis, and delineate the extent of the disease before surgery. If a proximal common bile duct obstruction is suspected and surgery is *not* being considered, ERCP or PTC can provide biliary tract drainage after insertion of a stent.[10] In general, ERCP with stent placement is the procedure of choice for the palliative treatment of malignant obstruction particularly if the obstruction is in the distal part of the common bile duct.[11]

## Liver biopsy

Liver biopsy is not indicated in acute hepatitis but is desirable if chronic hepatitis or cirrhosis is suspected. Biopsy helps to differentiate the different types of cirrhosis, such as Laënnec's cirrhosis, postnecrotic cirrhosis, primary biliary cirrhosis, hemochromatosis, and Wilson's disease.

In conclusion, I believe the approach to the jaundiced patient must be a stepwise one using the information initially obtained by the history, physical findings, and liver function tests. Recent advances in radiologic and endoscopic techniques have greatly improved our diagnostic accuracy and provided nonsurgical therapeutic options not available a decade ago.

## References

1. Weiss JS: The clinical importance of a protein-bound fraction of serum bilirubin in patients with hyperbilirubinemia, *N Engl J Med* 309:147-150, 1983.
2. Richter JM, Silverstein MD, Schapiro R: Suspected obstructive jaundice: a decision analysis of diagnostic strategies, *Ann Intern Med* 99:46-51, 1983.
3. Kaplan MM: Primary biliary cirrhosis, *N Engl J Med* 316:521-528, 1987.
4. Olson R, Danielsson A, Jarnerol G, et al: Prevalence of primary sclerosing cholangitis in patients with ulcerative colitis, *Gastroenterology* 100:1319-1323, 1991.
5. Lee YM, Kaplan MM: Primary sclerosing cholangitis, *N Engl J Med* 332:924-933, 1995.
6. Matzen P, Malchow-Moller A, Brun B, et al: Ultrasonography, computed tomography, and cholescintigraphy in suspected obstructive jaundice—a prospective comparative study, *Gastroenterology* 84:1492-1497, 1983.
7. Elias F, Hamlyn AN, Jain S, et al: A randomized trial of percutaneous transhepatic cholangiography with the Chiba needle versus endoscopic retrograde

cholangiography for bile duct visualization in jaundice, *Gastroenterology* 71:439-443, 1976.

8. Zimmin DS, Chang J, Clemett AR: Advances in the management of bile duct obstruction, *Med Clin North Am* 63:593-609, 1979.

9. Kozarek RA, Sanowski RA: Nonsurgical management of extrahepatic obstructive jaundice, *Ann Intern Med* 96:743-745, 1982.

10. Frank BB, and members of the patient care committee of the American Gastroenterological Association: Clinical evaluation of jaundice: a guideline of the patient care committee of the American Gastroenterological Association, *JAMA* 262:3031-3034, 1989.

11. Consensus of the American Society for Gastrointestinal Endoscopy: Endoscopic therapy of biliary and pancreatic disease, *Gastrointest Endosc* 37:117-119, 1991.

# Chapter 25

# *Ascites*

Karim A. Fawaz

Ascites, the accumulation of fluid in the abdominal cavity, is derived from the Greek word *askos,* which means a 'sack' or a 'bag'.[1] Many causes of ascites exist, but most cases, particularly in an urban setting, are attributable to chronic liver disease.

## HISTORY AND PHYSICAL EXAMINATION

Routine examination of the abdomen to detect ascites, though desirable, is not usually performed. So what features in the history and physical exam would make the physician check for ascites more carefully? The following are some of the important clues:

- A history of:
  Alcohol abuse or known chronic liver disease
  Malignancy
  Heart failure
  Hypothyroidism
  Nephrotic syndrome
  Rapid weight loss or weight gain with increase in abdominal girth
  Chronic recurrent pancreatitis or severe acute pancreatitis
- Physical findings of:
  Icterus, palmer erythema, spider angiomas, abdominal collateral veins, temporal or upper extremity muscle wasting
  Hepatomegaly or splenomegaly
  Distended neck veins, rales, hepatojugular reflux, peripheral edema
  Evidence of significant weight loss
  Protuberant abdomen or bulging flanks

In general, abdominal fluid accumulation of 1500 mL or more is needed for ascites to be detected by physical examination.[2] The absence of flank dullness in the supine position usually denotes the absence of ascites, whereas the presence of flank dullness indicates the need to perform the maneuvers necessary to detect shifting dullness, which is a much more reliable finding in the diagnosis of ascites than the presence of a fluid wave or puddle sign. An obese abdomen or dilated small bowel loops partially filled with fluid sometimes can be mistaken for ascites. If one is in doubt, it is preferable to obtain an abdominal ultrasonogram to document the presence of ascites, particularly if paracentesis is contemplated. As little as 100 mL of fluid can be detected by ultrasound.[3]

# ABDOMINAL PARACENTESIS

The location and technique of an abdominal paracentesis are important in making it a safe procedure. The most common complication of paracentesis is bleeding; fortunately it is rare even in the presence of coagulopathy. The safest location to insert a needle is in the midline below the umbilicus and above the urinary bladder. The midline is avascular, contrary to the flanks, which are vascular. Thus, unless there is a surgical scar or an evident collateral vein, I choose the midline for insertion of the needle after asking the patient to void and to assume a semireclining position. The manner in which the needle is introduced is important in patients with tense ascites who could develop continued leakage of fluid after the needle is removed; the use of the Z-tract technique minimizes leakage.[1] The Z-tract is created when one moves the skin about 2 cm inferiorly in relation to the abdominal muscle wall and then introduces the needle. When fluid begins to flow, the skin is released; so when the needle is removed, the skin assumes its original position and covers the needle entry site into the abdominal wall. If the needle is introduced straight without a Z-tract, it becomes easier for the fluid to leak out because of the straight pathway created.[1]

# ANALYSIS OF ASCITIC FLUID

## Gross appearance

The gross appearance of ascitic fluid sometimes is helpful in determining the cause of ascites. Sterile cirrhotic ascites is transparent and yellow tinged, infected ascitic fluid is cloudy, chylous ascites is milky, malignant ascites may be bloody (22% of malignant ascites is hemorrhagic[4]), and ascites secondary to a bile leak or hemorrhagic pancreatitis often is very dark.

## Protein

Traditionally ascites had been classified as transudate (protein less than 2.5 g/dL) or exudate (protein equal to or more than 2.5 g/dL).[5] Recently the serum-ascites albumin gradient has replaced the exudate-transudate concept. One measures the serum-ascites albumin gradient by subtracting the ascitic albumin (not the total protein) concentration from the serum albumin measured the same day. Patients with gradients of 1.1 g/dL or more have a 97% chance of having portal hypertension, whereas patients with a gradient of less than 1.1 g/dL do not have portal hypertension.[6] In contrast, the old exudate-transudate concept gave the correct classification of ascites in only 56% of instances.[6] The two main reasons for the discrepancy were (1) the low ascitic fluid protein concentration in spontaneous bacterial peritonitis (traditionally expected to be an exudate) and (2) the high ascitic fluid protein concentration in cardiac ascites (traditionally believed to be a transudate).[6]

I favor taking into consideration the serum-ascites albumin gradient as well as the total protein in the ascitic fluid. For example, both cirrhotic ascites and cardiac ascites have a serum-ascites albumin gradient of 1.1 g/dL or more, but if total ascitic fluid protein is measured, it is below 2.5 g/dL in cirrhotic ascites and 2.5 g/dL or more in cardiac ascites.

## White blood cell count
The total ascitic white blood cell (WBC) count and the absolute neutrophil count are important in the diagnosis of infected peritoneal fluid. Keep in mind that the WBC count in the ascitic fluid may increase after diuresis because the WBCs leave the peritoneal cavity more slowly than water does. In general, bacterial infection of the peritoneal fluid is associated with an increase in the absolute neutrophil count, except in tuberculous peritonitis where the increase is mainly in lymphocytes. I adhere to the following measurements of the absolute neutrophil count with respect to the likelihood of ascitic fluid bacterial infection: (1) no infection—neutrophil count less than 250 cells/$\mu$L, (2) definite infection—neutrophil count more than 500 cells/$\mu$L, (c) probable infection—neutrophil count 250 to 500 cells/$\mu$L.

## Culture
There is great variance in the reported sensitivity of bacterial cultures in detecting bacterial growth in ascitic fluid depending on the method of culture employed. The inoculation of agar plates is inferior to culturing ascitic fluid as if it were blood (blood culture method), and bedside inoculation of blood culture bottles has been shown to be superior to delayed inoculation in the laboratory.[7]

## Other tests
Cytology, amylase, bilirubin, and triglycerides are requested when malignancy, pancreatic ascites, bile leak, and chylous ascites respectively are suspected. Ascitic fluid glucose, lactate dehydrogenase, and pH determinations are rarely helpful, and I almost never order their measurement.

# CAUSES OF ASCITES

There are many causes of ascites (see box on p. 233), but liver cirrhosis is by far the major etiologic factor. In a series reported by Runyon[8] on the various causes of ascites in the United States, 81% had cirrhosis, 10% cancer, 3% heart failure, 2% tuberculosis, 1% pancreatic disease, 1% dialysis, and 2% other causes.

## Etiology of Ascites

### LIVER DISEASE

Cirrhosis
Fulminant hepatitis

### MALIGNANCY

Peritoneal carcinomatosis
Liver metastasis
Lymph node obstruction (chylous ascites)

### HEPATIC VEIN THROMBOSIS

### CARDIAC DISEASE

Heart failure
Constrictive pericarditis
Right atrial myxoma

### INFECTION

Bacterial
  Spontaneous
  Secondary
Tuberculosis
Fungal
*Chlamydia* bacteria in females

### PANCREATIC

### RENAL

Nephrotic syndrome
Ascites of dialysis

### MISCELLANEOUS

Bile leak
Eosinophilic gastroenteritis (serosal involvement)
Granulomatous peritonitis
Vasculitis (serositis)

## Cirrhotic ascites
### Pathophysiology

There are two theories of ascites formation in patients with cirrhosis: the *underfill* and *overflow* theories.[9] The underfill theory maintains that an alteration in hepatic and splanchnic hemodynamics causes lymph to ooze into the peritoneal cavity, resulting in a decrease in effective plasma volume and stimulating the kidney to increase sodium and water reabsorption. The overflow theory maintains that the primary event is renal sodium retention leading to plasma volume expansion and overflow of fluid into the peritoneum in a setting of altered hepatic and splanchnic hemodynamics.

The most recent explanation of ascites formation proposes a new pathophysiologic mechanism: peripheral arterial vasodilatation. Proponents of this theory believe that both the underfill and overflow mechanisms are in operation at different stages as illustrated in the following scheme: peripheral arterial vasodilatation → sodium and water retention → overflow of fluid from hepatic sinusoids in a setting of increased intrahepatic pressure → *ascites* → decreased effective intravascular volume → increased secretion of renin, aldosterone, and antidiuretic hormone → sodium and water retention → *ascites.*[10]

## Diagnosis

Sterile cirrhotic ascites is usually straw-colored and transparent. The serum-ascites albumin gradient is >1.1 g/dL, and the absolute neutrophil count is less than 250 cells/$\mu$L.

## Complications

**Spontaneous bacterial peritonitis (SBP).** Spontaneous bacterial peritonitis (SBP), a serious complication of cirrhotic ascites, is associated with a mortality as high as 30% in some series. The diagnosis should be suspected whenever there is an unexplained deterioration in liver function, renal function, or mental function even if there are no signs or symptoms of peritonitis. The standard of diagnosis is a positive ascitic fluid culture, but because of the differences in ascitic fluid culture methods employed in different hospitals (and hence different sensitivity and results), the absolute neutrophil count is critical as discussed earlier. In general, if there is high clinical suspicion of SBP and the absolute neutrophil count in the ascitic fluid is more than 250 cells/$\mu$L, I believe it prudent to treat the patients with antibiotics even if the ascitic fluid culture is negative. The bacteria most commonly cultured are gram-negative rods and gram-positive cocci (pneumococcus and streptococcus); anaerobes are not common. The choice of antibiotics before culture results are available should be directed accordingly.

**Hepatic hydrothorax.** Pleural effusions are not uncommon in patients with cirrhosis and ascites. The effusion is usually right-sided and unilateral but could be left-sided or bilateral. Fluid accumulates in the pleural cavity by direct extension of ascitic fluid through microscopic or macroscopic holes in the diaphragm. Some patients have barely detectable ascites in the face of a large pleural effusion. This phenomenon is explained by the preferential movement of fluid to the pleural space because of the presence of a negative intrathoracic pressure compared to the intra-abdominal pressure.

## Treatment

Restriction of dietary sodium intake and diuretic therapy are the usual mainstays of treatment. Restriction of water is not necessary unless there is an associated dilutional hyponatremia. The most effective regimen is a combination of spironolactone and furosemide with a reasonable starting daily dose being 100 mg of spironolactone and 40 mg of furosemide.[8] There is no evidence that divided doses are better than one dose. In general the presence of leg edema seems to protect against the development of prerenal azotemia secondary to diuretic use.

Some patients do not respond to diuretics or develop prerenal azotemia. What options are available for these patients? Other modalities include therapeutic paracentesis, peritoneovenous shunt, transjugular intrahepatic portosystemic shunt (TIPS), and liver transplantation. Therapeutic paracentesis (up to 5 liters) has been shown to be effective and safe with and without simultaneous intravenous albumin administration (8 g of albumin for every liter of ascitic fluid removed). The peritoneovenous shunt has fallen out of favor because of its high occlusion rate and the high risk of bleeding secondary to disseminated intravascular coagulation in patients whose disease is already associated with coagulation abnormalities. The TIPS procedure is a shunt between the hepatic vein and the portal vein that is accomplished in the radiology special procedure department under local anesthesia and fluoroscopic guidance. Physiologically, TIPS acts like a surgical side-to-side portacaval shunt. Originally devised to treat patients with variceal bleeding, TIPS recently has been used to treat diuretic-resistant ascites with a more than 50% success rate. The TIPS cannot be performed if there is an associated portal vein thrombosis because of technical problems or if there is significant hepatic encephalopathy because any type of portosystemic shunt will worsen encephalopathy.

## Malignant ascites
Malignant ascites caused by peritoneal carcinomatosis is formed by exudation of protein-rich fluid from the malignant cells studding the peritoneum. In patients with massive liver metastasis or large hepatocellular carcinoma, the mechanism of ascites formation remains unknown.[1] It is presumed that obstruction of the portal or hepatic veins causes portal hypertension, which may contribute to ascites formation. There is an interesting difference in the ascitic fluid analysis between the two main types of malignant ascites.[2] In peritoneal carcinomatosis the fluid cytology results are more likely to be positive, and the serum-ascites albumin gradient is less than 1.1 g/dL, whereas in space-occupying lesions of the liver, whether primary or metastatic, the cytology is more likely to be negative, and the serum-ascites albumin gradient is usually equal to or more than 1.1 g/dL.

## Cardiac ascites
The mechanism of ascites formation in cardiac ascites is leakage of fluid from congested hepatic sinusoids,[11] which is similar to the mechanism of ascites formation in cirrhosis where an elevated portal pressure causes high pressure in the sinusoids. Cardiac ascites is an exudate by the old definition but the serum-ascites albumin gradient is equal or more than 1.1 g/dL. It can be seen in patients with high or low output heart failure, constrictive pericarditis, and an obstructing right atrial myxoma.

## Other causes of ascites

Other causes include tuberculosis peritonitis (serum-ascites albumin gradient less than 1.1 g/dL and elevated WBC count with lymphocytosis), pancreatic ascites (serum-ascites albumin gradient less than 1.1 g/dL and elevated amylase in the ascitic fluid), bile leak (high bilirubin and bilious dark color), chylous ascites (white creamy ascitic fluid and high triglycerides), and nephrotic syndrome (serum-ascites albumin gradient less than 1.1 g/dL, proteinuria, elevated serum cholesterol).[6]

## References

1. Runyon BA: Ascites. In Schiff L, Schiff ER, editors: *Diseases of the liver,* ed 7, Philadelphia, 1993, Lippincott, pp 990-1015.
2. Cattau EL, Benjamin SB, Knuff TE, et al: The accuracy of the physical exam in the diagnosis of suspected ascites, *JAMA* 247:1164-1166, 1982.
3. Goldberg BB, Clearfield HR, Goodman GA, et al: Ultrasonic determination of ascites, *Arch Intern Med* 131:217-220, 1973.
4. Runyon BA: Paracentesis of ascitic fluid: a safe procedure, *Arch Intern Med* 146:2259-2261, 1986.
5. Cheson BD: Clinical utility of body fluid analysis, *Clin Lab Med* 5:195-208, 1985.
6. Runyon BA, Montano AA, Akriviadis EA, et al: The serum-ascites albumin gradient is superior to the exudate-transudate concept in the differential diagnosis of ascites, *Ann Intern Med* 117:215-220, 1992.
7. Runyon BA, Antillon MR, Akriviadis EA, et al: Bedside inoculation of blood culture bottles with ascitic fluid is superior to delayed inoculation in the detection of spontaneous bacterial peritonitis, *J Clin Microbiol* 28:2811-2812, 1990.
8. Runyon BA: Care of patients with ascites, *N Engl J Med* 330:337-342, 1994.
9. Levy M: Nephrology Forum: Hepatorenal syndrome, *Kidney Int* 43:737-753, 1993.
10. Schrier RW, Arroyo V, Bernardi M, et al: Peripheral arterial vasodilation hypothesis: a proposal for the initiation of renal sodium and water retention in cirrhosis, *Hepatology* 8:1151-1157, 1988.
11. Runyon BA: Cardiac ascites: a characterization, *J Clin Gastorenterol* 10:410-412, 1988.

# Part 4

# Renal Disease

## Chapter 26

### Hyponatremia and Hypernatremia

Richard A. Lafayette

Hyponatremia and hypernatremia, the most common electrolyte disturbances in hospitalized patients, indicate disturbances in *water* metabolism. Although disturbances in the serum sodium concentration often
coexist with disorders of sodium metabolism, the serum sodium concentration does *not* indicate the total body sodium content or the
extracellular fluid (ECF) volume. Mild hyponatremia and hypernatremia
rarely are associated with serious symptoms or complications and are
usually corrected by treatment of the underlying condition. However,
severe hyponatremia or hypernatremia can be life threatening and are
medical emergencies. The proper diagnosis and treatment require a
clear understanding of the factors that regulate osmolality and water metabolism.

Water constitutes approximately 60% of body weight. Cell membranes are freely permeable to water; thus the body fluid compartments
are in osmotic equilibrium. The normal range for serum osmolality is
280-295 mOsm/kg. In practice, it rarely is necessary to measure serum

osmolality as it can be estimated from the serum sodium concentration. Sodium (and an approximately equal concentration of anions), glucose, and urea are the most abundant solutes in the ECF. If the blood glucose and BUN concentrations are normal, the serum sodium concentration may be used to calculate serum osmolality as follows:

$$\text{Osmolality} = 2[\text{Na}^+] + [\text{Glucose}]/18 + [\text{BUN}]/2.8$$
$$\text{(mOsm/kg)} \quad \text{(mEq/L)} \qquad \text{(mg/dL)} \qquad \text{(mg/dL)}$$

$$\text{Osmolality} = 2[\text{Na}^+] + 90/18 + 14/2.8$$

$$\text{Osmolality} = 2[\text{Na}^+] + 10$$

In normal circumstances, the estimated serum osmolality approximates (within $\pm$ 10 mOsm/kg) the measured serum osmolality. Errors in this estimation may occur in two conditions: (1) if water is displaced from serum by increased concentrations of protein or lipid, or (2) if additional solute is present in serum. In the first case, the additional colloid may introduce an error in the measurement of serum solute concentrations; the value for sodium is artifactually low (pseudohyponatremia), leading to underestimation of serum osmolality, while the true value for osmolality is normal. The widespread use of ion-selective electrodes to measure serum sodium concentration (directly per unit of water) have made this problem much less likely. In the second case, the presence of additional solute raises plasma osmolality, draws water into the plasma, and lowers the serum sodium concentration. Such patients have true hyponatremia but are hyperosmolar and may require urgent treatment to reverse the underlying disorder. Hyperosmolar conditions are discussed in a later section of this chapter.

Osmolality is normally maintained within narrow limits by thirst, antidiuretic hormone (ADH), and the renal concentration mechanism.[1] A reduction in total body water from either decreased water intake or increased water loss leads to an increase in osmolality, which stimulates thirst and the release of ADH. These latter two factors in turn lead to increased water intake and decreased renal water excretion, respectively, thereby restoring total body water and serum osmolality to normal. Conversely, an increase in total body water from either increased intake or impaired excretion results in decreased osmolality, reduced thirst, and decreased ADH. The subsequent decreased water intake and increased water excretion reduce body water and raise serum osmolality to normal. Figure 26-1 shows the normal relationships between serum osmolality, plasma ADH, urine concentration, and urine volume.[2,3] In most patients, the cause of hyponatremia and hypernatremia can be diagnosed accurately from measurement of urinary osmolality and urine volume. The measurement of the ADH level is generally unnecessary.

## HYPONATREMIA

Hyponatremia, defined as a serum sodium concentration less than 135 mEq/L, is the most common electrolyte abnormality and affects

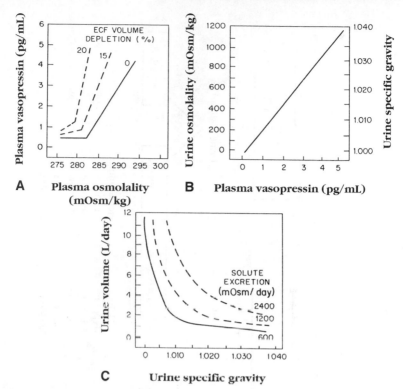

**Figure 26-1.** *Relationships between serum osmolality, plasma antidiuretic hormone level, urine concentration, and urine volume. The bold lines represent normal relationships. The dotted lines in panel A indicate altered relationships in ECF volume depletion. The dotted line in panel C indicates altered relationships in osmotic diuresis. Na, Sodium; OSM, osmolality; UUSM, urine osmolality; USG, urine specific gravity.* (Adapted from Robertson GI, Shelton RL, Athar S: *Kidney Int* 10:25, 1976.)

approximately 2.5% of hospitalized patients.[4] In most patients, the hyponatremia is mild to moderate (serum sodium between 120 and 135 mEq/L) and asymptomatic. Patients with severe hyponatremia (serum sodium less than 120 mEq/L), however, frequently have signs and symptoms of hyposmolality, including nausea, vomiting, diarrhea, confusion, and seizures, and they may develop permanent neurologic damage.[5] In patients with serious underlying medical illnesses, such as heart failure or cirrhosis, hyponatremia is associated with a more severe pathophysiologic disturbance and a poorer prognosis.[6] Regardless of the cause of severity of hyponatremia, rapid diagnosis is the key to successful treatment.

## Approach to the patient

A practical approach to the diagnosis of the cause of hyponatremia is shown in Fig. 26-2. Most patients with hyponatremia are hyposmolar;

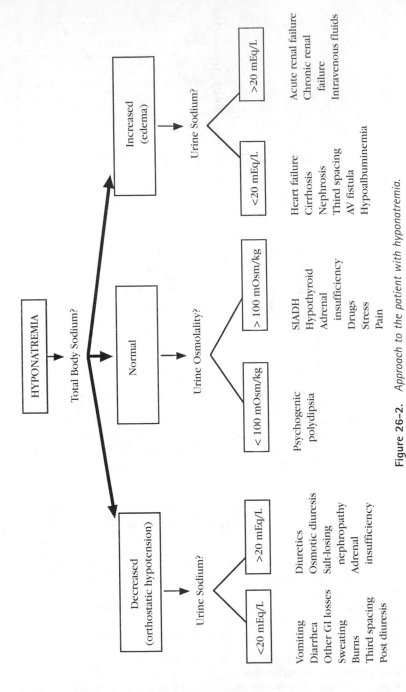

**Figure 26-2.** *Approach to the patient with hyponatremia.*

it is necessary only to measure serum osmolality if pseudohyponatremia or hyperosmolar conditions are suspected. In patients with hyposmolality, water intake has exceeded water excretion, resulting in a relative excess of water. Measurement of urinary specific gravity or, better, urine osmolality is necessary to determine whether the underlying pathophysiologic defect is excessive water ingestion (such as psychogenic polydypsia) or inadequate water excretion (such as SIADH). Nearly all patients with hyponatremia have impaired water excretion. As discussed above, an abnormality in the serum sodium concentration is not indicative of an abnormality in sodium metabolism or ECF volume. Nonetheless, disorders of sodium metabolism may cause water retention leading to hyponatremia. Therefore it is essential first to assess the state of ECF volume to determine the cause of inadequate water excretion. A recent history of fluid losses, diuretic use or weight loss, and physical findings of diminished skin turgor, orthostatic hypotension, or tachycardia usually indicate ECF volume depletion. In contrast, a recent history of fluid administration, weight gain, jugular venous distension, peripheral edema, pulmonary congestion, ascites, or pleural effusions virtually always indicate ECF volume expansion. It rarely is necessary to measure central venous or pulmonary capillary wedge pressures to confirm the diagnosis.

**Hyponatremia with normal or increased osmolality.** These disorders formerly accounted for up to 15% of cases of hyponatremia[4] and were recognized easily from the patient's history and clinical presentation. Hyponatremia attributable to hyperlipidemia or hyperproteinemia is encountered infrequently since the implementation of sodium-selective electrodes, which directly measures ion concentration. If hyponatremia is encountered in this setting, the serum osmolality is normal. Typically the serum sodium concentration is stable, there are no symptoms of hyposmolality, and serum concentrations of potassium, chloride, bicarbonate, BUN, and creatinine are proportionately reduced. In these patients, measurement of serum osmolality is necessary to confirm the diagnosis of pseudohyponatremia.

Patients with hyponatremia caused by the presence of another solute are often symptomatic from their underlying disorder and may have symptoms of hyperosmolality, including polyuria, thirst, lethargy, coma, or seizures. Moreover, they often have accompanying disorders in acid-base and potassium metabolism and abnormal renal function. These conditions are reviewed in the discussion of hyperosmolarity. In patients with hyponatremia caused by hyperglycemia, the serum sodium is reduced by 2 to 3 mEq/L for each 100 mg/dL elevation of the blood glucose above normal.

**Hyponatremia from excessive water intake.** Excessive water intake is a relatively rare disorder seen in patients with psychiatric disorders (psychogenic polydypsia).[7] If renal function is normal, maximal water excretion is 10 to 12 liters per day, or 400 to 500 mL per hour. Hyponatremia thus develops only if the rate of water ingestion exceeds this amount. Although it is extremely rare for a patient to drink this volume of water continuously, a transient binge of water drinking (2 or 3 gallons) may temporarily exceed the maximal rate of water excretion and lead to severe hyponatremia. (Of course, if renal water excretion is impaired, hyponatremia will develop with less extreme water intake.) Patients with psychogenic polydypsia can easily be identified by their history of excessive water drinking, polyuria, and very low values for urinary specific gravity or osmolality; ADH levels are significantly suppressed. BUN and serum creatinine concentrations are usually below normal. The diagnosis may be obscured if no history is available, either because of encephalopathy caused by severe hyposmolality or because of the patient's unwillingness to admit to the excessive water drinking behavior. The usual clinical picture may be further complicated by simultaneous ingestion of antipsychotic drugs that alter ADH release or by complications from self-induced vomiting or ingestion of cathartics or diuretics. Even in these patients, however, the response to treatment is usually characteristic. Treatment is restriction of water intake. If renal function is normal, polyuria will continue, and the serum sodium will rise rapidly. For example, if urine output is 400 to 500 mL/hour in a 70 kg patient, serum sodium concentration will rise from 110 to 120 mEq/L in 6 to 8 hours. Treatment with hypertonic saline is generally not indicated.

**Hyponatremia with ECF volume depletion.** ECF volume depletion causes approximately 20% of cases of hyponatremia in hospitalized patients.[4] Two pathophysiologic factors contribute to impaired water excretion: (1) direct stimulation of ADH release and (2) reduced renal perfusion with enhanced water reabsorption. The relationships between serum osmolality, ADH level, and ECF volume are shown in Fig. 26-1, *A* (2). For any level of serum osmolality, reduction in ECF volume results in a higher ADH level, a higher urine concentration, and a reduced rate of water excretion. If the intake of water exceeds the reduced water excreting capacity, hyponatremia develops.

The diagnosis is recognized by clinical features associated with ECF volume depletion and urinary osmolality greater than 150 mOsm/kg (specific gravity greater than 1.003). Measurement of urinary sodium concentration is helpful in establishing the route of ECF fluid losses. Urinary sodium concentration often exceeds 40 mEq/L if renal sodium wasting is ongoing, as in patients with renal diseases or adrenal insufficiency, or those taking diuretics. Urinary sodium concentration is less than 20 mEq/L if the losses are "nonrenal," as in patients with vomiting, diarrhea, gastrointestinal drainage, third-space losses, or heat exposure. Replacement of the ECF deficit with isotonic saline and correction of the underlying disorder will lead to correction of the hyponatremia. When ECF volume is restored, the ADH level will decline, renal blood flow will improve, and the excess water will be excreted. If hyponatremia is severe and symptoms arise, hypertonic saline should be administered.

**Hyponatremia with ECF volume expansion.** Signs of ECF volume expansion are found in approximately 20% of hospitalized patients with hyponatremia.[4] In congestive heart failure and liver disease, the two most common causes, the underlying renal pathophysiologic characteristics are similar to those found in patients with volume depletion. Altered systemic hemodynamics result in release of ADH and reduced renal perfusion, leading to impaired water excretion (in addition to impaired sodium excretion and edema). Hyponatremia develops late in the course of heart failure and cirrhosis and reflects severe circulatory abnormalities. It may develop earlier, however, as a consequence of diuretic administration. The diagnosis is usually clear cut. Urinary osmolality is greater than 150 mOsm/kg (specific gravity greater than 1.003), the patient has signs of ECF volume excess, the BUN is elevated, and serum creatinine also may be increased. Urinary sodium concentration is typically less than 20 mEq/L, unless diuretics are being administered. Management of these patients is difficult. In general, it is best to reduce diuretic dosage and restrict total water intake (oral and intravenous) to 1 liter per day. Definitive treatment must be directed at improving the underlying medical condition. For patients with heart failure, measures should be taken to improve cardiac output by augmenting myocardial contractility and optimizing afterload and preload. Converting enzyme inhibitors are helpful, but patients must be monitored for acute renal failure. For patients with cirrhosis, the options are limited. Fluid restriction should be maintained and diuretics continued at the lowest doses that maintain the patient's comfort. If hyponatremia is severe and symptomatic, hypertonic saline with increased dosage of diuretics may be administered judiciously. Although providing temporary improvement of hyponatremia, this regimen often worsens edema.

**Hyponatremia with normal ECF volume.** This disorder was first characterized by Schwartz and Bartter in 1957, who defined it as a syndrome of inappropriate ADH secretion (SIADH). Now SIADH is recognized as the most common cause of hyponatremia among hospitalized patients, accounting for approximately one third of cases.[4] The pathophysiologic characteristics of impaired water excretion are fundamentally different in two respects from the previous disorders: (1) ADH levels usually are elevated, but there is no physiologic stimulus for its release (that is, patients are not hyperosmolar and not volume depleted); and (2) renal perfusion is normal or increased; thus there is no stimulus for sodium retention. The cause of the disorder is excessive release of ADH from the pituitary of certain drugs (see the box on p. 244), endocrine, central nervous system, and pulmonary disorders, or from ectopic production of ADH by tumors. The disorder can be mimicked by drugs that increase the sensitivity of the kidney to ADH (clofibrate) or by selective impairment of the urinary dilution mechanism (thiazide diuretics). The clinical features include a urine osmolality of greater than 50 mOsm/kg (urinary specific gravity greater than 1.003) and apparently normal ECF volume. The serum concentrations of BUN, creatinine, and uric acid are usually low (reflecting increased renal perfusion, increased glomerular filtration, and decreased tubular reabsorption). Urinary sodium concentration is usually greater than 40 mEq/L, unless the patient is following a very low salt diet. Initial treatment is restriction of total water intake, usually to 1 liter or less per day. With this regimen, the hyponatremia and all other features of the disorder will resolve. Severe hyponatremia must be treated with hypertonic saline and diuretics as will be discussed.

## Drugs That Can Induce SIADH

### ANTIDIURETIC HORMONES

Vasopressin
Oxytocin

### THIAZIDE DIURETICS

### ANTIDEPRESSANTS AND ANTIPSYCHOTIC AGENTS*

Monoamine oxidase inhibitors
Tricyclic antidepressants
Tetracyclic antidepressants
Phenothiazines
Thioxanthines
Butyrophenones

### ANTICONVULSANTS

Carbamazepine

### ORAL HYPOGLYCEMICS

Chlorpropamide
Tolbutamide
Glyburide
Glipizide

### ANTINEOPLASTIC AGENTS

Vincristine
Cyclophosphamide

### ANALGESICS AND ANTI-INFLAMMATORY AGENTS*

Narcotic analgesics
Nonsteroidal anti-inflammatory drugs
Acetaminophen

### OTHERS

Clofibrate

*SIADH,* Syndrome of inappropriate antidiuretic hormone.
* They may also be related to the underlying stress or pain

If the underlying disease cannot be improved, long-term therapy to prevent the redevelopment of hyponatremia will be necessary. Although long-term water restriction is effective, most patients will not be compliant. Several alternative measures to increase renal water excretion have been developed.[8] The most useful method is administration of demeclocycline, which induces a mild urinary concentrating defect. Doses of 600 to 1200 mg/day are usually well-tolerated and effective. Mild azotemia may occur, but it is reversible upon reduction in the dose. Demeclocycline should not be used for the treatment of hyponatremia caused by heart failure or cirrhosis because renal failure has been reported as a complication of this therapy.

## Emergency treatment of severe hyponatremia

Severe symptomatic hyponatremia can result in permanent neurologic impairment or death.[5,9] Immediate treatment with hypertonic saline should be considered if serum sodium is less than 120 mEq/L and neurologic symptoms are present. The initial goal of therapy is to raise the serum sodium level rapidly (1 to 2 mEq/L per hour). Some authors have cautioned that this treatment may be associated with a devastating neurologic complication, central pontine myelinolysis, especially if the hyponatremia is chronic.[8,10] However, it appears that the development of this lesion may be associated with rapidly raising the serum sodium concentration to normal or elevated levels.[11] Because of the potential danger of rapid correction or overcorrection of hyponatremia, treatment with hypertonic saline should be administered cautiously, and serum sodium should be monitored frequently during therapy. Correcting the serum sodium rapidly to a point where the patient is no longer symptomatic or is in a safe range (such as 125 mEq/L) is an appropriate target. As discussed earlier, treatment with hypertonic saline usually is necessary only in patients with impaired water excretion. Administration of 200 to 400 mL of 3% saline (520 mEq/L) over 4 hours would be expected to raise the serum sodium level by 3 to 5 mEq/L in a typical 70 kg individual. In patients with ECF volume depletion, the restoration of ECF volume will reduce ADH secretion, improve renal perfusion, and increase water excretion, thus raising the serum sodium concentration to an even higher level. In patients with normal or expanded ECF, administration of hypertonic saline poses a risk of precipitating pulmonary congestion. In such patients, loop diuretics, such as furosemide 80 mg, should be administered intravenously to reduce ECF volume before infusion of hypertonic saline.[12] In addition, the water diuresis that results will further increase the serum sodium concentration. Repeat measurement of serum electrolytes should be obtained within 4 hours as a guide to further therapy.

# HYPERNATREMIA

Hypernatremia, defined as a serum sodium concentration greater than 145 mEq/L, always indicates hyperosmolality. Hyperosmolality is usually the result of reduced total body water, but in some cases it is the result of solute excess. Regardless of the cause, hyperosmolality is a potent stimulus to thirst; thus the development of significant hyperosmolality also indicates either a disorder of thirst or an inability to obtain water. Severe hyperosmolality (serum osmolality greater than 330 mOsm/kg) may lead to neurologic alterations, including delirium, coma, and permanent brain damage.[5,11] The causes of hyperosmolarity and the associated serum sodium concentrations are listed in Table 26-1. In this chapter, only those disorders associated with hypernatremia are discussed. Mild hypernatremia (serum sodium less than 155 mEq/L) that develops in postoperative or debilitated patients unable to obtain water usually poses no difficulty in recognition or treatment. Severe hypernatremia (serum sodium greater than 155 mEq/L) is associated with severe hyperosmolality and requires urgent diagnosis and therapy. Regardless of the severity, the cause of hypernatremia generally can be diagnosed quickly.

## Approach to the patient

The approach to the patient with hypernatremia is shown in Fig. 26-3 and should rapidly establish the diagnosis.[13] Measurement of urinary volume and urine osmolality (or urinary specific gravity) allows classification of hyperosmolar syndromes according to the pathophysiologic defect: impaired water intake, solute excess, or renal water losses. In patients with impaired water intake, renal water conservation is normal, resulting in a reduced volume of highly concentrated urine. In patients with solute excess, urinary solute excretion is elevated, the urine is isotonic with plasma, and the urine volume is increased. In patients with renal water losses, the urine is dilute or only slightly concentrated, and the urine volume is not increased. The cause of the renal defect is assessed by observation of the patient after administration of exogenous ADH. Measurement of the plasma level of ADH also can be helpful.

**Table 26-1.** *Causes of hyperosmolality*

| Condition | Associated serum Na$^+$ concentration |
|---|---|
| Hyperglycemia | Low |
| Mannitol administration | Low |
| High-protein feedings | Low |
| Ethanol | Normal |
| Methanol | Normal |
| Ethylene glycol | Normal |
| Severe renal failure (azotemia) | Normal or low |
| Sodium bicarbonate administration | High |
| Water deprivation | High |
| Neurogenic diabetes insipidus | High |
| Nephrogenic diabetes insipidus | High |

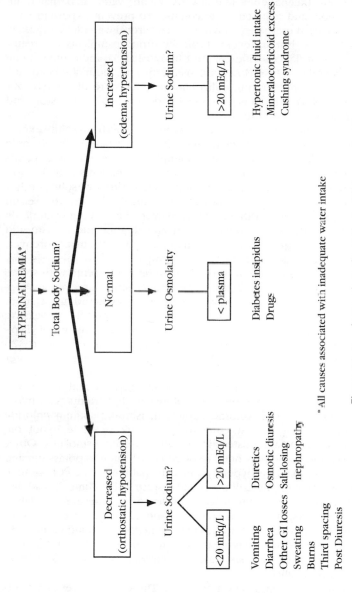

Figure 26-3. *Approach to the patient with hypernatremia.*

HYPERNATREMIA*

Total Body Sodium?

**Decreased** (orthostatic hypotension)

Urine Sodium?

<20 mEq/L | >20 mEq/L

Vomiting
Diarrhea
Other GI losses
Sweating
Burns
Third spacing
Post Diuresis

Diuretics
Osmotic diuresis
Salt-losing nephropathy

**Normal**

Urine Osmolality

< plasma

Diabetes insipidus
Drugs

**Increased** (edema, hypertension)

Urine Sodium?

>20 mEq/L

Hypertonic fluid intake
Mineralocorticoid excess
Cushing syndrome

*All causes associated with inadequate water intake

**Hypernatremia from inadequate water intake.** Inadequate water intake is the most common cause of hypernatremia. The diagnostic features include the patient's inability to obtain water, maximal urine concentration, and reduced urine volume. To prevent hypernatremia, water intake must increase when there is extrarenal water losses (gastrointestinal losses, burns, fever). Typically, urine osmolality is greater than 800 mOsm/kg (specific gravity 1.025 to 1.035), and urine volume is 500 mL per day or less. However, in elderly or malnourished patients, maximal urine concentrating ability may be reduced, resulting in higher urine volumes. Treatment is provision of adequate water to restore and maintain normal osmolality.

**Hypernatremia from solute excess.** Hypernatremia from solute excess results from either of two mechanisms: (1) Administration of hypertonic sodium salts directly raises serum sodium concentration and expands ECF volume. If renal function is impaired, these patients may develop ECF volume excess. (2) Administration or generation of solutes other than sodium raises serum osmolality and initially lowers the serum sodium concentration (Table 26-1). However, the ensuing osmotic diuresis impairs the renal concentration and dilution mechanism and leads to water losses and the development of hypernatremia. Moreover, the sodium and chloride losses that accompany osmotic diuresis may lead to extreme contraction of the ECF volume.[11] Patients with solute excess usually are easy to recognize. There is a history of recent development of diabetic hyperglycemia or hypertonic solute administration, such as saline, sodium bicarbonate, dextrose, high protein nasogastric tube feedings, intravenous hyperalimentation fluid, or mannitol. Typically, urine osmolality is similar to plasma, approximately 290 to 320 mOsm/kg (specific gravity 1.008 to 1.012), urine volume is greater than 2 liters per day, and solute excretion exceeds 800 mOsm daily. Treatment is discontinuation of solute administration, and in the case of diabetic hyperglycemia, provision of insulin. In patients with hypotension caused by ECF volume depletion, isotonic sodium chloride should be administered first. Once the vital signs are stable, hypotonic solutions should be administered to lower the serum osmolality. Other electrolyte losses also may need to be replaced, such as potassium and phosphorus in diabetic hyperglycemia. In patients with ECF volume expansion, ongoing solute diuresis will restore ECF volume, but administration of hypotonic solutions is necessary to lower serum osmolality. In these patients, hypotonic solutions should be given carefully to avoid pulmonary edema. Diuretics may be necessary to increase solute excretion but may further increase serum osmolality. If renal function is severely impaired, dialysis may be necessary to lower ECF volume and serum osmolality.

**Hypernatremia from renal water losses.** These renal water loss disorders are recognized by hypernatremia without increased solute excretion and failure to concentrate the urine maximally. They often can be diagnosed on the basis of typical clinical features and urinary concentrating ability. In many cases, accurate diagnosis requires performing an overnight water-deprivation test and administering exogenous

ADH (vasopressin). For a detailed discussion of the overnight water-deprivation test, see reference 6.

NEUROGENIC DIABETES INSIPIDUS. In neurogenic or central diabetes insipidus, pituitary secretion of ADH is absent or reduced. The most common causes of neurogenic diabetes insipidus are head trauma, neurosurgery, brain tumors (especially pituitary adenomas and craniopharyngiomas), and idiopathic disease of young adults. Many patients can be recognized by their neurologic and endocrine features. If ADH levels are extremely low (less than 1 pg/mL), urine osmolality is less than 150 mOsm/kg (specific gravity less than 1.003), and urine volume is 3 to 5 liters per day or more. If access to water is denied, rapid dehydration and severe hyperosmolality result. In these circumstances, the urine can become mildly concentrated but only to a urine osmolality of 400 mOsm/kg. In adults, this extreme defect is seen only in neurogenic diabetes insipidus. With milder defects in ADH secretion, ADH levels are higher than 1 pg/mL but are still abnormally low for the elevated serum osmolality. Urine osmolality may be as high as 400 mOsm/kg (specific gravity may be as high as 1.012), and urine volume as low as 2 to 3 liters per day. Clinically, these patients may be difficult to distinguish from patients with nephrogenic diabetes insipidus. To make the diagnosis, it is often necessary to perform an overnight water-deprivation test and assess the response to vasopressin. In neurogenic diabetes insipidus, the urine concentration rises only slightly after water deprivation but increases promptly after administration of vasopressin. Treatment is correction of the underlying disorder, if possible. Emergency treatment is subcutaneous administration of arginine vasopressin in oil (pitressin tannate) every 12 hours to maintain urine volume at approximately 3 liters per day. Long-term treatment is intranasal administration of short-acting lypressin (lysine vasopressin) or long-acting desmopressin (DDAVP) to maintain the desried urine volume, usually 2 to 4 liters per day. Partial defects in ADH excretion can be treated by chlorpropamide or clofibrate, which increases ADH release and the renal response to ADH, respectively.

NEPHROGENIC DIABETES INSIPIDUS. In nephrogenic diabetes insipidus, ADH levels are normal for the degree of hyperosmolality, but the urine concentration is not appropriately increased. Nephrogenic diabetes insipidus is the result of renal disorders that interfere with the urine concentration mechanism and the response to ADH. In adults, common causes are metabolic disturbances (hypokalemia and hypercalcemia), drugs (lithium compounds, demeclocycline, amphoteracin B, loop diuretics), and parenchymal renal diseases causing prominent tubulo-interstitial damage (see box on p. 250). In addition, a severe reduction in glomerular filtration rate (serum creatinine greater than 4 mg/dL) results in impaired urinary concentration and may lead to hypernatremia if water intake is reduced.

In most cases, the renal defect is not severe and urinary concentration may achieve osmolalities as high as 400 mOsm/kg (specific gravity 1.012). Thus urine volume is typically 2 to 3 liters per day. As discussed earlier, the diagnosis may be difficult to distinguish from mild neurogenic diabetes insipidus. In contrast to neurogenic diabetes insipidus,

---

**Renal Diseases Causing Nephrogenic Diabetes Insipidus through Tubulointerstitial Damage**
······································································

Acute pyelonephritis
Obstructive nephropathy
Acute tubular necrosis (recovery phase)
Sickle cell nephropathy
Sjögren's syndrome
Amyloidosis
Myeloma kidney, light-chain disease
Lead nephropathy

---

urinary concentration remains low even after an overnight water deprivation test and administration of vasopressin. Treatment is correction of the underlying cause of renal dysfunction, if possible. In more severe cases, thiazide diuretics (hydrochlorothiazide 100 mg/day) can be used to promote mild ECF volume contraction, which can increase urine concentration. With this regimen, urine osmolality can increase toward 300 and up to 400 mOsm/kg (specific gravity 1.012), and urine volume can be reduced to 2 to 4 liters per day.

## Repairing the water deficit

Whether it is the result of solute excess or water loss, hyperosmolality indicates a water deficit relative to the amount of solute. The magnitude of the water deficit is estimated from the patient's present weight and serum osmolality by application of the following formula:

(a) Present serum $[Na^+] \times (0.6 \times$ Present weight [kg] $= 140 \times$ ideal total body water

(b) $\dfrac{[\text{Present serum Na}^+] \times (0.6 \times \text{Present weight})}{140} = $ ideal total body water

(c) Water deficit $=$ ideal total body water $- 0.6 \times$ present weight

This calculation is based on the assumption that there has been *no* change in total body solute content. In hyperosmolality attributable to water deprivation and neurogenic and nephrogenic diabetes insipidus, this assumption is generally valid. In cases of solute excess and osmotic diuresis, however, this assumption is not valid. The solute gains or losses may be estimated by comparison of the patient's calculated normal weight with the actual weight before the development of hyperosmolality. As discussed above, repair of solute excess or deficit should begin before correction of the relative water deficit. The preferred solution for correcting the water deficit is 5% dextrose in water. If hyperosmolality has developed over several days, water administration should proceed slowly to prevent the development of cerebral edema. Not more than one half the water deficit should be infused during the first 24 hours.[2] The serum sodium should be measured at least every 12 hours during therapy.

## References

1. Berl T, Schrier RW: Disorders of water metabolism. In Schrier RW, editor: *Renal and electrolyte disorders,* Boston, 1992, Little, Brown.
2. Levey AS, Harrington JT: Polyuria. In Taylor RB, editor: *Difficult diagnosis,* Philadelphia, 1985, Saunders.
3. Robertson GL, Shelton RL, Athar S: The osmoregulation of vasopressin, *Kidney Int* 10:25, 1976.
4. Anderson RJ, Chung HM, Kluge R, Schrier RW: Hyponatremia: a prospective analysis of its epidemiology and the pathogenetic role of vasopressin, *Ann Intern Med* 102:164, 1985.
5. Arieff AI, Guisado R: Effects on the central nervous system of hypernatremic and hyponatremic states, *Kidney Int* 10:104, 1976.
6. Leier CV, Dei Cas L, Metra M: Clinical relevance and management of the major electrolyte abnormalities in congestive heart failure: hyponatremia, hypokalemia, and hypomagnesemia, *Am Heart J* 128:564, 1994.
7. Siegler EL, Tamres D, Berlin JA, et al: Risk factors for the development of hyponatremia in psychiatric inpatients, *Arch Intern Med* 155:953, 1995.
8. Schrier RW: Treatment of hyponatremia, *N Engl J Med* 312:1121, 1985.
9. Berl T: Nephrology Forum. Treating hyponatremia: damned if we do and damned if we don't, *Kidney Int* 37:1006, 1990.
10. Höjer J: Management of symptomatic hyponatremia: dependence on the duration of development, *J Intern Med* 235:497, 1994.
11. Arieff AI: Osmotic failure: physiology and strategies for treatment, *Hosp Pract* 23:173, May 1988.
12. Hartman D, Rossier B, Zohlman R, Schrier RW: Rapid correction of hyponatremia in the syndrome of inappropriate secretion of antidiuretic hormone: an alternative to hypertonic saline, *Ann Intern Med* 78:870, 1973.
13. Palersky PM, Blagrath R, Greenberg A: Hypernatremia in hospitalized patients, *Ann Int Med* 124:197, 1996.

# Chapter 27
## Hypokalemia and Hyperkalemia

Richard A. Lafayette

The normal serum potassium concentration is maintained between 3.5 and 5.0 mEq per liter. Hypokalemia occurs in nearly one third of all hospitalized patients and up to one half of acutely ill patients.[1] Hyperkalemia is less common but still occurs in approximately 10% of hospitalized patients.[2] Consultation is usually requested when the abnormality in serum potassium is severe, prolonged, or difficult to explain. Making the proper diagnosis is important because alterations in serum potassium often reflect serious underlying disorders or a complication of treatment. Furthermore, the resulting alteration in transmembrane potential may cause life-threatening complications, such as muscle paralysis and cardiac arrhythmias. This chapter focuses on the pathophysiology, diagnosis, and treatment of hypokalemia and hyperkalemia.

## PATHOPHYSIOLOGY OF DISORDERS OF POTASSIUM METABOLISM

The total body potassium content is approximately 50 mEq/kg or 3000 to 3500 mEq in adults. Potassium is the predominant intracellular cation, with an intracellular concentration of approximately 150 mEq/L. The majority of potassium resides in skeletal muscle. In contrast, only 2% of total body potassium is in the extracellular fluid. This distribution is maintained by active transport processes that are influenced by insulin levels, adrenergic nervous system activity, exercise, alterations in osmolality and acidity of the body fluids, drugs that affect membrane transport, and disorders that disrupt cell metabolism or cause cell lysis. Disorders of the serum potassium concentration result from either altered internal distribution, increased intake, or decreased excretion of potassium.[3,4]

The average American diet includes 50 to 125 mEq per day of potassium (equivalent to 2 to 3 g per day). Potassium is present in all animal and vegetable matter, especially meat, certain fruits (bananas, oranges, tomatoes), beans, coffee, and cocoa. Gastrointestinal losses average approximately 5 to 15 mEq per day but increase with diarrhea, chronic renal failure, and hyperaldosteronism. The remainder of dietary potassium (approximately 90% of dietary intake) is excreted in the urine. Renal excretion of potassium closely follows dietary intake, maintaining total body content and serum concentration of potassium stable at normal levels.

The kidney freely filters potassium at the glomerulus, totally reabsorbs the filtered load in the proximal tubule, and controls excretion by secretion in the distal tubule. The major sites of distal secretion are the distal convoluted tubule and the cortical collecting duct. Potassium excretion is regulated by alterations in the rate of potassium secretion. Urinary excretion of potassium can vary widely, from 5 to 1000 mEq per day under circumstances of severe depletion or loading of potassium. These extreme adaptations occur slowly, over days, as compared to the smaller, faster adaptation to daily dietary sodium intake. The major factors regulating renal potassium excretion are the aldosterone level, the urine flow rate, the distal delivery of sodium, and the serum potassium concentration.

Intravenous administration of 50 mEq of potassium, if it were confined to the extracellular space, would result in severe hyperkalemia. In fact, approximately 50% of the administered load is taken up by cells; thus the serum potassium rises by only 0.3 to 0.5 mEq/L. If potassium is administered over several days, increases in the renal and gastrointestinal excretion of potassium occur, and the rise in serum potassium is lower. Therefore, the rise in serum potassium after a load depends on the amount, the route and rate of administration, the transcellular distribution, and the renal excretion of potassium.

When potassium is withdrawn from the diet, renal excretion of potassium continues until there is a deficit of total body content and a reduction in the concentration of potassium in cells and extracellular fluid. Up to 3 weeks is required to maximize the renal conservation of potassium. Therefore, the decline in serum potassium depends on the extent of renal losses, the occurrence of gastrointestinal losses, and the factors influencing the transcellular distribution of potassium.

The relationship between the serum concentration and total body content of potassium varies in disorders of potassium metabolism. If the disorder is attributable to transcellular shifts, the total body content of potassium remains normal. However, in disorders where total body content is altered, the extent of change in serum potassium roughly correlates with the extent of deficit or excess (Table 27-1). The definitions of mild, moderate, and severe alterations in Table 27-1 are arbitrary but provide a framework for discussion of the etiology of hypokalemia and hyperkalemia. Notice that large deficits of total body potassium content must occur before moderate or severe hypokalemia develops. By contrast, severe hyperkalemia may result from relatively modest expansion of total body potassium content. Formal data on potassium excess in moderate or severe hyperkalemia are not available, but common clinical experience demonstrates that the administration of small amounts of potassium (about 100 mEq) to patients with mild hyperka-

**Table 27-1.** *Relation between serum potassium level and change in body potassium content*

| Severity | Serum concentration (mEqlL) | Approximate deficit or excess (mEq) |
|---|---|---|
| HYPOKALEMIA | | |
| | | *Deficit* |
| Severe | ~2.5 | 500-1000 |
| Moderate | 2.5-2.9 | 300-800 |
| Mild | 3.0-3.4 | ~300 |
| HYPERKALEMIA | | |
| | | *Excess* |
| Mild | 5.1-5.5 | 50-75 |
| Moderate | 5.9-6.0 | >100 |
| Severe | >6.0 | >100 |

lemia can result in the development of moderate or severe hyperkalemia.

# HYPOKALEMIA

## Consequences

Severe hypokalemia can lead to dysfunction in many organs. Impaired urinary concentration may lead to polyuria; impaired insulin secretion and hepatic gluconeogenesis can cause hyperglycemia; increased renal ammonia production can lead to hepatic encephalopathy. These effects are seen rarely without severe hypokalemia.

However, the most important effects of hypokalemia are on muscle and nerve function. With moderate hypokalemia, impaired gastrointestinal motility may occur. With even mild hypokalemia, cardiac abnormalities may develop. Electrocardiographic changes are common (Fig. 27-1) and ventricular arrhythmias can occur, especially in patients taking digoxin. The contribution of mild hypokalemia to arrhythmias after myocardial injury or in patients with underlying heart disease is not conclusively determined. Likewise, the absolute frequency of arrhythmias from hypokalemia in patients with normal cardiac function is unknown. However, it is unlikely that severe arrhythmias result from hypokalemia unless other factors are involved.[5,6] Hypokalemia and potassium depletion have been linked to a mild increase (3 to 5 mm Hg) in blood pressure, especially in hypertensive subjects.[7] Current studies continue to address the role of potassium in blood pressure regulation.

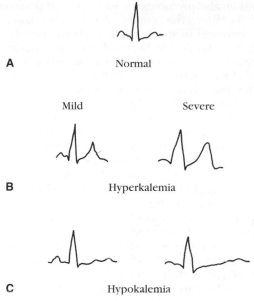

**A**          Normal

Mild          Severe

**B**          Hyperkalemia

**C**          Hypokalemia

**Figure 27-1.** *ECG changes in hypokalemia and hyperkalemia. A, Normal. In hyperkalemia, B, the T-wave becomes peaked, followed by loss of the p wave and prolongation of the QRS complex, approaching a "sine-wave" appearance as serum potassium increases. In hypokalemia, C, the QT interval is slightly prolonged and the ST segment is depressed. The QRS becomes prolonged as serum potassium decreases. (Adapted from Robertson GL, Shelton RL, Athan S: The Osmoregulation of vasopressin, vol 10, p. 25, 1976, Mosby.)*

## Causes
### Altered transcellular distribution

Shifting of potassium from extracellular fluid to inside the cell should be suspected as a cause of hypokalemia when there is a sudden decrease in serum potassium concentration by approximately 0.5 mEq/L without evidence of a recent loss of potassium. Up to 25% of patients with sudden hypokalemia have no obvious source of potassium losses, and in many of these patients hypokalemia resolves without therapy.[1] The major causes of transcellular shift of potassium are discussed below.

**Beta-adrenergic receptor stimulation.** Intravenous infusion of epinephrine to achieve physiologic "stress" levels leads to a temporary fall of serum potassium concentration by approximately 0.5 mEq/L. The magnitude does not appear to depend on the initial serum potassium concentration. The mechanism of the hypokalemia is movement of potassium into skeletal and liver cells that is mediated through the activation of beta$_2$-adrenergic receptors. Similar declines occur as the result of inhaled beta$_2$-agonists. Generally, no therapy is needed for the hypokalemia unless the patient also has potassium deficiency or the patient is at substantial risk for arrhythmias.

**Insulin.** Insulin also promotes the movement of potassium into liver and muscle cells. In fact, the combination of glucose and insulin results in a prompt lowering of the serum potassium concentration and is utilized as therapy for severe hyperkalemia. Hypokalemia caused by the transcellular shift of potassium associated with insulin occurs in two common clinical settings. In nondiabetic patients receiving large amounts of dextrose (as in parenteral nutrition), the resulting hyperinsulinemia can lead to hypokalemia. In the absence of renal failure, the administration of 80 to 100 mEq per day of potassium is recommended. In patients with diabetes and hyperglycemia, administration of insulin will lower both serum glucose and potassium levels. Potassium supplementation is not necessary for patients eating normally. However, in patients with severe hyperglycemia, potassium deficiency frequently occurs because of renal potassium losses, and moderate to severe hypokalemia can occur with insulin therapy. Repletion of 100 to 200 mEq of potassium is frequently necessary and can be started immediately unless the patient is initially hyperkalemic.

**Bicarbonate.** Acute elevation of the serum bicarbonate concentration results in a transcellular shift of hydrogen ions out of cells into extracellular fluid and a shift of potassium from extracellular fluid into cells. However, administration of sodium bicarbonate has variable effects on lowering serum potassium in patients with hyperkalemia. It is likely that the shift of potassium into cells is related to the bicarbonate concentration more than to the change in hydrogen-ion concentration because hypokalemia is not a feature of respiratory alkalosis.[8] The reduction in potassium concentration after sodium bicarbonate administration also is attributable to enhanced urine flow and enhanced availability of sodium and bicarbonate promoting renal potassium excretion.

**Hypokalemic periodic paralysis.** Hypokalemic periodic paralysis constitutes a rare group of disorders characterized by profound muscle weakness in the face of sudden moderate to severe hypokalemia.[9] It chiefly occurs as an inherited autosomal dominant trait. However, it has been reported as a rare complication of hypothyroidism, mainly in Orientals. Acute episodes can be treated with oral or intravenous administration of potassium in doses up to 120 mEq until the muscle weakness and hypokalemia resolve.

### Inadequate intake

The adaptation to reduced potassium intake occurs slowly. Thus, mild potassium deficiency and hypokalemia can result from reduced intake. In this setting, urine potassium losses should be minimal, with urine potassium excretion less than 20 mEq per day. Severe hypokalemia does not occur unless there are coexistent losses of potassium.

### Excessive losses

Potassium deficiency may result from increased losses of potassium from the gastrointestinal tract or from the kidney. If potassium deficiency is attributable to gastrointestinal losses, urinary potassium excretion should decrease to less than 20 mEq per day. By definition, if urinary potassium excretion exceeds this amount, hypokalemia is the result of renal potassium losses. Therefore, measurement of urinary potassium excretion distinguishes between hypokalemia caused by inadequate intake or gastrointestinal losses and hypokalemia caused by renal losses of potassium.

**Gastrointestinal losses.** The potassium content in stool can be as high as 30 to 50 mEq/L. Thus the large losses of potassium and bicarbonate that occur with severe diarrhea lead to hypokalemia and metabolic acidosis with a normal anion gap (see Chapter 28). The potassium content of gastric, biliary, and pancreatic secretions is much lower, only 5 to 10 mEq/L. The hypokalemia that results from vomiting or other types of gastric drainage is attributable to the renal potassium wasting that occurs in association with metabolic alkalosis.

## Renal losses

**Diuretics.** Except for the "potassium-sparing" diuretics, all diuretics increase the secretion of potassium into the distal nephron as a result of increased delivery of sodium chloride and the enhanced flow rate at this site.[6,10] The magnitude of potassium loss correlates well with the magnitude of sodium excretion. Diuretics such as thiazides and carbonic anhydrase inhibitors are mildly natriuretic and generally cause mild potassium deficiency. On the other hand, potent loop diuretics and osmotic agents can result in severe hypokalemia. The magnitude of the potassium deficiency also depends on the underlying disorder. In essential hypertension patients without edema, the diuretic-induced deficit is typically less than 200 mEq. In only 5% of patients does the potassium concentration decrease to less than 3.0 mEq/L.[10] However, in patients with edematous disorders such as congestive heart failure, cirrhosis, or nephrotic syndrome, where there is enhanced aldosterone levels, the potassium deficiency caused by diuresis is further augmented.

The treatment of hypokalemia caused by diuretics is based on the severity of the potassium deficiency. Prevention is often the best course, with the prescription of 80 to 120 mEq of potassium (with chloride) a day often necessary to prevent hypokalemia in edematous patients receiving diuretics. Patients treated with carbonic anhydrase inhibitors also can develop metabolic acidosis and can occasionally require replacement of bicarbonate as well as potassium supplements. In nonedematous patients the role of potassium supplementation is controversial. These patients are unlikely to develop significant complications or severe hypokalemia. However, potassium supplementation (or use of potassium-sparing diuretics) is warranted in patients who are taking digoxin, have symptoms related to hypokalemia, or have persistent potassium levels lower than 3.0 mEq/L. Treatment of these patients with 40 to 60 mEq per day of potassium is generally required to restore serum potassium to normal and to correct the potassium deficit. Additionally there is preliminary evidence indicating that hypertensive patients treated with diuretics who receive potassium supplementation may be better protected from long-term cardiovascular morbidity.[7]

**Chronic metabolic acidosis and metabolic alkalosis.** Urinary potassium excretion is increased in the majority of chronic metabolic acid-base disorders.[8] In metabolic acidosis, the increased excretion of anions such as salicylate, lactate, or ketoacid anions into the urine facilitates the secretion of potassium by the distal nephron, leading to hypokalemia. This phenomenon does not occur in metabolic acidosis caused by mineral acids such as ammonium chloride, arginine chloride, or hydrochloric acid or in the acidosis associated with acute or chronic renal failure. In these settings, the serum potassium is usually normal or elevated.[8] In metabolic alkalosis, volume depletion and chloride deficiency lead to increased reabsorption of sodium in the distal area of the nephron in exchange for potassium, leading to hypokalemia.[11] Treatment of hypokalemia in these settings includes correcting the underlying acid-base disorder and replacement of the potassium deficit. In metabolic acidosis, potassium should be provided with alkali; in metabolic alkalosis, potassium should be provided with chloride.

**Hyperaldosteronism.** The primary action of aldosterone on the distal tubule is to facilitate sodium reabsorption and to increase the secretion of potassium and hydrogen ions. Persistently high levels of aldosterone and other mineralocorticoids lead to potassium depletion, hypokalemia, and metabolic alkalosis. Numerous disorders lead to increased secretion of adrenal steroids and cause hypokalemia (Table 27-2). Primary hyperal-

**Table 27-2.** *Disorders of potassium metabolism caused by alterations in the renin-angiotensin-aldosterone system*

| Disorder | Hypokalemia | Hyperkalemia |
|---|---|---|
| Abnormal aldosterone secretion | Primary hyperaldosteronism<br>  Adrenal adenoma<br>  Adrenal hyperplasia<br>  Adrenal carcinoma<br>Exogenous adrenal steroids<br>  Licorice<br>  Iatrogenic | Primary hypoaldosteronism<br>  Congenital biosynthetic<br>  defect<br>  Addison's disease<br>Drugs<br>  Heparin<br>  Angiotensin-converting<br>  enzyme inhibition |
| Abnormal renin secretion | Hyperreninemic-<br>  hyperaldosteronism<br>  Congestive heart failure<br>  Cirrhosis<br>  Nephrotic syndrome<br>  Volume contraction<br>  Bartter's syndrome<br>  Malignant hypertension<br>  High renin-essential<br>  hypertension | Hyporeninemic-<br>  hypoaldosteronism<br>  Diabetes<br>  Renal diseases<br>  Prostaglandin synthetase<br>  inhibition<br>  Beta-adrenergic blocking<br>  agents |
| Abnormal ACTH secretion | Cushing's syndrome<br>Pituitary adenoma<br>Ectopic ACTH | |

dosteronism, characterized by mild to moderate hypokalemia, hypertension, and mild metabolic alkalosis, can be caused by an adrenal adenoma (Conn's syndrome), bilateral adrenal hyperplasia, or adrenal carcinoma. Women are affected more commonly and the usual age is from 30 to 50 years. The diagnosis can be made by demonstration of an elevated urine or plasma aldosterone level in association with a suppressed renin level. The renin level remains low despite maneuvers that normally stimulate renin release such as assumption of an upright posture or diuresis. By definition, secondary hyperaldosteronism is the result of increased plasma renin activity. The most common causes are disorders of extracellular volume status (congestive heart failure, cirrhosis, nephrosis, volume depletion, Bartter's syndrome), renal damage from malignant hypertension, and high renin hypertension. Glucocorticoid hormone activity, when elevated as in Cushing's syndrome, stimulates distal potassium excretion and can lead to hypokalemia. Treatment of the underlying condition and replacement of potassium resolves the hypokalemia. Spironolactone and other potassium-sparing diuretics prevent ongoing potassium losses in patients with primary hyperaldosteronism or with Cushing's syndrome. Agents that inhibit prostaglandin secretion reduce elevated renin levels and help to correct hypokalemia in patients with Bartter's syndrome. Long-term therapy with potassium supplements, 80 to 120 mEq per day, often is necessary in patients with secondary hyperaldosteronism.

**Renal tubular disorders.** Some drugs and diseases can cause hypokalemia by directly increasing renal tubular potassium excretion through a variety of mechanisms. These disorders include renal tubular acidosis, resolving acute tubular necrosis, postobstructive diuresis, multiple myeloma, light-chain nephropathy, and nephrotoxicity from amphotericin B and platinum. In addition to enhanced potassium excretion, tubular defects in sodium absorption and hydrogen ion secretion may also be observed. Acute myelogenous leukemia, hypomagnesemia, and administration of carbenicillin can cause hypokalemia without other tubular defects.

## Treatment of hypokalemia

The treatment of hypokalemia is determined by the severity and cause of the hypokalemia and by the patient's medical condition. As previously discussed, treatment is not usually necessary for mild, transient hypokalemia attributable to transcellular shift or to treatment of hypertension with thiazides. However, treatment should be provided if the serum potassium is less than 3.0 mEq/L or the patient is at risk for cardiac arrhythmias.

The other causes of hypokalemia require therapy to correct the hypokalemia and to replace the potassium deficit. Two types of therapy are available, potassium supplements and potassium-sparing diuretics. Potassium-sparing diuretics are not effective in raising the serum potassium quickly and are not indicated in the acute therapy of moderate to severe hypokalemia. Potassium supplements are more reliable. Mild hypokalemia caused by inadequate intake can be corrected with potassium-rich foods. Diuretic-induced hypokalemia should be corrected with potassium chloride, whereas hypokalemia caused by diarrhea and by renal tubular disorders with associated metabolic acidosis should be treated with alkalinizing potassium salts.

The route and speed of administration of potassium replacement depends on the patient's ability to tolerate oral and enteral medication, renal function, and the severity of the hypokalemia. Generally it is safer and easier to replace potassium orally with liquid solutions of 10% to 20% potassium chloride in doses of 40 mEq each. For prevention of hypokalemia, potassium tablets or potassium-sparing diuretics generally are well tolerated. For severe hypokalemia, potassium can be given intravenously. The concentration in the administered fluid should not exceed 60 mEq/L. The serum level of potassium should be carefully monitored after 80 to 100 mEq have been administered, and more than 200 mEq should not be given in 1 day. Higher rates of replacement rarely are needed but can be accomplished with 10 to 20 mEq of potassium chloride per 100 mL of intravenous fluid infused over 1 hour. The solution should be delivered through a central venous catheter or diluted into another intravenous line to prevent sclerosis of the vein. These doses are recommended only for the prevention of cardiac arrhythmias in patients with severe hypokalemia taking digoxin or during myocardial infarction. For life-threatening hypokalemia (serum potassium less than 2.0 mEq/L, ventricular arrhythmias, or paralysis) 30 to 40 mEq per hour can be infused with continuous monitoring of the electrocardiogram.[12] The serum potassium should be repeated after 2 to 3 hours.

The major risk of therapy is hyperkalemia. The prevalence of hyperkalemia is approximately 5% in hospitalized patients receiving potassium therapy; life-threatening hyperkalemia occurs in 0.4% of patients.[13] The risk of life-threatening hyperkalemia increases to 5% to 9% in patients over 50 years of age who have a BUN concentration greater than 50 mg/dL or receive both orally and intravenously administered potassium. The prevalence of hyperkalemia is approximately 10% in patients receiving potassium-sparing diuretics; life-threatening hyperkalemia occurs in 3%.[14] The risk increases dramatically if the patient has renal failure or is also receiving oral therapy. Thus potassium is the most commonly used potentially lethal drug in the hospital. These considerations argue for the judicious use of potassium supplements and potassium-sparing diuretics for the treatment and prevention of hypokalemia.

# HYPERKALEMIA

## Consequences

Hyperkalemia causes disturbances in cardiac and skeletal muscle. With severe hyperkalemia, parasthesias and weakness of the extremities can be followed by ascending symmetric flaccid paralysis, which can cause hypoventilation. Muscles of the head and neck as well as sensation are spared. However, the most serious complications of hyperkalemia are cardiac arrhythmias. Changes in the electrocardiogram (ECG) only roughly correlate with the degree of hyperkalemia. Nonetheless, because of the potential for life-threatening cardiac arrhythmias, the ECG is a crucial guide to the need for and urgency of treatment of hyperkalemia (see Fig. 27-1). In general, changes in the ECG occur when the serum potassium exceeds 6.0 mEq/L. Thereafter, the serum potassium can rise precipitously, and the progression from mild ECG changes to ventricular fibrillation can occur within minutes. Thus an ECG must be obtained in patients with severe hyperkalemia, and treatment must be initiated immediately if any changes of hyperkalemia are present.

## Causes: factitious hyperkalemia

In factitious hyperkalemia it is the serum potassium in the test tube, not in the patient, that is elevated. Potassium is released into the serum from white blood cells and from platelets during in vitro blood coagulation or in vitro lysis of red blood cells. Normally, the concentration of potassium in the serum exceeds the plasma concentration by 0.2 to 0.3 mEq/L. Major elevations of the serum potassium concentration can occur in patients with thrombocytosis (platelet counts greater than 800,000 per mm$^3$) or leukocytosis (white blood cell count greater than 100,000 per mm$^3$) attributable to in vitro blood coagulation. In this case, the concentration of potassium is elevated in serum but not in plasma. In vitro hemolysis is easily detected by examination of the serum after centrifugation. Of course, it is essential to differentiate in vitro hemolysis from in vivo hemolysis, which can cause true hyperkalemia. In factitious hyperkalemia, there are no ECG abnormalities, and treatment is unnecessary. The absence of ECG changes despite severe hyperkalemia should alert the physician to check for factitious hyperkalemia.

## Causes: altered transcellular distribution

Hyperkalemia attributable to a shift of potassium from cells to the extracellular fluid results from many causes.[4] Renal potassium excretion is enhanced by hyperkalemia. Thus the hyperkalemia caused by transcellular shifts is generally mild. The serum potassium concentration rarely exceeds 6.0 mEq/L unless there is a simultaneous reduction in renal potassium excretion. Typically the hyperkalemia caused by exercise, acidosis, and glucose infusion in diabetics is transient. Hyperkalemia caused by drugs is sustained as long as the drugs are continued.

**Exercise.** Potassium is released when muscle cells depolarize. Vigorous, prolonged exercise can result in a transient elevation of the serum potassium concentration by as much as 1 to 2 mEq/L with associated ECG changes.[15]

**Acidosis.** The hyperkalemia resulting from acidemia is highly variable and is related to the cause and severity of the acidosis.[8] Significant hyperkalemia occurs only in the setting of acute metabolic acidosis caused by the administration of mineral acids or in the setting of acute, severe respiratory acidosis (pH < 7.00). There is virtually no rise in the serum potassium concentration in acute lactic acidosis, ketoacidosis or in mild respiratory acidosis. As discussed above, chronic metabolic acidosis results in increased potassium excretion and can lead to hypo-kalemia.

**Glucose.** In healthy subjects, glucose infusion leads to the release of insulin, which stimulates cellular uptake of potassium and lowers serum potassium concentrations. In diabetics, however, infusion of 50 to 100 g of dextrose increases serum potassium concentrations by 0.2 to 2.0 mEq/L.[16] The mechanism for this hyperkalemia appears to be transcellular shift of potassium related to extracellular fluid hyperosmo-lality. Hyperkalemia occurs in diabetics with hyperosmotic coma through a similar mechanism. Glucose-induced hyperkalemia also can occur in diabetics after hypertonic dextrose therapy of presumed hypo-glycemic coma. Severe hyperkalemia may result if renal function is impaired from dehydration, hypoaldosteronism, or diabetic ne-phropathy.

**Beta-adrenergic inhibition.** Long-term therapy with beta-adrenergic blocking drugs results in dose-dependent mild hyperkalemia. The aver-age rise in serum potassium is 0.5 mEq/L, and the serum potassium rarely exceeds 6.0 mEq/L.[16] Severe hyperkalemia has been noted when these agents are used in conjunction with high potassium diets, vigor-ous exercise, diabetes, renal disease, and hypoaldosteronism. Since this effect occurs through inhibition of beta$_2$-adrenergic receptors, selective beta$_1$-adrenergic receptor blockers do not raise serum potassium levels and are a more appropriate choice for patients at risk for hyperkalemia.

**Other agents.** Succinylcholine, arginine monohydrochloride, and alpha-adrenergic stimulation raise serum potassium concentration and cause severe hyperkalemia in high-risk patients.[16] Massive digitalis over-dose (over 20 times the usual dose) may also cause severe hyperkalemia. Other agents can directly inhibit distal potassium secretion, such as pen-tamidine.[17]

**Hyperkalemic periodic paralysis.** Hyperkalemic periodic paralysis is defined by profound muscle weakness and hyperkalemia, and the de-gree of hyperkalemia is variable.[9] The condition occurs as an autosomal dominant trait with a typical age of onset of 5 to 10 years. Treatment is with oral glucose. If the hyperkalemia is severe, additional therapy may be necessary.

## Causes: excessive intake

Increased intake of potassium leads to increased renal tubular secretion and increased renal excretion of potassium. With normal renal function, severe hyperkalemia can occur only if the potassium load is very large or given rapidly. The potassium load can be exogenous, as in dietary potassium or prescribed potassium supplements, or endogenous, as in the case of massive cell lysis. Cell lysis is considered with this type of hyperkalemia because the extra potassium cannot shift back into the ruptured cells and must be excreted.

**Increased dietary intake.** Despite the fact that all food derived from animal or vegetable matter contains potassium, hyperkalemia from dietary sources is virtually impossible in the setting of normal kidney function. However, with severely reduced renal function, hyperkalemia is common unless dietary potassium is restricted. Daily potassium intake can be assessed by dietary recall or by measurement of a 24-hour urinary potassium excretion. Urinary potassium excretion closely reflects intake as long as the serum potassium concentration is stable and the patient is not greatly catabolic. In patients subject to hyperkalemia, potassium intake can be restricted to 50 to 75 (2 to 3 g) mEq per day. Further restriction is impractical because nearly all protein sources contain potassium.

Other dietary sources of potassium must also be considered. Salt substitutes frequently contain 15 to 75 mEq of potassium per teaspoon and have been implicated in the development of hyperkalemia in patients with inadequate excretion.[18] Other unusual sources include food supplements and herbal remedies.

**Potassium-containing medications.** Potassium chloride is the most common medicinal source of potassium. In a survey of hospitalized patients, it was implicated in nearly 100% of hyperkalemia. In contrast, hyperkalemia occurred in only 0.4% of patients not taking potassium chloride.[13] The risk of potassium-containing medications has already been discussed in the section on treatment of hypokalemia. Other medicinal potassium sources include alkalinizing potassium salts, potassium penicillin (1.7 mEq per million units), and blood (3 to 4 mEq of potassium per unit).

**Cell lysis.** Acute tumor lysis, rhabdomyolysis, and hemolysis result in the release of potassium from the lysed cells into the extracellular fluid. Occasionally, these disorders also can result in acute renal failure, which prevents rapid excretion of the potassium load and can result in severe elevations in serum potassium concentration. Even in the absence of renal failure, severe hyperkalemia has been reported, as in patients receiving chemotherapy with very large tumor burdens.[16] The hyperkalemia generally peaks in the first 24 hours, and aggressive treatment including dialysis may be necessary. Other complications from the release of intracellular contents include hyperphosphatemia, hyperuricemia, and metabolic acidosis. Prior administration of fluids, sodium bicarbonate, and allopurinol help reduce the incidence and severity of tumor lysis.

## Causes: inadequate excretion

In the majority of patients with clinically significant hyperkalemia, renal excretion of potassium is defective for various reasons.

**Chronic renal failure.** In chronic renal diseases, serum potassium is usually normal or only slightly elevated unless the renal function is severely impaired (glomerular filtration rate less than 15 mL/min). The principal mechanism maintaining potassium balance is increased distal potassium secretion.[4] An additional mechanism is enhanced colonic secretion of potassium. As glomerular filtration falls further, moderate to severe hyperkalemia is commonly observed. Restriction of dietary potassium to 50 mEq (2 g) per day is often successful in preventing severe hyperkalemia if the patient is compliant. However, adequate compliance is difficult to achieve, and the oral administration of the cation-exchange resin, sodium polystyrene sulfonate, 50 to 75 g per day, is occasionally necessary to prevent hyperkalemia. Each gram of resin binds approximately 1 mEq of potassium and releases 2 to 3 mEq of sodium, which can precipitate volume overload in patients with reduced renal function or congestive heart failure. If glomerular filtration is relatively well preserved, hyperkalemia indicates a defect in renal tubular function. Causes of defective tubular potassium secretion are discussed below.

**Acute renal failure.** Acute renal failure is associated with many derangements that can lead to severe hyperkalemia. They include reduced glomerular filtration rate, oliguria, enhanced catabolism, acidemia, and inadvertent administration of potassium chloride.[3] Hyperkalemia occurs in 50% of patients with acute renal failure and often requires dialysis for correction. In prerenal azotemia, measures that improve renal perfusion and function can promptly restore potassium balance and correct hyperkalemia.

**Hypoaldosteronism.** Hyperkalemia is the most common manifestation of hypoaldosteronism. Primary hypoaldosteronism is the result of adrenal disorders. Although rare, Addison's disease should be considered in all cases of hyperkalemia because life-threatening complications can be averted by hormonal therapy. A wide variety of conditions are associated with secondary hypoaldosteronism (see Table 27-2). Drug-induced hyperkalemia caused by inhibition of the renin-angiotensin-aldosterone axis is a common cause of hyperkalemia. Angiotensin-converting enzyme inhibitors, beta blockers, nonsteroidal anti-inflammatory drugs, heparin, and spironolactone are common agents that can cause hyperkalemia through this mechanism.[16] Hyporenin hypoaldosteronism, another important cause of hyperkalemia, tends to occur in older patients (mean age 65 years), with mild renal insufficiency in 70% and diabetes in 50%. Sustained hyperkalemia is found in approximately 75%, metabolic acidosis in 50%, and salt-wasting is rare.[19] Most patients are asymptomatic, but muscle weakness and arrhythmias occur in up to 25% of patients. These patients have normal glucocorticoid function, but 80% had low renin levels. The cause of suppressed renin remains unclear.

Treatment is recommended if serum potassium exceeds 5.5 mEq/L because of the risk of arrhythmia in these patients. Restriction of dietary potassium to 2 to 3 g (<75 mEq) per day is generally sufficient. If not, doses of furosemide at 40 to 80 mg per day (or equivalent doses of other loop diuretics) facilitates renal potassium excretion. Supplemental orally administered sodium chloride is occasionally needed to prevent volume depletion. Correction of the metabolic acidosis, if present, can help lower the serum potassium. Cation-exchange resins, if tolerated, also are helpful. Although pharmacologic doses of exogenous mineralocorticoid fludrocortisone (Florinef), 0.4 to 1.0 mg per day, reduces the serum potassium concentration, therapy often results in sodium retention that can cause weight gain, hypertension, and edema.

**Potassium–sparing diuretics.** Three major potassium-sparing diuretics exist, all of which inhibit sodium reabsorption and thereby reduce potassium secretion in the distal tubule. Spironolactone is a competitive inhibitor of aldosterone for binding to a cytosolic receptor in renal tubular cells. Amiloride and triamterene bind reversibly to the luminal membrane of distal tubule cells, block reabsorption of sodium, and inhibit potassium and hydrogen secretion independency of aldosterone. Amiloride is the most potent of the three diuretics. Spironolactone and triamterene are primarily used in combination therapy to prevent hypokalemia in patients treated with other diuretics. The major side effect of these agents is hyperkalemia. Patients who have renal insufficiency or who are receiving potassium therapy are at high risk for the development of severe hyperkalemia during treatment with these agents. Thus these drugs are best avoided in patients with renal insufficiency or diabetes and in patients taking other medications that put them at risk for hyperkalemia by impairing transcellular distribution, interfering with the renin-angiotensin system, or directly increasing serum potassium.

**Renal tubular secretory defects.** Hyperkalemia can result from renal parenchymal disease that directly affects tubular potassium secretion.[3] Frequently, these diseases also impair hydrogen-ion excretion and result in a hyperchloremic metabolic acidosis. Serum aldosterone levels are appropriately elevated for the level of potassium retention and hyperkalemia. The most common causes of these defects include sickle cell disease, obstruction, lupus nephritis, chronic transplant rejection, and chronic cyclosporin A or lithium toxocity. Treatment is to correct the underlying disorder, if possible. If not, dietary potassium restriction and loop diuretics often help maintain potassium balance and prevent serum potassium concentrations greater than 5.5 mEq/L. Exchange resins are sometimes necessary.

## Treatment of hyperkalemia

The major goal of treatment for hyperkalemia is to avoid cardiac arrhythmias, to restore the serum potassium concentration to normal, and to reduce any excess potassium content of the body. No treatment is needed for factitious hyperkalemia or mild hyperkalemia caused by a temporary shift in body potassium. In patients with normal renal function, it is unnecessary to stop converting enzyme inhibitors, beta blockers, nonsteroidal anti-inflammatory agents, or heparin for mild hyperkalemia. However, these patients should be warned to avoid sustained, vigorous exercise and excessive dietary potassium, salt substitutes, or potassium-sparing diuretics. Serum potassium should be monitored at regular intervals. Similarly, in patients with mild renal failure, dietary potassium restriction is not necessary unless their serum potassium is greater than 5.5 mEq/L. However, these patients should also be warned to avoid excessive potassium intake and to avoid drugs that might further reduce their potassium excretory capacity.

Moderate hyperkalemia (serum potassium 5.5 to 6.0 mEq/L) does not generally cause any ECG abnormalities. To avoid severe hyperkalemia, these patients should reduce potassium intake and discontinue any drugs that may be contributing. If the serum potassium continues to rise or the patient's medical condition is unstable, treatment should be initiated immediately to avoid a further, sometimes precipitous rise in serum potassium.

For severe hyperkalemia (serum potassium greater than 6.0 mEq/L), treatment must be initiated promptly. Three approaches are utilized to reduce the danger of severe hyperkalemia; they include (1) reversing the effect of hyperkalemia on cell membranes (calcium), (2) shifting the potassium into intracellular fluid (dextrose, insulin, alpha-adrenergic stimulants), and (3) removal of potassium from the body (loop diuretics, cation-exchange resins, dialysis). The treatment depends on the severity of the hyperkalemia and on the ECG findings. If the serum potassium concentration is 6.0 to 6.4 mEq/L and there are no ECG changes, the main goal is to remove potassium from the body; this can be accomplished with loop diuretics. Intravenous furosemide 40 to 80 mg, ethacrynic acid 50 to 100 mg, or bumetanide 1 to 2 mg is usually successful in causing a diuresis of 1 to 2 liters containing 75 to 100 mEq of potassium over 1 to 2 hours. In oliguric patients, loop diuretics frequently are not effective. Sodium polystyrene, 25 to 50 g, can be administered orally with 100 to 200 mL of 50% sorbitol solution. In patients who cannot take oral medications, the cation-exchange resin can be administered as an enema, and sorbitol is unnecessary. If the serum potassium concentration is 6.5 mEq/L or greater and the ECG changes are limited to peaked T waves, glucose 25 to 50 g (with regular insulin, 5 to 10 units in diabetics) should be administered intravenously. Therapy with inhaled beta agonists (such as albuterol 10 to 20 mg in 4 mL of saline by nasal inhalation over 10 minutes) also is successful in lowering the serum potassium by approximately 0.5 to 1.5 mEq/L.[20] Intravenous bicarbonate, 45 to 50 mEq, generally has a hypokalemic effect occurring between 30 minutes and 2 hours of administration. This effect is highly variable, especially in renal failure patients. As the bicarbonate is administered with a large sodium load, its use must be monitored carefully in patients with volume expansion. The above therapies do not dispose of the excess potassium stores and are only temporizing; thus therapy with loop diuretics or cation-exchange resins also should be initiated immediately. If the ECG shows QRS widening, it is essential to administer 10% calcium gluconate, 10 mL intravenously, immediately to prevent malignant arrhythmias; the calcium dose can be repeated in 10- to 15-minute intervals. The ECG must be continuously monitored until the QRS interval returns to normal. If the cause of hyperkalemia can be corrected, usually only one or two doses of diuretics or exchange resin are needed to return the serum potassium to less than 5.5 mEq/L. However, dialysis is needed if the response to therapy is inadequate, if the causes of the hyperkalemia cannot be corrected, or if the serum potassium is expected to rise again. During dialysis, the ECG and serum potassium should be monitored every 2 to 4 hours and therapy adjusted appropriately.

## References

1. Lawson DH, Henry DA, Lowe JM, et al: Severe hypokalemia in hospitalized patients, *Arch Intern Med* 139:978, 1979.
2. Shemer J, Ezra D, Modan M, Cabili S: Incidence of hyperkalemia among hospitalized patients, *Isr J Med Sci* 19:659, 1983.

3. Kaplan B, Batlle D: Regulation of potassium balance and metabolism. In Jacobson HR, Striker GE, Klahr S, editors: *The principles and practice of nephrology*, St. Louis, 1995, Mosby.

4. Tannen RL: Disorders of potassium balance. In Brenner BM, Rector FC Jr, editors: *The kidney*, Philadelphia, 1991, Saunders.

5. Kaplan NM, Carnegie A, Raskin P, et al: Potassium supplementation in hypertensive patients with diuretic-induced hypokalemia, *N Engl J Med* 312:746, 1985.

6. Tannen RL: Nephrology Forum. Diuretic-induced hypokalemia, *Kidney Int* 28:988, 1985.

7. Singh H, Linas SL: Potassium therapy of hypertension, *Miner Electrolyte Metab* 19:57, 1993.

8. Adrogue HJ, Madias NE: Changes in potassium concentration during acute acid-base disturbances, *Am J Med* 71:456, 1981.

9. Layzer RB: Periodic paralysis, *Ann Neurol* 11:547, 1982.

10. Kassirer JP, Harrington JT: Diuretics and potassium metabolism: a reassessment of the need, effectiveness and safety of potassium therapy, *Kidney Int* 11:505, 1977.

11. Gennari FJ, Cohen JJ: Role of the kidney in potassium homeostasis: lessons from acid-base disorders, *Kidney Int* 8:1, 1975.

12. Pullen H, Doig A, Lambie AT: Intensive intravenous potassium replacement therapy, *Lancet* 2:809, 1967.

13. Saggar-Malik AK, Cappuccio FP: Potassium supplements and potassium-sparing diuretics: a review and guide to appropriate use, *Drugs* 46:986, 1993.

14. Greenblatt JD, Koch-Weser J: Adverse reactions to spironolactone, *JAMA* 225:40, 1973.

15. Williams ME, Gervine EV, Rosa RM, et al: Catecholamine modulation of rapid potassium shifts during exercise, *N Engl J Med* 312:826, 1985.

16. Ponce SP, Jennings AE, Madias NE, Harrington JT: Drug-induced hyperkalemia, *Medicine* 64:357, 1985.

17. Kleyman TR, Roberts C, Ling BN: A mechanism for pentamidine-induced hyperkalemia: inhibition of distal nephron sodium transport, *Ann Intern Med* 122:103, 1995.

18. Ricardella D, Dwyer JD. Salt substitutes and medicinal potassium sources: risks and benefits, *J Am Diet Assoc* 85:471, 1985.

19. DeFronzo RA: Nephrology Forum. Hyperkalemia and hyporeninemic hypoaldosteronism, *Kidney Int* 17:118, 1980.

20. Allon M, Takeshian A, Shanklin N: Albuterol and insulin for treatment of hyperkalemia in hemodialysis patients, *Kidney Int* 43:212, 1993.

# Chapter 28

# *Acid-Base Disorders*

Richard A. Lafayette

The maintenance of normal body fluid acidity is vital to normal cellular function. Disturbances in acid-base balance frequently indicate the presence of severe underlying disorders. Furthermore, the presence of significant acidemia or alkalemia can have profound clinical consequences. This chapter reviews the diagnosis and management of acid-base disorders focusing on the primary disorders of metabolic acidosis, metabolic alkalosis, repiratiory acidosis, and respiratory alkalosis. Mixed acid-base disorders also are reviewed briefly.

## ACID–BASE PHYSIOLOGY

Body acidity is determined by the interaction of metabolic, renal, and pulmonary processes.[1] The Henderson-Hasselbalch equation relates the equilibrium concentrations of hydrogen ions ($H^+$), bicarbonate ($HCO_3^-$), and partial pressure of carbon dioxide in arterial blood. ($Pa_{CO_2}$) as follows:

$$[H^+] \ (nEq/L) = 24 \times Pa_{CO_2} \ (mm \ Hg)/[HCO_3^-] \ (mEq/L)$$

Given the normal values for $Pa_{CO_2}$ (40 mm Hg) and bicarbonate (24 mEq/L), the normal hydrogen-ion concentration is 40 nEq/L, or a pH of 7.40. It should be clear that alterations either in $Pa_{CO_2}$ or bicarbonate will result in changes in hydrogen-ion concentration and therefore pH. Primary alterations in $Pa_{CO_2}$ are defined as respiratory acid-base disorders. Primary alterations in bicarbonate concentration are defined as metabolic acid-base disorders.

Normal metabolic processes generate approximately 15,000 mmol of $CO_2$ each day that are excreted by the lungs. Normal $Pa_{CO_2}$ is maintained by alterations in the rate of alveolar ventilation that match alterations in the generation of $CO_2$. Deviations from normal indicate a disturbance in alveolar ventilation caused by dysfunction of the peripheral or central nervous system or by dysfunction of respiratory mechanics. In addition to $CO_2$, nonvolatile acids such as phosphoric acid, sulfuric acid, and ammonium are liberated into the body fluids, titrated by bicarbonate and other body buffers, and finally excreted by the kidneys. Approximately 1 mEq/kg of body weight of these acids are generated daily and thus must be excreted each day. A normal plasma bicarbonate concentration is maintained by renal filtration and reabsorption of bicarbonate and by excretion of acid into the urine, thereby regenerating the bicarbonate lost in buffering these acids. Deviations in the bicarbonate concentration indicate disorders in the rate of addition of acid to the buffer system or disorders of the renal tubular processes of bicarbonate reclamation and acidification of the urine.

In addition to primary alterations in the $Paco_2$ or bicarbonate, in each acid-base disorder there are secondary physiologic responses that serve to diminish the effect on hydrogen-ion concentration that would result from the primary disorder. In metabolic acidosis, the decrease in serum bicarbonate is immediately followed by a decline in the $Paco_2$ through increased alveolar ventilation. As a result, the increase in hydrogen-ion concentration is blunted (but not completely corrected). In metabolic alkalosis, the primary elevation in bicarbonate concentration is followed by an increase in the $Paco_2$, reducing but not normalizing the fall in hydrogen-ion concentration. In respiratory alkalosis, the primary decrease in the $Paco_2$ is followed by a secondary decline in the serum bicarbonate concentration. This reduction in bicarbonate increases the hydrogen-ion concentration back toward normal. In respiratory acidosis, the primary increase in the $Paco_2$ is followed by an increase in the serum bicarbonate concentration partially restoring the hydrogen-ion concentration toward normal but leaving it slightly increased. Thus the net change in hydrogen-ion concentration always reflects the primary acid-base disturbance.

In summary, each of the primary acid-base disorders is defined by a primary and secondary alteration in the $Paco_2$ and bicarbonate concentrations and by the resultant effect on the hydrogen-ion concentration (or pH). The direction of these changes and the magnitude are given in Tables 28-1 and 28-2.

## DIAGNOSTIC APPROACH TO ACID-BASE DATA

The best start in defining an acid-base disorder is to classify it according to the definitions in Table 28-1. An arterial blood sample is required

**Table 28-1.** *Definition of acid-base disorders*

| Disorder | Primary alteration | Secondary alteration | Overall effect on body acidity |
|---|---|---|---|
| Metabolic acidosis | ↓ $HCO_3$ | ↓ $Paco_2$ | ↑ H (↓ pH) |
| Metabolic alkalosis | ↑ $HCO_3$ | ↑ $Paco_2$ | ↓ H (↑ pH) |
| Respiratory alkalosis | ↓ $PaCO_2$ | ↓ $HCO_3$ | ↓ H (↑ pH) |
| Respiratory acidosis | ↑ $Paco_2$ | ↑ $HCO_3$ | ↑ H (↓ pH) |

**Table 28-2.** *Responses to primary acid-base disorders*

| Disorder | Response |
|---|---|
| Metabolic acidosis | $Paco_2$ decreases 1.25 mm Hg for every mEq/L $\Delta HCO_3$ ($\pm 5$ mm Hg) |
| Metabolic alkalosis | $Paco_2$ increases 0.75 mm Hg for every mEq/L $\Delta HCO_3$ ($\pm 5$ mm Hg) |
| Respiratory acidosis | |
| Acute | $HCO_3$ increases 1 mEq/L for every 10 mm Hg $\Delta Paco_2$ ($\pm 3$ mEq/L) |
| Chronic | $HCO_3$ increases 4 mEq/L for every 10 mm Hg $\Delta Paco_2$ ($\pm 4$ mEq/L) |
| Respiratory alkalosis | |
| Acute | $HCO_3$ decreases 2 mEq/L for every 10 mm Hg $\Delta Paco_2$ ($\pm 3$ mEq/L) |
| Chronic | $HCO_3$ decreases 4 mEq/L for every 10 mm Hg $\Delta Paco_2$ ($\pm 3$ mEq/L) |

to measure $Paco_2$ and pH. From these data, a value for serum bicarbonate can be calculated and is usually reported. The measured value for serum total $CO_2$ should be within 3 or 4 mEq of the calculated value. If not, there is a measurement error in one of the values, and the samples should be repeated.

The next step is to determine if the acid-base data indicate a simple (single) or mixed (multiple) acid-base disturbance. By using the formulas given in Table 28-2, one can calculate whether the secondary response is within the range of that expected for the primary disturbance. One note of caution is that even acid-base disturbances that appear to be primary can occasionally be caused by a mixed disorder.

The final step is to generate a differential diagnosis for each disorder. The most important cause of each disorder is given in subsequent sections of this chapter. History, physical examination, and review of fluid intake and output often are very helpful in narrowing the list of diagnostic possibilities. Additional laboratory data usually are necessary for definitive diagnosis. The partial pressure of oxygen in arterial blood ($PaO_2$) is measured as part of the arterial blood gas analysis and is essential in evaluating respiratory acid-base disorders. Serum electrolytes (sodium, potassium, chloride), renal function tests (BUN and creatinine), and urine pH should also be obtained in all patients. It is sometimes necessary to measure serum lactate, ketones, salicylate, urine electrolytes, or drug metabolites in blood and urine. Based on these results, initial therapy can be started. Further evaluation is necessary to confirm the presence of isolated renal tubular defects or adrenal diseases.

# METABOLIC ACIDOSIS

Normal metabolism generates a large number of hydrogen ions tending to reduce the serum bicarbonate concentration. Maintenance of the normal bicarbonate concentrate requires urinary excretion of this acid load. The normal response to a decrease in the serum bicarbonate is to reduce the urinary pH to minimal values (4.5 to 5.0) and to increase renal acid excretion. Metabolic acidosis is the result of increased production or intake of nonvolatile acids, reduced renal acid excretion, or loss of bicarbonate.[1,2] These disorders reduce serum bicarbonate concentration, acidify body fluids, and lead to a secondary increase in alveolar ventilation, reducing the $Paco_2$.

In differentiating the causes of metabolic acidosis, it is helpful to calculate the anion gap (AG), defined as:

$$AG = [NA^+] - ([Cl^-] + [HCO_3^-])$$

$[NA^+]$ and $[Cl^-]$ are the serum concentrations of sodium and chloride, respectively. The normal value for the anion gap is 8 to 12 mEq/L and results from the presence of negatively charged proteins, principally albumin. Table 28-3 lists the causes of metabolic acidosis with an increased anion gap and their typical features. Table 28-4 lists the causes of metabolic acidosis with a normal anion gap.

An increased anion-gap metabolic acidosis indicates addition, increased production, or retention of acid in association with anions other than chloride.[3] Usually, the specific disorder can be recognized by the clinical and laboratory features. Confirmation of the disorder by measurement of the specific anion usually is needed only in drug intoxications or for atypical cases of ketoacidosis or lacticacidosis.

A normal anion-gap metabolic acidosis indicates addition of an acid with chloride as the anion, loss of bicarbonate, or failure of renal acid excretion. The patient's history usually allows for the diagnosis of the precise cause. In more complex cases, the urine pH is a valuable clue to the cause of normal anion-gap metabolic acidosis. If acid is added to the body fluids or bicarbonate is lost from the gastrointestinal tract (diarrhea, small bowel, pancreatic or biliary drainage), renal acid excretion should be enhanced, and the urine pH will be less than 5.0. On the other hand, if the cause of the acidosis is the urinary loss of bicarbonate or other specific renal tubular defects, the urine pH is variable (4.5 to 7.5) and reflects the specific defect.[2,4]

To accurately measure the urinary pH, the urine should be tested immediately after collection and should be free of infection. The evaporization of $CO_2$ or the addition of ammonia (from urease-splitting bacteria) alkalinizes the urine and interferes with the interpretation of the urine pH. However, in most cases, the urine dipstick measurement of pH provides the appropriate information. In the case that the urinary pH is borderline (5.5), the urine can be recollected under oil and tested with a pH electrode.

Table 28-4 indicates changes in the serum potassium concentration that are helpful in differentiating the cause of normal anion-gap meta-

**Table 28-3.** *Causes of metabolic acidosis with an increased anion gap (anion gap >12 mEq/L)*

| Disorder | Causes of elevated anion gap | Clinical characteristics | Confirmatory tests |
|---|---|---|---|
| **KETOACIDOSIS** | | | |
| Diabetes | Acetoacetate, beta-hydroxybutyrate | Hyperglycemia, urine, and serum ketones strongly positive | Serum beta-hydroxybutyrate |
| Alcoholism | Beta-hydroxybutyrate | History of alcoholism, urine and serum ketones weakly positive | Serum beta-hydroxybutyrate |
| Starvation | Acetoacetate, beta-hydroxybutyrate | Mild acidosis, urine and serum ketones weakly positive | |
| **LACTIC ACIDOSIS** | | | |
| Renal failure | Lactic acid | Hypoxia, shock, tumor | Serum lactate |
| | Sulfate, phosphate, other endogenous anions | Increased BUN, creatinine | Serum creatinine >4 mg/dL |
| **DRUG INTOXICATION** | | | |
| Aspirin | Salicylate, endogenous anions | Primary respiratory alkalosis, tinnitus | Serum salicylate level |
| Ethylene glycol | Glycolate | Coma, seizures, renal failure, urine calcium oxalate crystals, increased osmolar gap | Serum ethylene glycol level |
| Methanol | Formate | Dimmed vision, abdominal pain, increased osmolar gap; distinctive breath odor | Serum methanol level |
| Paraldehyde | Unknown | | Serum paraldehyde level |

272

**Table 28–4.** *Causes of metabolic acidosis with a normal anion gap (anion gap ≤12 mEq/L)*

| Disorder | Urine pH | Serum potassium | Clinical characteristics |
|---|---|---|---|
| Diarrhea or intestinal fluid loss | ≤5 | Decreased | Appropriate history |
| Urinary-intestinal anastomosis | ≥6 | Decreased | History of treatment for obstruction, reflux |
| Renal tubular acidosis (RTA) | | | |
| Type I (distal) | >5 | Decreased | Serum creatinine normal, nephrolithiasis, bone disease, failure to acidify urine with acidification test |
| Type II (proximal) | ≤5 | Decreased | Serum creatinine normal, increased urine pH with alkalinization |
| Hyporeninemic hypoaldosteronism (type IV RTA) | ≤5 | Increased | Mild renal disease, diabetes, decreased renin, decreased aldosterone |
| Mild renal disease | ≤5 | Normal, increased | Serum creatinine, 2 to 4 mg/dL |
| Carbonic anhydrase inhibitors | >5 | Decreased | History of medication |
| Adrenal insufficiency | <5 | Increased | Decreased serum cortisol |
| Acid ingestion | ≤5 | Increased | History of treatment with acid |

bolic acidosis. Hyperkalemia is often present with adrenal insufficiency, hypoaldosteronism, type IV renal tubular acidosis, or the administration of hydrochloric acidosis. Hypokalemia is usually present with diarrhea and type I and type II renal tubular acidosis.

## Consequences and treatment of metabolic acidosis

In some circumstances, the acidosis itself has serious consequences and requires urgent therapeutic intervention in addition to specific treatment for the underlying disorder. The most important consequences include secondary hyperventilation, disturbances in myocardial function, systemic vasodilatation, and alterations in the serum potassium concentration. Most patients experience labored respirations if the systemic pH declines to less than 7.10 (serum bicarbonate concentration less than 12 to 14 mEq/L). In addition, depression in myocardial contractility and reduction in the threshold for ventricular fibrillation may occur when the pH is below 7.10. Based on these considerations, intravenous administration of sodium bicarbonate is recommended to raise the pH to this level.[2] It should be kept in mind that no definitive benefit of alkali therapy on clinical outcome has been demonstrated.[5] The following guidelines should be followed during therapy with sodium bicarbonate:

1. The dose of sodium bicarbonate should be estimated from the bicarbonate deficit and the rate of ongoing losses. The bicarbonate deficit is calculated as follows:

$$\begin{array}{cc} \text{Bicarbonate} & \text{Space of} & \text{(Target value} \\ \text{deficit} = \text{distribution} \times - \text{Current value)} \\ \text{(mEq)} & \text{(L)} & \text{(mEq/L)} \end{array}$$

Ongoing losses of bicarbonate are calculated as follows:

$$\begin{array}{l} \text{Bicarbonate loss (mEq/day)} = \text{Fluid loss (L/day)} \\ \times \text{Fluid } [HCO_3^-] \text{ (mEq/L)} \end{array}$$

These calculations provide a rough estimate only. Usually half of this dose should be administered initially, and repeat measurements should be obtained in 4 to 8 hours.

2. The space of distribution for administered bicarbonate is approximately 50% of body weight (0.5 L/kg). In extreme acidosis (pH less than 7.10), the space of distribution usually exceeds this value and may be as high as 80% to 100% of body weight.[6]

3. If the reduction in the $Paco_2$ is appropriate for the reduction in serum bicarbonate concentration, the target value for bicarbonate concentration should be 12 to 14 mEq/L. In patients with mixed acid-base disorders, the target value should be estimated from the Henderson-Hasselbalch equation and Table 28-2 and should be based on the assumption that the $Paco_2$ will not change initially.

4. Serum potassium generally declines during bicarbonate therapy. Potassium supplementation should begin immediately in hypokalemic patients and in normokalemic patients without renal failure.[7] Potassium therapy should be withheld initially in patients with hyperkalemia or in normokalemic patients with renal failure. In all circumstances, serum potassium should be monitored at 8- to 24-hour intervals during therapy. Further discussion of potassium therapy is included in Chapter 27.

5. "Overshoot alkalosis" frequently occurs during therapy as a result of three factors: (1) persistent hyperventilation caused by persistent cerebrospinal fluid acidosis that results from slow equilibration of administered bicarbonate between plasma and cerebrospinal fluid, (2) metabolism of organic anions (ketoacids, lactate) to bicarbonate after correction of the underlying condition, and (3) continuing renal acid excretion and regeneration of bicarbonate.

6. In lactic acidosis, bicarbonate administration may actually increase lactate production, and blood lactate levels may rise; however, this increase has not been shown to have deleterious clinical consequences.[8] Recent studies employing inhibitors of lactate formation (dichloroacetate) or alternative sources of buffer such as carbicarb have not demonstrated any clear advantage over bicarbonate.[9,10]

For these reasons it is important to limit bicarbonate therapy to cases of severe acidemia and not to exceed the target value of 12 to 14 mEq/L for the serum bicarbonate concentration.

## METABOLIC ALKALOSIS

Metabolic alkalosis is defined as a primary elevation in serum bicarbonate concentration. Although many disorders may lead to an increase in serum bicarbonate concentration, the alkalosis persists only if the increased bicarbonate concentration is sustained. In discussing metabolic alkalosis, the processes that initiate a rise in serum bicarbonate concentration must be distinguished from those that sustain it. This is especially important, since in metabolic alkalosis, unlike other acid-base disorders, the disorder can persist even after resolution of the initiating factors.

Metabolic alkalosis may be initiated by addition of bicarbonate, loss of hydrogen ions, or loss of chloride.[1,2] The most common causes of metabolic alkalosis include vomiting, nasogastric suction, diuretic administration, and antacid ingestion. These disorders raise the serum bicarbonate, alkalinize body fluids, and lead to a secondary decrease in ventilation. Two normal processes operate to reduce the elevated bicarbonate level. First, the ongoing generation of endogenous acids titrates bicarbonate. Second, the normal response to a primary increase in the serum bicarbonate concentration is a decrease in renal acid excretion. Therefore factors that may sustain the metabolic alkalosis include persistent bicarbonate administration or enhanced net renal acid excretion caused by increased secretion of mineralocorticoid hormones or by chloride depletion.

The patient's history usually discloses the factors that initiated the metabolic alkalosis. In distinguishing among the factors that sustain the alkalosis, measurement of urine pH and of chloride concentration provides valuable clues to the diagnosis and a rationale for treatment. Table 28-5 lists the causes of metabolic alkalosis on the basis of these measurements.

A urine pH greater than 6.0 discloses the presence of bicarbonate in the urine and indicates that alkali administration or vomiting may be ongoing. Because of the high rate of bicarbonate excretion that may be achieved by the normal kidney, metabolic alkalosis rarely results from alkali administration unless the glomerular filtration rate is impaired. It is important to note that other factors may raise the urine pH in patients with metabolic alkalosis. As discussed earlier, evaporation

**Table 28-5.** *Causes of metabolic alkalosis*

| Clinical disorder | Characteristics | Confirmatory tests |
|---|---|---|
| **ALKALI ADMINISTRATION (urine pH >6)** | | |
| Milk-alkali syndrome | Increased serum calcium | |
| Administration of large amounts of sodium bicarbonate | Hypertension | |
| Renal insufficiency | Increased serum creatinine | |
| **CHLORIDE RESPONSIVE (urine Cl <10 mEq/L)** | | |
| Gastric fluid loss | Decreased serum potassium | |
| Diuretic therapy | Decreased serum potassium | |
| After relief of hypercapnia | Decreased serum potassium | |
| Colonic villous adenoma | Decreased serum potassium | |
| **CHLORIDE RESISTANT (urine Cl >20 mEq/L)** | | |
| Primary hyperaldosteronism | Hypertension, decreased serum potassium | Increased aldosterone Decreased renin |
| Cushing's syndrome | Hypertension, hirsutism, decreased serum potassium | Cortisol |
| Bartter's syndrome | Decreased serum potassium | Increased aldosterone Increased renin |
| Idiopathic | Decreased serum potassium | |

of carbon dioxide or infection with urease-producing bacteria will alkalinize the urine. In addition, transient elevation of the urine pH may occur during vomiting and during alkali administration, even if the administered alkali is not responsible for sustaining the alkalosis. Thus the finding of an alkaline urine must be interpreted in light of the patient's clinical history.

A urine pH less than 6.0 indicates that ongoing renal acid excretion is the cause of sustained metabolic alkalosis. Measurement of the urine chloride concentration distinguishes two subgroups of disorders that differ in their pathogenesis and treatment. A urine chloride concentration less than 10 mEq/L indicates that the patient is ingesting a low-salt diet and that relative chloride deficiency is the cause of persistent renal acid excretion. These disorders are termed "chloride responsive" because of the prompt excretion of bicarbonate in the urine and resolution of the alklaosis when chloride is administered. In patients with metabolic alkalosis attributable to ongoing diuretic therapy, the urine chloride concentration is transiently elevated during the diuresis. However, the alkalosis is sustained even after the diuretic is discontinued unless chloride is provided. Severe metabolic alkalosis (serum bicarbonate concentration greater than 35 mEq/L) with low urine chloride is usually the result of drainage of gastric fluid or of diuretic therapy for edematous conditions. In contrast, metabolic alkalosis from diuretic administration in nonedematous subjects is usually relatively mild.

A value for urine chloride greater than 20 mEq/L indicates that the patient has adequate dietary chloride intake and that another factor, usually mineralocorticoid excess, is the cause of sustained renal acid excretion. These disorders are termed "chloride resistant" because treatment with chloride fails to improve the metabolic alkalosis and, in fact, may worsen the acid-base disorder. In most cases, the metabolic alkalosis is mild; hypokalemia is usually the more pronounced electrolyte abnormality.

## Consequences and treatment of metabolic alkalosis

In addition to specific treatment for the underlying cause of metabolic alkalosis, therapy to lower the serum bicarbonate may be indicated if the value exceeds 35 mEq/L. The rise in systemic pH in metabolic alkalosis is not usually extreme because of secondary hypoventilation. Indeed, the pH does not exceed 7.55 unless the serum bicarbonate concentration is greater than 50 mEq/L. Nonetheless, reduction of the serum bicarbonate concentration to less than 35 mEq/L is important because of the following considerations:

1. Secondary hypoventilation reduces alveolar oxygen tension. For patients with cardiopulmonary diseases, the resultant decline in the Pao$_2$ may result in clinically significant hypoxia.
2. Transient hyperventilation of even a modest degree strikingly raises systemic pH to severely alkaline values. For example, if serum bicarbonate concentration is 35 mEq/L, a reduction in the Paco$_2$ from the expected value of 47 to 35 mm Hg results in a rise in pH from 7.50 to 7.62. In fact, it follows from the Henderson-Hasselbalch equation that whenever the values for bicarbonate concentration and Paco$_2$ are equal, hydrogen concentration is 24 mEq/L and corresponds to a pH of 7.62. Extreme alkalemia may be associated with depression of consciousness, delirium, seizures, and tetany. The likelihood of hyperventilation is greatest in patients with cardiopulmonary or liver disease, with sepsis, and in the postoperative period circumstances in which metabolic alkalosis frequently occurs.
3. Increased urinary potassium excretion and potassium depletion are the consequence of virtually every cause of metabolic alkalo-

sis. In general, the degree of potassium depletion parallels the severity of the alkalosis although the acid-base disturbance is not directly the cause of the altered potassium metabolism. In patients with serum bicarbonate 35 to 40 mEq/L, the serum potassium is often 2.5 to 3.5 mEq/L, and the potassium deficit is 200 to 500 mEq. Furthermore, renal potassium conservation and repair of the potassium deficit cannot proceed until the underlying acid-base disorder is corrected. During treatment of metabolic alkalosis, it is important to assess the extent of the potassium deficit, to provide adequate potassium therapy, and to monitor the serum potassium concentration carefully.

The treatment for metabolic alkalosis caused by alkali administration is discontinuation of alkali therapy. If renal function is not severely impaired, the continuing alkaline diuresis rapidly lowers serum bicarbonate concentration. If hypercalemia is also present, as in the milk-alkali syndrome, treatment with sodium chloride and loop diuretics often improves renal function and aids in resolution of the alkalosis. This treatment increases urinary potassium excretion. Treatment with hydrochloric acid or its precursors is necessary (see below) only if renal function is severely reduced.

Chloride-responsive metabolic alkalosis requires provision of chloride to correct the acid-base disorder and to prevent further renal potassium wasting. The choice of the cation to accompany chloride depends on the severity of the cation deficits, the patient's tolerance to administered cations, and the severity of the alkalosis. As discussed, potassium chloride administration is usually necessary because of the accompanying potassium deficit. In patients with extracellular fluid depletion, sodium and potassium chloride should be prescribed in the diet or intravenously.[11] In edematous patients, it is necessary to continue sodium restriction and to administer potassium chloride alone. With correction of chloride depletion, renal acid excretion is reduced, and bicarbonate is excreted in the urine. However, if serum bicarbonate is greatly elevated or if renal function is impaired, several days may be required for serum bicarbonate to decline to an acceptable level. In these cases, more rapid lowering of serum bicarbonate may be achieved with infusion of hydrochloric acid.

In chloride-resistant alkalosis, by definition, treatment with chloride fails to improve both the alkalosis and the potassium deficit. Definitive treatment requires resolution of the underlying condition. Disorders of excess adrenal steroid secretion may be ameliorated by spironolactone, and Bartter's syndrome may improve after treatment with indomethacin. Treatment with large amounts of potassium chloride is sometimes helpful in idiopathic chloride-resistant metabolic alkalosis. The alkalosis is rarely severe, and treatment with hydrochloric acid is rarely necessary.

Extreme metabolic alkalosis (serum bicarbonate concentration greater than 45 mEq/L), regardless of the cause, should be treated by infusion of hydrochloric acid or one of its precursors. The dose of acid administered should be calculated to reduce the serum bicarbonate to approximately 35 to 40 mEq/L over an 8- to 24-hour interval. The space of distribution of administered acid may be assumed to be approximately 50% of body weight. Various acid solutions are available for intravenous infusion. Ammonium chloride (20 mg/mL) contains 350 mEq/L hydrogen ions and can be given at rates up to 500 mL per hour. Ammonium chloride is contraindicated in patients with liver disease. Arginine monohydrochloride (10%) contains approximately 500 mEq/L hydrogen ions and can be given at rates of 300 mL per hour if necessary. Serum potassium levels rise, however, and this therapy is contraindicated in patients with severe renal insufficiency. Dilute hydrochloric acid (0.1 to 0.15 N) contains 100 to 150 mEq/L hydrogen ions and may be given safely to patients with renal and liver diseases; however, because of its corrosive nature, it must be administered into a central vein. Hydrochloric acid is the preferable method of treatment if a central venous catheter is in place. As already discussed, serum potassium should be carefully monitored during therapy and acid-base status should be reassessed frequently.

# RESPIRATORY ALKALOSIS

Respiratory alkalosis, a primary decrease in the $Paco_2$, is synonymous with alveolar hyperventilation and is the most common acid-base disorder. In many cases, the abnormal pattern of respiration is easily detected by clinical observation. Often, however, these signs are overlooked, and hyperventilation is recognized only after an arterial blood gas measurement is performed. The primary decline in the $Paco_2$ alkalinizes body fluids and reduces renal acid excretion, thus leading to a secondary decline in serum bicarbonate concentration. Unlike the rapid respiratory response to metabolic acid-base disorders, the new steady-state levels for serum bicarbonate concentration and pH are achieved only 2 to 3 days after the primary change in the $Paco_2$.[7] Thus the duration of hyperventilation in patients with respiratory alkalosis may be estimated from the values for serum bicarbonate and pH, as shown in Table 28-2.

Under normal circumstances, the rate of alveolar ventilation is regulated by the brainstem respiratory center in response to changes in acidity and in oxygen tension in body fluids. Both hypoxemia and acidosis increase alveolar ventilation. However, these normal regulatory processes may be overridden by disorders of the central nervous system or of the pulmonary system and drugs that affect the respiratory center, thereby leading to hyperventilation despite normal $Pao_2$ and systemic pH.[12] As shown in the box on p. 280, respiratory alkalosis may be caused by a wide variety of disorders.

The approach to the diagnosis is first to determine if hypoxia is the cause of hyperventilation. Alveolar ventilation is stimulated by a decline in the $Pao_2$ to 60 mm Hg or less. The underlying causes of hypoxemia include ventilation-perfusion mismatching attributable to pulmonary diseases or to right-to-left (cyanotic) cardiac shunts. Tissue hypoxia caused by hypotension (especially when associated with sepsis) or by severe anemia (hemoglobin less than 30% of normal) also can result

## Causes of Respiratory Alkalosis

HYPOXIA

High altitude
Ventilation-perfusion mismatching
Right-to-left cardiac shunt
Hypotension
Severe anemia

CENTRAL NERVOUS SYSTEM MEDIATED

Pregnancy
Anxiety
Drugs and toxins (salicylates)
Neurologic diseases
Hepatic failure
Sepsis
Recovery from metabolic acidosis

PULMONARY DISEASES

Pulmonary edema
Interstitial lung disease
Pulmonary embolism
Pneumonia

MECHANICAL OVERVENTILATION

in hyperventilation, even if the $Pa_{O_2}$ is normal. Respiratory alkalosis is normally seen in people living at high altitude and is a result of the reduced atmospheric oxygen tension. In patients without hypoxia, hyperventilation is attributable either to stimulation of respiration by drugs or toxins, to central nervous system or pulmonary disorders, or to mechanical overventilation. It is important to note that respiratory alkalosis is a characteristic feature of normal pregnancy; the $Pa_{CO_2}$ falls to as low as 28 to 30 mm Hg in the third trimester. The hyperventilation of pregnancy has been ascribed to increased levels of progesterone.

## Consequences and treatment of respiratory alkalosis

Respiratory alkalosis occurs in a wide variety of clinical settings, ranging from normal adaptations and self-limiting anxiety to severe life-threatening disorders. In most cases the respiratory alkalosis itself is a harmless feature of the underlying condition. Reduced $Pa_{CO_2}$ causes cerebral vasoconstriction; consequently, mechanical hyperventilation is employed therapeutically in patients with acute neurologic disease to reduce cerebral edema. However, it is unknown whether the decline in cerebral blood flow is responsible for the central nervous system side effects of hyperventilation. Acute severe respiratory alkalosis is associated with paresthesias in the extremities, circumoral numbness, tightness in the chest, and, in some cases, seizures. Atrial and ventricular tachyarrhythmias may occur in patients with underlying ischemic heart disease. In contrast, there are few clinical manifestations attributable to chronic respiratory alkalosis.

Treatment should be directed at the underlying cause of the disorder. In patients with hypoxemia, elevation of the $Pa_{O_2}$ to 60 mm Hg should be sufficient to suppress the hypoxic respiratory drive and to raise the $Pa_{CO_2}$. In patients with anxiety attacks, one can raise the $Pa_{CO_2}$ transiently by instructing the patient to breathe in and out of a paper bag, thus raising the $Pa_{CO_2}$ in the inspired air. In patients with mechanical overventilation, ventilator settings for rate, tidal volume, or dead space should be adjusted to reduce the rate of alveolar ventilation. If the underlying disorder cannot be reversed (as in hepatic failure or central nervous system disease), there is little that can be done to suppress ventilation. Usually the alkalemia is not severe unless there is accompanying metabolic alkalosis. In cases of severe alkalemia attributable to mixed acid-base disorders, treatment of the alkalemia itself is best accomplished by treatment of the metabolic alkalosis.

# RESPIRATORY ACIDOSIS

Respiratory acidosis, a primary increase in the $Pa_{CO_2}$, is synonymous with alveolar hypoventilation. The adequacy of alveolar ventilation cannot be assessed on clinical gounds alone; the measurement of the $Pa_{CO_2}$ in an arterial blood sample is essential for an accurate diagnosis of respiratory acidosis. The rise in the $Pa_{CO_2}$ acidifies body fluids, secondarily increases renal acid excretion, and elevates serum bicarbonate concentration. The new steady-state levels for serum bicarbonate concentration and for pH are achieved 2 to 3 days after a primary change in $Pa_{CO_2}$. Thus acute and chronic respiratory acidosis may be distinguished by the values for serum bicarbonate, as shown in Table 28-2. This distinction is especially important for diagnosis and treatment.

The causes of respiratory acidosis include a variety of central and peripheral nervous system, thoracic, and pulmonary diseases that suppress the ventilatory response to $CO_2$ that impair respiratory mechanics, or that obstruct the airway (Table 28-6). Acute respiratory acidosis may result from any of these disorders and constitutes a medical emergency. The most common causes include airway obstruction from aspiration or asthma, depression of the respiratory center from drugs or toxins, severe pulmonary edema, cardiac arrest, cervical spinal cord transection, pneumothorax, and flail chest. Chronic respiratory acidosis is usually seen in patients with chronic obstructive or restrictive lung diseases, kyphoscoliosis, or neuromuscular diseases, and often persists despite therapy.

**Table 28-6.** *Causes of respiratory acidosis*

| Acute | Chronic |
|---|---|
| **AIRWAY OBSTRUCTION** | |
| Aspiration | Chronic obstructive pulmonary disease |
| Laryngospasm | |
| Bronchospasm | |
| Obstructive sleep apnea | |
| Drowning | |
| **RESPIRATORY CENTER DEPRESSION** | |
| General anesthesia | Obesity hypoventilation syndrome |
| Sedative-hypnotic drug overdose | |
| Central sleep apnea | |
| **CIRCULATORY CATASTROPHE** | |
| Cardiac arrest | |
| Severe pulmonary edema | |
| **NEUROMUSCULAR DEFECTS** | |
| Cervical spine transection | Poliomyelitis |
| Guillain-Barré syndrome | Multiple sclerosis |
| Myasthenia gravis crisis | Muscular dystrophy |
| Drugs or toxin (succinylcholine, | Amyotrophic lateral sclerosis |
| aminoglycosides) | Polymyositis |
| Myxedema | |
| **RESTRICTIVE DEFECTS** | |
| Pneumothorax | Kyphoscoliosis |
| Flail chest | Spinal arthritis |
| Pleural effusion | |
| Severe interstitial fibrosis | |
| Decreased diaphragmatic | |
| movement (ascites, obesity) | |
| **MECHANICAL UNDERVENTILATION** | |

Modified from Cohen JJ, Kassirer JP: *Acid base,* Boston, 1982, Little, Brown.

The approach to the diagnosis starts with examination of the patient's respiration. Infrequent shallow respirations in respiratory acidosis indicate depression of the brainstem respiratory center or neuromuscular disorders. It is especially important to discontinue or reverse drugs causing sedation or neuromuscular blockade. Tachypnea and signs of respiratory distress indicate thoracic disorders and obstructive or restrictive pulmonary diseases. The history, physical examination (including neurologic examination), and blood gas analysis (including measurement of the $Pao_2$) are usually sufficient to distinguish among the various causes of respiratory acidosis. In some cases, measurement of respiratory mechanics is also necessary. In contrast to metabolic acidosis, measurements of serum electrolytes, renal function, urinary pH, and urinary electrolytes usually do not help distinguish among the causes of respiratory acidosis.

## Consequences and treatment of respiratory acidosis

The most serious consequences of alveolar hypoventilation are hypoxia and central nervous system effects of hypercapnia. During acute hypoventilation, severe hypercapnia rarely develops because patients succumb to hypoxia before the $Paco_2$ can rise to extreme levels. If ventilation ceases abruptly, death from hypoxia occurs in less than 5 minutes. Thus, in the absence of supplemental oxygen, $Paco_2$ values greater than 80 mm Hg rarely occur. If, however, the $Pao_2$ is maintained by supplemental oxygen, the $Paco_2$ may rise to levels in excess of 100 mm Hg. The effects of hypercapnia include cerebral and peripheral vasodilatation and stimulation of the sympathetic nervous system. Clinical manifestations include anxiety, breathlessness, headache, disorientation, and confusion. With extreme hypercapnia ($Paco_2$ 70 to 100 mm Hg), depression of consciousness, asterixis, and coma may occur. Rarely, clinical signs of increased intracranial pressure including papilledema and focal neurologic findings occur. The effects of the $Paco_2$ on neurologic function are highly variable and are influenced by the prevailing $Pao_2$, the pH, the base-line level of $Paco_2$, and the rate of rise in $Paco_2$. Acute respiratory acidosis is accompanied by flushing, tachycardia, and diaphoresis; however, these manifestations are not present in chronic respiratory acidosis. Although supraventricular and ventricular tachycardias are common in patients with chronic respiratory acidosis attributable to chronic lung disease, it is likely that these arrhythmias are caused by the concomitant effect of hypoxia, bronchodilators, and digitalis, rather than by the elevated level of the $Paco_2$ directly.

Acute respiratory acidosis is a medical emergency. Supplemental oxygen and restoration of ventilation must be achieved at once. Mechanical ventilation must be initiated if the underlying disorder cannot be reversed within minutes.

In chronic respiratory acidosis related to obstructive airway disease, the degree of airway obstruction correlates poorly with the level of hypercapnia.[1] Chronic $CO_2$ retention reduces the sensitivity of the repiratory center to $CO_2$. Although provision of supplemental oxygen frequently is necessary for treatment of hypoxemia, elevation of the $Pao_2$ to values greater than 60 mm Hg may suppress hypoxic respiratory drive and further suppress ventilation. Therefore oxygen should be administered initially in a low dose (24% to 28%) to patients with chronic respiratory acidosis. Arterial blood gases should be sampled after 20 mintues to guide further oxygen therapy. Treatment of the underlying disorder may improve the $CO_2$ retention.

# MIXED ACID-BASE DISORDERS

A mixed acid-base disorder is defined as the coexistence of two or more primary (simple) acid-base disorders. As discussed earlier, a large number of medical conditions affect the $Paco_2$ and bicarbonate concentrations. Not surprisingly, the coexistence of these conditions frequently gives rise to a mixed acid-base disorder. Some examples of common mixed acid-base disorders include (1) severe pulmonary edema (lactic acidosis and hypoventilation), (2) sepsis (lactic acidosis and hyperventilation), (3) severe renal failure with vomiting (uremic acidosis and metabolic alkalosis), (4) salicylate intoxication (metabolic acidosis and hyperventilation), and (5) improvement after an exacerbation of chronic obstructive pulmonary disease (respiratory acidosis and metabolic alkalosis). Although the diagnosis of mixed acid-base disorders should be suspected in patients with multiple causes of acid-base disturbances, accurate diagnosis requires evaluation of arterial blood gas data and knowledge of the formulas in Table 28-2. If the secondary responses are not appropriate, a mixed disorder is present. However, the converse is not true: a mixed disorder may be present even if the data are consistent with a simple disorder.[2] For example, combined metabolic acidosis and alkalosis may appear as a simple metabolic acidosis or alkalosis, and combined acute respiratory acidosis and metabolic alkalosis may appear as a simple chronic respiratory alkalosis. In these cases the correct diagnosis is surmised from the clinical history, the temporal evolution of the acid-base abnormalities, consideration of the anion gap, and serum potassium concentrations.

In general, the treatment of mixed acid-base disorders should proceed in the same fashion as the treatment of the individual acid-base disorders that are present. It is important to remember that the coexisting primary disorders may have offsetting or aggravating effects on overall hydrogen-ion concentration. Therefore, special care is required to select target values for bicarbonate that will maintain pH in the desirable range during the administration of acid or alkali.

## References

1. Cohen JJ, Kassirer JP: *Acid base,* Boston, 1982, Little, Brown.
2. Madias NE: Fluid, electrolyte and acid-base disorders. In Jacobson HR, Striker G, Klahr S, editors: *The principles and practice of nephrology,* St. Louis, 1995, Mosby.
3. Gabow PA: Nephrology Forum. Disorders associated with an altered anion gap, *Kidney Int* 27:472, 1985.
4. Morris RC, Ives HE: Inherited disorders of the renal tubule. In Brenner BM, Rector FC, editors: *The kidney,* Philadelphia, 1991, Saunders.
5. Graf H, Leach W, Arieff AI: Evidence for a detrimental effect of bicarbonate therapy in hypoxic lactic acidosis, *Science* 227:754, 1983.
6. Garrella S, Dana CL, Chazan JA: Severity of metabolic acidosis as a determinant of bicarbonate requirements, *N Engl J Med* 289:121, 1973.
7. Fulop M: Serum potassium in lactic acidosis and ketoacidosis, *N Engl J Med* 300:1087, 1970.
8. Madias NE: Nephrology Forum. Lactic acidosis, *Kidney Int* 29:752, 1986.

9. Leung JM, Landow L, Franks M, et al: Safety and efficacy of intravenous carbicarb in patients undergoing surgery: comparison with sodium bicarbonate in the treatment of metabolic acidosis, *Crit Care Med* 22:1540, 1994.
10. Stacpole PW, Wright EC, Baumgartner TG, et al: A controlled trial of dichloroacetate for treatment of lactic acidosis in adults, *N Engl J Med* 327:1564, 1992.
11. Halperin ML, Scheich A: Should we continue to recommend that a deficit of KCl be treated with NaCl? A fresh look at chloride-depletion alkalosis, *Nephron* 67:263, 1994.

# Chapter 29
# *Diagnosis of Renal Insufficiency*

Richard A. Lafayette

Renal insufficiency is defined as a decline in glomerular filtration rate (GFR). It may occur acutely or be a chronic condition. This chapter focuses on the diagnosis of acute renal insufficiency; the management of acute and chronic renal insufficiency is discussed in the following chapter. Acute renal insufficiency is a frequent and serious problem among hospitalized patients. Despite the inexact relationship between serum creatinine concentration and GFR, a rise in serum creatinine concentration is the most reliable and readily available clinical indicator of an acute decline in renal function.[1,2] Consultation is frequently requested because of a sudden increase in the serum creatinine concentration during the monitoring of an acutely ill patient.

## HOSPTIAL-ACQUIRED RENAL INSUFFICIENCY

In a prospective survey of approximately 2000 patients admitted to the medical and surgical services of a large teaching hospital,[3] acute renal insufficiency was diagnosed in 5% of patients; 80% of episodes of renal insufficiency were acquired during the course of hospitalization. The prevalence of hospital-acquired acute renal insufficiency was higher in patients with preexisting renal insufficiency: it was 2.9% for patients with an initially normal serum creatinine concentration and 14% for patients with an initially elevated serum creatinine concentration. The major causes were reduced renal perfusion attributable to circulatory disturbances (42%), drug toxicity, particularly from aminoglycoside antibiotics and radiographic contrast (20%), or a combination of disorders occurring within 72 hours after surgery (18%) (Table 29-1). Fortunately, most episodes of renal insufficiency were mild; the rise in serum creatinine was greater than 3.0 mg/dL in only 19% of patients, and dialysis was necessary in only 8%. Mortality was approximately 30% and was related to the severity of acute renal insufficiency (Table 29-1). In patients with a rise in serum creatinine concentration of less than 3.0 mg/dL, mortality was 15%; in patients with a rise greater than 3.0 mg/dL, mortality was 65%. Despite the high mortality, only

**Table 29–1.** *Causes and mortality of hospital-acquired renal insufficiency*

| | Number of episodes | Percentage of total | Number of deaths | Mortality (%) |
|---|---|---|---|---|
| Decreased renal perfusion | | 42 | | |
| ECF volume contraction | 22 | | 2 | 9 |
| Severe heart failure | 18 | | 9 | 50 |
| Sepsis with hypotension | 10 | | 4 | 40 |
| Hypotension of unknown cause | 4 | | 4 | 100 |
| Therapeutic agents | | 20 | | |
| Aminoglycosides | 9 | | 1 | 11 |
| Contrast media | 16 | | 1 | 6 |
| Platinum | 1 | | 0 | 0 |
| Major surgery | | 18 | 3 | 13 |
| Heart surgery | 15 | | | |
| Aorta surgery | 3 | | | |
| Other surgery | 5 | | | |
| Urinary obstruction | 3 | 2 | 0 | 0 |
| Hepatorenal syndrome | 5 | 4 | 4 | 80 |
| Multifactorial | 4 | 3 | 0 | 0 |
| Miscellaneous and unknown | 14 | 11 | 4 | 29 |
| Total | 129 | 100 | 32 | 25 |

Data from Hou SH, Bushinsky DA, Wish JB, et al: *Am J Med* 74:243, 1983.
*ECF*, Extracellular fluid.

10% of deaths could be attributed to renal insufficiency itself as compared with the underlying disorder.

## DIFFERENTIAL DIAGNOSIS OF ACUTE RENAL INSUFFICIENCY

### Serum creatinine concentration

The interpretation of the serum creatinine concentration is complicated by several factors.[1,2] First, creatinine is excreted both by glomerular filtration and by tubular secretion; therefore the serum creatinine concentration is consistently below the value that would be obtained if creatinine were an ideal filtration marker. Second, creatinine generation is reduced in normal persons with reduced meat intake or with low muscle mass, such as vegetarians, thin women, and the elderly, and in patients who are chronically ill. Thus, even normal values for serum creatinine concentration may be associated with reductions in GFR to as low as 20 mL/min/1.73 m². As a result, the serum creatinine correlates only roughly with the absolute value of the GFR. Nevertheless, the finding of an elevated serum creatinine in the steady state is a near-certain indication that the GFR is reduced. An important exception to this rule is the elevation in serum creatinine that occurs without a reduction in the GFR because of interference by certain drugs or chemicals with tubular secretion of creatinine or with laboratory measurement of creatinine (Table 29-2).[1] Creatinine clearance (Ccr) is a more accurate estimate of GFR than serum creatinine is. Although the GFR may be reduced despite a normal value for creatinine clearance, a reduced value for creatinine clearance virtually always indicates a reduced GFR. Unfortunately, measurement of creatinine clearance requires collection of a timed urine sample, such as a 24-hour sample, which is usually difficult in sick, hospitalized patients. Alternatively, a variety of formulas and nomograms are available to allow one to predict creatinine clearance from the patient's steady-state serum creatinine concentration (Pcr), age, and weight. The formula derived by Cockcroft and Gault is particularly simple to use[4]:

**Men:** Ccr (mL/min) = 140 − Age (years) × Weight (kg)/ 72 × Pcr (mg/dL)
**Women:** Ccr (mL/min) = 140 − Age (years) × Weight (kg)/ 85 × Pcr (mg/dL)

However, predicting the GFR from formulas and nomograms also requires caution. First, because creatinine is excreted by both glomerular filtration and tubular secretion, creatinine clearance exceeds GFR at all levels of renal function. Second, the predicted value for creatinine

**Table 29-2.** *Causes of elevated serum creatinine without reduced GFR*

INHIBITION OF TUBULAR SECRETION OF CREATININE

Trimethoprim
Cimetidine

INTERFERENCE WITH MEASUREMENT OF CREATININE IN SERUM

Ketones (Jaffé reaction method)*
Cephalosporins (Jaffé reaction method)*
Flucytosine (iminohydrolysis method)†

* Jaffé reaction is utilized by ACA and SMAC autoanalyzers (Technicon instruments Corp., Tarrytown, N.Y.).
†The iminohydrolysis method is used by EKTACHEM autoanalyzers (Eastman Kodak Co., Rochester, N.Y.).

clearance exceeds the measured value in patients with obesity, edema, or severe renal insufficiency, in whom body weight is not an accurate estimate of creatinine generation. As a result, the predicted value for creatinine clearance may deviate substantially from the GFR. It is important to recall that patients with acute renal insufficiency are generally not in a steady state of creatinine balance; thus it is not appropriate to estimate GFR or to predict creatinine clearance from the serum level. If serum creatinine is rising, the serum creatinine overestimates the GFR.[5]

## Pathophysiologic classification of acute renal insufficiency

The causes of acute renal insufficiency are traditionally classified according to the mechanism of the decline in the GFR. Circulatory disturbances that reduce blood flow to the kidney, and consequently reduce the GFR, are termed "prerenal." Reduced renal blood flow can accompany states of extracellular fluid (ECF) volume excess (such as congestive heart failure) or volume depletion (such as dehydration consequent to severe diarrhea). By definition, "prerenal" disorders do not cause renal parenchymal damage, impaired tubular function, or appearance of tubular cells or casts in the urinary sediment; and most important, reversal of "prerenal" conditions restores renal blood flow, GFR, and serum creatinine concentration to their prior levels. Persistently reduced GFR after relief of "prerenal" conditions indicates, by definition, the presence of a concomitant "postrenal," or "renal," condition. Conditions that obstruct urine flow in the renal pelvis, ureters, or lower urinary tract are termed "postrenal." The resulting increase in pressure within the renal pelvis leads to hydronephrosis and a decline in the GFR. If obstruction persists for more than a few days, it may lead to impaired tubular function, parenchymal damage, and urinary sediment abnormalities, which may persist even after obstruction is relieved. Although successful treatment of "postrenal" conditions relieves the obstruction and raises the GFR, recovery of glomerular and tubular function may be delayed or incomplete. In addition, concomitant "prerenal" or "renal" conditions may be responsible for persistent renal insufficiency after relief of obstruction. The "renal" causes of acute renal insufficiency include primary renal diseases and systemic diseases that affect the kidneys. These conditions damage renal parenchyma, reduce the GFR, impair tubular function, and cause urinary sediment abnormalities. The most common "renal" causes of acute renal insufficiency are ischemic and drug-induced acute tubular necrosis. Other renal parenchymal diseases are included in the box on p. 290. Patients with acute renal insufficiency often have multiple disorders. Accurate diagnosis requires consideration of all potential causes of reduced GFR, differentiation of acute and chronic renal insufficiency and careful interpretation of selected diagnostic tests.

## Differentiation of acute and chronic renal insufficiency

Acute and chronic renal insufficiency are differentiated by the cause and course of the disorder and by measurement of kidney size. The causes of

## Renal Parenchymal Diseases Causing Acute Renal Insufficiency

GLOMERULAR DISEASE: Crescentic glomerulonephritis (acute and rapidly progressive glomerulonephritis)

### Low serum complement

Systemic lupus erythematosus
Poststreptococcal glomerulonephritis
Subacute bacterial endocarditis
"Shunt" nephritis
Essential mixed cryoglobulinemia
Idiopathic membranoproliferative glomerulonephritis

### Normal serum complement

Polyarteritis nodosa
Hypersensitivity vasculitis
Henoch-Schönlein purpura
Wegener's granulomatosis
Visceral abscess
Goodpasture's syndrome
IgA-IgG nephropathy
Idiopathic crescentic glomerulonephritis

## TUBULOINTERSTITIAL DISEASE

### Severe interstitial inflammation

Severe pyelonephritis
Drug-induced allergic interstitial nephritis
Drug-induced toxic interstitial nephritis

### Mild interstitial inflammation

Acute tubular necrosis
Papillary necrosis
Myeloma kidney
Hypercalcemic nephropathy
Uric acid nephropathy

## VASCULAR DISEASE

Hemolytic-uremic syndrome
Malignant nephrosclerosis
Scleroderma
Atheroembolism
Cortical necrosis
Infarction

acute renal insufficiency have been discussed above. The principal causes of chronic renal insufficiency are listed in the box on p. 292. Notice that acute tubular necrosis, the most common cause of acute renal insufficiency, is not listed because it rarely causes permanent reduction in renal function. The course of acute renal failure is traditionally divided into three phases: a phase of injury during which the pathophysiologic events are initiated that lead to the decrease in the GFR, a maintenance phase during which the reduction in GFR is sustained, and a recovery phase during which the GFR gradually improves. The maintenance phase is characterized by a rapid rise (over a few days) in serum creatinine concentration; if the reduction in GFR is severe, clinical manifestations of uremia may appear. In addition oliguria and serious derangements in fluid and electrolyte balance occur in more than one half of patients.[6] The recovery phase is frequently heralded by diuresis, with falling values for serum creatinine following immediately or within a day or two.

Chronic renal insufficiency, like acute renal insufficiency, is initiated by a phase of parenchymal injury. If the injury is sustained, a phase of progression ensues, during which further decline in GFR occurs. Progression frequently occurs despite apparent resolution of the initial injurious process. Eventually, severe renal insufficiency develops, manifested by uremia. The phase of progression is characterized by a slow rise (over several weeks to many years) in serum creatinine concentration. However, because of remarkable adaptations in nephron function, oliguria and serious disorders of fluid and electrolyte metabolism are generally absent until the GFR has fallen below a range of 10 to 15 mL/min.[7]

Chronic renal disease leads to fibrosis and atrophy of renal parenchyma with concomitant reduction in kidney size. Kidney size is usually normal or slightly enlarged in acute renal insufficiency. As discussed below, assessment of kidney size by ultrasound examination is a valuable diagnostic procedure in the evaluation of patients with renal insufficiency.[6]

It is typical for patients with chronic renal insufficiency to exhibit an asymptomatic elevation in serum creatinine, mild hyperkalemia, metabolic acidosis, hyperphosphatemia, and hypertension, with minimally expanded extracellular fluid (ECF) volume. Review of past records would indicate that serum creatinine had been abnormal for several months or years, and if serum creatinine is approximately 4 mg/dL or greater, renal ultrasound examination is likely to reveal small kidneys with reduced cortical thickness. In contrast, patients with acute renal insufficiency typically would have a recent increase in serum creatinine concentration in the setting of an acute medical illness, frequently associated with ischemia-inducing or nephrotoxic procedures. Moreover, many of these patients would manifest oliguria, ECF volume overload, hyponatremia, severe hyperkalemia, or severe metabolic acidosis. Kidney size and cortical thickness would be normal.

## DIAGNOSTIC TESTS

Further evaluation of the patient with acute renal insufficiency includes the following diagnostic tests.

## Renal Parenchymal Diseases Causing Chronic Renal Insufficiency

### GLOMERULAR DISEASE

Diabetes mellitus
Systemic vasculitis
  Systemic lupus erythematosus
  Polyarteritis nodosa
  Wegener's granulomatosis
  Henoch-Schönlein purpura
Amyloidosis, light-chain nephropathy, other fibrillary diseases
HIV nephropathy
Drug-induced diseases
  Heroin, gold, penicillamine, captopril
Idiopathic diseases
  Membranous nephropathy
  Focal glomerulosclerosis
  Membranoproliferative glomerulonephritis
  IgA-IgG nephropathy

### TUBULOINTERSTITIAL DISEASE

Drug-induced diseases
  Analgesic nephropathy
  Allergic interstitial nephritis
Sickle cell nephropathy
Multiple myeloma, light-chain nephropathy
Hypercalcemia
Vesicoureteral reflux nephropathy
Postobstructive nephropathy
Urinary tract stones
Urinary tract infections
Bacterial infections (associated with obstruction, reflux, stones, sickle cell
  disease)
Tuberculosis

### VASCULAR DISEASE

Benign or malignant nephrosclerosis
Atheroembolism
Renal artery stenosis
Scleroderma
Sequelae of hemolytic-uremic syndrome
Postpartum renal failure

### HEREDITARY DISEASE

Hereditary nephritis (Alport's syndrome)
Polycystic kidney disease
Medullary cystic disease

## Assessment of renal perfusion

**Diagnosis of reduced renal perfusion.** Renal blood flow is reduced by conditions that lower systemic blood pressure or increase renal vascular resistance. Even if systemic blood pressure remains within the normal range, an increase in renal vascular resistance leads to a depression in renal perfusion and GFR. Unfortunately, no single item of the patient's history, physical examination, or laboratory data provides a foolproof assessment of renal perfusion. The box below includes disorders that are often associated with reduced renal perfusion. Assessment of the status of ECF volume is most important. In particular, evidence of ECF volume depletion should be carefully sought; the presence of one or more findings listed in the box on p. 294 usually is associated with a reduction in renal blood flow.

**Response to a volume challenge.** The patient's response to a rapid intravenous infusion of isotonic solution (volume challenge) provides important diagnostic information. The purpose of a volume challenge is to increase intravascular volume, central venous pressure, pulmonary capillary wedge pressure, and cardiac output and thereby to increase renal perfusion. If reduced renal perfusion is the cause of reduced GFR ("prerenal" disorders), the improvement in renal perfusion raises the GFR, increases urine flow, and lowers serum creatinine concentration. If reduced renal perfusion is not the cause of reduced GFR ("postrenal" or "renal" disorders), no improvement occurs in the GFR, urine flow, or serum creatinine concentration.

A volume challenge should be administered to patients with acute renal insufficiency in whom a prerenal disorder is suspected unless there are signs of intravascular volume excess (increased central venous pressure, pulmonary capillary wedge pressure, or pulmonary edema). A volume challenge can be cautiously administered even to patients with ECF volume excess in whom intravascular volume depletion is suspected (as in patients with burns or gastrointestinal ileus). In all cases, it is necessary to monitor the systemic hemodynamic response to the volume challenge as well as the renal response. In patients with overt ECF volume depletion, administration of isotonic saline is not

---

### Clinical Settings Associated with Reduced Renal Perfusion

Hypotension
Decreased cardiac output
Hemorrhage
Greatly reduced serum albumin concentration
Congestive heart failure
Cirrhosis
Gastrointestinal ileus
Burns
Decreased extracellular fluid volume

## Causes and Findings in Extracellular Fluid (ECF) Volume Depletion

### CAUSES OF ECF VOLUME DEPLETION

Increased fluid losses
  Vomiting
  Diarrhea
  Drainage of stomach, intestinal, pancreatic, or biliary fluid
  Profuse sweating
Diuretic therapy
Reduced fluid intake
  Fluid restriction
  Dietary salt restriction

### SIGNS OF ECF VOLUME DEPLETION

Orthostatic hypotension
Fluid intake less than fluid output
Recent weight loss
Reduced skin turgor
Dry oral mucous membranes and axillary skin
Reduced central venous pressure
Reduced pulmonary capillary wedge pressure
Response to volume challenge (see text)

only a diagnostic test of the cause of acute renal insufficiency, it also is the appropriate therapy. Monitoring of the supine and sitting blood pressure and pulse is a sufficient measure of the systemic hemodynamic response. In patients with apparently normal or increased ECF volume, further measurements are required in performing a volume challenge. In addition to monitoring pulse and blood pressure, a catheter should be inserted for measurement of central venous or pulmonary capillary pressure every 15 minutes during the volume challenge. Patients with apparently normal ECF volume should receive 300 to 1000 mL of isotonic saline over one half to 2 hours. Patients with ECF volume excess should *not* receive saline because they already have a surfeit of salt and water; instead they can receive 12.5 to 25 g of "salt-poor" albumin. An increase in arterial and venous pressure during the volume challenge indicates that sufficient fluid has been administered to alter the systemic hemodynamic profile. An improvement in urine flow and serum creatinine concentration indicates that the renal insufficiency is attributable to reduced renal perfusion and that definitive measures should be undertaken to improve renal perfusion. Whether these measures should include further administration of intravenous fluids depends on the underlying disorder. No improvement in urine flow or serum creatinine, despite improvement in the systemic hemodynamic profile, indicates that renal insufficiency is not attributable to intravascular volume depletion and that "postrenal" or "renal" disorders should be considered.

## Urine volume and pattern of urination

The normal average urine volume (1 to 2 liters per day) is only the tiny fraction of the glomerular filtrate (150 to 180 liters per day) that is not reabsorbed by the renal tubules. Assuming a normal upper limit of urinary concentration of 1200 to 1400 mOsm/kg (urinary specific gravity approximately 1.030), and assuming a normal solute load of approximately 600 mOsm per day, urine volume cannot decline to less than 400 mL per day if the GFR is normal. Consequently the finding of urine volume less than 400 mL per day, defined as oliguria, is a definite indication of reduced GFR. In approximately two thirds of patients with acute renal insufficiency, however, the urine volume remains normal because of a reduction in both GFR and tubular reabsorption (nonoliguric acute renal insufficiency). Urine volume less than 50 mL per day, defined as anuria, is the result of severe reduction in GFR and is suggestive of total obstruction, bilateral renal vascular occlusion, or specific severe renal diseases including acute glomerulonephritis, cortical necrosis, and hemolytic uremic syndrome. Although anuria occurs infrequently as a result of acute tubular necrosis (ATN), because it is the most frequent cause of acute renal insufficiency, ATN remains the most frequent cause of anuria. The decline in GFR, frequency of complications, and mortality are greater in patients with oliguria and anuria than in patients with normal urine volume.[8,9]

The pattern of urination often is normal in patients with acute renal insufficiency. Symptoms during urination may indicate lower urinary tract abnormalities associated with obstruction. Similarly, erratic intervals between urination or widely varying urine volumes may indicate partial obstruction, even in patients who are asymptomatic. Rectal and pelvic examinations should be performed on all patients with acute and chronic renal insufficiency to detect mass lesions that could cause obstruction of the lower urinary tract.

## Dipstick and urine sediment examination

"Dipstick" testing of the urine for protein and hemoglobin is easily and accurately performed by hospital laboratories. However, there is no substitute for the careful examination of the urine sediment by the consulting physician. In both acute and chronic renal disorders, the presence of significant proteinuria (2+ or greater), renal tubular cells, cellular or coarsely granular casts, or fat in the urine is diagnostic of parenchymal renal damage.[10] In acute renal sufficiency, these findings are suggestive of either an acute "renal" condition or an acute "prerenal" or "postrenal" condition superimposed on a chronic "renal" condition. Moreover, the types of cells and casts are suggestive of the type of pathologic process involving the renal parenchyma (Fig. 29-1). For example, red blood cells and red blood cell casts are seen in acute glomerulonephritis and rarely in vascular diseases, which also involve the glomeruli, such as hemolytic-uremic syndrome and malignant nephrosclerosis; white blood cells and white blood cell casts usually

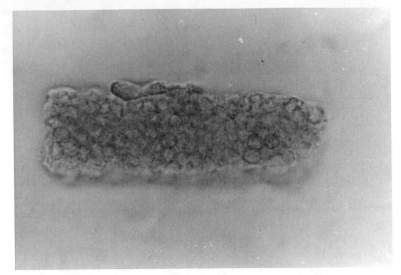

**A**

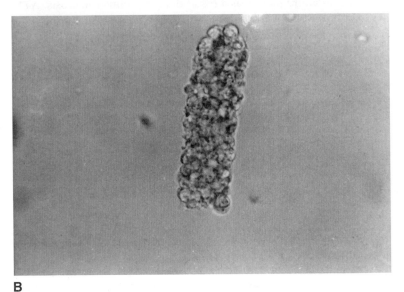

**B**

**Figure 29-1.** *Urinary sediment. A, Red blood cell cast. B, White blood cell cast.*

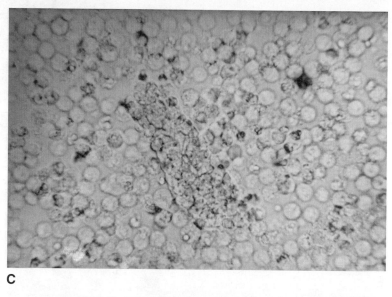

C

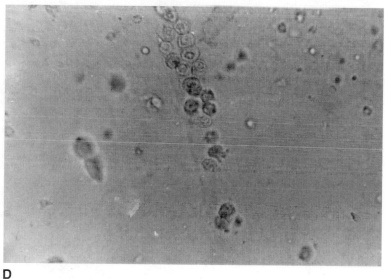

D

**Figure 29–1.** *(continued) C, White blood cells and white blood cell cast. D, Renal tubular epithelial cell casts.*

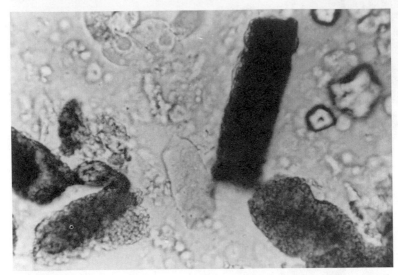

E

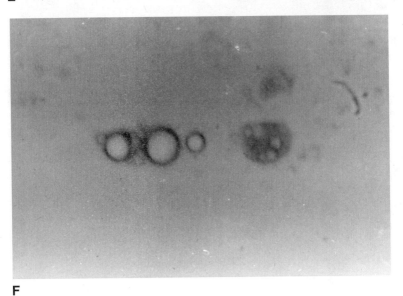

F

**Figure 29-1.** *(continued) E, "Muddy brown," coarse granular cast. F, Oval fat body and free fat.*

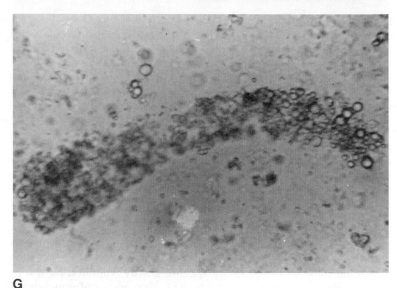

G

Figure 29-1. (continued) G, Fatty casts. (B, from Gennari FJ, Kassirer JP: Laboratory assessment of renal function. In Early LE, Gottschalk CW, editors: Strauss and Welt's Diseases of the kidney, Boston, 1979, Little, Brown.)

indicate an inflammatory tubulointerstitial disease, such as acute pyelonephritis or allergic interstitial nephritis; tubular cells, tubular cell casts, and coarsely granular casts are seen in all forms of acute renal damage, but they are the principal findings in acute tubular necrosis and are found in the urine sediment in 70 to 80% of patients with this disorder.[11]

The results of the urine sediment examination permit an orderly, focused approach to further diagnostic testing. The approach to patients with acute glomerulonephritis relies on identification of whether the patient has a systemic disease and the measurement of serum complement.[12] Expectations for serum complement for the most important causes of acute glomerulonephritis are given in the box on p. 290. The approach to patients with inflammatory tubulointerstitial diseases includes obtaining a urine culture, measurement of eosinophil count, and assessment of possible allergic or toxic reactions to recently administered drugs.[12] Identifying the likely ischemic or toxic insult that caused parenchymal damage is the best approach to patients with acute tubular necrosis. The most difficult diagnostic problems arise in two circumstances: (1) The urinary sediment is only mildly abnormal: the patient may have either mild acute tubular necrosis, a noninflammatory tubulointerstitial disorder, or a "prerenal" condition. (2) The urinary sediment contains red blood cells, renal tubular cells, and granular casts, but no red blood cell casts: The patient may have either acute glomerulonephritis, a vascular disease, an inflammatory tubulointerstitial disease, or a combination of diseases. These circumstances occasionally require a renal biopsy to define the disorder and to guide therapy.

## Urinary specific gravity

Careful interpretation of the urinary specific gravity in acute renal insufficiency contributes valuable information on the status of tubular function. In "prerenal" conditions, reduced renal perfusion leads not only to reduced GFR but also to increased reabsorption of sodium and water from tubular fluid. The resulting urine has an increased concentration of nonreabsorbable solutes (such as creatinine and urea) and therefore the specific gravity is greater than serum. Patients with acute obstruction or acute glomerulonephritis also may have preserved tubular function and concentrated urine. By contrast, in most "renal" conditions, tubular and glomerular function both are impaired; thus the urine is not concentrated (specific gravity 1.010 to 1.012). Similarly, tubular function is impaired soon after the development of renal obstruction; consequently the urine usually is not concentrated in chronic "postrenal" conditions. Thus the finding of concentrated urine (specific gravity greater than 1.015) in acute renal insufficiency indicates preserved tubular function and usually is diagnostic of a "prerenal" condition.

The usefulness of the urinary specific gravity is limited by several factors. Diuretics impair urinary concentration and are frequently administered to patients with acute renal insufficiency. Consequently, in patients who have been treated with diuretics within the previous 12 to 24 hours, urine specific gravity may remain 1.010 to 1.012 even if acute renal insufficiency is attributable to reduced renal perfusion. Urinary specific gravity is raised by the presence of small solutes in high concentration, such as glucose or mannitol, by large amounts of high molecular weight solutes, such as protein, or by heavy solutes, such as radiographic contrast. If these solutes are present, urinary specific gravity may be elevated even if the concentrating ability of the tubules is impaired.[9]

## Ultrasound examination

A renal ultrasonogram should be obtained in patients in whom the cause of acute renal insufficiency is not determined by assessment of renal perfusion, urine volume, pattern of urination, and urinalysis. The principal uses of the ultrasound examination are to detect obstruction and to measure kidney size. Hydronephrosis is detected on the ultrasonogram as the presence of enlarged kidneys with echolucent clusters within the central renal echoes, corresponding to dilated calyces within the renal pelvis (Fig. 29-2). Ultrasound is highly sensitive in detecting these abnormalities but may not demonstrate the cause of the obstruction.[7] The absence of hydronephrosis on ultrasound examination usually eliminates obstruction as the cause of renal insufficiency. In patients with hydronephrosis, the site and cause of obstruction are sometimes visible on the ultrasound exam. Additionally, a postvoiding view of the bladder should be obtained to determine if there is bladder-outlet obstruction.

As mentioned earlier, kidney size is normal (11 to 12 cm in length) in most patients with acute renal insufficiency. Small kidneys indicate that renal disease is chronic, whereas large kidneys are found in only

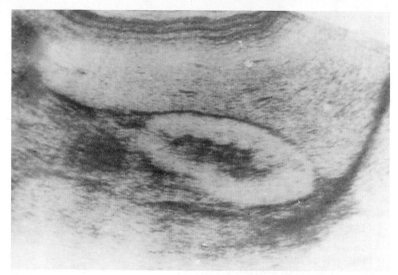

**A**

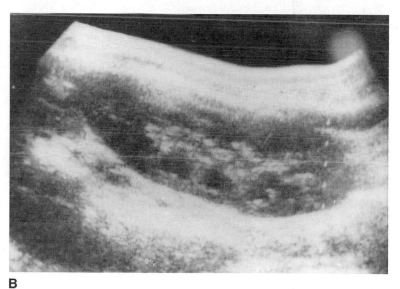

**B**

**Figure 29-2.** *Renal ultrasonogram. Normal features, A, include peripheral homogeneous thick cortex (white) and central heterogeneous fluid-filled calyces (black). Notice that individual calyces cannot be visualized. In acute hydronephrosis, B, features include normal cortex (gray) and dilated calyces (grey areas within central white).*

a few specific diseases. Causes of considerable kidney enlargement include obstruction and polycystic kidneys. Mild kidney enlargement may be seen in diabetes, acute glomerulonephritis, acute pyelonephritis, and renal infiltration by tumor (especially lymphoma).

## Urine chemistries and urinary diagnostic indices

Measurements of urine sodium concentration, fractional excretion of sodium, and the ratio of urine to serum concentration of creatinine are useful to confirm the diagnostic impression based on the investigations discussed above.[14] The fractional excretion of sodium (FENa), may be calculated from the concentrations of sodium (Na) and creatinine (cr) in samples of serum and urine obtained at approximately the same time. The fractional excretion of sodium is defined as the percentage of filtered sodium that is excreted in the urine. Filtered sodium is calculated as the product of the serum sodium concentration and the GFR (as assessed by creatinine clearance).

$$\text{FENa (\%)} = \frac{\text{Na excreted}}{\text{Na filtered}} \times 100\%$$

$$\text{FENa (\%)} = \frac{\text{Urine Na (mEq/L} \times \text{Urine flow (mL/min)}}{\text{Serum Na (mEq/L)} \times \text{Ccr (mL/min)}} \times 100\%$$

$$\text{FENa (\%)} = \frac{\text{Urine Na (mEq/L)} \times \text{Serum cr (mg/dL)}}{\text{Serum Na (mEq/L)} \times \text{Urine cr (mg/dL)}} \times 100\%$$

In "prerenal" conditions, in acute obstruction and in acute glomerulonephritis, tubular function is intact, the concentration of sodium is low (<20 mEq/L), the fractional excretion of sodium is low (<1%), and the ratio of urine to serum concentration of creatinine is high (>40). By contrast, in most renal and postrenal conditions, tubular function is impaired, urinary concentration of sodium is high (>40 mEq/L), the fractional excretion of sodium is high (>1%), and the ratio of urine to plasma concentration of creatinine is low (<20).

**Table 29–3.** *Urine chemistry analyses and urinary diagnostic indices in acute renal insufficiency*

|  | Prerenal conditions | Oliguric acute tubular injury | Nonoliguric acute tubular injury | Postrenal conditions |
|---|---|---|---|---|
| Urine Na (mEq/L) | 18 ± 3 | 68 ± 5 | 50 ± 5 | 68 ± 10 |
| FENa (%) | 0.4 ± 1 | 7 ± 1 | 3 ± 1 | 6 ± 2 |
| Urine-to-serum creatinine ratio | 45 ± 6 | 17 ± 2 | 17 ± 2 | 16 ± 4 |

Data from Miller TR, Anderson RJ, Linas SL, et al: *Ann Intern Med* 89:47, 1978. Values are presented as mean ± standard deviation.

Representative values for urine chemistry analytes and urinary diagnostic indices for several causes of acute renal insufficiency are listed in Table 29-3.[14]

## References

1. Levey AS, Perrone RD, Madias NE: Serum creatinine and renal function, *Ann Rev Med* 39:465, 1988.
2. Shemesh O, Goldbetz H, Kriss JP, Myers BD: Limitation of creatinine as a filtration marker in glomerulopathic patients, *Kidney Int* 28:830, 1985.
3. Hou SH, Bushinsky DA, Wish JB, et al: Hospital-acquired renal insufficiency: a prospective study, *Am J Med* 74:243, 1983.
4. Cockcroft DW, Gault MH: Prediction of creatinine clearance from serum creatinine, *Nephron* 16:31, 1976.
5. Kassirer JP: Clinical evaluation of kidney function: glomerular function, *N Engl J Med* 285:385, 1971.
6. Brivet FG, Kleinknecht DJ, Loirat P, et al: Acute renal failure in intensive care units. Causes, outcome, and prognostic factors of hospital mortality: a prospective multicenter study, *Crit Care Med* 24:192, 1996.
7. Doherty FJ: Ultrasound of the kidney. In Jacobson HR, Striker GE, Klahr S, editors: *The principles and practice of nephrology*, St. Louis, 1995, Mosby.
8. Anderson RJ, Linas SL, Berns AS, et al: Non-oliguric acute renal failure, *N Engl J Med* 296:1134, 1977.
9. Myers BD, Moran SM: Hemodynamically mediated acute renal failure, *N Eng J Med* 314:97, 1986.
10. Yager HM, Harrington JT: Urinalysis and urine electrolytes. In Jacobson HR, Striker GE, Klahr S, editors: *The principles and practice of nephrology*, St. Louis, 1995, Mosby.
11. Levinsky NG, Alexander EA, Venkatachalam M: Acute renal failure. In Brenner BM, Rector FC Jr, editors: *The kidney*, Philadelphia, 1981, Saunders.
12. Madaio MP, Harrington JT: The diagnosis of acute glomerulonephritis, *N Engl J Med* 309:1299, 1983.
13. Appel GB, Kunis CL: Acute tubulo-interstitial nephritis. In Cotran RS, Brenner BM, Stein JH, editors: *Contemporary issues in nephrology 10: Tubulointerstitial nephropathies*, New York, 1983, Churchill Livingstone
14. Miller TR, Anderson RJ, Linas SL, et al: Urinary diagnostic indices in acute renal failure: a prospective study, *Ann Intern Med* 89:47, 1978.

# Chapter 30

# *Management of Renal Insufficiency*

Richard A. Lafayette

Renal insufficiency, a decrease in the glomerular filtration rate (GFR), may be acute or chronic. The diagnosis of acute and chronic renal insufficiency is discussed in the previous chapter. In this chapter, the management of acute and chronic renal insufficiency is described. Discussion of the management of end-stage renal disease, defined as a decrease in the GFR to a level that is not compatible with life, is not included in this chapter because it requires dialysis and other specialized procedures. Before we proceed, it is necessary to review the clinical manifestations of acute and chronic renal insufficiency.

## CLINICAL MANIFESTATIONS

The signs and symptoms of renal insufficiency are determined by the severity of the decrease in the GFR. The normal value for the GFR in adults is approximately 125 mL/min. Patients with a GFR above 20 to 25 mL/min generally have few symptoms attributable to renal insufficiency, whereas if the GFR is below a range of 5 to 10 mL/min, the full cluster of uremic symptoms appears. Manifestations that may be seen in both acute and chronic renal insufficiency include pericarditis, gastrointestinal symptoms, and encephalopathy, particularly if the serum urea nitrogen concentration is greater than 100 mg/dL. In addition to the severity of renal insufficiency, the duration also influences clinical manifestations.

In acute renal insufficiency, serious derangements in fluid and electrolyte balance are common. As discussed in the previous chapter, oliguria, extracellular fluid (ECF) volume overload, hyponatremia, severe hyperkalemia, severe metabolic acidosis, or hyperphosphatemia occur in more than one half of patients. By contrast, in chronic renal insufficiency, serious fluid and electrolyte disturbances are uncommon unless the GFR is severely reduced. Symptoms that occur more commonly in patients with a long duration of renal insufficiency include nausea, vomiting, weight loss, pruritus, peripheral neuropathy, osteodystrophy, and metastatic calcifications.

Whether renal insufficiency is acute or chronic, severe and persistent manifestations of uremia constitute a medical emergency, and a nephrologist should be consulted at once to arrange for dialysis. Thus the first responsibility of the consulting internist in patients with renal insufficiency is to assess their need for dialysis. Indications for initiation of dialysis are given in the box below.

# SPECIFIC GOALS OF MANAGEMENT

The goals of management of patients with renal insufficiency are as follows:

1. Identify and treat reversible causes of renal insufficiency.
2. Prevent complications of renal insufficiency.
3. In acute renal insufficiency, provide general supportive care until recovery of renal function.
4. In chronic renal insufficiency, delay progression of renal functional decline.

---

### Indications for Dialysis in Renal Failure

**INDICATIONS ARISING COMMONLY IN ACUTE AND CHRONIC RENAL FAILURE**

Pericarditis
Anorexia
Nausea
Vomiting
Hiccups
Lethargy
Seizures

**INDICATIONS ARISING MOST COMMONLY IN ACUTE RENAL FAILURE**

Extracellular fluid volume overload
Hyponatremia
Severe hyperkalemia
Severe metabolic acidosis
Hypermagnesemia

**INDICATIONS ARISING MOST COMMONLY IN CHRONIC RENAL FAILURE**

Weight loss
Pruritus
Peripheral neuropathy

# REVERSIBLE CAUSES OF RENAL INSUFFICIENCY

Systematic evaluation of patients with renal insufficiency must be undertaken to detect all treatable causes of renal disease. Potentially reversible conditions are listed in the box below. Reversible causes are more frequently encountered in patients with acute renal insufficiency. Nonetheless, patients with chronic renal insufficiency frequently suffer acute reductions in their GFR. Detection and reversal of superimposed causes of renal insufficiency may permit partial recovery of renal function and

---

## Reversible Causes of Renal Insufficiency

### "PRERENAL CONDITIONS"

ECF volume depletion
Congestive heart failure
Nonsteroidal anti-inflammatory agents
Hyperviscosity syndromes

### "POSTRENAL" CONDITIONS

Bladder-outlet obstruction
  Prostatic enlargement
  Pelvic malignancy
Ureteric obstruction (bilateral)
  Urinary tract stones
  Papillary necrosis
  Retroperitoneal malignancy

### RENAL CONDITIONS

Glomerular disease
  Postinfectious glomerulonephritis
  Systemic vasculitis
  Preeclampsia
Tubulointerstitial diseases
  Urinary tract infection
  Drug toxicity
  Drug allergy
  Hypercalcemia
  Tumor lysis
Vascular diseases
  Malignant hypertension
  Hemolytic-uremic syndrome
  Renal artery stenosis

delay the onset of total renal failure. The differential diagnosis of these conditions is discussed in the previous chapter.

In addition, it is important to avoid further insults to renal function because the risk of acute renal insufficiency from diagnostic procedures and therapeutic agents is much greater in patients with reduced renal function. If possible, depletion of ECF volume, intravenous radiographic contrast, aminoglycoside antibiotics, nonsteroidal anti-inflammatory agents, and cisplatin should be avoided in patients with renal insufficiency.

# PREVENTION OF COMPLICATIONS

Successful prevention of complications of renal insufficiency depends on prescription of appropriate dietary and fluid restrictions, adjustment of drug dosages, and as discussed earlier, timely initiation of dialysis.

## Dietary and fluid restrictions

The goal of dietary and fluid management in patients with renal insufficiency is to maintain the volume and composition of body fluids close to normal.[1] Initial evaluation of the patient requires measurement of weight, physical examination to determine the status of ECF volume, assessment of dietary intake, and the serum and urine measurements as shown in the box below. The dietary prescription is formulated on the basis of this assessment as well as the severity and duration of renal insufficiency.[2,3] The assistance of a skilled nutritionist is essential in

---

### Serum and Urine Measurements in Patients with Renal Insufficiency

| SERUM | URINE |
|---|---|
| Creatinine | Creatinine |
| Urea nitrogen | Urea nitrogen |
| Sodium | Sodium |
| Potassium | Potassium |
| Chloride | Protein |
| Bicarbonate | |
| Calcium | |
| Phosphorus | |
| Magnesium | |
| Albumin | |
| Transferrin | |
| Glucose | |
| Triglycerides | |
| Cholesterol | |

assessment of dietary intake and design of a dietary regimen that fulfills the prescription. An approach to patients with acute and chronic renal insufficiency is summarized below and in Table 30-1. Chronic renal insufficiency is described first because the dietary and fluid prescription is simpler than in acute renal insufficiency.

## Chronic renal insufficiency

As discussed earlier, the manifestation during the progressive phase of chronic renal insufficiency is retention of nitrogenous wastes, such as creatinine and urea. Hypertension, disorders of calcium metabolism, phosphorus retention, and mild elecrolyte and acid-base disorders are common, but serious disturbances of fluid and electrolyte balance are not usual. Serum albumin and transferrin concentrations are normal unless nephrotic syndrome, nutritional deficiency or another chronic illness is present. Abnormalities in carbohydrate and lipid metabolism are frequent and manifest as hypertriglyceridemia. Serum glucose and cholesterol concentration usually are normal.

If serum urea nitrogen concentration is greater than 70 to 80 mg/dL, dietary protein intake can be restricted to 0.6 g/kg of lean body weight per day, with more than one half of the dietary allowance composed of high biologic value protein, such as meat and eggs.[1] Energy intake should be prescribed to maintain lean body weight, usually approximately 35 kcal/kg per day. The proportion of calories derived from fat and carbohydrate should be adjusted to maintain lipid levels as close to normal as possible. A fluid restriction is not necessary.

Patients with chronic renal insufficiency do not absorb dietary calcium adequately because of deficient renal production of the active form of vitamin D (1,25-dihydroxycholecalciferol). As a result, negative calcium balance and diminished bone calcium content are universal findings. If serum creatinine is greater than approximately 4 mg/dL, it is advisable to prescribe a calcium supplement, usually calcium carbonate, 500 mg two or three times daily with meals, except in special situations as described below.

The serum phosphorus can often be maintained below 5 mg/dL by dietary restriction and by prescription of phosphorus-binding antacids. Restriction of dietary protein usually results in concomitant reduction in phosphorus intake and serum phosphorus concentration. However, persistent elevation requires further reduction in dietary intake by restriction of foods rich in phosphorus such as dairy products and cola-colored soft drinks and by prescription of phosphorus binders, either calcium carbonate or aluminum hydroxide at initial doses of 500 to 1000 mg three times daily with meals. Because aluminum is not completely excreted in patients with renal insufficiency, it is preferable to prescribe binders containing calcium rather than aluminum. However, if serum calcium is greater than 11.0 mg/dL or if serum phosphorus exceeds 6 to 7 mg/dL, aluminum hydroxide is preferred over calcium carbonate because of the risk of serious hypercalcemia and metastatic calcification. Magnesium-containing antacids are contraindicated because of risks of magnesium accumulation and hypermagnesemia.

**Table 30-1.** *Dietary and fluid prescription in acute and chronic renal insufficiency*

| | Chronic renal insufficiency | Acute renal insufficiency |
|---|---|---|
| **Fluid** | No restriction | Restrict intake based on measured losses to maintain extracellular fluid volume and serum sodium concentration |
| **Protein** | Restriction to 0.6 g/kg/day (50% as high biologic value) | Provide adequate intake to maintain nitrogen balance or minimize amount of negative balance (often 1.0 g/kg/day) |
| **Energy** | 35 kcal/kg/day to maintain body weight; adjust proportion of carbohydrate and fat to maintain serum glucose and lipids | At least 1500 kcal of carbohydrate per day; if possible 40 to 50 kcal/kg/day |
| **Calcium** | Calcium carbonate, 1000 to 1500 per day | No supplements unless serum calcium <8.0 mg/dL |
| **Phosphorus** | Calcium carbonate or aluminum hydroxide to maintain serum phosphorus ≤5.0 mg/dL | Aluminum hydroxide to maintain serum phosphorus ≤6.0 mg/dL |
| **Sodium** | No restriction unless hypertension or edema | Restrict intake to measured losses or 2 g per day |
| **Potassium** | No restriction unless serum potassium ≥5.5 mEq/L | Restrict intake to measured losses or 2 g per day |
| **Alkali** | Calcium carbonate or sodium bicarbonate to maintain serum bicarbonate ≥18 mEq/L | Sodium bicarbonate to maintain serum bicarbonate >18 mEq/L |

If blood pressure is elevated, dietary sodium should be kept under 3 g (130 mEq) per day. It is important to note that some patients with chronic renal insufficiency cannot fully conserve sodium. Sharp reductions in dietary sodium may result in a negative sodium balance and ECF volume depletion, possibly leading to further deterioration in renal function. If blood pressure is normal, sodium restricton need not and should not be advised. Instead, dietary sodium content should be estimated from diet records and urinary sodium excretion, and this amount should be prescribed.

Dietary potassium intake can be assessed by the same methods. If serum potassium is normal, patients should be instructed in the potassium content in their diet, and the amount of potassium that they are currently ingesting should be prescribed. If serum potassium is greater than 5.5 mEq/L, dietary potassium should be restricted to 2 to 3 g (50 to 75 mEq) per day. If hyperkalemia persists, cation-exchange resins, such as Kayexalate 25 to 75 g per day, or loop diuretics, such as furosemide 40 to 80 mg per day, may be prescribed. Kayexalate contributes approximately 2 mEq of sodium per 1 g and may contribute to ECF volume expansion. On the other hand, diuretics may result in ECF volume depletion. Careful monitoring for these complications is essential.

Treatment of metabolic acidosis is warranted if serum bicarbonate is below approximately 18 mEq/L. Alkali, 25 to 50 mEq per day, should be prescribed, either as additional calcium carbonate (10 mEq per 500 mg tablet) or sodium bicarbonate (8 mEq per 650 mg tablet).

## Acute renal insufficiency

Different dietary and fluid restrictions are necessary in patients with acute renal insufficiency because, as discussed above, it is frequently accompanied by serious fluid and electrolyte disturbances.[2,3] Throughout the maintenance and recovery phases, preservation of fluid balance is of the utmost importance. If the ECF volume is increased, oral and intravenous fluids should be restricted or witheld, and vigorous therapy with loop diuretics should be employed. On the other hand, if ECF volume is depleted, isotonic fluid must be administered. If ECF volume appears normal but the serum sodium concentration is low, oral fluids should be restricted to 500 mL per day, and all intravenous solutions should be isotonic. If the patient is euvolemic with a normal serum sodium concentration, the combined oral and fluid intake should be restricted to the amount that is excreted by renal and extrarenal routes. Extrarenal fluid loss is attributable to insensible water loss, generally approximately 500 mL per day. Insensible losses are increased in patients with high fever or burns. Additional extrarenal fluid losses also occur through the gastrointestinal tract, as in patients with vomiting, nasogastric drainage, or diarrhea. In patients with increased extrarenal losses, the fluid allowance must be increased.

The dietary sodium and potassium prescription should be based on measured sodium and potassium losses in urine and other fluids. Typically, in the absence of oliguria or gastrointestinal fluid losses, sodium and potassium should be restricted to 2 g per day each

(85 mEq and 50 mEq, respectively). Potassium-sparing diuretics should be avoided, and nondietary sources of potassium also must be restricted (see Chapter 27). The allowance of sodium and potassium should be increased for patients with gastrointestinal fluid losses.

Guidelines for protein intake are controversial.[3] Patients with acute renal failure are catabolic. Although a low-protein diet may maintain low serum urea nitrogen concentrations, it also contributes to negative nitrogen balance. It is probably best to provide adequate protein and essential amino acids even if it requires earlier or greater dialytic support. Energy needs are higher than in patients with chronic renal insufficiency and range from 40 to 50 kcal/kg per day. However, because of the anorexia that typically accompanies acute renal insufficiency, it is difficult for patients to achieve this intake. At a minimum, 1500 kcal per day, including at least 20 g of essential amino acids, should be provided because of the beneficial effect on preventing complications.[3,4]

It is usually not necessary to modify energy intake on the basis of serum lipid levels or to provide supplementary calcium during acute renal insufficiency. Short-term treatment of hyperphosphatemia and metabolic acidosis can be accomplished with aluminum hydroxide and sodium bicarbonate, respectively, rather than with calcium carbonate.

During the recovery phase of acute renal insufficiency, it is necessary to increase allowances of fluid, sodium, and potassium. Protein restriction may be lifted, and aluminum hydroxide may be discontinued as serum concentrations of urea nitrogen and phosphorus decline. It may be necessary to continue alkali therapy or potassium restriction temporarily.

## DRUG PRESCRIBING IN RENAL INSUFFICIENCY

Metabolism and excretion of many drugs are altered in renal insufficiency. Proper drug prescribing requires knowledge of the usual routes of elimination, alterations in patients with reduced renal function, the approximate level of renal function in the patient under consideration, and the method of dose adjustment, if any, that is necessary for that level of renal function. Comprehensive reviews of this subject are available and should be consulted before prescription of any and all drugs for patients with renal insufficiency.[5,6]

Drug elimination by the kidneys occurs by glomerular filtration, tubular secretion, and cellular metabolism. Drugs that are hydrophilic, not bound to plasma proteins, and having molecular weight below approximately 10,000 daltons are available for glomerular filtration. Examples include sulfonamides, penicillins, most cephalosporins, aminoglycosides, aspirin, normeperidine (a metabolite of meperidine), digoxin, allopurinol, methotrexate, and cisplatin. Tubular secretion of other low-molecular-weight anions and cations, such as cimetidine, trimethoprim, probenecid, hippuric acid, phenobarbital, diuretics, and radiographic contrast mediums, contributes significantly to their renal excretion. Moreover, renal tubular cells are the site of metabolism of several peptides, including insulin. In renal insufficiency, excretion or degradation of these substances is reduced. Consequently, reduction of dosage is necessary to achieve and maintain therapeutic levels and to avoid toxicity.

Dosage may be reduced either by reduction of the amount but maintenance of the same interval between doses, by lengthening the interval between doses but maintenance of the same amount, or by a combination of methods. In general, all methods are acceptable for most agents. Most references provide the appropriate dose reduction or interval change according to the level of renal function estimated from creatinine clearance. As discussed in the previous chapter, estimation of creatinine clearance in the steady state is possible from the serum creatinine and the formula of Cockcroft and Gault. Wherever possible, serum drug levels also should be measured directly. As discussed in the previous chapter, if serum creatinine is not stable but is rising, renal function should not be estimated from this formula. Instead creatinine clearance should be assumed to be less than 10 mL/min, and drug levels should be monitored frequently.[7]

# SUPPORTIVE MEASURES DURING ACUTE RENAL INSUFFICIENCY

In "prerenal" and "postrenal" causes of acute renal insufficiency, the maintenance phase continues until the underlying cause of reduced GFR is corrected. In acute tubular necrosis, the most common "renal" cause of acute renal insufficiency, no treatment is available for the renal disease itself: the duration of the maintenance phase is from a few days to 6 to 8 weeks. In other parenchymal renal diseases, the duration depends on the efficacy of treatment. For the treatment of specific diseases, refer to general nephrology textbooks.

Despite advances in nutritional and dialytic support, mortality of acute tubular necrosis remains greater than 50%.[8] The principal causes of death are related to the underlying illness that precipitated the renal injury. Potentially preventable causes of death include infections and upper gastrointestinal hemorrhage. Careful monitoring of sites of infection (wounds, urinary tract, and respiratory tract), minimizing invasive procedures, and removing indwelling catheters can aid recovery. For prevention of upper gastrointestinal hemorrhage, routine prophylactic regimens (at adjusted dosages) are recommended.

The hallmark of the recovery phase is an early increase in urine volume, sometimes leading to polyuria, and a gradual decline in serum creatinine concentration. Serious fluid and electrolyte disturbances also may arise during this phase because of incomplete recovery of glomerular and tubular function. If the patient survives, full recovery of renal function is the rule in acute tubular necrosis, many acute tubulointerstitial diseases, and reversible "prerenal" and "postrenal" conditions. Unfortunately, effective treatment is not available for many of the glomerular and vascular diseases that cause acute renal insufficiency; hence renal function may not recover fully, and patients may be left with chronic renal insufficiency.

# DELAYING PROGRESSION OF CHRONIC RENAL INSUFFICIENCY

As discussed above, during the progression phase of chronic renal insufficiency, patients are typically asymptomatic. Efforts at treatment during this phase should focus on delaying the progressive decline in kidney function. Many studies have suggested that dietary and medical intervention can slow the progression of renal insufficiency. In type I diabetics, blood pressure control aiming for levels lower than 135/85 mm Hg retards the progression of renal insufficiency.[9] Angiotensin-converting enzyme inhibitors confer a further progression-delaying effect independent of their effects on blood pressure.[10] Strict glycemic control has been effective in slowing progressive renal disease regardless of the stage of diabetic nephropathy.[11] Finally, a low-protein diet, restricted to 0.6 to 0.8 g/kg per day also appears to be efficacious in retarding the progression rate of diabetic nephropathy.[12] These therapies simply slow and do not arrest the rate of progression; however, utilized together, they may keep patients away from renal replacement therapy for significant periods of time. It is likely that type II diabetics might experience similar benefits, but similar studies have not been performed to the same extent as of yet.

In nondiabetics, there is less evidence for successful therapies. Nonetheless, recent studies suggest a benefit of dietary protein restriction in subgroups of patients with chronic renal insufficiency, including proteinuric, black, and rapidly progressing subjects.[13,14] The majority of studies utilizing aggressive control of blood pressure ($<135/85$ mm Hg) demonstrate significant reductions in the rate of progression of renal insufficiency.[9,13] Angiotensin-converting enzyme inhibition therapy also appears promising in reducing proteinuria and retarding progression in nondiabetics with chronic renal insufficiency.

Thus it is crucial to identify patients at risk for chronic renal insufficiency very early, perhaps before their renal function is even impaired. They are likely to benefit from early, aggressive therapy as outlined above. Eventually, with the development of novel therapies, they may actually avoid progressive renal dysfunction.

## References

1. Mitch WE, Walser M: Nutritional therapy of the uremic patient. In Brenner BM, Rector FC Jr, editors: *The kidney,* Philadelphia, 1991, Saunders.
2. Druml W: Nutritional management of acute renal failure. In Jacobson HR, Striker GE, Klahr S, editors: *The principles and practice of nephrology,* St. Louis, 1995, Mosby.
3. Kopple JD: Acute renal failure: conservative, non-dialytic management. In Glassock RJ, editor: *Current therapy in nephrology and hypertension 1984-1985,* Philadelphia, 1984, BC Decker.

4. Toback FG: Amino acid treatment of acute renal failure. In Brenner BM, Stein JH, editors: *Contemporary issues in nephrology 6: Acute renal failure,* New York, 1980, Churchill Livingstone.

5. Brater DG: Dosing regimens in renal disease. In Jacobson HR, Striker GE, Klahr S, editors: *The principles and practice of nephrology,* St. Louis, 1995, Mosby.

6. Shuler CL, Bennett WM: Principles of drug usage in dialysis patients. In Nissenson AR, Fine RN, editors: *Dialysis therapy,* Philadelphia, 1993, Hanley & Belfus.

7. Maher JF: Pharmacological aspects of renal failure and dialysis. In Drukker W, Parsons PM, Maher JF, editors: *Replacement of renal function by dialysis,* Boston, 1991, Martinus-Nijhoff.

8. Brezis M, Rosen SE, Epstein FH: Acute renal failure. In Brenner BM, Rector FC Jr, editors: *The kidney,* Philadelphia, 1991, Saunders.

9. Odrizzi L, Rugiu C, DeBiase V, Maschio G: The place of hypertension among the risk factors for renal function on chronic renal failure, *Am J Kidney Dis* 21:119, 1993.

10. Breyer JA, Hunsicker LG, Bain RP, Lewis EJ, and Collaborative Study Group: Angiotensin converting enzyme inhibition in diabetic nephropathy, *Kidney Int* 45:S156, 1995.

11. The Diabetes Control and Complications Trial Research Group: Effect of intensive therapy on the development and progression of diabetic nephropathy, *Kidney Int* 47:1703, 1995.

12. Zeller K, Whittaker E, Sullivan L, et al: Effect of restricting dietary protein on the progression of renal failure in patients with insulin-dependent diabetes mellitus, *N Engl J Med* 324:78, 1991.

13. Klahr S, Levey AS, Beck GJ, et al: The effects of dietary protein restriction and blood pressure control on the progression of chronic renal disease, *N Engl J Med* 330:877, 1994.

14. Pedrini MT, Levey AS, Lan J, Chalmers TC, Wang PH: The effect of dietary protein restriction on the progression of diabetic and non-diabetic renal diseases: a meta-analysis, *Ann Int Med* 124:627, 1996.

# Chapter 31

# *Renal Stones*

Richard A. Lafayette

Urinary tract stones affect 0.5% of the general population. The most common clinical presentation, passage of a ureteral stone, is manifest by colic, microscopic hematuria, and a calcification on plain film of the abdomen. Approximately 15% to 20% of patients with a stone will require hospitalization and instrumentation of the urinary tract because of prolonged pain, persistent obstruction, or development of infection.[1] In addition to the acute morbidity of recurrently passing stones, chronic renal damage and renal failure may develop. Remediable metabolic abnormalities contribute to stone formation in up to 80% of patients with recurrent urinary tract stones.[1] Thus a metabolic work-up should be undertaken in all patients with recurrent stones to determine the cause of the disorder and to guide therapy for prevention of further stones. In patients who have only had a single stone, the prevalence of metabolic abnormalities is equally high, and these patients have a high risk (50% to 70%) of recurrent stones.[2] Based on these observations, evaluation of patients who have had only one stone is also advisable. For all patients, the work-up begins with the identification of the chemical composition of the stone.

## TYPES OF URINARY TRACT STONES

Most urinary tract stones form in the kidney. Stones that form in the bladder and prostate are usually the consequence of either an indwelling catheter or chronic prostatic infection. This chapter is a discussion of stones that form only in the kidney. Table 31-1 lists the chemical composition of the principal types of renal stones, their prevalence, roentogenographic appearance, and the urinary pH that favors their formation. These characteristics help to identify the type of stone even before it is passed. Renal stones are the result of formation and growth of crystals in supersaturated urine. Fig. 31-1 shows the characteristic appearance of crystals in the urinary sediment. Two major factors contribute to stone formation: (1) an abnormally high concentration of ions in the urine and (2) an imbalance of promoters and inhibitors of urinary crystallization. Table 31-2 lists the most important abnormalities of urinary composition that lead to stone formation and the major

**Table 31-1.** *Types of renal stones*

| Chemical composition | Prevalence (% of stones) | Roentgenographic appearance | Urinary pH |
|---|---|---|---|
| Calcium | 70.6 | | |
|   Calcium oxalate | 25.4 | Opaque, round | Any |
|   Calcium phosphate | 7.4 | Opaque, round or branched | >7.5 |
|   Mixed calcium | 37.8 | Opaque, round | Any |
| Struvite (magnesium-ammonium phosphate and calcium phosphate) | 21.5 | Opaque, round Lucent (if no calcium) | >7.5 |
| Uric acid | 5.4 | Lucent, round or branched | <6.0 |
| Cystine | 3.5 | Opaque, round or branched | <7.5 |

Data from Preminger GM, Pak CYC: Nephrolithiasis. In Jacobson HR, Striker GE, Klahr S, editors: *The principles and practice of nephrology,* St. Louis, 1995, Mosby.

causes of each abnormality. Calcium stones are the most common renal stones and are associated with the greatest number of metabolic abnormalities. In the following sections of this chapter, the pathogenesis and treatment of recurrent urinary stones are discussed. The less common types of stones (struvite, cystine, and uric acid) are discussed briefly first. Then calcium stones are discussed in more detail.

## Struvite stones

The crystallization of calcium, magnesium, and ammonium with phosphate occurs only in the presence of elevated urine pH (see Table 32-1). Elevated urine pH (>7.0) is the result of increased concentration of ammonia attributable to infection with bacteria that produces urease, an enzyme that hydrolyzes urea to ammonia (a strong base) and carbon dioxide. Bacteria that produce urease include *Klebsiella, Proteus, Pseudomonas,* and rarely *Escherichia coli.* Patients with struvite stones invariably have a history of recurrent infections with these bacteria and have alkaline urine but usually do not have other metabolic abnormalities.

Medical therapy for struvite stones is unsatisfactory. In principle, effective antibiotic therapy should eradicate the source of urease, lower the concentration of ammonium, and reduce the abnormally high urine pH. However, antibiotic therapy is rarely effective because bacteria persist within the substance of stones that remain in the renal pelvis.

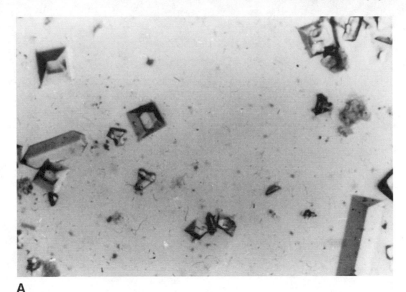

**Figure 31-1.** *Crystals in urine sediment. A, Triple phosphate (struvite) crystals with typical oblong and rectangular shapes. B, Cystine crystals with typical hexagonal shape. (A from Gennari FJ, Kassirer JP: Laboratory assessment of renal function. In Early LE, Gottschalk CW, editors: Strauss and Welt's Diseases of the kidney, ed 3, Boston, 1979, Little, Brown.)*

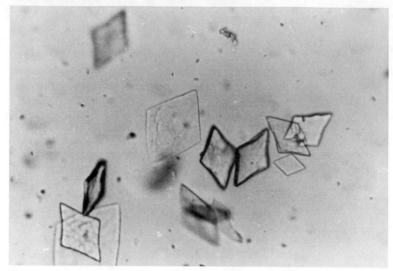

C

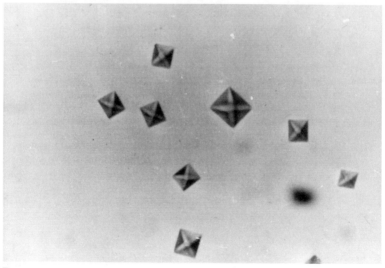

D

**Figure 31-1.** *(continued) C, Uric acid crystals with typical diamond shape. D, Calcium oxalate crystals with typical square shape and "envelope" pattern. (D from Gennari FJ, Kassirer JP: Laboratory assessment of renal function. In Early LE, Gottschalk CW, editors: Strauss and Welt's* Diseases of the kidney, *ed 3, Boston, 1979, Little, Brown.)*

**Table 31-2.** *Metabolic abnormalities associated with renal stones*

| Abnormality | Definition | Types of stone | Causes |
|---|---|---|---|
| Low urine volume | <1 L/day | Contributes to formation of all stones in susceptible persons | Poor intake, chronic diarrhea, vigorous exercise, hot environment |
| Alkaline urine pH | >7.5 | Struvite<br>Calcium phosphate | Infection, distal renal tubular acidosis |
| Persistently acid urine pH | <6.0 | Uric acid | Diarrhea, high protein intake, gout, idiopathic |
| Hyperuricosuria | >800 mg/day (men)<br>>750 mg/day (women) | Uric acid<br>Calcium oxalate | High protein intake, gout, myeloproliferative disorders |
| Hypercalciuria | >300 mg/day (men)<br>>250 mg/day (women) | Calcium oxalate<br>Calcium phosphate | Hypercalcemia, distal renal tubular acidosis, increased dietary calcium intake, idiopathic |
| Hyperoxaluria | >50 mg/day | Calcium oxalate | Gastrointestinal disease, pyridoxine deficiency |
| Hypocitraturia | <320 mg/day | Calcium oxalate | Distal renal tubular acidosis, chronic diarrhea, urinary tract infection, thiazide diuretics, idiopathic |
| Cystinuria | >400 mg/day | Cystine | Homozygous cystinuria |
|  | >60–300 mg/day | Cystine | Heterozygous cystinuria |

Persistence of infected stones causes episodes of recurrent pyelonephritis, sepsis, and parenchymal renal damage and can culminate in renal failure. Chronic therapy with antibiotics may be prescribed to reduce the risk of bacteremia, but it is not successful in preventing growth and recurrence of stones or in preventing renal damage. The primary therapy for struvite stones is the complete surgical removal of all stone fragments. However, struvite stones are incompletely removed or recur after 30% of renal lithotomies. The efficacy of stone removal is dramatically improved by postoperative antibiotics and irrigation of the renal pelvis with hemiacidrin (Renacidin, an acid solution of magnesium and organic acids that promotes stone dissolution) through a nephrostomy tube for 2 to 30 days until stone fragments are no longer visible on renal tomograms and urine is sterile. Using this approach, one investigator has reported that only one of 46 patients with struvite stones developed a recurrence within a mean follow-up interval of 7 years.[3] Experience with lithotripsy using percutaneous methods or extracorporeal shock waves demonstrates successful fragmentation and passage of struvite stones in 90% of patients.[4] These techniques do not always permit complete removal of all stone fragments, and recurrence is well recognized. Prolonged therapy with antibiotics, high fluid intake, and potassium citrate improves the success rate. A chemical inhibitor of bacterial urease, acetohydroxamic acid, also has been used to treat struvite stones. After oral administration, the agent is absorbed, and in patients with normal renal function, it is excreted unchanged in the urine. In one small clinical trial, acetohydroxamic acid and suppressive antibiotics retarded the growth of stones, prevented the appearance of new stones, and reduced the necessity for surgical intervention in treated patients compared to patients receiving only suppressive antibiotics.[5] However, stones did not dissolve, and half the patients had side effects that required reduction in dosage or discontinuance of the drug. In view of the need for long-term therapy and the high rate of side effects, acetohydroxamic acid is of limited usefulness. It should be prescribed only for patients in whom surgery or lithotripsy is not advised and in whom continuous antibiotic therapy has failed to prevent stone growth and recurrence. Moreover, it should not be used in patients with serum creatinine concentration greater than 3.0 mg/dL because of reduced renal excretion and the possibility of a higher risk of side effects.

## Cystine stones

Recurrent formation of cystine stones is the major complication of the metabolic disorder cystinuria. In this autosomal recessive disorder, homozygotes display a pronounced defect in renal tubular and intestinal transport of the cationic amino acids, cystine, ornithine, lysine, and arginine (COLA). The genetic defects have recently been described and are located on chromosome 2.[6] Reduced renal tubular reabsorption of the filtered amino acids results in excessive urinary excretion. Cystine is the least soluble of these amino acids and precipitates if the concentration exceeds 300 mg/L. As shown in Table 31-2, in homozygotes and some heterozygotes, the urine is saturated with cystine unless the urine volume is high. Recurrent urinary stones are the only clinical complications of cystinuria. Serum levels of the four amino acids are slightly low, but growth and nutrition of affected children appear normal. The prevalence of homozygous cystinuria is approximately one in 7000 infants. The diagnosis of cystinuria is usually made by the detection of cystine in a urinary stone. As shown in Table 31-1, the prevalence of cystine stones is only 3% to 4%. Approximately half of stones formed by patients with cystinuria contain other salts; thus it is important to examine all urinary stones for the presence of cystine. Furthermore 5% to 10% of stones formed by patients with cystinuria do not contain cystine. The diagnosis can also be made by measurement of cystine in the urine (by the nitroprusside test) or by detection of cystine crystals in the urine sediment. The nitroprusside test for cystine detects heterozygotes as well as homozygotes and should be performed on all patients with recurrent urinary tract stones; the test is also positive in patients with ketosis. Cystine crystals may be seen in the urine sediment if the concentration of cystine exceeds 250 mg/L; examination of the first morning urine specimen increases the likelihood of detecting the cystine crystalluria. Heterozygotes are sometimes detected. In patients with a positive nitroprusside test or urine sediment examination, the 24-hour excretion of cystine should be measured.

All homozygotes, as well as heterozygotes who have formed stones, should be treated. The first goal of treatment is to increase the water intake to a range of 5 to 7 liters per day to reduce the urinary concentration of cystine to less than 300 mg/L at all times. Adherence to a strict regimen of high water intake can prevent further stone formation. Sodium restriction also diminishes cystine excretion. Alkalinization of the urine to pH >7.4 with bicarbonate, citrate, or carbonic anhydrase inhibitors greatly increases the solubility of cystine and is useful for the many patients who cannot maintain a sufficiently high water intake to prevent recurrent stones. Compliance with alkalinizing agents is not always ideal because of abdominal side effects. Administration of D-penicillamine ($\beta,\beta$-dimethylcysteine) in dosage of 1 to 2 g daily in 3 or 4 divided doses also is effective. This agent undergoes sulfhydryl-disulfide exchange with cystine to form the mixed disulfide of penicillamine and cysteine, which is 50 times more soluble than cystine. During therapy with penicillamine, urinary cystine excretion is reduced, and urinary stones dissolve. Because of the high frequency of side effects, penicillamine should be used only in patients who have developed recurrent stones despite attempts at alkalinization of the urine or in patients who have suffered previous complications that have resulted in nephrectomy or renal insufficiency. Tiopronin (mercaptopropionyl-glycine) and captopril also interact with cystine to make it more soluble. Captopril therapy can reduce free cystine excretion by 50%.[7] Finally, if chronic renal failure develops from recurrent stones, renal transplantation is effective therapy. Recurrence does not occur because the transplanted kidney handles cystine normally.

## Uric acid stones

Uric acid, formed by the oxidation of hypoxanthine by the enzyme xanthine oxidase, is the end product of purine catabolism. The usual excretion of uric acid is approximately 600 to 1000 mg per day, of which one third is excreted into the gastrointestinal tract and metabolized by bacteria by a process called *uricolysis;* the remaining two thirds is excreted in the urine. Under normal conditions, urine is supersaturated with uric acid. The most common causes of uric acid stones are hyperuricosuria and persistently low urine pH. Hyperuricosuria is found in only one third of patients with uric acid stones. In the steady state, the major determinant of the urinary excretion of uric acid is the rate of production of uric acid. Hyperuricosuria and formation of uric acid stones may result from increased dietary purine intake, increased purine turnover as occurs in primary gout, or accelerated cell turnover as occurs in chronic hemolysis or in the tumor lysis syndrome. Interestingly, the prevalence of calcium oxalate stones also is increased in patients with hyperuricosuria and gout (see below).

Uric acid excretion may be decreased by restriction of foods rich in purines (especially meat) and by administration of allopurinol, a competitive inhibitor of xanthine oxidase. The usual dose of allopurinol is 300 mg per day, but up to 900 mg per day may be prescribed for short periods of time, as in preparation for chemotherapy of lymphoma or leukemia. During therapy with allopurinol, there is a decline in serum and urine levels of uric acid, and there is a concomitant increase in the levels of xanthine and hypoxanthine. However, because the latter compounds are far more soluble than uric acid, urinary stone formation is reduced. Persistently low urine pH is found in most patients with uric acid stones. Low pH greatly increases the tendency for uric acid to crystallize in urine. At lower values for urine pH, more uric acid is in the form of undissociated acid, and the risk of crystallization is increased. If urine is persistently acid, crystals grow and stones form. At higher values for pH ($>6.0$), far less undissociated uric acid is present, and uric acid crystals dissolve. One important cause of persistently low urine pH and uric acid stones is chronic diarrhea. Loss of water and bicarbonate in stool leads to reduced urine volume, increased net acid excretion, and low urine pH. Another cause of persistently low urinary pH is increased dietary protein intake, which results in increased net acid excretion and decreased urine pH. In other patients, including some patients with primary gout, urine pH is low even though net acid excretion is normal because a lower proportion of acid is excreted as ammonia and a higher proportion is excreted as titratable acidity. The cause of reduced ammoniagenesis in these patients is not understood. Whatever the cause of persistently low urinary pH, oral administration of alkali, such as sodium bicarbonate 40 to 60 mEq per day, results in intermittent excretion of alkaline urine and increased solubility of uric acid. Maintenance of a high urine volume also reduces urine concentration of uric acid. Finally, even if uric acid excretion is not excessive, treatment with allopurinol is effective in lowering uric acid excretion and in preventing recurrent stone formation in patients with persistently low urine pH. Allopurinol dose must be adjusted for renal function, and monitoring for side effects is essential.

## Calcium stones

As shown in Table 31-1, most calcium stones are composed of calcium and oxalate. Normal urine is saturated with calcium and oxalate, and calcium oxalate crystals may be found during examination of urinary sediment. These findings indicate that formation of calcium and oxalate stones may be the result of excessive excretion of calcium or oxalate

**Table 31–3.** *Summary of metabolic abnormalities and treatment in patients with calcium stones*

| Metabolic abnormality | Prevalence (%) | Treatment* |
|---|---|---|
| Hypercalciuria | | |
| Primay hyperparathyroidism | 5 | Surgery |
| Renal tubular acidosis | 1 | Alkali |
| Other causes† | 6 | Treat primary disorders |
| Idiopathic | 32 | Thiazide |
| Hyperoxaluria (enteric) | 5 | Treat primary disorder Low oxalate diet |
| Hyperuricosuria | 15 | Allopurinol |
| Hypercalciuria and hyperoxaluria | 14 | Thiazide and allopurinol |
| Hypocitraturia | 19–63 | Citrate |

Data may overlap with those of other conditions. Data from Preminger GM, Pak CYC: Nephrolithiasis. In Jacobson HR, Striter GE, Klahr S, editors: *The principles and practice of nephrology*, St. Louis, 1995, Mosby; Coe FL, Parks JH, Asplin JR: The pathogenesis and treatment of kidney stones, *N Engl J Med 327:1141, 1992.*
* Increased water intake should be included in therapy for all conditions.
† Causes include Paget's disease, sarcoidosis, vitamin D ingestion, increased calcium intake.

or the result of an imbalance in promoters and inhibitors of crystallization in urine that usually maintain the urinary tract free of stones. As shown in Table 31-3, one or more treatable disorders are present in 80% or more of patients with calcium stones.[8] The following sections of this chapter are a description of these disorders and their treatment. The box below describes the suggested metabolic evaluation for patients with calcium stones.

| Metabolic Evaluation for Patients with Calcium Stones | |
|---|---|
| SERUM | URINE (24-hour collection) |
| Calcium | Volume |
| Uric acid | pH |
| Sodium, chloride, bicarbonate, potassium | Creatinine |
| | Calcium |
| | Uric acid |
| | Oxalate |
| | Citrate (if no other abnormalities are present) |

# ABNORMALITIES ASSOCIATED WITH CALCIUM STONES

## Hypercalciuria

Hypercalciuria is defined as urinary calcium excretion greater than 300 mg per day in men or 250 mg per day in women (see Table 31-3). Other definitions include calcium excretion greater than 4 mg/kg of body weight per day or greater than 140 mg/g of urinary creatinine per day in both sexes. It is important that 24-hour urine samples for measurement of urinary calcium be collected while the patients are at home and eating their usual diets. Increased urinary excretion of calcium may result from increased filtration of calcium by the renal glomerulus, decreased reabsorption of calcium by the renal tubule, or both. Increased glomerular filtration of calcium occurs only if the serum calcium concentration is elevated. Decreased tubular reabsorption of calcium occurs in a variety of conditions, including distal renal tubular acidosis and increased dietary calcium intake. In most patients with hypercalciuria, no cause can be found; this condition is defined as *idiopathic hypercalciuria.*

**Hypercalcemia.** Renal stones occur in several conditions that cause both hypercalciuria and hypercalcemia. Serum calcium concentration should be measured as part of the evaluation of patients with a history of even a single calcium stone. The most common cause of hypercalcemia, hypercalciuria, and renal stones is primary hyperparathyroidism. The incidence of stones in this disorder ranges from 40% to 80% in various reports and is increased by high dietary calcium intake and high levels of vitamin D. Renal stones may occasionally complicate other disorders in which hypercalciuria and hypercalcemia occur, such as sarcoidosis, vitamin D intoxication, hyperthyroidism, Cushing's syndrome, Paget's disease, and immobilization. In some cases, the hypercalcemia may be minimal or even transient. Correction of the underlying disorder is required to correct the hypercalcemia and hypercalciuria. Interestingly, not all disorders causing hypercalcemia are associated with hypercalciuria and renal stones. Renal stones are not usually seen in patients with hyperparathyroidism associated with chronic renal failure because glomerular filtration rate and urinary calcium excretion are reduced. In patients with hypercalcemia caused by advanced malignancy, renal stones are also uncommon, perhaps because of the short survival of the patients affected and the reduced glomerular-filtration rate seen in association with severe hypercalcemia.[9] Also, renal stones do not complicate familial hypocalciuric hypercalcemia. In this disorder, the primary defect appears to be increased tubular reabsorption of calcium resulting in hypercalcemia and hypocalciuria.[10]

**Distal renal tubular acidosis.** Distal renal tubular acidosis is a rare disorder characterized by a non anion gap metabolic acidosis, a defect in urinary acidification (inability to lower urinary pH below 5.3), normal glomerular filtration rate, osteopenia, hypercalciuria, and recurrent formation of calcium phosphate renal stones.[11] Measurements of serum electrolytes and urine pH usually are sufficient to detect distal renal tubular acidosis. In some patients, however, the metabolic acidosis may be mild, and serum bicarbonate concentration may be in the normal range; nonetheless the urine pH is consistently elevated. An exogenous acid load can be administered to expose the defect in urinary acidification. The cause of hypercalciuria in distal renal tubular acidosis is not understood. Some authors hypothesize that metabolic acidosis directly reduces renal tubular reabsorption of calcium and that reduced bone mineral content is secondary to increased renal calcium loss. Other investigators suggest that the hypercalciuria is a secondary effect of the liberation of calcium from bone as a result of buffering retained acid by alkali in bone mineral. In addition to hypercalciuria, other alterations in urine composition contribute to stone formation in distal renal tubular acidosis. These include increased urinary pH and decreased urinary citrate excretion, which decrease the solubility of calcium and phosphate in urine. Treatment with alkali (sodium bicarbonate or potassium citrate, 40 to 60 mEq per day) raises serum bicarbonate, reduces urinary calcium excretion, raises urinary citrate excretion, and reduces the risk of stone recurrence.

**Increased dietary calcium intake.** The relationship between dietary calcium intake and urinary calcium excretion is shown in Fig. 31-2. Within the normal range of intake from 600 to 1200 mg per day, urinary calcium excretion is approximately 100 to 250 mg per day and is not influenced greatly by alterations in dietary calcium. The relative constancy of urinary calcium excretion throughout the normal range of intake is attributable, in part, to regulation of intestinal calcium

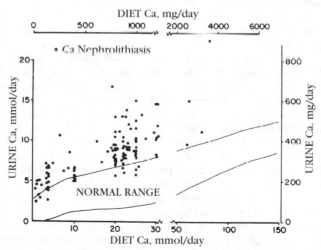

**Figure 31–2.** *Dietary and urinary calcium in normal humans and patients with calcium nephrolithiasis and idiopathic hypercalciuria. (Reprinted by permission of* The New England Journal of Medicine, *from Lemann J, Adams N, Gray R: Urinary calcium excretion in human begins,* N Engl J Med *301:535–541, 1979, Massachusetts Medical Society.)*

absorption by vitamin $D^{12}$. At low levels of calcium intake, the level of vitamin D and the fraction of ingested calcium that is absorbed are high. At high levels of intake, the level of vitamin D, and the fraction of calcium absorbed are reduced. The amount of calcium absorbed is approximately equal to the amount of calcium excreted in the urine; thus calcium balance is maintained. If excessive calcium is consumed, as in dairy products, antacids, or vitamin and mineral supplements, the level of vitamin D and the fraction of calcium absorbed decline, yet the absolute amount of calcium that is absorbed by the intestine and excreted in the urine is excessive. The resulting hypercalciuria is associated with an increased risk of stone formation. Patients with hypercalciuria should be referred to a nutritionist for estimation of their dietary calcium intake. If their dietary intake is excessive (that is, greater than a range of 1000 to 1200 mg per day), they should be advised to restrict dairy products and to discontinue taking antacids and vitamin-mineral supplements that contain calcium. Compliance with the treatment regimen can be assessed by subsequent measurement of urinary calcium excretion. Recently, it has come under question whether further dietary restriction might actually increase the risk for symptomatic kidney stones perhaps by increasing oxalate absorption.[13] A prospective study demonstrated increased risk of a first symptomatic stone when dietary calcium intake was less than 600 mg per day. Thus calcium restriction should be suggested only for patients with excessive calcium intakes.

Idiopathic hypercalciuria. Idiopathic hypercalciuria affects 5% of the general population. The prevalence of renal stones among individuals with this disorder is approximately 4%, compared to 0.5% in the general population. The disorder may be familial, is detectable in childhood, and presents as recurrent episodes of gross hematuria without apparent passage of urinary stones. There are no other complications of the disorder. As shown in Fig. 31-2, intestinal calcium absorption and urinary calcium excretion are increased at all levels of dietary calcium intake. Thus patients with idiopathic hypercalciuria appear to have two disorders that result in maintenance of calcium balance: increased excretion and increased absorption of calcium.

Two major hypotheses have been put forward to account for the alterations in calcium metabolism in idiopathic hypercalciuria: In "renal hypercalciuria" it is hypothesized that a primary reduction in tubular reabsorption of calcium leads to hypercalciuria and tends to lower serum calcium concentration, thereby raising parathyroid hormone, vitamin D, and intestinal absorption of calcium. In "absorptive hypercalciuria" it is hypothesized that a primary increase in either vitamin D or intestinal calcium absorption tends to raise serum calcium concentration, thereby lowering parathyroid hormone and renal tubular reabsorption of calcium and increasing urinary calcium excretion. In both disorders the serum calcium concentration is within the normal range. Although it is possible to distinguish between renal and absorptive hypercalciuria, in clinical practice, making this distinction is difficult and is usually not necessary. Several treatments for idiopathic hypercalciuria have been proposed. Thiazide diuretics are most commonly employed. In doses equivalent to hydrochlorothiazide 25 to 50 mg twice daily, urinary calcium excretion is reduced by approximately one half, and the rate of formation of new stones is reduced by approximately 90%. There are probably two mechanisms of action by which thiazide diuretics reduce calcium excretion. First, by inducing mild contraction of the extracellular fluid volume, thiazides stimulate proximal tubular filtrate reabsorption, including sodium and calcium reabsorption. This effect is blunted if extracellular fluid volume contraction is prevented by excessive dietary sodium intake. Second, thiazides appear to directly stimulate distal tubular reabsorption of calcium. Short-term effects of thiazides include a transient increase in serum calcium concentration because of increased serum protein concentration consequent to volume contraction. Serum ionized calcium concentration remains normal. Other side effects of thiazide diuretics include a 1% incidence of skin rash and a 10% incidence of nonspecific symptoms that resolve after reducing the dosage to once daily. Routine potassium supplementation is not necessary.

Factors associated with recurrent stone formation during treatment for idiopathic hypercalciuria include lower urine volume and higher (but normal) urinary calcium excretion. Patients should be encouraged to maintain a high urine volume (2 to 3 l. per day) and to restrict dietary sodium intake to 2 to 3 g (approximately 85 to 125 mEq) per day if necessary in order to decrease urinary calcium excretion to less than 2.5 mg/kg of body weight per day. Another potential explanation for recurrent stone formation during treatment may be reduced urinary citrate excretion (see below). The effects of long-term treatment with thiazide diuretics on calcium balance in idiopathic hypercalciuria remain unknown. In renal hypercalciuria, it is expected that calcium balance will be maintained with reduced calcium excretion and absorption. In absorptive hypercalciuria it is possible that a positive calcium balance could develop as a result of reduced excretion in the face of persistently increased absorption of calcium. However, studies of patients treated with thiazides for hypercalciuria (some of whom probably had absorptive hypercalciuria) have not revealed persistent hypercalcemia, soft-tissue calcification, osteosclerosis, or other evidence of a positive calcium balance. More studies are required to confirm the long-term effects of the calcium balance.

As an alternative to thiazide diuretics for absorptive hypercalciuria, some investigators have proposed oral administration of cellulose phosphate, an ion-exchange resin that complexes intestinal calcium, reduces intestinal calcium absorption, and consequently reduces urinary calcium excretion. When used as a single agent, cellulose sodium phosphate, 10 to 15 g per day in divided doses, reduces urinary calcium excretion. However, the frequency of stone formation is not reduced, perhaps because of decreased absorption and excretion of magnesium and increased absorption and excretion of oxalate, which both increase the risk of recurrent stone formation. When combined with a low-calcium, low-oxalate diet supplemented with magnesium, cellulose sodium phosphate does reduce stone recurrence.[14] Another alternative is therapy with inorganic phosphate salts (orthophosphates), including potassium phosphate ($K_2HPO_4$) and sodium phosphate ($Na_2HPO_4$). The mechanism of action of orthophosphates is not clear. There is a slight decline in urinary calcium excretion, which may be the consequence of elevated parathyroid hormone and reduced vitamin D that results with the rise of serum inorganic phosphorus concentration. In addition, the urinary excretion of pyrophosphate (an inhibitor of calcium oxalate crystallization) is increased during phosphate administration. In doses of approximately 2 g of elemental phosphorous per day in 3 or 4 divided doses, inorganic phosphate is effective in reducing recurrent stone formation. However, diarrhea occurs frequently, and 10% of patients are unable to tolerate the drug, even in reduced dosage. Phosphate should not be administered to patients with a reduced glomerular filtration rate.

Finally, protein intake stimulates calcium excretion in the urine, probably through increased acid production. Thus protein restriction (approximately 0.75 to 1.0 g/kg per day) is helpful in reducing urine calcium excretion as well as reducing urate excretion and in alkalinizing the urine. Furthermore, potassium citrate therapy, perhaps by alkalinizing the blood, also is effective in reducing daily calcium excretion and is a useful agent in hypercalciuric recurrent stone formers.

In summary, a therapeutic regimen employing thiazide diuretics with a high fluid intake and moderate sodium and protein restriction appears to be the most effective, least complicated, and safest strategy for prevention of recurrent stones caused by idiopathic hypercalciuria.

## Hyperoxaluria

Although most calcium stones contain oxalate, increased oxalate excretion is rarely found in patients with recurrent calcium stones (see Tables 31-2 and 31-3). Oxalate, a low-molecular-weight organic acid derived principally from the metabolism of ascorbic acid, glycine, and other amino acids, is freely filtered at the renal glomerulus and also is secreted by the tubule. Normally, endogenous oxalate accounts for 80% to 85% of urinary oxalate; the remaining 10% to 15% of urinary oxalate is the result of intestinal absorption of dietary oxalate. The most important cause of hyperoxaluria is increased intestinal absorption of oxalate as a result of gastrointestinal diseases; this condition is defined as enteric hyperoxaluria. Other causes of hyperoxaluria are rare, including excessive consumption of dietary oxalate or oxalate precursors (such as ascorbic acid), pyridoxine deficiency, or genetic metabolic disorders (primary hyperoxaluria).

**Enteric hyperoxaluria.** Oxalate is absorbed primarily in the small bowel by passive processes. Normally, only 5% of dietary oxalate is absorbed because it is complexed with calcium in the bowel lumen. In a variety of gastrointestinal disorders, increased oxalate absorption is associated with hyperoxaluria and recurrent calcium oxalate stones. These include regional enteritis, bacterial overgrowth, blind-loop syndrome, nontropical sprue, small bowel resection or bypass, pancreatitis or pancreatectomy, and biliary tract disease.[15] In enteric hyperoxaluria, the colon appears to be the site of increased oxalate absorption. Two hypotheses have been advanced to explain the increased oxalate absorption in gastrointestinal disorders: (1) with steatorrhea, fatty acids form complexes with calcium, thus decreasing the availability of calcium to form complexes with oxalate, which then becomes available for absorption in the colon; (2) with bile salt malabsorption, colonic mucosa is injured and becomes more permeable to oxalate. The frequency of stones in these disorders is variable, approximately 25% after intestinal bypass and 5% in inflammatory bowel disease. In addition to hyperoxaluria, other factors may contribute importantly to stone formation in gastrointestinal diseases. Mild metabolic acidosis and reduced urine volume, urine pH, and magnesium and citrate excretion are often found as a result of chronic diarrhea. Treatment includes prescription of a high fluid intake and a low oxalate diet as well as specific measures to control steatorrhea and bile salt diarrhea. Metabolic acidosis, magnesium depletion, and hypocitraturia should be treated if present. Allopurinol also may be prescribed to reduce urinary acid excretion as described previously.

## Hyperuricosuria

Increased urinary excretion of uric acid is found in approximately 30% of patients with calcium stones. In approximately half of patients with hyperuricosuria, hypercalciuria is also present (see Table 31-3). One hypothesis for the pathogenesis of calcium stones in these patients is heterogeneous nucleation of calcium stones by crystals of uric acid or monosodium urate that has formed as a result of hyperuricosuria. Another hypothesis is that crystals of uric acid or monosodium urate absorb macromolecules that normally inhibit the growth of calcium oxalate crystals. The most frequent cause of hyperuricosuria in patients with recurrent calcium stones is excessive dietary purine intake. A minority of patients have mild hyperuricemia, and in some patients the hyperuricosuria is the result of primary gout. Treatment of hyperuricosuria with a low-protein diet and allopurinol 100 mg twice daily is effective in reducing uric acid excretion by 30% and reducing the rate of stone formation by 90%. In patients with both hypercalciuria and hyperuricosuria, treatment with a combination of thiazides, allopurinol, and a low-purine diet is effective in reducing formation of recurrent stones.

## Hypocitraturia

Citric acid, an intermediate in the Krebs' tricarboxylic acid cycle, is a low-molecular-weight organic acid that inhibits the growth of calcium oxalate crystals in urine. Citrate is filtered by the renal glomerulus and reabsorbed by the tubule. Citrate excretion is reduced during metabolic acidosis (including renal tubular acidosis), chronic diarrhea, urinary tract infection, and treatment with thiazide diuretics. Recently it has been recognized that a large minority of patients with calcium stones have reduced urinary citrate excretion. In some patients, hypocitraturia is the only identifiable metabolic abnormality.

In one report, 15 patients with idiopathic hypocitraturia as the sole metabolic abnormality were treated with potassium citrate 60 mEq per day in three divided doses.[16] An additional 10 patients with hypocitraturia and hypercalciuria were also treated with potassium citrate alone. In these 25 patients, urinary citrate excretion rose into the normal range, and the frequency of recurrent stone formation decreased by 90%. Twelve other patients with hypocitraturia and either hypercalciuria or hyperuricosuria underwent treatment with a combination of potassium citrate and either hydrochlorothiazide or allopurinol. Citrate excretion was increased to normal, and stone recurrence was reduced. In another study, 13 patients with hypercalciuria and hypocitraturia had recurrent stones, despite reduction of urinary calcium excretion during treatment with thiazide diuretics.[17] Addition of potassium citrate raised urinary citrate excretion and reduced the rate of stone formation by 90%. Minor side effects of therapy included diarrhea and nausea. Thus it appears that some patients with recurrent calcium oxalate stones have idiopathic hypocitraturia and that treatment with potassium citrate is simple, safe, and effective in restoring urinary citrate excretion to normal and reducing the risk of stone recurrence. Based on these data it is advisable to measure urinary citrate excretion in patients with calcium oxalate stones who do not have hypercalciuria or hyperuricosuria and in patients who do have these disorders but who have recurrent stone formation despite thiazide or allopurinol treatment. Patients with hypocitraturia should be treated with potassium citrate, 40 to 80 mEq per day, to raise citrate excretion to normal. The medication is best tolerated when given as a solid preparation during meals.

## No apparent metabolic disorder

Approximately 25% of patients with recurrent calcium oxalate stones studied by Coe and colleagues had normal serum and urinary measurements of calcium, oxalate, and uric acid.[1] It is hypothesized that these patients had an imbalance between promoters and inhibitors of crystallization that account for stone formation. Presumably, some, but not all, of the patients had hypocitraturia; however, the data on urinary citrate excretion in these patients have not been reported. Other inhibitors that might be abnormally low include magnesium, pyrophosphate, or the anionic protein CGI (14,000 daltons). Additional potential causes of stone formation in this group might be habitually low urine volume or pH. Although the cause of recurrent stones in these patients is unknown, empiric treatment with a combination of thiazides and allopurinol is successful in lowering the excretion of calcium and uric acid by 15% to 30% and reducing the rate of stone formation by 80%.[2] Presumably by reducing the concentrations of calcium and uric acid one lessens the risk of recurrent stones. One report demonstrates successful therapy with allopurinol alone in a dose of 300 mg per day.[18] Whether thiazide diuretics alone would be equally successful is not known. Because of the morbidity of stones, it seems reasonable to prescribe both agents for patients who form recurrent stones without an apparent metabolic disorder.

## References

1. Preminger GM, Pak CYC: Nephrolithiasis. In Jacobson HR, Striker GE, Klahr S, editors: *The principles and practice of nephrology.* St. Louis, 1995, Mosby.

2. Coe FL, Parks JH, Asplin JR: The pathogenesis and treatment of kidney stones, *N Engl J Med* 327:1141, 1992.
3. Silverman DE, Stamey TA: Management of infection stones: the Stanford experience, *Medicine* 62:44, 1983.
4. Kahnoski RJ, Lingeman JE, Coury TA, et al: Combined percutaneous and extracorporeal shock wave lithotripsy for staghorn calculi: an alternative to anatrophic nephrolithotomy, *J Urol* 135:679, 1986.
5. Williams JJ, Rodman JS, Peterson CM: A randomized double-blind study of acetohydroxamic acid in struvite nephrolithiasis, *N Engl J Med* 311:760, 1984.
6. Oras E, Arber N, Aksentijevich I, et al: Localization of a gene causing cystinuria to the chromosome 2p, *Nat Genet* 6:415, 1994.
7. Perazella MA, Buller GK: Successful treatment of cystinuria with captopril, *Am J Kidney Dis* 21:504, 1993.
8. Millman S, Strauss AL, Parks JH, Coe FL: Pathogenesis and clinical course of mixed calcium oxalate and uric acid nephrolithiasis, *Kidney Int* 22:366, 1982.
9. Muggia FM, Heinemann HO: Hypercalcemia associated with neoplastic disease, *Arch Intern Med* 73:281, 1970.
10. Marx SJ: Familial hypocalciuric hypercalcemia, *N Engl J Med* 303:810, 1980.
11. Coe FL, Parks J: Stone disease in hereditary distal renal tubular acidosis, *Ann Intern Med* 93:60, 1980.
12. Lemann J, Adams ND, Gray RW: Urinary calcium excretion in human beings, *N Engl J Med* 301:535, 1979.
13. Curhan GC, Willett WC, Rimm EB, Stampfer MJ: A prospective study of dietary calcium and other nutrients and the risk of symptomatic kidney stones, *N Engl J Med* 328:833, 1993.
14. Pak CYC: A cautious use of sodium cellulose phosphate in the management of calcium nephrolithiasis, *Invest Urol* 19:187, 1981.
15. Obialo CI, Clayman RV, Matts JP, et al: Pathogenesis of nephrolithiasis post-partial ileal bypass surgery, *Am J Kidney Dis* 17:370, 1991.
16. Pak CYC, Fuller CY: Idiopathic hypocitraturic calcium oxalate nephrolithiasis successfully treated with potassium citrate, *Ann Intern Med* 104:33, 1986.
17. Pak CYC, Peterson R, Sakhaee K, et al: Correction of hypocitraturia and prevention of stone formation by combined thiazide and potassium citrate in the therapy in thiazide-unresponsive hypercalciuric nephrolithiasis, *Am J Med* 79:284, 1985.
18. Ettinger B, Tang A, Citron J, et al: Randomized trial of allopurinol in the prevention of calcium oxalate calculi, *N Engl J Med* 315:1386, 1986.

# Chapter 32

# *Recurrent Urinary Tract Infections*

Richard A. Lafayette

Urinary tract infection is a major cause of morbidity in the United States. Evaluation and treatment of urinary tract infection result in approximately 7 million office visits and a cost of over one billion dollars per year. Although most common in young, sexually active women, urinary tract infection occurs in other patient populations, especially when there is a urinary tract disorder. This chapter is a review of the approach to urinary tract infections in women and men and suggests a guide to therapy and further evaluation.

## URINARY TRACT INFECTIONS IN WOMEN

**Uncomplicated infection.** Women are much more susceptible to urinary tract infection than men, attributable, at least in part, to the anatomic nature of the female urethra. The typical presentation of dysuria, frequency, urgency, or suprapubic pain in an otherwise healthy, sexually active woman leads to the proper suspicion of cystitis. Generally easy to differentiate from vaginitis or acute urethral syndrome, the presence of pyuria (often with hematuria) by dipstick or on urine examination is sufficient to make a diagnosis of cystitis.[1,2] When the presentation is atypical, the diagnosis can be confirmed by an abnormal urine culture demonstrating $\geq 10^2$ colony-forming units/ mL. The etiologic agents and response to therapy are predictable. Typical bacterial causes of urinary tract infection are listed in Table 32-1. In considering all the factors involved in therapy such as cost, efficacy, and side effects, there are multiple approaches to drug therapy. Seven-day regimens are highly effective in eradicating infection but are costly, are likely to have side effects, and alter vaginal flora. Single-dose regimens are less costly and have fewer side effects but are generally less effective. There has arisen general agreement that therapy for 3 days with broad-spectrum antibiotics known to eradicate the usual

**Table 32-1.** *Typical causes of urinary tract infection*

| Agent | Approximate frequency |
|---|---|
| **UNCOMPLICATED URINARY TRACT INFECTION** | |
| *Escherichia coli* | 80% |
| *Proteus mirabilis* | 10-15% |
| *Staphylococcus saprophyticus* | 5% |
| Other Enterobacteriaceae | <5% |
| Enterococci | <5% |
| Group B streptococci | <5% |
| Chlamydiae | <5% |
| **COMPLICATED URINARY TRACT INFECTION** | |
| *Escherichia coli* | 20% |
| *Klebsiella* | 10-20% |
| Enterobacteriaceae | 10-20% |
| *Pseudomomas aeruginosa* | ≈10% |
| *Serratia* | ≈10% |

bacteria provides the ideal combination of safety and efficacy.[3,4] Recommended empiric therapy for cystitis is listed in Table 32-2.

It often is quite difficult to differentiate cystitis from pyelonephritis because the clinical feature overlaps. Typically, some flank pain or costovertebral angle tenderness is present in pyelonephritis. However, up to 30% of apparently simple urinary tract infections have upper tract involvement. When pyelonephritis is suspected, urine and blood cultures should be obtained in case empiric therapy proves unsuccessful. *Escherichia coli* remains the most common bacterial agent, and pyelonephritis can be treated safely in nonpregnant outpatients, as long as nausea and vomiting are absent and the patient does not appear clinically ill. Regimens for empiric therapy of pyelonephritis are listed in Table 32-2. Symptoms generally resolve in 2 or 3 days, and it is prudent to continue therapy for 10 to 14 days. Routine evaluation for anatomic abnormalities is not indicated after uncomplicated pyelonephritis. However, persistent fever of continuing illness should lead to a search for complicated infection with ultrasound or CT scanning, and hospitalization with treatment utilizing intravenous antibiotics should be initiated.[4]

Pregnancy requires a different, more conservative, approach to urinary tract infection. Uncomplicated cystitis should be assessed by urine culture, and therapy should be extended for 7 days with agents that do not affect fetal development, such as ampicillin or trimethoprim-sulfamethoxazole. Cure should be documented by follow-up urine culture. Pyelonephritis should be treated aggressively with hospitalization

**Table 32-2.** *Suggested empiric therapy for urinary tract infection*

| Infection (manifestation) | Antibiotic | Dose | Duration (days) |
|---|---|---|---|
| **CYSTITIS** | | | |
| (Women) | Trimethoprim-sulfamethoxazole | 160/800 mg bid | 3 |
| | Ofloxacin | 200 mg bid | 3 |
| | Norfloxacin | 400 mg bid | 3 |
| | Ciprofloxacin | 250 mg bid | 3 |
| | Cefixime | 400 mg qd | 3 |
| | Amoxicillin | 250 mg tid | 7[†] |
| (Pregnancy) | Cefpodoxime proxetil | 100 mg bid | 7 |
| | Trimethoprim-sulfamethoxazole | 160/800 mg bid | 7 |
| (Men) | Same as above | | 7 |
| **PYELONEPHRITIS** | | | |
| (Oral) | Trimethoprim-sulfamethoxazole | 160/800 mg bid | 14 |
| | Ofloxacin | 300 mg bid | 14 |
| | Norfloxacin | 400 mg bid | 14 |
| | Ciprofloxacin | 500 mg bid | 14 |
| | Cefixime | 400 mg qd | 14 |
| (Intravenous)* | Trimethoprim-sulfamethoxazole | 160/800 mg bid | 14 |
| | Ofloxacin | 300 mg bid | 14 |
| | Norfloxacin | 400 mg bid | 14 |
| | Ciprofloxacin | 500 mg bid | 14 |
| | Cefixime | 400 mg qd | 14 |
| | Gentamycin | 5 mg/kg gd | 14 |
| | Ceftriaxone | 1-2 g qd | 14 |
| | Ticarcillin-clavulanate | 3.1 g tid | 14 |

* For clinically serious infections, it can be changed to oral therapy when clinically improved, but it should be adjusted to appropriate antibiotic once culture is available.
† High chance of resistance.

and administration of parenteral antibiotics such as aminoglycosides or ceftriaxone until therapy can be based on culture results.

**Recurrent infections.** As stated above, it is common for women to have recurrent cystitis. In fact, over 20% of women with an initial diagnosis of cystitis will have recurrent infection. It is important to differentiate patients whose first infection was inadequately eradicated and is relapsing from patients who are experiencing recurrent bouts with new infection. Relapse generally occurs in the first week after discontinuance of therapy with antibiotics and can be identified if a follow-up culture yields the same organism seen in the first infection. Relapse often indicates poor compliance or infection with a resistant organism. However, it also can be a clue to unsuspected pyelonephritis or to structural abnormalities of the urinary tract including vesicoureteral reflux, bladder or ureteral diverticuli, nephrolithiasis, and neuromuscular disorders of the urinary tract (associated with diabetes, spinal cord injury, multiple sclerosis, or drugs). Relapses require longer therapy, often 4 to 6 weeks. Furthermore, careful consideration should be given to evaluation of the urinary tract for anatomic abnormalities.

Recurrent infections attributable to new infection generally occur several months after the prior infection. Risk factors include genetic predisposition, sexual activity, the use of barrier contraception, wiping the perineum back to forwards, oral contraceptives, holding back urine flow, and, of course, bacterial virulence factors. In general, these infections can be managed successfully the same as a first episode of uncomplicated cystitis with 3-day regimens. However, recommendations to limit the risk factors above, as possible, may limit the recurrence rate. The routine use of cranberry juice (which has weak antimicrobial properties), one large glass per day, also may reduce the risk of recurrent infection. Postmenopausal women also have an increased risk of recurrent infection related to changes in vaginal flora. Estrogen creams can reduce the risk in this population.

If urinary tract infection still recurs at a rate greater than twice per year despite a change in these habits, medical prophylaxis is reasonable. Agents that change urinary pH (acidifying agents such as methenamine) are not highly effective. Agents such as quinolones or trimethoprim-sulfamethoxazole, taken once or alternated daily, have proved highly effective with little evidence of resistance over many years of experience. However, discontinuing these regimens is generally associated with resumption of infections. An alternative therapy for women with recurrent infection associated with sexual activity is "prophylaxis" only on the days they have sexual intercourse. In patients who can identify their own infections, another option is to have the patient start treatment on her own as soon as any symptoms arise. This therapy is safe and effective and also results in lower cost as compared to continuous prophylactic regimens.

**Complicated urinary tract infections.** Urinary tract infections should be considered complicated anytime they occur in a subject with an anatomically abnormal urinary tract, the patient is immunosuppressed, or the infection is caused by resistant organisms. High fevers, renal dysfunction, intractable nausea and vomiting, or sepsis are all signs suggestive of complicated infection. Typical causitive organisms are listed in Table 32-1. Complicated infections must be investigated with a urine culture to tailor antibiotic therapy to appropriate agents that will reach high concentrations in the urine. Although oral therapy with quinolones and trimethoprim-sulfamethoxazole can be effective, intravenous therapy often is required. Empiric antibiotics need to have broad and efficient gram-negative bacterial coverage; therapy generally is required for at least 2 weeks. Failure of clinical response should prompt an investigation to find and correct any anatomic problem that may prevent eradication of infection.

# URINARY TRACT INFECTION IN MEN

Urinary tract infections are quite rare in otherwise healthy, young men. However, uncomplicated infections can occur and generally are caused by the same organisms that cause urinary tract infection in women. Typical symptoms of suprapubic discomfort, dysuria, and frequency generally occur. However, sometimes men can present with an acute urethritis syndrome with a discharge. Risk factors for uncomplicated urinary tract infection include lack of circumcision, homosexual activity, and sexual intercourse with a partner colonized with uropathogens. Immunosuppression, either from HIV infection or medications, is an important additional risk factor.

Empiric treatment is a 7-day course of a quinolone or trimethoprim-sulfamethoxazole. Success rates approach 100%, and it is unnecessary to proceed to any evaluation of the urinary tract unless relapse occurs.[5] Recurrent urinary tract infection in men should prompt an evaluation for anatomic abnormalities and lead to the initiation of therapy for complicated urinary tract infection. In older men, it always is important to consider prostatitis as a cause for apparent urinary tract infection. Differentiation by physical exam is generally straightforward. However, it occasionally is necessary to compare the results of urine culture before and after prostatic massage. Treatment of acute prostatitis (again using quinolones, trimethoprim-sulphamethoxazole, or trimethoprim alone) is urgent because there is a high risk of gram-negative bacterial sepsis. Hospitalization and parenteral therapy are needed for acutely ill patients. Treatment for 4 to 6 weeks is usually necessary to eradicate the infection.

# ASYMPTOMATIC URINARY TRACT INFECTION

Asymptomatic urinary tract infection always has been an area of great concern regarding the risk for symptomatic infection and the associated risk of death. Studies in nursing-home subjects have demonstrated increased mortalities in subjects with abnormal urine cultures ($>10^5$ colony-forming units/mL).[6] However, population-based therapy has not demonstrated any benefit in the routine treatment of asymptomatic bacteriuria, an indication that bacteriuria may be simply a marker of comorbidity. The only patient populations that do benefit from therapy of asymptomatic bacteriuria are pregnant women and patients who are to have urologic surgery because they are at high risk from complications from their infection. Otherwise, the routine treatment of asymptomatic bacteriuria cannot be advocated.

# URETHRAL CATHETER–
# ASSOCIATED INFECTION

The use of urethral catheters is associated with a high rate of urinary tract infections. In the United States, greater than a million cases of infection per year are believed to occur as a result of indwelling catheters, and such catheters are the most frequent source of gram-negative bacteremia.[7]

The ideal treatment for catheter-associated infections is prevention. Catheters must be placed under sterile conditions and optimally are drained into sealed collecting devices. The seal should be broken as infrequently as possible. The catheter should be maintained as necessary, and every opportunity to use alternative methods of urine drainage, such as intermittent catheterization, should be employed. Although systemic antibiotics can prevent or delay catheter-associated infection, the cost and side effects are not attractive. Prophylactic therapy generally is not employed except for short-term use in very high risk settings.

Symptomatic infection occurs frequently and is documented by the abnormal culture of $\geq 10^2$ colony-forming units/mL. The infection is frequently polymicrobial. Catheters can form biofilms that protect bacteria from antimicrobial agents. Thus catheters should be changed (if not discontinued) during therapy for infection. Therapy should be similar to that given for complicated urinary tract infections, and patients must be monitored for evidence of sepsis. Asymptomatic bacteriuria occurs in virtually all patients with long-standing catheters; however, routine treatment is not advocated in this setting because of the high rate of recurrence and the lack of clinical evidence that treatment reduces complications.[8]

## References

1. Hooton TM: A simplified approach to urinary tract infection, *Hosp Pract* 30:23, 1995.
2. Carroll KC, Hale DC, Von Boerum DH, et al: Laboratory evaluation of urinary tract infections in an ambulatory clinic, *Am J Clin Pathol* 101:100, 1994.
3. Hooton TM, Johnson C, Winter C, et al: Single-dose and three-day regimens of ofloxacin versus trimethoprim-sulfamethoxazole for acute cystitis in women, *Antimicrob Agents Chemother* 35:1479, 1991.
4. Stamm WE, Hooton TM: Management of urinary tract infection in adults, *N Engl J Med* 329:1328, 1993.
5. Lipsky BA: Urinary tract infections in men: epidemiology, pathophysiology, diagnosis and treatment, *Ann Intern Med* 110:138, 1989.
6. Dontas AS, Kasviki-Charvarti P, Papanayiotou PC, Marketos SG: Bacteriuria and survival in old age, *N Engl J Med* 304:939, 1984.
7. Kreger BE, Craven DE, Carling PC, McCabe WR: Gram-negative bacteremia. III. Reassessment of etiology, epidemiology and ecology in 612 patients, *Am J Med* 68:332, 1980.
8. Warren JW, Anthony WC, Hoopes JM, Muncie HL: Cephalexin for susceptible bacteriuria in afebrile, long-term catheterized patients, *JAMA* 248:454, 1982.

# Pulmonary Disease

## Chapter 33

### Management of Asthma

Leonard Sicilian

The definition of asthma has always been the most controversial of the obstructive lung diseases. The intermittent nature of the disease had long been observed. Early scientific data focused on spasm of the bronchial smooth muscle. Recent data increasingly support the basic nature of asthma as an inflammatory disease of the airway of which bronchospasm is only a component.[1,2] The currently accepted definition states that asthma has the following characteristics: (1) airway obstruction that is reversible (not completely in some) either spontaneously or with treatment, (2) airway inflammation, and (3) increased responsiveness to a variety of stimuli.[3]

## ASTHMA MORTALITY

There are estimated to be greater than 10 million patients in the United States with asthma. Despite better understanding of the mechanisms and mediators of this disease, there has been a steady rise in asthma-related deaths over the last 10 to 15 years. These deaths (some 6000 per year) are disturbing not only because they occur in young people who usually have the disease, but also because it is a treatable disease from which few people if any should die. This paradox of increasing mortality in the face of increasing knowledge also spills over to the other aspects of asthma care. Hospitalizations, including emergency department visits, have increased, and as such have driven up the cost of asthma care. In addition, the deaths are not evenly distributed across the population, with higher death rates for blacks and children in urban areas.[4]

The cause of this increased mortality has not clearly been elucidated. Overuse of beta-adrenergic agonist bronchodilators administered through metered-dose inhalers (MDI) has been implicated in some studies.[5] Closer examination of the data does not appear to support a causal relationship and excess beta-adrenergic agonist MDI use may just be a marker for severe and uncontrolled disease.[6,7] Review of asthmatics who have died or nearly died from their disease indicated that even when these patients were being seen by their primary physician assessment of optimum clinical care and self-management showed these areas to be inadequate.[8] For a variety of reasons many of these patients delay receiving medical care during an acute attack, and death ensues.[8,9]

## ASTHMA INITIATIVES

In an attempt to obtain more information about asthma, and especially to stem the rising tide of deaths, several national and international efforts were set in motion. The best known of these was the National Asthma Education Program (NAEP). The report of the expert panel convened by this group was supposed to begin to bridge the gap between what we knew about asthma and how we managed the disease.[3] The essential message of this group was that asthma was a heterogeneous disease that varies from patient to patient and within the same patient over time. As a result, patient management needed to be individualized within a larger framework. Most important, the patient was targeted as being a major force in the management of his or her own disease. The patient along with his or her primary physician was urged to know the severity of the disease by subjective and objective measurements, to understand the triggers of acute attacks, and to develop an individualized strategy of therapy that could be adjusted as needed, based on changes in the symptoms and functional status. Communication and education were the major building blocks of this relationship between the asthmatic and the physician.

The publication of guidelines 5 years ago has generated some controversy. Individuals and groups in many instances have latched onto certain aspects of the guidelines and have given them a prominence the authors likely never intended. One glaring example is the almost obsessive use of hand-held peak-flow meters as the "one thing" that will improve asthma management. The NAEP guidelines when read carefully suggest several tools and strategies to be used to optimize management. The physician and patient partnership should decide which work best in the ongoing treatment of the asthmatic.[10]

The NAEP guidelines focused on four components of asthma care: (1) objective measurements of assessing the severity of disease and outcomes of therapy, (2) pharmacologic management aimed at inflammation in the airways, (3) environmental controls, and (4) patient education. It is impossible to cover the entire range of these recommendations, but I will attempt to highlight those approaches and newer developments that have helped most in my day-to-day management of asthma.

## SEVERITY AND OUTCOMES

Although many asthmatics can tell when their disease is worsening, this does not apply to all patients. It is unclear whether this inability to detect a deterioration in respiratory status is a result of chronic symptoms, which the patients learn to ignore, or a lack of education resulting in the patients being unaware of the importance of worsening symptoms. In any case, either or both have been implicated in asthma deaths.[9] The NAEP guidelines identify three categories of severity in asthma that should serve as markers for control of the disease. They are simply mild, moderate, and severe (Table 33-1). Ideally all asthma patients should be kept asymptomatic or at least in the mild category. Thus the categories are important as an educational tool to teach patients which symptoms are unacceptable. This implies that a change to a more severe category will also trigger an escalation of therapy. The goal of this therapy is to return the patient to a lower level of severity or abolish symptoms altogether. Thus the physician and patient not only can rapidly identify worsening of disease, but also can have specific goals to achieve in therapy (such as reducing nocturnal symptoms from daily to less than once per week). This requires an open channel of communication between physician and patient. Communication can include specific written instructions on increased medication use, emergency procedures, and phone numbers. In fact, in a very cooperative and trustworthy patient, a sophisticated and intense regimen of home treatment can be given in a time-limited fashion for safe control of symptoms and for help in preventing unnecessary utilization of the emergency department.[3]

It can be seen from Table 33-1 that several factors contribute to a level of asthma severity. Peak expiratory flow rate (PEFR) measurements as made by a hand-held peak-flow meter is only one method. PEFR is clearly the link between the objective realm of pulmonary physiology and the subjective symptoms and therefore may be of great benefit. It can be applied to establish a patient's "personal best" peak flow, which can be used not only to signify optimal function, but also to signal a patient that he or she is deteriorating and a change in therapy is needed. Indeed it may be a valuable tool to monitor the efficacy of changes in medication. This can help identify which drugs work best for a particular patient in either the outpatient, emergency, or inpatient setting.

**Table 33-1.** *Characteristics of asthma by severity*

| Characteristics | Mild | Moderate | Severe |
|---|---|---|---|
| Exacerbations | ≤1 or 2 times/week | >1 or 2 times/week<br>ED or office visit <3 times/year | Daily symptoms<br>ED or office visits >3 times/year<br>Hospitalization >2 times/year |
| Symptom frequency | Few between exacerbations | Often present | Continuous though may be low grade |
| Nocturnal symptoms | <1 or 2 times/month | 2 or 3 times/week | Almost nightly |
| Exercise tolerance | Good<br>May not tolerate vigorous activity | Diminished | Poor<br>Limitation of routine activity |
| School or job attendance | Good | Occasional absence | Poor |

| | | | |
|---|---|---|---|
| Pulmonary function | PEFR >80% predicted<br><20% variability<br>Spirometry normal<br>>15% improvement with inhaled bronchodilators | PEFR 60% to 80% predicted<br>20% to 30% variability<br>Spirometry shows airflow obstruction<br>>15% improvement with inhaled bronchodilators | PEFR <60% predicted<br>>30% variability<br>Spirometry shows substantial airflow obstruction<br>Does not improve to normal with inhaled bronchodilators |
| Response/duration of therapy | Regular therapy usually for short-term only<br>12- to 24-hour response to addition of medication<br>No use of oral corticosteroids | Regular therapy required most of the time<br>Periodic addition of medication including oral corticosteroids for days to weeks | Continuous therapy required occasionally with oral or high-dose inhaled corticosteroids |

ED, Emergency department; PEFR, peak expiratory flow rate.

Patients in the severe asthma category are clearly at increased risk for hospitalization and death. Any patient whose symptoms place him or her chronically or frequently in the moderate or severe category should be managed with the help of a pulmonary specialist or allergist if the major triggers of asthma are allergic in nature. Table 33-2 lists other situations where referral is indicated.

# PHARMACOLOGIC MANAGEMENT

The key to pharmacologic management is not just to know the action and dosage of commonly used drugs, but also to apply them in a step-wise fashion.[3] This means to increase the amount and type of drug used as a patient moves to a higher severity level and once the patient has become asymptomatic or returns to the base-line function, to reduce that medication. It is clear that the more medication used the greater is the chance of side effects; however, the primary physician should not hesitate to escalate both the type and dose of medication to prevent deterioration.

The physician should know both what medications work for his or her individual patients and what written (preferably) management plan should be given to the patient so that worsening asthma can be treated quickly. This will allow the patient to begin therapy without waiting for phone calls or explaining the patient's history to covering physicians. However, the patient must be responsible for contacting the physician once this additional therapy is begun. Since no two asthma exacerbations are exactly alike even in the same patient, modification of dose and duration of therapy will always be necessary. Although this frequent communication may at times seem like overkill, the improved care, diminished costs of emergency department visits, and potential benefit

**Table 33-2.** *Guidelines for referral to a specialist*

| | |
|---|---|
| For diagnosis: | Initial pulmonary function testing |
| | Specialized pulmonary testing, such as: |
| |     Methacholine challenge |
| |     Exercise testing |
| |     Allergy or irritant testing |
| For management assistance: | $\geq$2 hospitalizations in last year |
| | $\geq$3 emergency visits in last year |
| | Continuous use of oral corticosteroids |
| | Prior ICU admission or intubation |
| | Psychiatric or psychosocial problems |
| | Poor response to routine changes in medication for exacerbation |
| | Experimental or toxic drug use |

of reducing time lost from work or school far outweigh the perceived inconvenience.

For mild asthma, therapy can often begin with use of a beta-adrenergic agonist metered-dose inhaler (MDI) on an as-needed basis or before an activity that is known to cause bronchospasm (such as exercise or exposure to cold air). Although my experience as a subspecialist is biased, this is not the usual situation. Very often these drugs need to be administered regularly three or four times a day. In these instances and certainly in any patient with moderate or severe disease an anti-inflammatory drug should be added. The most commonly used anti-inflammatory drugs are the inhaled corticosteroids. Although many brands are available, they all appear to have similar efficacy. Initial use of two to four puffs twice a day is usually adequate in mild or moderate disease. Both cromolyn sodium and nedocromil sodium MDI's are non-steroidal anti-inflammatory drugs that can also be used. Occasionally for refractory moderate or severe asthmatics both drug categories may be used at the same time. The exact mechanism of action of these types of drugs in asthma is unknown.

Patients with chronic moderate asthma will usually require regular use of an inhaled beta-adrenergic agonist and an anti-inflammatory agent with the majority of recent data pointing to the anti-inflammatory agent as the primary drug of choice. Recently a long-acting beta-agonist, salmeterol xinafoate, has become available as an MDI.[11] Its advantages are twofold. First the twice-a-day dosing schedule should improve patient compliance, and, second, it appears to decrease airway hyperreactivity, a feature short-acting beta-agonists lack.[12] By the same token, it cannot be used for relief of acute symptoms, and therefore patients using this drug must have their short-acting MDI available at all times for emergent use. This property also makes the use of salmeterol xinafoate less helpful as an additional medication during exacerbations. It is my practice to add this drug (two puffs twice a day) to patients when their symptoms are stable and then to try to reduce and discontinue the shorter-acting beta agonist.

Sustained-release theophylline is also recommended for exacerbations of mild asthma or regular use in patients with moderate or severe disease. This drug was in disfavor for most of the last 10 to 15 years because of concerns about excess toxicity. The cause of this was inappropriately high dosing. Currently 200 to 300 mg twice a day of sustained-release theophylline by mouth will give both bronchodilator and some (theoretical) anti-inflammatory effect in most patients. At these doses, serum levels need not be regularly monitored, and levels need not exceed 12 mg/mL. Sustained-release theophylline is also helpful as a single-dose bedtime medication to control nocturnal symptoms.

If combination and increased dosage of the above-mentioned drug do not control the exacerbation and return the patient to a lower level of severity, orally administered steroids must be used. They should be started early when other medication does not work quickly and continued on a short and tapering course over 5 days to 4 weeks depending on severity of symptoms and rapidity of resolution.

A complete discussion of the drug therapy of asthma is impossible in this setting, and the NAEP guidelines review them in detail.[3] The physician must be aware of several new drugs that are under investigation for use in asthma.[13,14] It is unlikely that any single agent will be effective for all patients. The clinician must also remember, especially in adults, that whenever there is an exacerbation of asthma that responds poorly to step therapy, other precipitating illnesses must be considered. Most commonly these are infections, heart failure or cardiac ischemia, gastroesophageal reflux disease, or subtle environmental allergies. Clearly, patients who show poor response to standard aggressive therapy should be managed with a pulmonary specialist.

## ENVIRONMENTAL CONTROLS

Triggering of the inflammatory response in asthma is commonly a result of allergen exposure. Therefore control of these exposures by either avoidance or reduction in magnitude is important in the management of asthma. It is not necessary as an initial step to have patients undergo extensive intradermal allergy testing. A simple screening history will often alert the physician to the possible allergen or source of allergen in most patients. Once a potential source is identified, the specific allergen (or irritant) can be characterized, controlled, or eliminated. Table 33-3 lists a simple screening tool to assess the possible role of allergens in an asthmatic patient.

Exposure to an allergen once identified can be avoided or controlled. Avoidance of outdoor activity during times of high airborne-pollen levels coupled with augmentation of drug therapy may be very helpful in reducing seasonal asthma. Indoor allergen control is often more difficult because it not only entails avoidance behavior but also often requires a change in life-style. There are no "hypoallergenic" dogs or

**Table 33-3.** *Screening for allergy in asthma*

| Asthma symptoms | Possible agents |
| --- | --- |
| Seasonal asthma or association with seasonal rhinitis | Pollens, molds |
| Asthma on contact with a pet or a home with a pet | Animal dander |
| Asthma with housecleaning or indoor dusty environment | House dust, mites, molds |
| Asthma at the workplace or on return to workplace after weekend or vacation | Need specific job history, such as polyvinyl chloride (PVC), toluene diisocyanate (TDI) |

cats, and thus, if asthma is precipitiated by danders of these animals, ideally the pets should be removed from the home. Often pet owners will not do this, and in those circumstances the pet should be kept out of the asthmatic's bedroom at the very least. If house dust mites are the offending agent, carpeting, if any, should be removed, mattresses and pillows encased in plastic, humidity level lowered, and vacuum cleaners with high-efficiency particulate air (HEPA) filters should be used. Needless to say, this may present an unusual hardship for some families. Although not allergenic in nature, cigarette smoke is a common irritant that can precipitate asthma exacerbations. Having household smokers quit or move outside to "light up" may be the single most difficult environmental control measure.

Occupational asthma is beyond the scope of this chapter, but the principles of avoidance and control remain the same. In some instances the physician needs to enlist the help of public agencies such as local departments of public health or the federal Occupational Safety and Health Administration (OSHA) to aid in environmental control in the workplace.

# PATIENT EDUCATION

Perhaps the greatest thrust of the NAEP guidelines is the proper education of the patient and making him or her an active partner in the management of his or her asthma. A physician's knowledge of pathophysiology and pharmacology in asthma is of little use if the patient has no understanding of his or her own disease. Information alone passed on to the patient is useless. The physician and other members of the health care team must develop in each patient with asthma, not only the skills to manage the disease, but also the confidence that he or she can do this well. The patient must be encouraged to communicate freely with the physician, for this feedback is the only way management can be fine tuned. All aspects of asthma care are fair game, ranging from simple instruction on the proper use of MDIs to enlisting family and school support for the adolescent asthmatic. One protocol will not work for all patients.[3,10] The rigorous monitoring of peak flow, which may be very helpful in one patient, may be marginally beneficial for a patient who needs to understand what allergens trigger his attacks or who needs reassurance that the medications are nonaddicting. Older women may be concerned about whether prolonged inhaled steroid use will accelerate osteoporosis. Currently there is no answer to that question, but a physician who recognizes this concern and works with the patient to allay fears and arrange follow-up study is likely to have a well-managed and compliant patient.

At this point in time it is hard to say what effect this emphasis on comprehensive management of asthma will have on the health care system beyond the individual patient. We all hope to see a reduction in mortality. Preliminary information from patients enrolled in a comprehensive therapeutic and educational program appears to show a significant decrease in high-cost emergency department management and lower indices of severity of disease.[15]

## References

1. Holgate S: Mediator and cytokine mechanisms in asthma, *Thorax* 48:103-110, 1993.
2. Horwitz RJ, Busse WW: Inflammation and asthma, *Clin Chest Med* 16:583-602, 1995.
3. National Heart, Lung and Blood Institute: National Asthma Program Expert Panel Report. Guidelines for the diagnosis and management of asthma, *J Allergy Clin Immunol* 88:425-534, 1991.
4. Sly MR: Changing asthma mortality, *Ann Allergy* 73:259-268; 1994.
5. Spitzer WO, Suissa S, Ernst P, et al: The use of beta agonists and the risk of death and near death from asthma, *N Engl J Med* 326:501-506, 1992.
6. Fahy JV, Boushey HA: Controversies involving inhaled beta agonists and inhaled corticosteroids in the treatment of asthma, *Clin Chest Med* 16:715-734, 1995.
7. Suissa S, Ernst P, Bovin JF, et al: A cohort analysis of excess mortality in asthma and the use of inhaled beta agonists, *Am J Respir Crit Care Med* 149:604-610, 1994.
8. Campbell DA, McLennan G, Coates JR, et al: A comparison of asthma deaths and near fatal asthma attacks in South Australia, *Eur Respir J* 7:490-497, 1994.
9. Strunk RC: Death due to asthma: new insight into sudden unexpected deaths, but the focus remains on prevention, *Am Rev Respir Dis* 148:550-552, 1993.
10. Kohler CL, Davies LS, Bailey WC: How to implement an asthma education program, *Clin Chest Med* 16:557-566, 1995.
11. Pearlman DS, Chervinsky P, LaForce C, et al: A comparison of salmeterol with albuterol in the treatment of mild to moderate asthma, *N Engl J Med* 327:1420-1425, 1992.
12. Sears MR, Taylor DR, Print CG, et al: Regular inhaled beta-agonist treatment in bronchial asthma, *Lancet* 336:1391-1396, 1990.
13. Barnes PJ: New drugs for asthma, *Eur Respir J* 5:1126-1136, 1992.
14. Rennard SI, Floreani AA: Nonstandard and potential future therapies for asthma, *Clin Chest Med* 16:735-744, 1995.
15. Dzyngeal B, Kesten S, Chapman KR: Assessment of an ambulatory care asthma program, *J Asthma* 31:291-300, 1994.

# Chapter 34

# *The Solitary Pulmonary Nodule*

## Leonard Sicilian

The solitary pulmonary nodule (SPN) ("coin lesion") is defined roentgenographically as a discrete spherical or oval density located completely within the lung parenchyma and measuring not greater than 3 cm in diameter. The single lesion may have smaller satellite nodules and may also have an irregular border. Original descriptions of SPNs set their size at up to 6 cm in diameter, but more recent data indicate that lesions greater than 3 cm are almost always malignant and therefore do not require the same type of evaluation.[1] Studies before 1975 indicated about 60% of all SPNs were benign.[2,3] The majority were infectious granulomas (many healed), with hamartomas, arteriovenous malformations, cysts, and miscellaneous entities making up the remaining small percentage. Of the 40% of SPNs that are malignant, approximately 10% represent a metastatic lesion from an extrapulmonary primary cancer. Currently studies show an almost even split, with selected studies showing up to 75% of SPNs being malignant.[4] In areas of the United States where fungi are endemic, the percentage of benign SPN's may still be high. Therefore it is important for the primary physician to be aware that the work-up of an SPN may vary based on geographic location.

The goal of evaluation of a patient with SPN is to determine whether the lesion is malignant or benign. The presumption always has been that a malignant lesion discovered when small is curable. Indeed, early surgical series reported a cure rate of up to 85%. More recent data, however, reveal overall only a 30% to 50% 5-year survival. This difference in outcome may be attributable to the fact that, theoretically, there are about 30 doublings of a single tumor cell necessary for a nodule to reach a size of 1 cm. Therefore even small nodules represent established disease, and presumably microscopic metastatic spread accounts for the lower cure rates found in the recent literature.[5] Nevertheless, it is clear that the chance of survival in malignant SPNs is significantly greater than 15% to 20% 5-year survivals for lung cancer in general. This fact, coupled with the usually low mortality and morbidity of resection of a small lung lesion, forces the clinician to begin to think of surgery whenever an SPN is discovered.

If this goal of differentiation between benign and malignant could easily be accomplished, unnecessary surgery could be avoided for benign SPNs, and malignant disease could be rapidly removed. This strategy by definition would not only expose the patient to the lowest risk but also be the most cost effective. Unfortunately there are very few criteria that make an SPN easy to diagnose on first presentation. Certain patterns of calcification and absence of growth when compared to those on a chest roentgenogram greater than 2 years old are the only currently accepted indicators of benign disease. The radiographic appearance of malignancy and the physician's ability to predict this varies over a wide range. Table 34-1 lists the characteristics associated with the increasing likelihood of malignancy in an SPN. The following discussion of the clinical, roentgenographic, and biopsy evaluation of the patient with an SPN should aid the physician in making appropriate decisions regarding the nature of the lesion and its management.

**Table 34–1.** *Factors associated with the probability of malignancy of a solitary pulmonary nodule*

| Probability | Clinical characteristics | Management |
|---|---|---|
| Low | Nodule observed to develop in 3 weeks or less<br>Central, diffuse, laminar, popcorn calcification on roentgenogram<br>No change in size compared to that on chest roentgenogram 2 years or more old | No further evaluation necessary |
| Indeterminate | Noncalcified nodules in nonsmoker less than 35 years old<br>Speckled or eccentric calcification<br>Noncalcified nodule of undermined age | Close observation versus resection: densitometry, biopsy, decision analysis may be helpful |
| High | New noncalcified nodule in smoker more than 35 years of age<br>Growth noted compared to prior chest roentgenogram<br>Prior pulmonary or extrapulmonary cancer | Immediate biopsy or resection usually necessary |

# CLINICAL EVALUATION

The cause of an SPN rarely is discovered from information obtained by history and physical examination alone. The one exception is an acute or subacute lung injury (such as pneumonia, an infarct, a hematoma, a rounded atelectasis) that heals in the shape of a lung nodule. Here the physician can follow clinically and roentgenographically the formation of the SPN from its inception and therefore can be certain of its cause. Short of this unusual situation, less than 25% of SPNs are discovered by the symptoms they cause. A thorough history and physical examination can detect systemic disease that may involve the lung (such as rheumatoid arthritis with an associated rheumatoid lung nodule). A prior history of extrapulmonary primary cancer is important since an SPN in this setting is likely to be a metastatic lesion in two thirds of cases.[2] Despite this observation, patients too often have an expensive metastatic work-up done on the assumption that all pulmonary nodules represent metastatic disease. Routine radionucleotide scans, gastrointestinal series, and mammograms result in finding an extrathoracic primary cancer in less than 10% of cases in the absence of signs and symptoms discovered by routine laboratory and physical examination (such as bone pain, blood in stool, abnormal liver functions, and breast lumps). It is more cost efficient to seek another cancer after resection of the SPN if the histologic pattern is diagnostic of a nonlung primary cancer.

Excluding x-ray evaluation, the work-up of an SPN is limited. Skin tests or complement-fixation studies for granulomatous disease are most helpful only if the results are negative. A positive reaction or result, though clearly indicating exposure, does not ensure that there is a relationship between the SPN and that exposure. Thus a negative test in the immunocompetent patient effectively eliminates that disease from the differential diagnosis. Sputum must be submitted for cytologic and culture examination in cases where the patient spontaneously produces sputum; these simple inexpensive tests yield a specific diagnosis in up to 25% of patients. Because of the low yield, however, it is not worthwhile to induce sputum in patients who do not produce it spontaneously.

Perhaps the most valuable single piece of clinical information is the patient's age. Large series have shown an extremely small percentage (3%) of malignancies in individuals less than 35 years of age.[2,3] Thus an asymptomatic SPN in a nonsmoker less than 35 years of age would be strongly suggestive of a benign lesion. Although the SPN should not be forgotten, young patient age allows the physician at least the opportunity to observe the patient over time to determine if the lesion is static or growing.

# ROENTGENOGRAPHIC EVALUATION

The roentgenographic evaluation of an SPN is the cornerstone of patient management. Pulmonary nodules can be detected at a size of 3 to

5 mm on good-quality films.[6,7] Remember that the lesion should be visible on both the anteroposterior and the lateral projections. If not, consideration must be given to an extrathoracic structure (such as nipple, skin tag, or nevus).

The size of the lesion has some importance. SPNs greater than 3 cm in diameter are benign less than 5% of the time.[1] Lesions less than 8 mm have been reported to be benign in a high percentage of cases. However, as our ability to detect nodules improves, physicians need to be wary of any "small" nodule and, at a minimum, place the patient in a close observation category.

The growth of an SPN, as noted in successive chest films, is another important factor. Lesions that have remained static for greater than 2 years are almost always benign and additional work-up can be avoided. Nodules that double in size in less than 3 weeks are also benign and, in most cases, represent acute infectious processes. Between these two extremes lies a vast array of doubling times of tumors and some granulomas.[4] Unfortunately, doubling times of tumors cannot be applied prospectively as a way to follow small suspicious nodules. Thus, earlier chest films are of great importance in determining prior presence or growth of a nodule. Old chest roentgenograms must be retrieved and reviewed. Reliance on reports alone is poor practice because lesions missed on initial reading (10% to 30%) can often be found in retrospect.[3,4]

Calcification is the best roentgenographic evidence of a benign lesion. The pattern of calcification can be central, laminar (bull's-eye), diffuse, or popcorn in appearance. The only patterns of calcification that are questionable for malignancy are eccentric and speckled calcifications. With these patterns, malignancy has been found in up to 6% of cases.[4,8] In this situation it is reasonable to observe closely or perform a closed biopsy before surgical resection is considered.

The greatest advance in the evaluation of an SPN has been the application of computerized tomography (CT) of the chest. The chest CT scan, more sensitive than plain x-ray in picking up and defining nodules,[9] should be performed in all cases of SPN when the plain films and clinical information do not clearly indicate a benign lesion. The CT scan can more easily detect (1) multiple nodules that are suggestive of metastatic disease, (2) calcification, and (3) mediastinal abnormalities that are suggestive of metastasis and that therefore need staging if resection of the SPN is planned. For all intents and purposes the CT scan has obviated the need for fluoroscopy or linear tomography in the evaluation of SPNs.

Increasingly, work has been done using the CT scan density of the SPN (densitometry) to determine whether the lesion is benign.[10] It is believed that microscopic calcification in a benign nodule can be detected by CT scan as an increased density (above a certain value when compared to water density) in instances where macroscopic calcification cannot be visualized.

Currently the use of densitometry is being modified and improved to yield more specific results. The density of an SPN can be measured in comparison to a phantom of known "benign" density,[11] by high-resolution CT scan (HRCT),[12] or by a combination of both methods. In fact, Khouri and associates[13] using a combination of densitometry and transthoracic needle biopsy were able to identify accurately almost 88% of lesions found to be benign at the time of resection. Positron emission tomography (PET), magnetic resonance imaging (MRI), and contrast-enhanced CT scanning have all been reported to help distinguish benign from malignant SPNs.[14] These latter modalities, though unproved, actually do more than measure density and may give insight into the metabolic and vascular properties of the nodule, information that may ultimately be more specific in identifying the nature of the SPN.

It goes without saying that the use of these radiographic studies should be in conjunction with a radiologist who is experienced in performing and interpreting these procedures. Should the results of such studies indicate a "benign" SPN, the patient should be placed in a close observation category at a minimum and follow-up study should require enlistment of the help of a pulmonary specialist.

## BIOPSY EVALUATION

Transthoracic needle aspiration biopsy and bronchoscopic transbronchial biopsy have a variable role in the evaluation of the SPN. They are not always a necessary part of the work-up, though both procedures are safe with acceptable morbidity and little or no mortality. One or both usually are considered if the evaluation previously outlined has not revealed a clearly benign lesion.

Transthoracic needle aspiration (TNAB) under CT guidance is the method of choice for smaller peripheral lesions and yields positive results in better than 90% of cancers. The ability of TNAB to diagnose a specific benign condition is somewhat harder to assess though it is clearly the information needed to avoid thoracotomy. Recent studies have emphasized the concept of a "specific negative" TNAB.[1,13,14] Here the biopsy specimens did not always show a specific benign disease (such as fungus) but at the time of resection were found to be negative for cancer approximately 85% of the time. This is not so simple as it sounds, since success is highly dependent on the expertise and experience of both the performer and the pathologist. In addition the following criteria must be fulfilled: (1) The needle must be visualized to be in the lesion by CT scan. (2) An adequate amount of material must be obtained. Therefore several passes may be needed, and the pathologist must confirm adequacy before the procedure is terminated. (3) The tissue obtained is not normal lung. (4) No endobronchial lesion is present. (5) There is no suspicion of cancer after interpretation by the pathologist. Even if all these criteria are fulfilled, it is suggested that the patient be placed on a close observation schedule and not dismissed as having a "benign" process.

TNAB is not without its risks. Twenty percent to 34% develop pneumothorax, of which 5% to 14% will require closed-chest tube drainage. An additional 2% to 14% will have hemoptysis.[1] Because of this, TNAB is contraindicated in patients who are uncooperative, have a coagulopathy or advanced emphysema, are experiencing severe respiratory distress or cough, have a contralateral pneumonectomy, or have pulmonary hypertension.

Transbronchial biopsy and brushing under fluoroscopic guidance is less sensitive for small peripheral lesions but has the same yield for nodules larger than 2 cm or more central lesions. Bronchoscopy has the added advantage of allowing evaluation of the central airways in patients with SPN who have concomitant airway symptoms of cough, hemoptysis, or wheezing with or without stridor. The appearance of the relationship of the SPN to the bronchus entering it seen on thin-section CT may help in deciding whether transbronchial biopsy or brush specimens will yield a diagnosis.[1] When the bronchus is cut off by the SPN or penetrates it or is narrowed by the nodule, the likelihood of establishing the diagnosis is high. Since fiberoptic bronchoscopy with transbronchial biopsy has a much lower complication rate than TNAB does, the CT information may be helpful in selecting which procedure to pursue. The primary clinician should always enlist the assistance of a pulmonary specialist to help in these decisions.

If clinical and x-ray evaluation of the SPN indicate a moderate or high suspicion of malignancy without evidence of metastatic spread, closed biopsy procedures often are bypassed in favor of an open excisional biopsy or resection. Excision should be performed in these cases, whether the closed biopsy is positive or negative for malignancy. However, either of these procedures may be quite helpful in avoiding thoracotomy and should be done in cases where metastatic disease is suspected or where thoracotomy is contraindicated because of poor pulmonary function. In these instances, a closed biopsy that is diagnostic of metastatic cancer can obviate the need for surgery in the former setting and provide information regarding prognosis in the latter.

## CLOSE OBSERVATION

Often the clinician is faced with the difficult situation where the SPN cannot readily be placed in the high or low probability of cancer category.[15] Similar difficulty arises when the characteristics of the SPN place it in the high-probability group, but the patient is a poor risk for either closed biopsy or surgery (such as a patient with severe cardiac or pulmonary disease or coagulopathy). In these instances, the physician may opt to monitor the patient closely. Follow-up examinations should be at least every 3 months. A plain chest roentgenogram or preferably a CT scan at each visit is necessary for evaluation of any change in the nodule. Should the patient develop symptoms in the interim, he should be instructed to contact the physician immediately for reevaluation.

Unfortunately there are few data in the literature on which to base an estimation of the increased risk of a localized resectable cancer becoming metastatic during a period of observation. Therefore it should be made clear to the patient that some risk of missing a cancer is involved, that the problem must not be ignored, and that close follow-up study is mandatory. Even though close observation alone is at times the most appropriate management, it also may be the most anxiety-producing approach for both the patient and the physician.

Decision analysis has been offered as a way to help quantitate the uncertainties of choosing a strategy in this indeterminate category.[4] The first thing that needs to be obtained are predictive factors that are clinical or roentgenographic characteristics that help determine the likelihood or probability of cancer in an SPN.[4,16,17] These factors include age, smoking history, size and edge characteristics of the SPN, the base-line prevalence of malignancy in an SPN (for example, this will be lower in areas of endemic mycoses), and information from nodule densitometry. This information can be obtained from published litera-ture, but the physician must be aware of bias in reported studies and attempt to eliminate these before establishing a usable prior probability of cancer.[17] Studies using this approach show that decision analysis is better than using a single criterion (such as densitometry) alone in predicting which SPNs are malignant. However, when decision analysis has been applied to the choice of management strategies (close observa-tion versus biopsy and observation versus biopsy and excision versus immediate excision), the utility is not very high.[15] That is, over a wide range of probabilities there was very little survival benefit noted from any strategy. Thus it is still recommended that issues of patient prefer-ence and surgical risk combined with specialist input be major factors in the primary physician's recommendation to a patient in these indeter-minate cases.[18,19]

# THERAPY

If the SPN cannot be proved to be benign and if close observation is not chosen because of a high suspicion of malignancy, the only treatment is complete excision. As in any thoracotomy with lung resection, com-plete preoperative pulmonary evaluation, including function testing, is necessary to determine if the patient can tolerate the procedure and to assess the probability of postoperative pulmonary impairment.

If CT scans show evidence of mediastinal abnormality in the pres-ence of SPN, a staging procedure should be performed to rule out metastatic disease. Staging can be done preoperatively by means of mediastinoscopy or a small anterior intercostal incision or it can be done intraoperatively by direct visualization and examination of the mediastinum. Flexible bronchoscopy should be performed preopera-tively in all patients with airway symptoms to rule out a central tumor, which would necessitate a change in the extent of surgery or would possibly indicate nonresectability.

Surgical mortality ranges from 0.3% for resection of a benign nodule to about 9% in patients requiring lobectomy or pneumonectomy who are older than 70 years. The average mortality is 3% to 4%.[4] Less invasive video-assisted thoracoscopic surgery (VATS) is being used with increas-ing frequency to resect peripheral SPNs. However, at this time it is unknown whether VATS resection will offer the same survival as standard resection[18] or will be more cost effective and have lesser morbidity than a standard thoracotomy.[20]

At thoracotomy or VATS, the SPN should not be biopsied but excised in total. A frozen section should be performed; if a malignancy is found, a curative resection of that lobe or segment (depending on pulmonary function) can then be performed if indicated.

Figures 34-1 and 34-2 summarize the management of an individual with an SPN. Figure 34-1 is most applicable to patients with a low probability of malignancy. Figure 34-2 shows a scheme for those cases where the probability of malignancy is indeterminate or high. At present, there are no data that favor one plan of action over the other. As always, the clinician must individualize each patient and make the best decision based on the specific facts of the case.

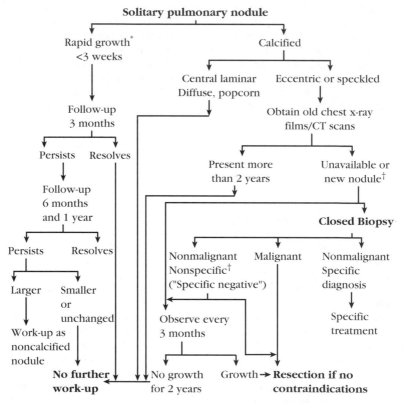

*Must have recent base-line normal x-ray film
†Either subsequent choice is acceptable

**Figure 34-1.** *Management of a patient with a solitary pulmonary nodule with a low probability of malignancy.*

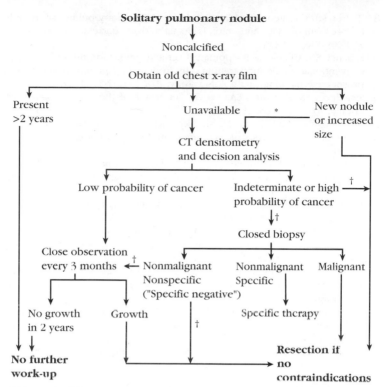

**Figure 34–2.** *Management of a patient with a solitary pulmonary nodule with an indeterminate or high probability of malignancy.*

*Optional pathway if patient refuses or resection contraindicated
†Either pathway acceptable based on clinical setting and patient preference

## References

1. Viggiano RW, Swensen SJ, Rosenow II EC: Evaluation and management of solitary and multiple pulmonary nodules, *Clin Chest Med* 13:83-95, 1992.
2. Lillington GA: The solitary pulmonary nodule, *Am Rev Respir Dis* 110:699-707, 1974.
3. Lillington GA: Pulmonary nodules: solitary and multiple, *Clin Chest Med* 3:361-367, 1982.
4. Lillington GA: Management of solitary pulmonary nodules, *Disease-A-Month* 37:274-318, 1991.
5. Weiss W, Boucot KR: The prognosis of lung cancer originating as a round lesion. Data from the Philadelphia Pulmonary Neoplasm Research Project, *Am Rev Respir Dis* 116:826-836, 1977.
6. Radke JR, Conway WA, Eyler WR, Kvale PA: Diagnostic accuracy in peripheral lung lesions, *Chest* 76:176-179, 1979.
7. Kundel HL: Predictive value and threshold detectability of lung tumors, *Radiology* 139:25-29, 1981.

8. Zwirewich CV, Vedal S, Miller RR, Müller NL: Solitary pulmonary nodule: high-resolution CT and radiologic-pathologic correlation, *Radiology* 179:469-476, 1991.

9. Schaner EG, Chang AE, Doppman JL, et al: Comparison of computed and conventional whole lung tomography in detecting pulmonary nodules: a prospective radiologic-pathologic study, *AJR* 131:51-54, 1978.

10. Siegelman SS, Zerhouni EA, Leo FP, et al: CT of the solitary pulmonary nodule, *AJR* 135:1-13, 1980.

11. Zerhouni EA, Boukadoum M, Siddiky MA, et al: A standard phantom for quantitative CT analysis of pulmonary nodules, *Radiology* 149:767-773, 1983.

12. Khan A, Herman PG, Vorwerk P, et al: Solitary pulmonary nodules: comparison of classification with standard, thin section and reference phantom CT, *Radiology* 179:477-481, 1991.

13. Khouri NF, Meziane MA, Zerhouni EA, et al: The solitary pulmonary nodule, assessment, diagnosis and management, *Chest* 91:128-133, 1991.

14. Swensen SJ, Brown LR, Colby TV, Weaver AL: Pulmonary nodules: CT evaluation of enhancement with iodinated contrast material, *Radiology* 194:393-398, 1995.

15. Cummings SR, Lillington GA, Richard RJ: Managing solitary pulmonary nodules: the choice of strategy is a "close call," *Am Rev Respir Dis* 134:453-460, 1986.

16. Cummings SR, Lillington GA, Richard RJ: Estimating the probability of malignancy in solitary pulmonary nodule: a Bayesian approach, *Am Rev Respir Dis* 134:449-452, 1986.

17. Gurney JW: Determining the likelihood of malignancy in solitary pulmonary nodules with Bayesian analysis: Part I. Theory, *Radiology* 186:405-413, 1993.

18. Lillington GA, Caskey CI: Evaluation and management of solitary and multiple pulmonary nodules, *Clin Chest Med* 14:111-120, 1993.

19. Gurney JW, Lyddon DM, McKay JA: Determining the likelihood of malignancy in solitary pulmonary nodules with Bayesian analysis: Part II. Application, *Radiology* 186:415-422, 1993.

20. Hazelrigg SR, Nunchuck SK, Landreneau RJ, et al: Cost analysis for thoracoscopy: thoracoscopic wedge resection, *Ann Thorac Surg* 56:633-635, 1993.

# Chapter 35

## Care of the Mechanically Ventilated Patient

Alexander C. White

Leonard Sicilian

Intubation and mechanical ventilation have become the standard of care for patients with respiratory failure in the intensive care unit. Over the past 25 years the mechanical ventilator has evolved from a relatively simple device that delivered a preset tidal volume to a sophisticated computerized piece of equipment. In this chapter we discuss the routine management of the intubated and mechanically ventilated patient and the complications of these therapeutic interventions.

## INTUBATION

Establishing an airway forms an essential part of resuscitation both in the field and in the hospital. Intubation of the trachea, if it can be done safely, is the most effective method of protecting the airway, ensuring adequate oxygenation and providing assisted ventilation.

The most common indications for intubation include (1) relief of upper airway obstruction, (2) protection against aspiration of oropharyngeal secretions or gastric contents in patients with impaired mental status or with neuromuscular diseases, (3) enhanced clearance of secretions in patients with ineffective cough, and finally (4) mechanical ventilation in patients with hypoxemic or hypercapnic respiratory failure refractory to other less invasive forms of treatment. Once a decision has been made to intubate a patient it should be performed by someone skilled in the procedure to minimize complications. Adequate oxygenation and ventilation can usually be achieved by use of a mask respirator, supplemental oxygen, and an oropharyngeal airway. Sedation is required for intubation unless the patient is obtunded and minimally responsive. A short-acting benzodiazepine such as midazolam (Versed, 1 to 5 mg, intravenously) usually is sufficient. To perform a safe intubation, occasionally it is necessary to paralyze the patient briefly, using a muscle relaxant such as pancuronium (Pavulon, 0.06 to 0.15 mg/kg).

An individual intubation attempt should last no longer than 1 minute, while oxygenation is being monitored using a finger oximeter. Prolonged attempts at intubation may result in either severe hypoxemia, causing grand mal seizures, or intense vagal stimulation, causing brady-cardia and a reduction in cerebral perfusion. If intubation is not success-ful, the patient should be reoxygenated with the bag and mask for 2 to 3 minutes before one reattempts the procedure. It may be necessary to intubate under direct vision. This is best accomplished by placement of the endotracheal tube over a flexible fiberoptic bronchoscope, pass-ing the bronchoscope through the vocal cords and advancing the endo-tracheal tube over the bronchoscope directly into the trachea. The bronchoscope then is removed, and the airway is established. Once the patient is intubated, the chest should be auscultated immediately and the presence of exhaled carbon dioxide ($CO_2$) confirmed using a colorimetric $CO_2$ monitor.[1]

Intubation of the right mainstream bronchus, one of the most com-mon complications of intubation, can be suspected from greatly re-duced breath sounds on the left side compared to the right side. Persis-tent intubation of the right mainstream bronchus may result in hypoxemia because of either inadequate overall ventilation or shunting of blood through the underventilated left lung causing a ventilation-perfusion (V/Q) mismatch, pneumothorax (because all the ventilator volume will be delivered to only one lung), respiratory alkalosis with subsequent predisposition to cardiac arrhythmias, and an inability to suction secretions from the left lung, predisposing the patient to atelec-tasis and pneumonia.[2] The endotracheal tube should be repositioned and a chest roentgenogram taken to confirm that the distal end of the endotracheal tube is 2 to 3 cm above the carina. The proximal endotracheal tube should be marked at this optimal position at the gum, lip, or anterior nares so that any movement can be easily observed and corrected.

The route of intubation (orotracheal, nasotracheal, or a tracheos-tomy) must be individualized. When rapid establishment of an airway is the major goal, orotracheal intubation is the procedure of choice. In patients with suspected or diagnosed cervical spine injury, the cervical spine first must be immobilized. Nasotracheal intubation without neck manipulation or emergency tracheostomy then can be performed to avoid further damage to the cervical spinal cord.[3] Orotracheal intuba-tion allows one to use an endotracheal tube with a large internal diameter facilitating suctioning and reducing airway resistance. These two factors are useful in patients with preexisting chronic bronchitis or emphysema, the former because secretions are usually a major prob-lem and the latter because the added airway resistance resulting from a small tube may cause respiratory muscle fatigue during weaning. We recommend the placement of at least an 8-mm internal-diameter tube in all patients. Tubes with less than a 7-mm internal diameter greatly increase airway resistance and limit the ability to suction secretions from the lower respiratory tract.[4]

Nasotracheal tubes have the advantage of stability with a lower incidence of accidental extubation or right mainstream bronchus intu-bation. The size of the nasal passage limits the internal diameter of the tube size to a maximum of 7 to 7.5 mm. Epistaxis is a common complication of nasotracheal intubation but usually is self-limiting unless the patient has a coagulopathy. As a result, nasotracheal intubation usually is avoided in patients with thrombocytopenia and abnormal coagulation times. Sinusitis (maxillary or sphenoidal) and otitis media are other potential complications seen with nasotracheal intubation and also in patients with nasogastric tubes[5]; fever and facial and ear pain should all be suggestive of the diagnosis. Bedside sinus films are usually enough to make the diagnosis, but occasionally sinus computerized tomography or sinus aspiration is necessary. Diabetic and immunocompromised patients are at risk of fungal infections in the sinuses, which may be both difficult to treat and life threatening.

In the successfully intubated patient, a sudden loss of expired volumes associated with reduced airway pressure may be attributable to tube dislodgment or cuff leak. When this occurs with an orotracheal or nasotracheal tube, the tube should be repositioned correctly or, if the cuff is at fault, a new endotracheal tube inserted. In the case of a tracheostomy tube, it may not be possible to replace the tube if the tract is not mature (that is, less than 72 hours old), and in this case, temporary orotracheal intubation should be performed.

Kinking or blockage of the tube with secretions causes elevation of the peak inspiratory pressure delivered by the ventilator. It usually can be corrected by manipulation or repositioning of the tube and by suction, respectively. Aseptic technique must be followed whenever suction catheters are utilized to clear secretions from the lower respiratory tract.

Tracheomalacia and tracheal stenosis, caused by excessive cuff pressure on the tracheal wall, are much less common since the advent of high-volume, low-pressure cuffs. However, it is important to adhere to the correct inflation pressures for endotracheal tubes; that is, the cuff pressure must be below the capillary filling pressure of the trachea, which is less than 25 mm Hg. This goal can be accomplished by attachment of an aneroid manometer to the external cuff port and reading of the cuff pressure directly (two to three times per day) to determine if the cuff inflation is in the safe range.

Finally, tracheostomy tubes usually are reserved for elective placement in those patients who require permanent or prolonged intubation. At one time tracheostomy was performed on any patient intubated for more than 72 hours. Now, because of new tube material and cuff construction, orotracheal or nasotracheal tubes may remain in position for 3 to 4 weeks without the need for tracheostomy. We recommend early tracheostomy in patients with acute or chronic neuromuscular disease who will need prolonged ventilatory support. We assess patients whose long-term outlook is unclear at the end of 2 weeks. If it appears that extubation will not be accomplished in the next 7 to 10 days, we schedule the patient for an elective tracheostomy.

Table 35-1 lists the advantages and disadvantages of the three routes of intubation. One can see that for short periods of intubation, other than tracheostomy, there is little difference among the options. For long-term intubation, these differences may become important. Endotracheal and tracheostomy tubes bypass the normal pulmonary defense

**Table 35-1.** *Comparison of the routes of intubation*

|  | Endotracheal | Nasotracheal | Tracheostomy |
|---|---|---|---|
| Ease of tube placement | Good with experience | Good with experience | Poor; need controlled surgery |
| Tube stability | Fair | Good | Good |
| Access to lower respiratory tract | Good | Good | Good |
| Resistance to breathing | Varies depending on tube size | Most; usually smaller tube | Least |
| Patient acceptance and communication | Poor to fair | Fair | Good |

mechanisms and predispose the ventilated patient to aspiration of material from the nasopharynx. When an intubated patient develops dyspnea, hypoxemia, and radiographic changes in the dependent part of the lung, aspiration pneumonia must be suspected. Care of the oral cavity and oropharynx and good aseptic technique when suctioning help prevent aspiration. Ventilator-associated pneumonia occurs in up to 20% of patients who require mechanical ventilation and may be attributable in part to aspiration. The diagnosis can be difficult to make on clinical grounds alone, and in some instances, the use of a protective specimen brush is helpful in identifying the pathogenic organism or organisms.[6]

# MECHANICAL VENTILATION

Mechanical ventilation seeks two main goals: the first is to ensure an arterial partial pressure of oxygen ($Pao_2$) of >60 mm Hg to prevent end-organ damage from hypoxemia, and the second is to avoid further lung damage from the process of mechanical ventilation itself. Previous attempts to maintain a normal partial pressure of carbon dioxide ($Pao_2$) have been tempered by a growing awareness of barotrauma because of the process of ventilation itself. Barotrauma is lung injury produced by high inflation pressures needed to maintain a set tidal volume in the lung that has low compliance (such as adult respiratory distress syndrome, ARDS) and results in lung overinflation (that is, volutrauma), which produces pneumomediastinum and pneumothorax. Pneumothorax probably is attributable to excessive alveolar pressure resulting in overdistension and rupture of alveoli (usually in the setting of reduced lung compliance). Pneumothorax occurs in 3% to 5% of patients undergoing positive-pressure ventilation and is more common in those with gram-negative bacterial or *Pneumocystis carinii* pneumonia and in those requiring positive end-expiratory pressure (PEEP) (usually greater than 7.5 cm $H_2O$); it is also a potential complication of internal jugular or subclavian central line placement. Physical examination usually is insufficient to detect small pneumothoraces. Therefore chest roentgenograms is mandatory, both on a daily basis and when there is any change in the patient's cardiopulmonary status. If a pneumothorax is seen, intercostal chest tube drainage usually is mandatory because the risk of tension pneumothorax in this situation is high.

Once a patient is intubated, we usually begin mechanical ventilation either in the assist control mode (A/C mode: every breath is machine-assisted) or in the intermittent mandatory ventilation mode (IMV mode: patient can breath spontaneously between breaths) with a rate of 8 to 12 breaths per minute, tidal volume ($V_T$) of 6 to 10 mL/kg, fraction of inspired oxygen ($Fio_2$) of 1.0, and inspiratory flow of 60 L/min.[7] These two modes of mechanical ventilation are the commonest used in the modern ICU. Two important differences between these modes of ventilation exist: the IMV mode is associated with increased work of breathing, which can be reduced by the use of pressure support with every spontaneous breath (it augments the $V_T$ on each spontaneous breath). The A/C mode can produce respiratory alkalosis if the spontaneous respiratory rate is high because every breath is assisted. Most clinicians will add positive end-expiratory pressure (PEEP) of 5 cm $H_2O$ in all patients to try and prevent atelectasis. In patients with ARDS requiring $Fio_2$ greater than 0.6, higher levels of PEEP may be needed to increase resting lung volumes and maintain alveolar patency. The increased resting lung volume may allow the $Fio_2$ to be reduced below 0.5 and may reduce the toxic effects of oxygen on the lung parenchyma. The complications associated with PEEP are discussed later. After the institution of mechanical ventilation, oxygenation can be monitored by use of a pulse oximeter (provided that a good signal can be obtained). In addition, a blood gas value always should be checked within 30 minutes of intubation to allow the $Fio_2$ and PEEP to be adjusted to maintain a $Pao_2$ of greater than 60 mm Hg. An arterial line should be inserted in all patients in whom a prolonged period (greater than 48 hours) of mechanical ventilation is anticipated because regular blood gas analysis is essential in monitoring the patient.

# ALTERNATIVE MODES OF MECHANICAL VENTILATION

There is a growing awareness that mechanical ventilation itself may produce lung injury. The mechanism of injury is unclear but may be caused by shear stress on the lung parenchyma from high airway pressures that overdistend lung units.[8] This concept of overdistension of lung tissue has led to the term "volutrauma." In addition, the injury tends to occur more in the compliant normal lung segments compared with the abnormal segments. Attempts made to minimize ventilator-induced lung injury are discussed in the following section.

**Permissive hypercapnia.** It appears unnecessary to keep the $Paco_2$ normal because most patients appear to tolerate higher $Paco_2$ levels, even up to 90 to 100 mm Hg. Patients with cerebrovascular disease are an exception to this because $CO_2$ is a powerful vasodilator and can increase intracranial pressure. Therefore permissive hypercapnia should not be used in this population. These observations have resulted in the use of controlled hypoventilation with permissive hypercapnia in some patients.[9] The $V_T$ and respiratory rate are reduced to a level that allows the $Paco_2$ to rise to less than 100 mm Hg while ensuring adequate oxygenation and keeping peak airway pressures less than 45 cm $H_2O$. Over 3 to 4 days, renal acid excretion will increase, bringing the pH back toward normal. If the pH remains below 7.2, bicarbonate can be administered intravenously carefully. We use this mode of ventilation in patients who are at risk of barotrauma, such as patients with ARDS with low lung compliance as evidenced by consistently high peak inspiratory pressures (PIPs) (greater than 45 to 50 cm $H_2O$). As lung compliance improves, the patient can gradually be converted to more conventional ventilation to facilitate extubation.

**Inverse-ratio ventilation.** In conventional ventilation the inspiratory-to-expiratory time (I : E) ratio is usually kept at 1 : 2. By prolonging the inspiratory time (that is, "inverting the ratio," with I : E ratio of 4 : 1) one can reduce the peak airway pressures while increasing the mean airway pressure. Inverse-ratio ventilation promotes a gradual reduction in the shunt fraction over hours and days (probably through the production of auto-PEEP) and limits parenchymal injury through the slower inspiratory airflow.[8] Inverse-ratio ventilation can be delivered in either a volume-cycled or pressure-cycled manner. This mode of ventilation is very uncomfortable for patients because of the prolonged inspiratory time and requires sedation and usually paralysis. This mode of ventilation should be reserved for patients who have impaired oxygenation despite high $Fio_2$ and PEEP as occurs in ARDS.

**Pressure–cycled ventilation.** Patients can be ventilated using a set $V_T$ or with a fixed pressure. The advantage of pressure-cycled ventilation is that a limit is set to the pressure the lung parenchyma is exposed, thus avoiding barotrauma.[10] This limit is usually less than 45 cm $H_2O$. The $V_T$ will vary with each breath, and patients commonly develop a mild respiratory acidosis from hypoventilation (see the preceding discussion of permissive hypercapnia). Pressure-cycled ventilation is used with inverse-ratio ventilation in the fibroproliferative phase of ARDS when lung compliance is very low (less than 0.02 L/mm Hg).

Data indicate that repositioning the patient (supine, left lateral, and right lateral) can improve oxygenation, presumably by the use of gravity to improve perfusion of lung units.[11] Prone-position ventilation can be done but requires special expertise.

High-frequency ventilation[12] and extracorporeal-membrane oxygenation[13] are alternative modes of ventilation that are used in very specialized circumstances.

# VENTILATOR MANAGEMENT

The ventilator itself is a frequent source of complications. The intubated and mechanically ventilated patient is dependent on the machine for respiration, especially if sedation and paralytic agents are used. Ventilator failure (including alarms, tubing, valves, and circuitry) can seriously impair the patient's respiratory status and if not rapidly corrected may lead to death. The best way to avoid and treat ventilator problems is to have alert and knowledgable bedside personnel present at all times. For this reason each patient in the MICU should have a designated nurse, and the ventilator (including tubing and other equipment) should be checked by a respiratory therapist at least once per nursing shift. The nurse and therapist should check the ventilator more frequently if necessary. A basic hourly checklist should include $Fio_2$, $V_T$, intermittent mandatory ventilation/synchronized intermittent mandatory ventilation (IMV/SIMV) rate, PIP, PEEP, and alarms. Ventilator malfunctions include mechanical failure, alarm failure, overheating of inspired air, and ventilator alarm left in the off position. Repeated sounding of the alarm unfortunately remains the commonest reason for the alarm being switched off and should not be permitted. Any alarm warrants immediate evaluation of both patient and ventilator rather than the alarm being considered a nuisance and simply switched off. Of the items being serially monitored, changes in PIP, compliance (static and dynamic), $V_T$, PEEP, and ABG levels are most important.

A sudden rise in airway pressure may be attributable to increased airway resistance or reduced pulmonary compliance. Airway resistance can be increased by malposition or blockage of the endotracheal tube or by bronchospasm. Lung compliance may be reduced by pneumothorax, pneumomediastinum, or pulmonary edema. The diffuse alveolar damage produced by ARDS can severely reduce compliance.

Sudden loss of $V_T$ can be noted when a discrepancy is detected between the measured exhaled $V_T$ and that $V_T$ set to be delivered by the ventilator. This results in impaired alveolar ventilation, and the $Paco_2$ rises. Loss of $V_T$ is usually caused by tube malposition (that is, partial extubation) or cuff leak, as previously discussed.

Positive end-expiratory pressure (PEEP) increases transpulmonary pressure at end-expiration and increases the functional residual capacity (FRC)[14] of the lung. Reduced FRC is often a significant factor in acute pulmonary disease and results in systemic hypoxemia from ventilation-perfusion (V/Q) mismatch. PEEP improves oxygenation through its effect on FRC. By improving the FRC, PEEP also improves lung compliance (though excessive PEEP can paradoxically reduce compliance), explaining the usefulness of PEEP in ARDS.

High levels of PEEP may lead to a reduction in cardiac output because of reduced venous return secondary to increased intrapleural pressure and by a direct mechanism of unknown cause.[15] In this setting patients should have a pulmonary artery catheter placed to monitor cardiac filling pressures and cardiac output. The information obtained can be used to optimize tissue oxygen delivery. We generally use the lowest level of PEEP that maintains the $Pao_2$ at 70 mm Hg and aim to keep the $Fio_2$ less than 0.5 and a cardiac index greater than 2.2 L/min/m$^2$. Data indicate that keeping the $Fio_2$ below 0.5 reduces the risk of hyperoxia-related lung injury. If the combination of PEEP and mean pulmonary airway pressure are greater than 45 cm $H_2O$, we switch to pressure-cycled ventilation to minimize barotrauma. High PEEP levels (greater than 12.5 cm $H_2O$) produce unreliable pulmonary capillary wedge pressure readings when the catheter is exposed to high alveolar pressure, resulting in a divergence of wedge and left atrial pressures (that is, the wedge pressure may be read as higher than it actually is). Other effects of PEEP include sodium retention and changes in atrial natriuretic peptide production. Hyponatremia also can occur from increased antidiuretic hormone production.

"Auto-PEEP," a phenomenon that occurs in patients with obstructive airways disease is caused by incomplete exhalation of the delivered lung volume resulting in an increase in alveolar pressure at end-expiration.[16] The amount of pressure can increase with successive breaths to the point that lung compliance is reduced and cardiac output is compromised. In the modern ventilator the level of auto-PEEP is easily measured and should be monitored closely in patients with COPD or asthma who are being ventilated. One can reduce auto-PEEP by lowering the $V_T$ or by increasing the exhalation time (by increasing the inspiratory flow rate or reducing the respiratory rate). When auto-PEEP is suspected as a cause of hypotension or reduced cardiac output, the ventilator should be disconnected and the patient ventilated with a bag and mask until the situation is clarified.

## MONITORING THE PATIENT

Successful management of the ventilated patient demands careful monitoring of both the respiratory and the cardiac status.[17] The physician must ensure adequate gas exchange while minimizing the risks of positive pressure. Even though a vast array of sophisticated equipment can be employed to aid in achieving this goal, direct patient observation by the nurse or physician and the interpretation of the arterial blood gas (ABG) levels remain the mainstays. Thus any new monitoring device must improve our ability to accurately measure pulmonary and cardiac function, thereby leading to improved gas exchange and ventilation of our patients.[18,19]

Table 35-2 lists the four different levels of monitoring. Physical examination (level I) and intermittent monitoring (level II) are most widely used. Although this approach clearly is "low tech" given today's electronics, auscultation of the chest is still the quickest way to detect a pneumothorax, and respiratory rates greater than 30 to 40 breaths per minute (counted at the bedside) actually correlate very well with more invasive measurements of respiratory muscle fatigue. The drawback to monitoring by physical examination is that physical signs of end-organ damage occur in the later stages of injury. For example,

**Table 35-2.** *Monitoring of intubated and ventilated patients*

| Level of monitoring | Advantages | Disadvantages |
|---|---|---|
| **LEVEL I** | | |
| Physical examination | Always available | Physical changes of end-organ damage occur late in critical illness |
| **LEVEL II** | | |
| Intermittent arterial blood gas levels<br>Chest roentgenogram<br>Spirometry and mechanics (FVC, MIF, $V_E$, $V_D$, Cdyn, Cst, $R_{aw}$) | Widely available<br>May be automated<br>Equipment simple | Changes occur between measurements<br>Some tests require patient cooperation<br>Measurement "crude" compared to controlled laboratory setting |
| **LEVEL III** | | |
| Continuous pneumotachygraphy<br>Capnography ($PET_{CO_2}$)<br>Oximetry ($Sa_{O_2}$)<br>Skin/transcutaneous ($P_{O_2}$, $P_{CO_2}$, pH)<br>Breath-sound analysis<br>Diaphragmatic EMG<br>Esophageal balloon | Automated<br>Reduces some invasive measurements<br>Detects trends early | Not always available<br>Frequent calibration and equipment check<br>Clinical usefulness still unproved |
| **LEVEL IV** | | |
| Computer | Rapid processing and display of data plots trends | Limited availability<br>Costly<br>Clinical usefulness still unproved |

*Cdyn,* Dynamic compliance; *Cst,* Static compliance; *EMG,* electromyography; *FVC,* forced vital capacity; *MIF,* maximal inspiratory force; *PET_{CO_2},* end tidal partial pressure of carbon dioxide; *$R_{aw}$,* airway resistance; *$Sa_{O_2}$,* oxygen percent saturation in the arteries; *$V_D$,* dead space volume; *$V_E$,* respiratory minute volume.

hypoxia is far advanced by the time it results in a change in heart rate or rhythm, blood pressure, or level of consciousness.

The arterial blood gas (ABG) measurement is the most useful and widely used form of intermittent monitoring of ventilated patients. This monitoring level also includes serial chest roentgenograms and serial measures of pulmonary mechanics used to determine lung compliance and testing the ability of the patient to breath spontaneously. Clearly the major disadvantage of intermittent monitoring is that changes can occur between measurements, thereby going undetected.

Continuous monitoring (level III), now becoming increasingly available, may be less invasive than intermittent monitoring in some instances. The accuracy of continuous monitoring devices (such as finger oximetry) is dependent on frequent quality checks and calibrations, but their clinical efficacy (defined as improvement in patient outcome) has not been proved. Finally, computer monitoring (level IV) is becoming increasingly popular. At present, the role of computerized equipment is to instantaneously gather, process, and display data derived from all levels of monitoring devices. In the future, direct feedback control may be available. In these instances, the computer may directly activate changes (such as changes in ventilation rate or inspired oxygen concentration) based on computation from the monitored data (such as $Paco_2$ and $Pao_2$). In patients monitored by these "high tech" approaches, the physician and nurse must resist the tendency to "care for" the equipment rather than the patient. "High tech" monitoring is truly beneficial to the intubated and ventilated patient only when it facilitates optimum decision making and frees the caretakers for more patient contact. Data collection obviously should not be an end point itself.

# OTHER ASPECTS OF MANAGEMENT

**Sedation.** Intubation and mechanical ventilation usually require some form of sedation. This can usually be achieved with a short-acting benzodiazepine such as lorazepam (Ativan). Concomitant alcohol withdrawal in the ventilated patient presents a clinical challenge. These patients may require large doses of benzodiazepines to achieve adequate sedation until the autonomic effects of alcohol withdrawal wear off. In other patients morphine is needed both to sedate and to relieve discomfort; in some circumstances it can be delivered as a continuous infusion. Haloperidol in addition to being a potent antipsychotic agent also is useful as an anxiolytic and does not cause respiratory depression or hypotension. The extrapyramidal side effects of this drug can be a problem, especially in the elderly. Fortunately the neuroleptic malignant syndrome is a rare complication of this drug but needs to be considered in the appropriate clinical setting.[20]

**Muscle paralysis.** Occasionally it is necessary to paralyse a patient to improve patient-and-ventilator synchrony. The usual clinical setting is a patient with ARDS in whom high concentrations of oxygen and levels of PEEP are needed to achieve an adequate $Pao_2$. Patients who are being ventilated using inverse ratio always should be adequately sedated and paralyzed because the sensation of respiration in this mode of ventilation is very uncomfortable. Pancuronium and vercuronium are the usual agents used. Paralytics should be discontinued at least every 24 hours to assess their continued need and to evaluate the patient's neurologic status. Prolonged muscle weakness, a recently recognized complication of neuromuscular paralysis in the critically ill, may be made worse by steroids.[21]

**Stress ulcer prophylaxis.** Respiratory failure and mechanical ventilation are well-recognized risk factors for stress gastritis. The mechanism of stress bleeding is not clear but appears to be related to breakdown of the mucosal defenses, possibly because of disuption of gastric mucosal blood flow. For short-term intubation and mechanical ventilation an $H_2$ blocker (such as ranitidine) or sucralfate is adequate. In patients in whom mechanical ventilation is prolonged, sucralfate is probably superior because alkalinization of gastric secretions has been associated with increased incidence of nosocomial pneumonia.[22]

**Deep venous thrombosis prevention.** Pulmonary embolism carries a significant mortality. With few exceptions all intubated and mechanically ventilated patients in the ICU should receive deep venous thrombosis prophylaxis. Heparin, 5000 units subcutaneously twice a day, or intermittent pneumatic venous compression boots in patients at risk of bleeding are the standard of care at present.

**Daily care.** Ventilated patients should be examined twice daily and more often if clinically indicated. Patient data are recorded hourly on a flow sheet and reviewed with other staff by the attending physician. In the awake patient, symptoms can be evaluated by direct questions, and in the intubated patient, letter boards can be useful to improve communication. Daily examination must include all intravenous and arterial line sites, pressure areas, calves, and eyes for evidence of ulceration. Daily weight and input and outflow charts are essential to monitor fluid status. With few exceptions a chest roentgenogram should be obtained every day to check the positions of the endotracheal tube (should be 2 cm above the carina or opposite the fourth thoracic vertebra on a well-centered anteroposterior chest roentgenogram), pulmonary artery catheter, and central lines. Pulmonary infiltrates should be monitored by serial chest roentgenograms and in patients requiring PEEP or with poor compliance pneumothorax or pneumomediastinum assiduously looked for.

With a respiratory therapist, the ventilator should be checked and the settings agreed on. Other settings that need to be checked every 8-hour shift include $Fio_2$, peak inspiratory pressures, tubing, alarms, and humidifier heat and water levels. All patients should have their static and dynamic compliance checked daily; in weaning patients, pulmonary mechanics (inspiratory force, $V_T$, and pulmonary capillary blood volume $[V_C]$), and a rapid shallow breathing index ($f/V_T$) should be monitored.

The frequency of blood testing is dictated by the clinical condition of the patient, and it is difficult to offer firm guidelines. We believe that blood gases should be checked 30 minutes after the initiation of mechanical ventilation and then at least daily. Further blood gas analyses may be needed if changes are made in the ventilator settings.

# SUMMARY

Optimal management of the intubated and mechanically ventilated patient is challenging and requires an understanding of ventilators and an awareness of the many potential problems. Close monitoring of the patient and anticipation of problems are essential to optimize outcome.

## References

1. Anton WR, Gordon RW, Jordan TM, et al: A disposable end-tidal $CO_2$ detector to verify endotracheal intubation, *Ann Emerg Med* 20:271-275, 1991.
2. Zwillich CW, Pierson DJ, Creach GE, et al: Complications of assisted ventilation: a prospective study of 354 consecutive episodes, *Am J Med* 57:161-170, 1974.
3. Einarsson O, Rochester CL, Rosenbaum S: Airway management in respiratory emergencies, *Clin Chest Med* 15(1):13-34, 1994.
4. Katkov WN, Ault MJ: Endotracheal intubation in massive hemoptysis: advantages of the orotracheal route, *Crit Care Med* 17:968, 1989.
5. Pedersen J, Schurizek BA, Melsen NC, Juhl B: The effect of nasotracheal intubation on the paranasal sinuses, *Acta Anaesthesiol Scand* 35:11-13, 1991.
6. Jourdain B, Novara A, Joly-guillou M, et al: Role of quantitative cultures of endotracheal aspirates in the diagnosis of nosocomial penumonia, *Am J Respir Crit Care Med* 152:241-246, 1995.
7. Kollef MH, Schuster DP: The acute respiratory distress syndrome, *N Engl J Med* 332(1):27-37, 1995.
8. Shanholtz C, Brower R: Should inverse ratio ventilation be used in adult respiratory distress syndrome? *Am J Respir Crit Care Med* 149:1354-1358, 1994.
9. Feihl F, Perret C: Permissive hypercapnia. How permissive should we be? *Am J Respir Crit Care Med* 150:1722-1737, 1994.
10. Abraham E, Yoshihara G: Cardiorespiratory effects of pressure controlled inverse ration ventilation in severe respiratory failure, *Chest* 96:1356-1359, 1989.
11. Langer M, Mascheroni D, Marcolin R, Gattinoni L: The prone position in ARDS patients: a clinical study, *Chest* 94(1):103-107, 1988.
12. Carlon GC, Howland WS, Ray C, et al: High frequency jet ventilation: a prospective randomized evaluation, *Chest* 84:551-559, 1983.
13. Zapol WM, Snider MT, Hill JD, et al: Extracorporeal membrane oxygenation in severe acute respiratory failure: a randomized prospective study, *JAMA* 242:2193-2196, 1979.
14. Petty TL: The use, abuse and mystique of positive end-expiratory pressure, *Am Rev Respir Dis* 138:475-478, 1988.
15. Pick RA, Handler JB, Friedman AS: The cardiovascular effects of positive end-expiratory pressure, *Chest* 82:345-350, 1982.
16. Pepe PE, Marini JJ: Occult positive end-expiratory pressure in mechanically ventilated patients with airflow obstruction, *Am Rev Respir Dis* 126:166-170, 1982.
17. Bone RC: Monitoring respiratory function in the patient with adult respiratory distress syndrome, *Semin Respir Med* 2:140-150, 1981.
18. Fallat RJ: Respiratory monitoring, *Clin Chest Med* 3:181-194, 1982.
19. Prakash O, Meij S, Zeelenberg C, van der Borden B: Computer based patient monitoring, *Crit Care Med* 10:811-822, 1982.
20. Rampertaap MP: Neuroleptic malignant syndrome, *South Med J* 79:331-336, 1986.

21. Hansen-Flaschen J, Cowen J, Raps EC: Neuromuscular blockade in the intensive care unit: more than we bargained for, *Am Rev Respir Dis* 147:234-236, 1993.
22. Tryba M: Prophylaxis of stress ulcer bleeding: a meta-analysis, *J Clin Gastroenterol* 13(suppl 2):S44-S55, 1991.

# Chapter 36

# *Recurrent Pulmonary Infections*

Douglas T. Phelps
Leonard Sicilian

The internist frequently is asked to evaluate and care for patients with multiple pulmonary infections.[1-5] Recurrent pneumonia is defined by two or more episodes of parenchymal infection with intervening wellness (no symptoms or complete clearing of the roentgenogram) for at least 1 month. Recurrent pneumonia, defined in this manner, is not uncommon and most often can be attributed to comorbidity that is readily apparent.[1-5] It comes as no surprise to the internist that heart failure, chronic obstructive pulmonary disease, alcoholism, and diabetes are the "big four" of such comorbidities. But, because pneumonia also results from several less common but serious host abnormalities, it triggers the need for detailed, thoughtful investigation.

We find it helpful to view host defects that affect the normally sterile lower respiratory tract as primarily mechanical or immunologic. Mechanical defects are those conditions in which increased influx or diminished bulk removal (as by cough) of pathogens results in a contaminated environment more susceptible to infection. In patients with immunologic defects, the frequency or duration of lower tract contamination may not be altered but the immune system that prevents episodic contamination from infecting tissues is weakened. Either or often both of these mechanisms cause recurrent pulmonary infections (RPI). Many common medical conditions that cause mechanical contamination or immune deficiency are associated with RPI (see box). In addition to common conditions there are a few special mechanical and immune conditions that are noted for their tendency to present with RPI. These "occult" conditions include endobronchial obstruction, cystic fibrosis (CF), hypogammaglobulinemia, primary ciliary dyskinesia (PCD), chronic granulomatous disease (CGD), and compliment deficiency. In this chapter we review some of these unusual diagnoses and outline a standard diagnostic approach (Table 36-1).

372

**Common Conditions Associated with Recurrent Pneumonia**

........................................................................

MECHANICAL

Chronic obstructive pulmonary disease (COPD)
Congestive heart failure (CHF)
Asthma
Chronic sinusitis
Sarcoidosis*
Cerebral vascular accident
Pulmonary tuberculosis*
Kyphoscoliosis
Epilepsy
Bronchiectasis*
Pulmonary resection
Systemic lupus erythematosus (SLE)
Pulmonary fibrosis*
Silicosis

IMMUNE

Alcoholism
Diabetes mellitus
Splenectomy
AIDS*
Malignancy
Systemic steroid use
Hemoglobinopathy

*Designates diagnoses that can cause bronchiectasis.

## THRESHOLD FOR WORK-UP

The decision to work up a patient for mechanical or immunological defects that cause recurrent lower respiratory tract infections should be based on the severity (such as frequency of pneumonia) of the recurrent disease and the presence or absence of an underlying comorbid condition. It is natural, for example, to have a higher suspicion in younger patients who seemingly are otherwise healthy. In some studies, 89% to 93% of adults admitted for pneumonia at least three times in 11 years had some underlying illness.[1-5] Since the majority of the underlying illnesses that predispose to RPI (see box) are evident on a thorough history and physical exam, most evaluations will require little additional cost. In one Swedish series, 85% of 90 patients with recurrent pneumonia had predisposing diseases identified without special exams or tests. If we reclassify the reported diseases to those that might be

**Table 36–1.** *Algorithm for evaluating patients presenting with recurrent pulmonary infections*

| | | |
|---|---|---|
| **Entry Definition** | >3 RPI/2 yrs × 2 yrs<br>>2 pneumonias/10 yrs | |
| | ↓ Yes | |
| **Obstruction Risk** | pneumonias in same location<br>or history c/w foreign body<br>or hemoptysis | — Yes → Refer for bronchoscopy |
| | ↓ No | |
| **Predisposing<br>medical illness**<br>(see box on p. 373) | -alcoholism<br>-diabetes<br>-chronic lung disease<br>-congestive heart failure | — Yes → Optimize medical<br>management |
| | ↓ No | |
| **Preliminary Testing** | HIV<br>&<br>HRCT chest | HIV neg.<br>Bronchiectasis in 1 lobe → Refer for bronchoscopy<br>HIV pos. → Evaluate for **AIDS**<br>defining criteria |
| | HIV neg ↓ Bronchiectasis<br>in multiple lobes | |
| **Secondary Testing** | Quantitative IgM, IgG, IgA<br>Quantitative IgG$_{subclasses (1-4)}$ | — Abnormal → **Immunoglobulin<br>Deficiency**<br>refer to Immunology/<br>Hematology |
| | ↓ Normal | |

**Optional Testing**

infertility, pancreatic dysfunction, fam hx → Sweat Cl⁻ iontophoresis
  ↓ Normal
  → >60 mEq/L repeatedly → **Cystic Fibrosis** refer to pulmonary/CF specialist

infertility, sinusitis, otitis, fam hx → Sperm motility, Nasal mucosa biopsy (EM& phase contrast microscopy)
  ↓ Normal
  → Abnormal motility, Abnormal microtubules → **Dysmotile Cilia Syndrome** genetic counseling, refer to pulmonary specialist

pyoderma, arthritis, pharyngitis → Nitroblue tetrazolium test, PMN function studies
  ↓ Normal
  → Abnormal → **Chronic Granulomatous Disease or PMN functional disorder**

$C_3$, $C_4$, $CH_{50}$
  ↓ Normal
  → Abnormal → **Complement deficiency or dysfunction**

**Follow up Testing**

Quantitative IgM, IgG, IgA repeated 2–3 times /several months
  ↓ Normal
  → Abnormal → **Common Variable Immunodeficiency**

IDIOPATHIC BRONCHIECTASIS
-training/support, pulm toilet
-consider cycling antibiotics

*AIDS*, Acquired immunodeficiency syndrome; *HIV*, human immunodeficiency virus; *HRCT*, high-resolution, thin-section computerized tomography; *Ig*, immunoglobulin; *RPI*, recurrent pulmonary infections.

missed on a routine evaluation, no more than 28 of the 90 patients (31%) would have had "occult" reasons for RPI. Based on these figures we expect no more than 15% to 31% of patients with three pneumonias in a decade to require special investigation. Therefore, in patients with no obvious reason for RPI, we recommend special evaluation after the occurrence of three pneumonias in 10 or fewer years. Working patients up after a second pneumonia may be warranted in younger patients or in situations in which other infections (such as sinusitis, otitis, dermatitis), other complaints (such as constitutional symptoms, infertility, hemoptysis, chronic copious sputum production), or the severity or duration of the pneumonias are suggestive of underlying disease.

## NOT ALL FEVERS WITH INFILTRATES ARE PNEUMONIA

Defining an episode of pneumonia is sometimes difficult. Histories and records outlining acute fever, cough, purulent sputum, an infiltrate, pathogens in the sputum, and resolution with antibiotics are probably the best criteria. The greater the number of these findings, the greater is the specificity for pneumonia. Special caution is warranted for diagnoses that mimic pneumonia such as pulmonary embolism and infarction (PE), hypersensitivity pneumonitis (HSP), Wegener's granulomatosis, allergic bronchopulmonary aspergillosis (ABPA), and bronchiolitis obliterans with organizing pneumonia (BOOP). In each, the lack of a convincing response to antibiotics, the lack of purulent sputum (PE, HSP), or an unusual course (Wegener's, PE, ABPA, BOOP) should help distinguish these diagnoses from pneumonia.

## MECHANICAL DYSFUNCTION AND BRONCHIECTASIS

Mechanical protection from infection is achieved through a filtering action by the nasopharynx, larynx, branching bronchial passages, and bronchial mucus. Mucociliary escalator action, reflex bronchospasm, and cough expel potential pathogens that do penetrate the filters and lodge in constitutive mucus. If organisms are retained, tight bronchial and alveolar epithelial junctions hinder penetration into tissue. Pathogen retention results from an overload of normal clearance mechanisms, defects in these mechanisms, or both. Sinusitis and aspiration are very common, and sometimes there are occult mechanical causes of RPI where the filters (larynx, nasopharynx) are overwhelmed or defective. Clearance defects can result from abnormal sputum viscosity (as seen in cystic fibrosis), abnormal bronchial anatomy (bronchiectasis or obstruction), or dysfunctional cilia.

Bronchiectasis is the prototype of severe clearance difficulties. Chronic inflammation damages bronchial cartilage and converts the stiff conduits into dilated pouches that trap secretions during a cough. Stagnation and infection further impair mucociliary clearance by causing metaplasia of ciliated to nonciliated bronchial epithelium. A setup for vicious cycling, bronchiectasis causes and results from repeated pulmonary infection. Commonly it first develops in segments or lobes that are atelectatic for long intervals. The localized bronchiectasis that results may manifest only as recurrent discrete infections. Pneumonias affecting the area may be separated by months or years without any intervening symptoms belying the chronic nature of the disease.[6] When localized disease is present, it often affects the left lung (left-to-right ratio 9:7) or the middle lobe, presumably because of their smaller airway caliber. The important causes of localized bronchiectasis are endobronchial malignancy or carcinoid, foreign bodies (Fig. 36-1) and right middle lobe syndrome. This differential diagnosis makes localized bronchiectasis probably the single most important cause of RPI. Localized disease caused by the conditions mentioned above and even localized postinflammatory bronchiectasis like that seen after *Bordetella pertussis* pneumonia often can be cured with local resection.

Frequently, however, more than one lobe is bronchiectatic and bilateral disease occurs in one third of all patients. There are many congenital and acquired causes of nonlocalized bronchiectasis. Acquired bronchiectasis can result from aspiration, fungal infection (such as ABPA), whooping cough, or several viral pneumonias. Congenital forms are acquired as sequelae of CF, hypogammaglobulinemia, pulmonary sequestration, or truly developmental abnormalities (such as Williams-Campbell bronchial cartilage deficiency). Bronchiectasis of the upper lobes often is caused by granulomatous disease (such as sarcoid, tuberculosis) and may have hemoptysis as a prominent symptom. The primary symptoms of lower lobe disease are chronic cough and purulent sputum production, which may be positional. The quantity and character of the sputum are quite variable. Amounts may vary with time and can range from 20 to 500 mL per day. Similar to localized disease, diffuse bronchiectasis results in a vicious cycle of stagnation and inflammation that can lead to functionless fibrotic lung.[7]

The incidence of anatomic bronchiectasis may be quite high; up to 40% of patients with acute pneumonia may transiently have some bronchiectasis.[8] On the other hand, the prevalence of symptomatic bronchiectasis appears not to be so high. Many attribute a decline in bronchiectasis to the modern antibiotic era, whereas others hypothesize that antibiotics have resulted in less severe disease. Nonetheless, bronchiectasis is a prominent cause of RPI.

The diagnosis of bronchiectasis is made on clinical grounds with radiographic confirmation. Plain chest roentgenograms are normal 10% of the time.[7] When chest films are abnormal, they may reveal clusters of cystic spaces 5 to 10 mm in diameter, ring shadows (or "tram lines") representing the thickened bronchial walls, atelectasis, or the characteristic dilated bronchi with mucus impaction (finger-glove pattern). Unfortunately, although plain films often show abnormality, their specificity is poor. Confirmation often requires high-resolution, thin-section (1.5 to 3 mm per slice) computerized tomography (HRCT)[9] (Fig. 36-2).

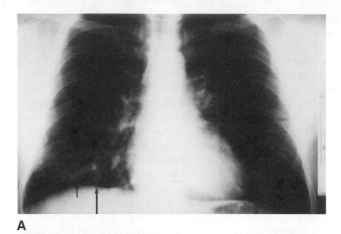

**Figure 36-1.** *Roentgenograms of a 27-year-old patient with an 18-year history of chronic sputum production and recurrent pneumonia. The chest roentgenogram, **A**, shows the finger-glove pattern of mucus-impacted bronchi in the right lower lobe (arrows). The high-resolution computerized tomographic scan (HRCT), **B**, confirms localized bronchiectasis with severe mucus impaction. Only after curative lobectomy and recovery of a plastic cap from the lower lobe of the bronchus did the patient recall a choking episode at 9 years of age.*

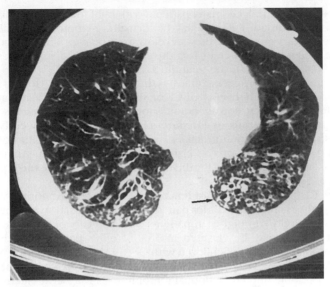

**Figure 36-2.** *HRCT example of diffuse idiopathic bronchiectasis. Bilateral multilobar changes of proximal and distal bronchial wall thickening and dilatation. Dilated bronchi extend subpleurally (arrow) and are associated with early parenchymal fibrosis.*

The aim of finding and treating nonlocalized bronchiectasis is to reduce recurrent infection and the resulting fibrosis of lung parenchyma. Usually there is no specific treatment for the underlying cause (except for hypogammaglobulinemia), so the brunt of therapy is aimed at controlling secretions and limiting infection. Postural drainage and chest physical therapy remain the mainstays of "pulmonary toilet." Antibiotics active against *Haemophilus influenzae* and *Streptococcus pneumoniae* should be used (possibly at increased doses) when there is a change in the amount of sputum or breathlessness.[10] Although there are no definitive studies, we believe that prophylactic alternating antibiotics (such as tetracycline, trimethoprim sulfamethoxizole taken 1 to 2 weeks per month) reduce secretions and exacerbations in selected patients.

## CYSTIC FIBROSIS

Cystic fibrosis (CF) is a condition where abnormal mucus results in abnormal mechanical clearance, infection, and severe progressive bronchiectasis. A well-known autosomal recessive disorder, it usually is diagnosed in childhood when severe respiratory infections and pancreatic insufficiency cause a failure to thrive. Because of multiple different mutations and variable penetrance of the affected CF transmembrane conductance regulator (CFTR) gene, there is a broad range of severity in this affliction. Indeed, many patients with mild forms escape diagnosis until adulthood. Patients may be virtually asymptomatic until the late teen-age years when they develop a chronic productive cough. These milder forms generally lack the gastrointestinal disturbances that are so characteristic of the infantile presentation.[11]

There may be no specific clues to the diagnosis of CF. Helpful leads may include a family history of CF or sibling illness and death, atopy, or infertility. Strong consideration should be given to patients with *Staphylococcus aureus* or *Pseudomonas aeruginosa* (especially mucoid strains) in the sputum. Likewise, diffuse streaky densities on the chest roentgenogram or the classic cystic changes with pulmonary fibrosis with a predilection for the upper lobes should raise the possibility of CF.

The CF diagnostic standard remains the sweat test. Abnormal values are not always reliable in older patients because normal sweat chloride values generally run higher in patients over 20 years of age. Likewise, sweat sodium may be elevated in 35% of older patients and in the asymptomatic parents of children with CF (that is, heterozygote). Nonetheless, sweat chloride values above 60 to 80 mEq/L are consistent with CF in the adult, and conventional iontophoresis for sweat electrolytes remains the standard for diagnosis. In adults, high values always should be repeated to establish the diagnosis. Low values in the absence of edema (which may give false-negative results) often are sufficient to exclude the diagnosis. The test should be performed in a laboratory that does at least 100 tests per year. Because laboratory error is the most common cause of false-positive results, the choice of centers greatly affects diagnostic accuracy.[12]

Therapy for CF is highly specialized and has dramatically changed in the past 5 to 10 years. Although pulmonary toilet and antibiotics are still the mainstays of treatment, sophisticated treatment protocols, lung transplantation, and the development of gene therapy make CF a disease best suited to the subspecialist.

# PRIMARY CILIARY DYSKINESIA

Primary ciliary dyskinesia (PCD) was first described as "immotile cilia syndrome" in 1976 in a group of patients with frequent infections involving the sinuses, middle ear, and respiratory tract. Infertility and situs inversus also are occasionally seen as part of the affliction and remind us that Kartagener's syndrome (situs inversus, bronchiectasis, and sinusitis) is the prototype of this anomaly. This familial syndrome results from ultrastructural microtubule defects in cilia and most of the time in sperm. A rare disorder, it affects approximately 1 in 15,000 to 30,000 individuals.

Primary ciliary dyskinesia often evades diagnosis until the second or third decade of life. Although situs inversus would be an immediate clue to the diagnosis, it is not always present. More frequently the diagnosis is made during evaluations for infertility or recurrent sinopulmonary infections. Several modalities allow the clinician to screen or measure abnormal mucociliary structure and clearance. The most useful exam is performed directly by means of small brush and curettage biopsies of the nasal or bronchial mucosa. Fresh samples can be examined for motility, and fixed specimens can be analyzed by electron microscopy for ultrastructural abnormalities. The most sensitive, readily available test is phase-contrast microscopy for motility; the simplest screening specimen in males is semen analysis looking at sperm motility.[13] There is no available treatment.

# IMMUNE DEFENSE

Pulmonary immune defense is complex and often iatrogenically or environmentally impaired. Mediators of inflammation normally sequester the infection, recruit cellular elements, and facilitate removal of the offending organisms. Neutrophils, lymphocytes, and macrophages play important roles in the prevention or limitation of pulmonary infection. Intact immunity depends on adequate cell numbers and function. Phagocytes need to chemotax, ingest, and then kill in order to abort seeded infections. Nonphagocytic cells (such as lymphocytes) initate and modulate cellular behavior and the humoral responses that assist in the localization and destruction of organisms and engorged phagocytes.

The network can break down on many levels, and the majority of RPI patients have pharmacologic (steroids), nutritional (malnutrition or alcohol), metabolic (diabetes), or malignant (leukemia or lymphoma) reasons for immunodeficiency. On the other hand, immunodeficient patients without obvious disease may require a sophisticated diagnostic evaluation. If obvious disease (such as those listed above), splenectomy, and hemoglobinopathies are removed from the differential diagnosis, then HIV infection, immunoglobulin deficiency, and neutrophil or complement dysfunction are primary considerations. Of these, immunoglobulin deficiency and HIV infection are far and away the most common diagnosis in the 1990s.

# IMMUNOGLOBULIN DEFICIENCY

The most prevalent immunoglobulin deficiency is a selective reduction in IgA. Its estimated incidence is about 1 in 500 patients with a male-to-female ratio of 2 : 1. Although many IgA-deficient patients are asymptomatic, as many as 70% suffer from RPI and develop bronchiectasis and emphysema. In addition, patients often have associated gastrointestinal (GI) problems (celiac or inflammatory bowel disease), autoimmune disorders, pernicious anemia, rheumatoid arthritis, lupus, chronic hepatitis), or allergies (asthma, allergic rhinitis, eczema). Furthermore, IgA-deficient patients have an increased incidence of GI and pulmonary tumors.[14]

Common variable immunodeficiency usually is diagnosed in adulthood. This acquired disorder presents in the fourth to seventh decade as a depression in one or all of the immunoglobulin classes. The onset is abrupt and affects males and females equally. IgG is the most commonly depressed class, but levels may wax and wane. The pathophysiologic feature is believed to be a maturation defect of B lymphocytes. Depressed immunoglobulin synthesis results in frequent infections, especially with encapsulated organisms. Affected areas include the lungs, sinuses, middle ear, and GI tract (especially with *Giardia* organisms). Cough, copious sputum, and frequent pneumonias (most with several per year) are the most common complaints, and bronchiectasis may occur in as many as 69% of such patients.[15] As with IgA deficiency, there is an increased incidence of autoimmune disorders and malignancies in these patients, with tumors of the GI tract, lungs, and lymphatic system representing the leading cause of death.

IgG and combined IgA-IgG deficiencies, congenital or acquired, are less common than IgA deficiency and similarly present with recurrent infections of the lungs or sinuses. Serum protein electrophoresis (SPEP) may provide a clue to immunoglobulin deficiency but cannot reliably exclude it because compensatory increases in IgM may mask other gamma globulin deficiency. Quantitative immunoglobulin analysis specifically measures each class of immunoglobulin but similarly can overlook subclass deficiency. The IgG class is composed of four subclasses ($IgG_{1-4}$), and reduced levels of a single subclass of IgG can lead to recurrent infection. Because subclasses 3 and 4 constitute only 10% of the total IgG level, a specific subclass deficiency easily may be overlooked if evaluation is limited to quantitative immunoglobulin analysis alone.[17] Therefore, for patients with suspicious histories for RPI, sinusitis, or bronchiectasis, we recommend quantitative immunoglobulins (IgM, IgG, IgA, IgD, IgE) and IgG subclasses levels. Several determinants may be necessary if common variable deficiency is suspected before this disorder can be excluded.

Early diagnosis of immunoglobulin deficiency is of particular importance because specific therapy is possible. In the case of IgG deficiency and common variable immunodeficiency, periodic infusion of gamma globulin has been shown to reduce the morbidity of recurrent infections.[15,18] Monthly infusions or intramuscular injections, empiric or adjusted for IgG levels between 200 and 500 mg/L, are aimed at reducing symptoms and suppurative infections. Unfortunately, IgA cannot be replaced. Since secretory IgA is produced locally, systemic infusion is not helpful, and there is a high incidence of anaphylactic reaction to immunoglobulin in IgA-deficient patients.

# PHAGOCYTIC CELL DYSFUNCTION AND COMPLEMENT DEFICIENCY

Disorders of phagocyte function usually are diagnosed in childhood but occasionally presentation may be delayed until early adult life. Phagocyte dysfunction may come from quantitative or qualitative inadequacies. The problems with reduced numbers of phagocytes are self-evident and manifest routinely in patients with certain hematologic malignancies and in those receiving cancer chemotherapy. Since phagocyte function encompasses chemotaxis, ingestion, and intracellular killing, potential qualitative defects are broad and complex. Abnormal chemotaxis is most commonly seen in disorders such as Chédiak-Higashi syndrome or the "lazy leukocyte" syndrome; it is most unusual for these to present in adulthood.

Intracellular killing of phagocytized organisms is fundamental to phagocyte function. Disorders of impaired intracellular killing include, again, Chédiak-Higashi syndrome, myeloperoxidase deficiency, and chronic granulomatous disease (CGD). Of these, CGD, a hereditary disease transmitted by X-linked or autosomal recessive inheritance, may occasionally present in the second or third decade of life. The most common adult presentation is pulmonary fibrosis. These patients recall recurrent bouts of necrotizing pneumonias, dermatitis, polyarthritis, or glomerulonephritis. Catalase-positive organisms such as staphylococci, *Escherichia coli, Aerobacter,* or *Klebsiella* are typical pathogens. Physical examination may show lymphadenopathy and hepatosplenomegaly, whereas blood studies typically demonstrate leukocytosis and hypergammaglobulinemia. Because phagocyte hydrogen peroxide production is impaired in CGD, this condition is easily screened for with an in vitro nitroblue tetrazolium test. Normal phagocytes ingest this compound and reduce it by means of reactive oxygen species to a blue-black substance. PMNs that fail to accumulate blue-black particles are consistent with the diagnosis of CGD.[2]

Complement plays a synergistic role with the phagocyte. Complement defects can stem from consumption or inadequate production. Functional abnormalities in or low levels of C3, C5, or C3b may result in recurrent pneumonias, ear and sinus infections, sepsis, and meningitis. The pathogens encountered with complement deficiency are similar to those seen in phagocyte dysfunction; pyogenic organisms and fungi predominate. The best screening tests are total hemolytic complement ($CH_{50}$) serum titers and quantitative $C_3$ and $C_5$ levels.[2]

Specific therapies for complement deficiency and phagocytic cell dysfunction are not available.

## HUMAN IMMUNODEFICIENCY VIRUS INFECTION

HIV infection is the most important addition to the differential diagnosis of RPI in the last decade.[19] In recent years recurrent bacterial infection has earned the status of an AIDS-defining illness, and idiopathic bronchiectasis has been reported in many patients.[20] Little is understood about the pathogenesis of bronchiectasis in these patients, but hypotheses include direct viral effects and the sequelae of recurrent or severe infections. HIV's place in the differential diagnosis of RPI is still evolving. Because of increasing prevalence, we believe HIV infection must be seriously considered in all patients with idiopathic RPI.

*References*

1. Ekdahl K, Braconier JH, Rollof J: Recurrent pneumonia: a review of 90 adult patients, *Scand J Infect Dis* 24(1):71, 1992, and Crofton J: Bronchiectasis. II: Treatment and prevention, *Br Med J* 19:783, 1966.

2. Fraser RG, Paré JAP, Paré PD, et al: *Diagnosis of diseases of the chest,* ed 3, Philadelphia, 1989, Saunders, p 774.

3. Kirtland SH, Winterbauer RH: Slowly resolving, chronic, and recurrent pneumonia, *Clin Chest Med* 12(2):303, 1991.

4. Roth RM, Gleckman RA: Recurrent bacterial pneumonia: a contemporary perspective, *South Med J* 78(5):573, 1985.

5. Winterbauer RH, Bedon GA, Ball WC Jr: Recurrent pneumonia: predisposing illness and clinical patterns in 158 patients, *Ann Intern Med* 70:689, 1969.

6. Croton J: Bronchiectasis. II: Treatment and prevention, *Br Med J* 19:783, 1966.

7. LeRoux BT, Mohlala ML, Odell JA, Whitton ID: Suppurative diseases of the lung and pleural space. Part II: Bronchiectasis, *Curr Probl Surg* 23:95, 1986.

8. Bachman AL, Hewitt WR, Beckly HC: Bronchiectasis: a bronchographic study of sixty cases of pneumonia, *Arch Intern Med* 91:78, 1953.

9. Phillips MS, Williams MP, Flower CDR: How useful is computed tomography in the diagnosis and assessment of bronchiectasis? *Clin Radiol* 37:321, 1985.

10. Stockley RA: Bronchiectasis: a management problem? *Br Dis Chest* 82:209, 1988.

11. Tomashefski JF, Christoforidis AJ, Abdullah AK: Cystic fibrosis in young adults, *Chest* 57(1):28, 1970.

12. Wood RE, Boat TF, Doershuk CF: Cystic fibrosis, *Am Rev Respir Dis* 113:833, 1976.

13. Rossman CM, Lee RMKW, Forrest JB, Newhouse MT: Nasal ciliary ultrastructure in patients with primary ciliary dyskinesia compared with that in normal subjects and in subjects with various respiratory diseases, *Am Rev Respir Dis* 129:161, 1984.

14. Ammann AJ, Hong R: Selective IgA deficiency: presentation of 30 cases and a review of the literature, *Medicine* 50:223, 1971.

15. Dukes RJ, Rosenow EC III, Hermans PE: Pulmonary manifestations of hypogammaglobulinemia, *Thorax* 33:603, 1978.

16. Hermans PE, Díaz-Buxo JA, Stobo JD: Idiopathic late-onset immunoglobulin deficiency: clinical observations in 50 patients, *Am J Med* 61:221, 1976.

17. Beck CS, Heiner DC: Selective immunoglobulin $G_4$ deficiency and recurrent infections of the respiratory tract, *Am Rev Respir Dis* 124:94, 1981.

18. Roifman CM, Lederman HM, Lavi S, et al: Benefit of intravenous IgG replacement in hypogammaglobulinemic patients with chronic sinopulmonary disease, *Am J Med* 79:71, 1985.

19. Chechani B, Allam AA, Smith PR, et al: Bronchitis mimicking opportunistic lung infection in patients with human immunodeficiency virus infection/AIDS. *NY State J Med* 92:197, 1992.

20. Holmes A, Trotman-Dickenson B, Edwards A, et al: Bronchiectasis in HIV disease, *Q J Med* 85(307):875, 1992.

# Chapter 37

# *Diagnosis and Management of Active Tuberculosis*

Ronald L. Ciubotaru
Leonard Sicilian

Major epidemiologic changes in the prevalence of tuberculosis in the United States have necessitated the addition of this chapter to the current edition of *Consultations in Internal Medicine.* From 1953 to 1985 the number of cases of tuberculosis decreased from 84,304 to 22,201.[1] During this period, the majority of cases were caused by reactivation of old infections. Transmission of new infection to infants and children decreased substantially, and in many areas of the country fewer than 1% of children entering school had positive tuberculin reactions.

In sharp contrast, since 1985 there has been an increase of 20% in reported cases of tuberculosis. This excess was seen mostly in Hispanics, blacks, and persons 25 to 44 years of age.[1] The increase was most pronounced in cities with a high incidence of HIV infection; in some inner-city tuberculosis clinics, 40% of all patients infected with tuberculosis were HIV positive. Persons born in foreign countries now represent 25% of all new cases of tuberculosis, and young children also have fallen victim, with a 19% increase in children younger than 4 years of age and a 40% increase in children 5 to 14 years of age.

HIV infection currently is the greatest known risk factor for reactivating latent tuberculosis infection. The estimated risk for developing tuberculosis in a tuberculin-positive individual who develops HIV infection is an extraordinary 7% to 10% per year. Development of overt disease in other tuberculin-positive patients within the first 2 years after infection is about 4% per year.[2] Development of disease can occur throughout the lifetime of an individual; however, clinically evident tuberculosis will eventually occur in 5% to 15% of all individuals who are infected with the organism.[1,3] Overt disease may be manifested either by progression of the original focus of infection or by the appearance of pulmonary or extrapulmonary disease months or years after the initial infection. Most active diseases in adults represent reactivation of an infection acquired earlier. In areas in which eradication of disease was most successful, however, adults increasingly are being seen with primary tuberculosis.

385

In persons infected with HIV, the diagnosis of tuberculosis often precedes the diagnosis of AIDS. The diagnosis of tuberculosis may be difficult in the AIDS population because anergy on skin testing is common. In addition, the roentgenographic presentation of lower-lobe infiltrates and hilar adenopathy in a patient with HIV carries a large differential diagnosis. Lastly, there have been reports of tuberculosis with a normal roentgenogram in this population. Extrapulmonary and disseminated disease also are much more common in HIV-infected patients.

In the remainder of this chapter, we provide a concise and orderly way to approach the increasingly complex topic of the diagnosis and treatment of active tuberculosis. The terminology used to describe tuberculous infection and treatment can be quite confusing. Accordingly we have tabulated a glossary of the common terms used (see following two boxes).

# DIAGNOSIS OF ACTIVE PULMONARY TUBERCULOSIS

Effective tuberculosis control requires prompt identification of active cases, institution of appropriate therapy, and assurance of completion of therapy. Case finding, however, remains the cornerstone of effective control. The most important factor in making an early diagnosis of tuberculosis is a high clinical index of suspicion. Physicians must be

---

## Classification of Tuberculosis

**Class 1. Tuberculosis exposure; no evidence of infection**
a. History of significant exposure
b. Negative tuberculin skin test

**Class 2. Tuberculosis infection; no disease**
a. Positive tuberculin skin
b. Normal chest roentgenogram
c. Negative culture for tuberculosis (if done)

**Class 3. Tuberculosis; clinically active**
a. Positive culture
   or
b. Clinical or radiologic signs compatible with tuberculosis and a positive tuberculin skin test

**Class 4. Tuberculosis; not clinically active**
a. Radiologic evidence of pulmonary tuberculosis
b. Positive tuberculin skin test
c. No clinical signs or symptoms compatible with progressive tuberculosis
d. Negative culture for tuberculosis (if done)

## Treatment Terminology

| | |
|---|---|
| **Phase 1. Initial therapy** | Directed at killing rapidly growing bacilli inside and outside the host's macrophages |
| **Phase 2. Continuation therapy** | Directed at killing those organisms initially dormant within the host's macrophages and thus not killed during the initial phase of therapy |
| **Prophylactic treatment** | Medication given during the infection with the intent to kill all the infecting organisms before the immune response occurs. If it is effective, the individual will never have a positive tuberculin test |
| **Preventive treatment** | The continuation phase given to an individual whose immune system is strong enough to serve in the place of the initial phase of therapy |

aware of the patient groups at special risk for tuberculosis (see box below). Persistent cough, fever, nightsweats, weight loss, and hemoptysis are suggestive of tuberculosis. After a thorough history and physical examination, the first diagnostic steps in persons suspected of having active

## Patients at Risk for Developing Active Tuberculosis

1. Low socioeconomic status (especially the homeless)
2. Age (early years of life and late adolescence/early adult, absolute number increased in geriatrics)
3. Ethnicity (such as Southeast Asia, Hispanics)
4. Genetics (monozygotic more than dizygotic concordance)
5. Medical conditions: silicosis, diabetes mellitus, chronic renal failure (especially dialysis patients), chronic interstitial lung disease, pulmonary alveolar proteinosis, gastrectomy, jejunoileal bypass, pulmonary cancer
6. Immunocompromised patients: hematologic malignancy, HIV, immunosuppressive agents, malnutrition
7. Close contacts of known cases of active tuberculosis (as in nursing homes with health care professionals)

tuberculosis should be a tuberculin skin test followed by a chest roent-genogram and sputum examination for mycobacteria if indicated.

## Clinical manifestations

Although nonspecific, the clinical manifestations of tuberculosis vary between primary and postprimary disease (reactivation disease).

### Primary disease

Most patients with primary disease are asymptomatic. When symptoms occur, they manifest as fever, cough, anorexia, weight loss, excessive perspiration, chest pain, lethargy, and dyspnea. Erythema nodosum occasionally is seen. Hematogenous dissemination of tuberculosis seen in primary tuberculosis rarely causes symptoms. If progressive disease ensues, more severe symptoms referable to the particular organ systems involved may develop.

Lab data pointing to the primary disease include a recent tuberculin conversion associated with bronchopulmonary, pleural, or lymph node involvement on chest roentgenogram. Pleural fluid and sputum usually test negative on smear and culture; accordingly the diagnosis is best confirmed by histopathologic or pleural biopsy culture results.

### Postprimary tuberculosis

Clinically apparent disease develops in 2% to 3% of tuberculin-positive individuals with normal chest roentgenograms.[1,4] Annual checkups of patients considered to have inactive disease without other risk factors, therefore, are not recommended. Patients should be instructed, however, to seek medical attention if symptoms develop. Symptoms, when present, are usually nonpulmonary; these include fatigue, weakness, anorexia, and weight loss. A contact history may be obtained in some cases. Direct questioning may elicit a history of recent onset nonproductive or mildly productive cough, occasionally associated with hemoptysis. Pleuritic chest pain and fever may be the presenting complaint. Hoarseness indicates laryngeal involvement and usually is associated with a positive sputum culture and a very high infectivity. Shortness of breath is uncommon. One third to one half of patients are febrile when first seen. The fever is low grade and usually occurs in the afternoon and evening. Its presence correlates with cavitation and far advanced, smear-positive disease.

Physical exam may reveal apical crackles. In patients with endobronchial dissemination, diffuse crackles and ronchi may be heard. A pleural rub or findings of a pleural effusion may be noted. Detecting abnormalities on a screening chest roentgenogram is the most common presentation of postprimary tuberculosis. Most are inactive. Most patients do not have a history suggestive of prior active disease. Some will recount a history of a protracted course of a prior pneumonia and persistent pleuritic pain and fever.

The clinical presentation of miliary tuberculosis is quite different. The onset is insidious, with the mean duration of symptoms of 8 to 16 weeks.[5] Cough, weight loss, weakness, anorexia, and night sweats are common. Headache and abdominal pain may indicate meningeal and peritoneal involvement, respectively. Tuberculin skin test is negative at least 25% of the time. Without treatment the cause of death is respiratory failure. Miliary tuberculosis may be diagnosed by a high clinical suspicion and supportive clinical presentation and roentgenographic pattern. Therapy should be instituted immediately. Definitive diagnosis then may be sought by transbronchial or even open lung biopsy. The yield of bone-marrow aspiration and biopsy is disappointing, ranging from 16% to 33%.

In the United States extrapulmonary tuberculosis is seen in the elderly, blacks, and patients with AIDS. Fever of unknown origin is the common presentation. Perhaps the most common site of extrapulmonary tuberculosis in adults is genitourinary. Sterile pyuria, hematuria, and albuminuria in a patient who has pulmonary tuberculosis always should raise suspicion of genitourinary tract tuberculosis. The female genital tract may be involved with infection presenting as pelvic pain, salpingitis, oophoritis, and menstrual disturbances. Bone and joint involvement, seen commonly in the past, particularly with spinal involvement (Pott's disease), rarely is seen today.

**Laboratory testing.** The standard 5 tuberculin-unit skin test is negative in the first few weeks of infection and positive thereafter. Anergy exists in immunocompromised states, either disease or iatrogenically induced. Appropriate criteria for defining a positive skin reaction depend on the population being tested (Table 37-1).

**Sputum smears and culture.** Sputum examination is an essential component of any diagnostic evaluation of pulmonary tuberculosis. Sputum is the most easily obtainable source of organisms. A smear showing acid-fast bacilli is diagnostic in the appropriate clinical setting and is sufficient reason to begin therapy while awaiting final culture results. Definitive diagnosis, however, requires culture of the organism. Levy and colleagues[6] reported sensitivity and specificity for sputum smears of 53.1% and 99.8%, respectively, and they found that for both smear and culture 95% of the positive results were obtained by examination of three sputum samples. Other studies have corroborated these findings. The yield of sputum cultures for detecting *Mycobacterium tuber-*

**Table 37-1.** *Criteria for positive skin test*

| Induration Size (mm) | Patient Population |
| --- | --- |
| >5 | Adults and children with HIV infection or other immunocompromised states |
| | Frequent contacts of infectious cases |
| | Patients with fibrotic lesions on chest roentgenogram |
| >10 | Adult and children at risk for acquiring tuberculosis (see bottom box on p. 387) |
| | All infants and children younger than 4 years of age |
| >15 | Persons without a defined risk factor |

*culosis* is greater than direct sputum examination, but the delay in obtaining results remains a problem. Levy and colleagues[6] reported a sensitivity and specificity for sputum cultures of 81.5% and 98.4%, respectively in a group of 435 patients. Again patients with cavitary disease (96%) were more likely to have positive cultures than patients with focal infiltrates (70%).[7] Smear-negative, culture-positive results occur in 25% of patients and in 5% to 10% of far-advanced cavitary disease. In patients where a diagnosis is suspected but sputum is not available, fiberoptic bronchoscopy is recommended. A similar high yield as noted just above results when smears and cultures are taken from a combination of brushings, washings, and biopsies.

Advances in culture technology should aid in the rapid and accurate diagnosis of pulmonary tuberculosis. There are enhanced broth-based culture detection and identification systems available. The most widely used system is the BACTEC system, in which a radioactive-labeled palmitic acid is used as substrate and in the presence of viable mycobacteria is metabolized to radioactive carbon dioxide ($CO_2$).[8,9] This $CO_2$ can be quantitated and used to detect the presence of mycobacteria well before conventional techniques would be positive. Definitive rapid identification of mycobacteria is available with species-specific nucleic acid probes. The combination of genetic probes and BACTEC can identify a positive culture in less than 2 weeks. Other methods of rapid diagnosis including serology and amplification of mycobacterial DNA with *polymerase chain reaction* (PCR) are being studied. At present their place in establishing the clinical diagnosis is undetermined.

For patients in whom the diagnosis is suspected but whose smear results are negative, one alternative is to begin therapy and wait for culture results. Treating patients in this manner has been the approach of many experienced chest physicians, and undoubtedly many patients have been cured. It also is likely that many such patients did not have tuberculosis and were treated unnecessarily. A recent investigation of *presumptive therapy* of patients with negative smear results indicated that half of such patients actually have disease.[10] Although *presumptive therapy* is valid and a justifiable approach for many patients, compliance tends to be more reliable if a firmly established diagnosis is presented to the patient. Thus, we believe that it is more appropriate to establish a definitive diagnosis as early as possible. The problems of AIDS and multidrug-resistant tuberculosis make this latter approach more reasonable.

**Fiberoptic bronchoscopy.** We believe that fiberoptic bronchoscopy is of use when sputum smears are negative and when there is a wider range of diagnostic possibilites (such as cancer and fungus). In addition, it may hasten the diagnosis in patients who are at high risk of adverse drug reactions from antituberculous chemotherapy, in whom presumptive therapy may be risky.

**Chest roentgenogram.** Parenchymal abnormalities associated with tuberculosis can be varied. The pattern of lung involvement seems to differ between primary and postprimary forms of disease. Moreover, the chest roentgenogram in the HIV population has a tendency to encompass the characteristics of both of these disease stages.

PRIMARY TUBERCULOSIS. In children, the upper lobes are affected slightly more than the lower lobes, but there are no significant differences between left or right lungs or between anterior and posterior segments.[11] Adults present with a much higher incidence of lower lobe involvement. The typical roentgenographic pattern, that of air-space consolidation (pneumonia), tends to be homogeneous in nature with ill-defined margins. Cavitation is seen in communities where the disease was introduced relatively recently but is rarely seen in communities with high prevalence. Evidence of miliary spread is very uncommon. Complete resolution is the rule usually within 6 months to 2 years after institution of therapy. However, some scarring or calcification is not uncommonly seen in long-term follow-up patients. Hilar or paratracheal lymph node enlargement is common and tends to distinguish primary from postprimary tuberculosis. In adults, adenopathy may be the presenting roentgenographic abnormality in primary disease.[11] Resolution of the adenopathy seems to parallel the parenchymal radiographic resolution. Atelectasis caused by tracheobronchial disease can be present. The anterior segment of the upper lobe and the medial segment of the middle lobe are most affected. This is a less-frequent finding in adults. Pleural effusion can be seen in 10% of children and 40% of adults.[11] It is most common among adolescents and young adults. However, there is evidence that pleural effusions can be seen in reactivation disease as well.

POSTPRIMARY (REACTIVATION) DISEASE. Postprimary disease has a tendency to involve the apical and posterior segments of the upper lobes. Only rarely will it affect the anterior segment solely, a feature that is useful in differentiating it from other granulomatous diseases or cancer. The superior segment of the lower lobes is affected in 5% to 10% of patients.[12] Several radiographic patterns may be identified in postprimary disease. Airspace consolidation reflects local exudative tuberculosis. Opacities are indistinct and homogeneous, and the bronchovascular markings of the ipsilateral hilum are accentuated. The shadows may disappear rapidly after institution of chemotherapy. Adenopathy is distinctly uncommon but may be present. Cavitation occurs in 50% of patients. The cavity wall may be thin or thick and may contain a fluid level up to 20% of the time. With adequate therapy the cavity may disappear but sometimes persists as an air-filled cystic space.

Sharply defined nodular shadows, usually irregular in contour, represent the chronic fibrocaseous form of tuberculosis lung involvement. Healing occurs by replacement of the granulation tissue by fibrous tissue and resultant cicatrization. The reduction in lung volume may become evident by elevation of the hilum and in some cases bulla formation. Numerous widely and uniformly distributed discrete and pinpoint opacities represent the miliary pattern of tuberculous infection. It usually takes 6 weeks from the time of dissemination to its appearance on the chest roentgenogram. In the absence of adequate therapy, the milia may grow and become confluent presenting a "snowstorm" appearance. With appropriate therapy, roentgenographic clearing may be rapid. Acute respiratory failure is a potential complication of miliary tuberculosis. A round or oval opacity commonly situated in the upper lobes, right more than left, is typical of a tuberculoma.[13] They range from 1 to 4 cm in diameter and are smooth and sharply defined. Satellite lesions may be identified in as many as 80% of patients. These are small discrete shadows in the immediate vicinity of the main lesion. The majority of these lesions remain stable over long periods of time, and many calcify. The larger the lesion the more likely it is to be active. Bronchiectatic changes may be localized to the apical and posterior segments of an upper lobe.

In summary, the diagnosis of pulmonary tuberculosis still rests on a high clinical suspicion combined with radiographic findings and the results of sputum examination. Empiric therapy of smear-negative cases is reasonable in some instances, but we favor a more aggressive approach to diagnosis (that is, bronchoscopy with transbronchial biopsy) in most cases. An aggressive approach definitely should be used in patients where a wide range of diagnostic possibilities exist and in patients considered most likely to suffer adverse effects from antituberculosis therapy. Techniques of molecular biology, especially PCR, offer promising noninvasive approaches to diagnosing active tuberculosis. Their clinical role is undetermined at present, however.

# THERAPY FOR ACTIVE TUBERCULOSIS

In the years since antituberculosis chemotherapy has become available, data accumulated in many clinical trials have resulted in three basic principles upon which treatment is based: (1) regimens must contain multiple drugs to which the organisms are susceptible; (2) the drugs must be taken regularly; (3) drug therapy must continue for a sufficient period of time. Control of tuberculosis depends on more than just the science of chemotherapy; only within the framework of the overall clinical and social management of patients and their contacts can chemotherapy be successful. An organized and smoothly functioning network of primary and referral services based on cooperation between clinical and public health officials, between health care facilities and community outreach programs, and between the private and public sectors of health care is essential.

The aim of therapy is to provide the safest and most effective regimen in the shortest period of time.[4,14] The proper initial phase of therapy is crucial for preventing the emergence of drug resistance. The particular regimen used becomes irrelevant if the drugs do not enter the patient's body. Promoting and monitoring the patient's adherence to the program are essential for success. All patients should be asked routinely about their compliance, and sporadic pill counts and urine drug tests may be necessary to monitor drug ingestion. Compulsive record keeping on drug pickups and clinic attendance is imperative. Communication of missed appointments by the patient and appropriate public health official must be done in a timely fashion. Several organizational strategies have been implemented to improve patient adherence. These include (1) setting clinic hours and location to suit the patient's needs; (2) directly observed therapy in clinic, home, workplace, or other location; and (3) the offering of incentives and enablers such as food, carfare, and babysitting services.

Studies performed during the past 45 years have allowed the following generalizations to be made:

1. Isoniazid (INH) should be used for the duration of whatever regimen is used, unless there are contraindications to its use, or the organism is resistent to the drug. INH posesses the best profile in terms of effectiveness, low frequency of side effects, and cost of any antituberculosis agents.
2. For regimens 6 months in duration, isoniazid and rifampin are essential for the total duration of therapy.
3. Pyrazinamide, given initially, improves the efficacy of regimens of less than 9 months in duration.
4. Substituting ethambutol or streptomycin for pyrazinamide in the initial phase decreases the effectiveness of a regimen.
5. After an initial daily phase of treatment as short as 2 weeks, intermittent administration of appropriately adjusted doses of the drugs produces results equal to those of daily administration. Regimens of four drugs given three times weekly throughout the course of treatment gives equally good results in adults. Although there are no good data for children in terms of three-times-weekly dosing, experience with other intermittent regimens indicates they would be equally efficacious.

The preceding guidelines apply to culture-sensitive organisms. Initial resistance remains low in some parts of the United States (<4% to isoniazid). Outbreaks of multiple drug–resistant strains have been re ported with increasing frequency, however.[15,16] These organisms have been resistant to isoniazid, rifampin, and frequently ethambutol and other agents as well. These outbreaks are particularly common among HIV patients and their contacts, in which rapid progression of disease is most common. It is essential that physicians initiating therapy for tuberculosis be aware of the prevalence of drug resistance in their communities and of the epidemiologic features of persons most likely to be harboring these organisms. Drug-susceptibility testing should be done on all newly diagnosed cases. Access to a laboratory that can both identify the organism and determine the susceptibility pattern in a timely fashion is mandatory. The box on p. 394 summarizes the current treatment recommendations.

**Adverse reactions.** Base-line measurements of hepatic enzymes, bilirubin, creatinine, complete blood count, and platelet count should be performed. If pyrazinamide is included in the regimen, uric acid should be added to the preceding profile. Patients receiving ethambutol should have a base-line visual acuity test and a red-green color-perception examination, though toxicity is unusual in doses less than 15 mg/kg/day. Base-line tests other than visual acuity are not required in children. All patients should be routinely monitored clinically for adverse effects of chemotherapy. At least monthly appointments with medical personnel to address symptoms of common side effects of the medicines are

## Summary of Treatment Protocols
· · · · · · · · · · · · · · · · · · · · · · · · · · · · · · · · · · · · · · · · · · · · · · · · · · · · · · · · ·

### 1. SIX-MONTH REGIMEN: PREFERRED TREATMENT FOR SUSCEPTIBLE ORGANISMS

2 months with isoniazid, rifampin, pyrazinamide (UNTIL CULTURE RESULTS ARE AVAILABLE) followed by

4 months with isoniazid and rifampin (if organisms are sensitive).

If suspected that there is >4% chance of resistance to isoniazid, ethambutol should be added in adults, and streptomycin in children who are too young to have visual acuity testing.

This four-drug 6-month regimen is effective even when the infecting organism is isoniazid resistant.

In HIV-1 positive patients it is crucial to assess clinical and bacteriologic response. If necessary, therapy should be prolonged as judged on a case by case basis.*

### 2. NINE-MONTH REGIMEN: PYRAZINAMIDE CONTRAINDICATED

Isoniazid and rifampin.

If > 4% CHANCE OF RESISTANCE TO ISONIAZID, ethambutol should be added in adults and streptomycin in children too young for visual acuity testing.

If isoniazid RESISTANCE IS DEMONSTRATED ON CULTURE, rifampin and ethambutol should be continued for a minimum of 12 months.

### 3. DIRECT-OBSERVED THERAPY

The Denver regimen

Consider its use in all patients but especially in patients where lack of compliance is an issue.

2 weeks of daily isoniazid, rifampin, pyrazinamide, and streptomycin or ethambutol (as per protocol 1), followed by 6 weeks of twice-weekly high dosages of the same drugs, followed by 4 months of twice-weekly high doses of isoniazid and rifampin.

### 4. MULTIPLE-DRUG RESISTANCE

Therapy must be individualized based on susceptibility testing. Consult a TB expert.

### 5. EXTRAPULMONARY TUBERCULOSIS

For adults manage according to the principles and with the drug regimens outlined above.

For children with miliary tuberculosis, bone or joint tuberculosis, or tuberculous meningitis, a minimum of 12 months of therapy is suggested.

### 6. PEDIATRIC TUBERCULOSIS

Managed as adults except in the circumstances mentioned above.

*In all cases a TB expert should be consulted if the patient is symptomatic or smear or culture has positive results after 3 months.

encouraged. All patients with base-line laboratory abnormalities should have follow-up tests during therapy. If base-line laboratory tests were normal, no further tests are required, unless symptoms should develop.

## SPECIAL CONSIDERATIONS IN TREATMENT

**Extrapulmonary tuberculosis.** The principles that underlie the treatment of pulmonary tuberculosis also apply to extrapulmonary tuberculosis. Despite the lack of comparable carefully controlled trials, however, increasing clinical experience indicates that short courses of 6 to 9 months of therapy are effective.[4,17] As previously mentioned, miliary pattern, bone and joint involvement, and meningeal involvement warrant a minimum of 12 months of therapy. Several points to keep in mind include the following: First, bacteriologic evaluation of extrapulmonary tuberculosis often is impossible because of the site of disease; second, adjunctive therapies such as surgery and corticosteroids are more commonly required, as in the treatment of constrictive pericarditis and spinal cord compression from Pott's disease; third, steroids are of proved efficacy in preventing cardiac constriction from tuberculous pericarditis and in decreasing the neurologic sequelae of tuberculous meningitis.

**Pregnancy and lactation.** In a pregnant woman with tuberculosis it is essential that effective therapy be given immediately. Untreated tuberculosis is a far greater hazard to a pregnant woman and her fetus than therapy is.[18] Tuberculosis is not an indication for termination of pregnancy. Initial therapy should include isoniazid and rifampin. Ethambutol should be added unless the risk of isoniazid resistance is low. In the United States, pyrazinamide is not routinely used because of the lack of data on its teratogenicity. Internationally, pyrazinamide is used routinely in therapy. Isoniazid, rifampin, and ethambutol all cross the placenta, but they have not proved to be teratogenic. Pyridoxine is recommended for pregnant women receiving isoniazid. Streptomycin is the only drug documented to have harmful effects on the fetus by interfering with ear development, and it may cause congenital deafness. This toxic side effect is presumably shared by kanamycin, and capreomycin though this presumption has not been definitively proved. The effects of ethionamide and cycloserine are not known; however, they should be avoided if possible. Breast feeding should not be discouraged because only small concentrations of antituberculous agents are found in breast milk. Accordingly, drugs in breast milk should not be considered effective therapy for tuberculous infection or disease in the nursing infant.

## FIRST-LINE DRUGS IN CURRENT USE

**Isoniazid (INH).** Isoniazid is the ideal agent, being bactericidal, relatively nontoxic, easily administered, inexpensive, and highly active against *Mycobacterium tuberculosis.* Absorption from the gastrointestinal tract is nearly complete. The drug penetrates into all body fluids and cavities, producing therapeutic levels in all locations. The recommended dose is 3 to 5 mg/kg, up to a maximum of 300 mg/day (supplied as 150 mg capsules).

Hepatitis is the most consistent toxic effect of INH, and the rate of hepatitis increases with age.[19] In a study of 13,838 patients the following rates were seen when INH was used as a single agent: 0% for those younger than 20 years of age, 0.3% for patients between 21 and 34 years of age, 1.2% for those between 35 and 49 years of age, and 2.3% for patients between 50 to 64 years of age. Alcohol consumption has been identified as a major risk cofactor.[14]

Peripheral neuropathy is associated with INH use and most likely is caused by interference with pyridoxine metabolism. In persons more prone to this side effect, such as patients with diabetes, uremia, alcoholism, and malnutrition, supplemental pyridoxine should be given. Pregnant women and persons with a seizure disorder also should receive pyridoxine supplementation. Mild or major central nervous system side effects are common with isoniazid. Seizures, optic neuritis, memory impairment, and muscle twitching have been reported. Hypersensitivity reactions, agranulocytosis, anemia, and thrombocytopenia occur rarely. Drug-induced lupus with positive antinuclear antibodies may be seen. Disulfiram-like reactions also are seen with INH use. INH has monoamine oxidase inhibitor (MAOI) activity. Therefore foods with tyramine and histamine should be avoided. Lastly, INH may cause hyperglycemia and poor glucose control in patients receiving hypoglycemics orally.

Concurrent use of phenytoin increases the serum concentration of both drugs. Thus monitoring and appropriate adjustment of phenytoin dosage is required.

**Rifampin (RIF).** Rifampin is bactericidal, relatively nontoxic, easy to administer, quickly absorbed from the gastrointestinal tract and penetrates well into tissues and cells, even though it is 75% protein bound. It penetrates into the cerebrospinal fluid only when the meninges are inflamed. A single daily dose of 600 mg/day should be used (supplied as 300 mg capsules). Gastrointestinal upset is the most common adverse reaction. Symptoms include heartburn, nausea, vomiting, epigastric distress, cramps, and diarrhea. Other reported reactions include skin eruptions, hepatitis, cholestatic jaundice, and thrombocytopenia. In general the frequency of these reactions is quite low.

RIF induces the hepatic microsomal enzymes, and so it accelerates the clearance of drugs metabolized by the liver. These agents include methadone, warfarin, glucocorticoids, estrogens, oral hypoglycemic agents, digitoxin, antiarrhythmic agents (quinidine, verapamil, mexiletene), theophylline, anticonvulsants, ketoconazole, and cyclosporin A. RIF may interfere with the efficacy of the birth-control pill. Concomitant antacid administration may reduce the absorption of RIF. Probenecid and cotrimoxizole have been reported to increase the level of RIF. In adults, intermittent doses of RIF larger than 10 mg/kg may be associated with thrombocytopenia, an influenza-like syndrome, hemolytic anemia, and acute renal failure; these reactions are uncommon at the recommended doses. RIF is excreted in urine, tears, sweat, and other body fluids, rendering such fluids orange. Patients should be warned of this side effect in advance and of the possible permanent discoloration of soft contact lenses and clothing.

**Pyrazinamide (PZA).** Pyrazinamide, bactericidal in an acid environment, is active against organisms in macrophages, presumably because of the acid environment within the cell. PZA penetrates well into most tissues, including the cerebrospinal fluid. A single dose of 15 to 30 mg/kg should be taken daily (supplied as 300 mg capsules). The most important adverse reaction associated with its use is its liver toxicity. There does not appear to be a significant increase in hepatotoxicity when it is added (in a dose of 15 to 30 mg/kg) for the initial 2 months of therapy with INH and RIF. Hyperuricemia occurs frequently, occasionally accompanied by arthralgias, but acute gouty attacks are uncommon. Salicylates provide symptomatic relief of pyrazinamide-associated arthralgias. Skin rash and gastrointestinal intolerance are occasionally seen. Liver function tests and uric acid levels should be checked.

**Ethambutol (EMB).** In usual doses ethambutol generally is considered to be bacteriostatic; higher doses used for intermittent therapy may have a bactericidal effect. The drug, easily administered, has a low frequency of adverse effects. The drug accumulates in patients with renal insufficiency. Cerebrospinal fluid penetration is weak, even in the presence of inflamed meninges. The recommended dose is 15 mg/kg as a single daily dose (supplied as 100 mg tablets). The most frequent adverse effect is retrobulbar neuritis. Symptoms include blurred vision, scotomas, and red-green color blindness. A dose-related toxicity, it occurs in less than 1% of patients given the standard daily dose of 15 mg/kg but increases with a daily dose of 25 mg/kg. The frequency of ocular side effects is increased in patients with renal failure. Visual symptoms commonly precede a measurable decreased visual acuity. Accordingly, monthly ophthalmologic exams are required. In children too young to have an accurate assessment of their visual acuity and red-green color discrimination, EMB should not be used.

**Streptomycin (SM).** Streptomycin, bactericidal in an alkaline environment, must be given parenterally because it is not absorbed from the gastrointestinal tract. Excretion is almost entirely renal; its dosage thus must be reduced in renal insufficiency. The drug has good tissue penetration, but cerebrospinal fluid penetration is seen only in the presence of meningeal irritation. A single intramuscular dose of 15 mg/kg daily (maximum of 1 g/day), or 25 to 30 mg/kg twice weekly (maximum of 1.5 g/day) are the most common regimens. Vestibular ototoxicity, the most common serious adverse effect, usually results in vertigo, but hearing loss may occur. Ototoxicity is enhanced in the presence of other ototoxic agents. Audiometric and caloric exams at base-line time and during therapy are required.

The incidence of nephrotoxicity is less than that seen with kanamycin and capreomycin. Preexisting renal failure or concomitant use with other nephrotoxic agents increases its renal toxicity. Other reported side effects include facial paresthesias, rash, fever, eosinophilia, urticaria, and angioneurotic edema. Persons older than 60 years have an

**Table 37-2.** *Second line antituberculous chemotherapeutic agents*

| Drug | Dose | Side Effects | Comments |
|------|------|--------------|----------|
| *para*-Aminosalicylic acid (PAS) | 150 mg/kg (max. 10–12 g/day) | GI: nausea, vomiting, diarrhea<br>Hepatic: hepatitis (uncommon)<br>Hypersensitivity: 5%–10% | Monitor liver function tests monthly. If fivefold or greater increase, the medicine should be discontinued. |
| Ethionamide | 15–20 mg/kg (max. 1 g/day) | GI: nausea, vomiting, loss of appetite<br>Hepatic: hepatitis<br>Other: arthralgias, impotence, dermatitis, hypothyroidism, metallic taste, gynecomastia | |
| Cycloserine | 15–20 mg/kg (max. 1 g/day) | Neuropsychiatric: most common including psychosis, seizures, peripheral neuropathy, especially with concurrent ioniazid use | Patients with a neuropsychiatric history are at greater risk. Pyridoxine supplementation (150 mg/day). |
| Capreomycin | 15-30 mg/kg (max. 1 g/day) IM | Neurologic: toxic to eighth cranial nerve causing hearing loss in 3.2% to 9.4%<br>Renal: tubular dysfunction common | Audiogram at base-line time and every other month thereafter. |

| Drug | Dose | Side effects | Monitoring |
|---|---|---|---|
| Amikacin | 15 mg/kg IM or IV | Renal toxicity common, electrolyte abnormalities. Other: vestibular dysfunction, hearing loss, circumoral numbness | Watch renal funtion and electrolytes. Andiogram at base-line time and every other month. |
| Quinolones | Ciprofloxicin, 750 mg bid Ofloxacin, 400 mg bid | GI: Distress, nausea Hepatic: elevated liver function tests Hypersensitivity: uncommon; generally well tolerated | Monitor theophylline levels. Antacids affect absorption. |
| Rifabutin | 300 mg/day | GI: distress Hepatic: hepatitis uncommon Hypersensitivity: uncommon | |
| Clofazamine | 50–100 mg/day | GI: distress common Other: skin and eye discoloration, life-threatening organ damage caused by crystal deposition | |

increased incidence of ototoxicity and nephrotoxicity. As such, physicians should try to avoid its use in this age group. A cumulative dose of more than 120 g should not be given unless there are no other therapeutic options.

# SECOND-LINE DRUGS

By definition, second-line antituberculous chemotherapy agents have a lower ratio of therapeutic efficacy to toxicity than first-line drugs have. Some of the newer agents have been used successfully to treat other common infections and have been noted to be helpful in the treatment of *Mycobacterium tuberculosis* infection. However, the experience with their use when first-line agents fail or are contraindicated is limited. Thus the patient must be followed closely. In general, any patient receiving second-line agents or newer antibiotics should be managed by a pulmonary and tuberculosis specialist. These agents are listed in Table 37-2 along with their doses and adverse effects.

## References

1. American Thoracic Society: Control of tuberculosis in the United States, *Am Rev Respir Dis* 146:1623, 1993.
2. Glassroth J, Robbins AG, Snider DE Jr: Tuberculosis in the 1980s, *N Engl J Med* 302:1441, 1980.
3. Davies BH: Infectivity of tuberculosis, *Thorax* 35:481, 1980.
4. American Thoracic Society: Treatment of tuberculosis and tuberculosis infection in adults and children, *Am J Respir Crit Care Med* 149:1359-1374, 1994.
5. Munt PW: Miliary tuberculosis in the chemotherapy era: with a clinical review in 69 American adults, *Medicine* 51:139, 1972.
6. Levy H, Feldman C, Sacho H, et al: A reevaluation of sputum microscopy and culture in the diagnosis of pulmonary tuberculosis, *Chest* 95:1193, 1989.
7. Greenbaum M, Beyt BE, Murray PR: The accuracy of diagnosing tuberculosis at a large teaching hospital, *Am Rev Respir Dis* 121:477, 1980.
8. Middlebrook G, Reggiardo Z, Tigertt WD: Automatable radiometric detection of growth of *Mycobacterium tuberculosis* in selective media, *Am Rev Respir Dis* 115:1066, 1977.
9. Schluger NW, Rom WN: Current approaches to the diagnosis of active pulmonary tuberculosis, *Am J Respir Crit Care Med* 149:264-267, 1994.
10. Gordin FM, Slutkin G, Schecter G, et al: Presumptive diagnosis and treatment of pulmonary tuberculosis based on radiographic findings, *Am Rev Respir Dis* 139:1090, 1989.
11. Choyke PL, Sustman HD, Curtis AM, et al: Adult onset pulmonary tuberculosis, *Radiology* 148:357, 1983.
12. Berger HW, Granada MG: Lower lung field tuberculosis, *Chest* 65:522, 1974.
13. Sochocky S: Tuberculoma of the lung, *Am Rev Tuberc* 78:403, 1958.
14. Peres-Stable EJ, Hopewell PC: Chemotherapy of tuberculosis, *Semin Respir Med* 117:991, 1978.
15. Iseman MD, Madsen LA: Drug resistant tuberculosis, *Clin Chest Med* 10:341, 1989.

16. Centers for Disease Control and Prevention: Transmission of multidrug-resistant TB among immuno-compromised persons in a correctional system: New York, *MMWR* 41:507, 1991.

17. Dutt AK, Stead WW: Treatment of extrapulmonary tuberculosis, *Semin Respir Infect* 4:225, 1989.

18. Snider DE, Layde RM, Johnson MW, Lyle MA: Treatment of tuberculosis during pregnancy, *Am Rev Respir Dis* 122:65, 1980.

19. Kopanoff DE, Snider DE, Caras GJ: Isoniazid related hepatitis, *Am Rev Respir Dis* 117:991, 1978.

# Chapter 38

# Advanced Chronic Obstructive Pulmonary Disease

Ayman O. Soubani
David S. Lazarus

Chronic obstructive pulmonary diseases (COPD) constitute a range of disorders of the airways and lung parenchyma, with most patients having some combination of chronic bronchitis and emphysema. In addition, there may be bronchospasm, decreased diffusion capacity, hypoxemia, or hypercapnia. The prevalence of COPD has remained constant at 110 out of 1000 men but has increased steadily in women over the past 15 years to reach the same level.[1] Mortality attributable to COPD has increased 36% over the past 15 years and is now the fourth leading cause of death in the United States. Overall, the 3-year survival rate of all patients with COPD is 40% to 65%, depending on age and the degree of obstruction.[2] Although curative therapies do not exist, there are new modalities of therapy that may improve or stabilize pulmonary function in moderately to severely affected patients.

A working definition of COPD is the presence of a fixed reduction in expiratory airflow with gas trapping caused by a loss of elastic recoil within the airways. Pathologically, destruction of lung parenchyma, hypertrophy of airway smooth muscle cells, and excessive production of sputum contribute to the obstructive ventilatory defect. Clinically this is manifested during pulmonary function testing (PFT) by a reduced forced expiratory volume in the first second ($FEV_1$) with a relatively preserved forced vital capacity (FVC), resulting in a decreased $FEV_1$/FVC ratio. The degree of airway obstruction is based on the percentage decrease in the $FEV_1$ relative to a predicted value[3] (Table 38-1). For the purposes of this chapter, *advanced* COPD is considered to be a "moderately severe" obstruction or worse. In some patients, however, the degree of clinical impairment does not correlate well with the degree of obstruction found during PFT. In this subset of individuals, advanced COPD is considered to include failure of conventional therapy, greatly deranged arterial blood gases, frequent hospitalizations or urgent office visits, or symptoms out of proportion to the degree of

**Table 38-1.** *Criteria for assessing severity of chronic obstructive pulmonary diseases (COPD)*

| Severity of Obstruction | Criteria |
|---|---|
| Normal | $FEV_1$/FVC within 95% CI<br>VC within 95% CI |
| Mild obstruction | $FEV_1$/FVC < lower limit of normal and % predicted $FEV_1$ <100 and ≥70 |
| Moderate obstruction | % predicted $FEV_1$ <70 and ≥60 |
| Moderately severe obstruction | % predicted $FEV_1$ <60 and ≥50 |
| Severe obstruction | % predicted $FEV_1$ <50 and ≥34 |
| Very severe obstruction | % predicted $FEV_1$ <34 |

*$FEV_1$,* Forced expiratory volume in the first second; *FVC,* forced vital capacity; *95% CI,* lower limit of normal, below the 95% confidence interval; *VC,* vital capacity.

airway obstruction. Large-scale studies of many therapies used for advanced COPD only now are being conducted. Until these results are available, therapies that improve functional activity and sense of well-being are advocated for selected patients.

## MEDICAL THERAPY

### Routine therapy
The mainstays of routine therapy for COPD are inhaled beta-adrenergic receptor agonists and anticholinergic agents because of their bronchodilator and antisecretory actions.[4] Theophylline, which has mild bronchodilating effects and may augment respiratory muscle function, also may be used. Patients without response to bronchodilators during repeated pulmonary function testing, however, often have minimal response to these drugs.

### Use of corticosteroids
Corticosteroids often are used in patients with advanced disease, though the efficacy of this therapy is controversial. A recent meta-analysis of corticosteroid trials for advanced COPD determined that $FEV_1$ improved in only 10% of treated patients as compared to placebo-treated patients.[5] Some patients may have a 10% to 20% increase in $FEV_1$ after treatment with oral steroids. This, however, represents a very small absolute improvement because of the severe nature of the underlying obstruction. Many patients feel subjectively better without

objective evidence of improvement because of the psychotropic effects of steroids. Because no study has demonstrated improved survival attributable to steroid use in patients with COPD, the small degree of improvement in a subset of patients must be balanced against the many risks of steroid use, especially in the elderly.

Our approach is to employ a trial of oral steroids in stable outpatients who have a significant bronchodilator response (that is, a >20% improvement in $FEV_1$ either immediately after inhaled bronchodilators or after 2 weeks of outpatient bronchodilator therapy) and who have not improved after treatment with maximal inhaled therapy and orally administered theophylline. Spirometry is repeated after 3 to 4 weeks of 40 to 60 mg/day of prednisone or equivalent. Patients with a >20% improvement in airflow rates then continue long-term or intermittent steroid therapy, using the lowest dose possible. Inhaled steroids may be an alternative for a few patients, but, overall, these preparations are ineffective in patients with advanced COPD. The utility of intravenous steroids in acutely ill patients is unproved and should be reserved for the 10% to 15% patients with known bronchodilator responses.

## Long-term oxygen therapy

Patients with advanced COPD and hypoxemia have a poor prognosis. The use of continuous oxygen is the only therapy proved to increase survival in these patients.[6] The goal of oxygen therapy should be improvement in oxygen delivery to vital tissues, not just a fixed level of partial pressure of oxygen ($Pao_2$) in arterial blood. Oxygen delivery is dependent on cardiac output and on the amount and saturation of hemoglobin. Increases in oxygen saturation above 90% to 92%, therefore, offer little benefit but do increase complications and cost.

Two multicenter trials proved conclusively that long-term oxygen therapy (LTOT) improved survival[7,8] in patients with a resting $Pao_2$ <55 mm Hg, or a $Pao_2$ <59 mm Hg with concomitant pulmonary hypertension, a hematocrit above 55, or peripheral edema (Fig. 38-1). Mortality decreased significantly in the group using oxygen continuously for at least 19 hours daily, compared to patients receiving only nocturnal oxygen. Pulmonary hypertension (defined as a mean right ventricular systolic pressure >35 mm Hg) is also an independent risk factor for death from COPD.[6] Doppler echocardiography is an accurate method to estimate pulmonary arterial pressure and should be performed in patients with a resting $Pao_2$ <60 mm Hg.

The current indications for LTOT and the standard Medicare criteria for reimbursable oxygen therapy are summarized in Table 38-2. Nearly all patients should undergo arterial blood gas analysis at least once during this period for evaluation of both oxygen and carbon dioxide levels. The dose of oxygen used should be sufficient to raise the resting $Pao_2$ to a range of 60 to 65 mm Hg (hemoglobin saturation of 90% to 95%), provided that respiratory acidosis does not occur. If hemoglobin desaturation still occurs while the patient is sleeping or exercising, the oxygen flow rate should be increased by 1 L/min during those activities.

In patients who do not meet the criteria for LTOT but develop hemoglobin desaturation during sleep or exercise, oxygen supplemen-

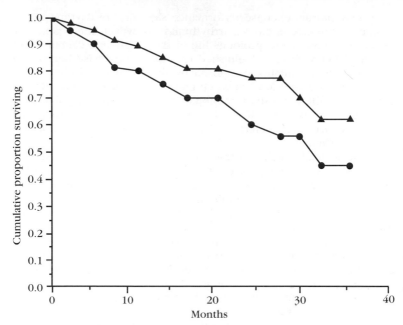

**Figure 38-1.** *Results of the Nocturnal Oxygen Therapy Group: Continuous or nocturnal oxygen therapy in hypoxemic chronic obstructive lung disease study, demonstrating improved survival when continuous oxygen (triangles) was used, compared to nocturnal only oxygen use (circles). (From Reference 7 with permission.)*

**Table 38-2.** *Criteria for use of supplemental oxygen*

| Indications | Requirements |
|---|---|
| Pao$_2$ ≤55 mm Hg or O$_2$ sat. ≤88% on room air *or* | Optimal medical management before certification for LTOT |
| Pao$_2$ 56 to 59 mm Hg *or* | |
| O$_2$ sat. 89% and one choice of ECG evidence of cor pulmonale *or* erythrocytosis (hematocrit >56%) | Measurement of arterial blood gases or hemoglobin saturation by a "qualified" lab |
| Pao$_2$ ≥60 mm Hg *or* O$_2$ sat. >90% with "compelling justification" | Completion of form HCFA-484 by the physician |

*HCFA-484*, Health Care Financing Administration form 484; *LTOT*, long-term oxygen therapy; *sat.*, saturation.

tation may improve exercise performance, sleep quality, daytime performance, and reduce nocturnal arrhythmias.[9] However, there is no evidence that oxygen use prolongs life in these patients. Patients with advanced COPD have a diminished capacity for exercise because of the mechanical limitations imposed by the airways and chest wall, rather than by a lack of oxygen. Often there is a cardiac limitation to exercise as well, because of pulmonary hypertension, cor pulmonale, or concomitant ischemic heart disease. These limitations, rather than a decreased $Pao_2$, often increase the sense of dyspnea on exertion and impair mobility.

In the acute setting, supplemental oxygen is given to increase $Pao_2$ to at least 60 mm Hg, equivalent to an arterial oxygen saturation of at least 90%. However, increasing $Pao_2$ beyond 65 mm Hg (hemoglobin saturation above 92% to 95%) minimally increases oxygen delivery and may impair hypoxic ventilatory drive, leading to hypoventilation and carbon dioxide ($CO_2$) retention.

Home oxygen is provided using refillable liquid oxygen containers, oxygen concentrators, or compressed gas in tanks. Liquid oxygen containers are portable but are more expensive and need frequent service to replenish the oxygen. The other two sources are cheaper but are not portable. The best method to deliver oxygen is by nasal prongs. Use of an on-demand flow device can substantially reduce wastage and prolong portable tank usage time. The long-term usefulness and reliability of these devices have not been established, however. A transtracheal oxygen catheter, inserted through the cricoid cartilage under local anesthesia, may reduce oxygen usage up to 50%; this approach is particularly useful for patients requiring high oxygen-flow rates. Transtracheal oxygen delivery may also improve the patient's self-image, increasing compliance and social interaction. However, this method also requires humidification and daily saline irrigation. In addition, bleeding, local irritation, pneumothorax, subcutaneous emphysema, and inadvertent catheter removal are potential complications.

## Alpha-1 antitrypsin replacement therapy

Alpha$_1$-antitrypsin (AAT) deficiency causes severe COPD in a small number of patients.[10] The disease is caused by mutations in the AAT gene that impair release of AAT from hepatocytes, resulting in a severely diminished plasma level of the enzyme. The normal function of AAT is to inactivate neutrophil elastase; therefore, AAT deficiency allows destruction of vital connective tissues in the lung. Panacinar emphysema results, often in the lower lung fields, with the most severe disease occurring in smokers. Patients who develop emphysema between 30 and 45 years of age should be investigated for AAT deficiency, especially if there is evidence of concomitant liver disease, or a history of prolonged neonatal jaundice. The first step should be measurement of serum AAT levels by an experienced laboratory; a true level below 11 $\mu$M is considered abnormal. Patients with low AAT levels should then have their AAT genetic phenotype analyzed. A normal phenotype is PiMM, whereas the usual mutant phenotypes are PiZZ, PiZ-null or Pi null-null. Although there have not been any controlled studies of

AAT replacement therapy, strong consideration should be given to treating patients whose serum AAT level is <11 $\mu$M with a mutant phenotype and advanced obstructive disease on PFT. AAT is replaced by use of intermittent infusions of human enzyme (Prolastin, Miles Pharmaceuticals, West Haven, Conn.) purified from pooled plasma. The dose given should increase serum levels above the critical threshold level of 11 $\mu$M. Although this therapy is safe, hepatitis B vaccination and HIV testing are performed before the initiation of therapy, as with use of any human blood product.

## Mucolytic therapy

Chronic bronchitis is characterized by excessive production of thick mucus. The increased viscosity of this sputum is partially attributable to the presence of extracellular DNA released by destroyed neutrophils during inflammatory or infectious processes. Traditional mucolytic therapies using iodinated glycerol or $N$-acetylcysteine are not effective in the management of chronic bronchitis. Recombinant human DNase (Pulmozyme, Genentech, South San Francisco, Calif.) may reduce these secretions to a less viscous state, facilitating access of antibiotics to airway pathogens, reducing bacterial colonization, decreasing the frequency of acute pulmonary exacerbations, and improving overall pulmonary function. Clinical trials have been published only in the cystic fibrosis population, demonstrating mild to moderate benefit.[11] Studies in patients with advanced COPD are still ongoing. The long-term benefit and cost effectiveness of this therapy therefore remain unclear.

# NONINVASIVE METHODS OF VENTILATION

Patients with advanced COPD and hypercapnia attributable to respiratory muscle fatigue may be helped using noninvasive methods of ventilation. In addition, those with pronounced dyspnea, nocturnal symptoms, or frequent hospitalizations for acute COPD exacerbations may benefit from a trial of noninvasive ventilation attempting to rest their respiratory muscles, lower arterial $CO_2$ levels, and improve the sensation of dyspnea.

## Continuous positive airway pressure (CPAP)

Positive airway pressure (usually 2.5 to 10 cm $H_2O$) is delivered by face or nasal mask during both inspiration and expiration. The patient must perform a substantial amount of work to generate airflow using this method. In theory, adding positive airway pressure during expiration will prevent dynamic airway collapse and therefore decrease the volume of air-trapping at end expiration. CPAP can also decrease atelectasis resulting from pneumonia, airway secretions, or pulmonary edema, thereby improving oxygenation, and may improve cardiac function in the setting of congestive heart failure. CPAP may be detrimental to some patients, especially those with respiratory muscle weakness, decreased level of consciousness, or risk of aspiration. The increased expiratory work of breathing may not be tolerated by some patients.

## Intermittent positive-pressure ventilation (IPPV)

In this method, positive pressure is generated using small portable ventilators that introduce fixed levels (5 to 20 cm $H_2O$) of inspiratory pressure when the patient initiates an inspiratory effort. The inspiratory flow provided by the ventilator overcomes some of the resistive properties of the lung, decreasing the work of breathing required of the patient. Newer models (BiPAP, Respironics, Monroeville, Penna.) can provide both inspiratory and expiratory pressures. The addition of expiratory pressure may prevent dynamic airway collapse and reduce air-trapping, as in CPAP. Some studies have shown that patients with severe COPD, especially those with chronic hypercapnic respiratory failure, may benefit from long-term IPPV. In one study, nine of 13 patients decreased their respiratory rates, heart rates, and $Paco_2$ and improved their physical activity after 2 months of therapy.[12] However, a crossover, randomized trial of IPPV during sleep versus conventional therapy did not show a difference in pulmonary function, respiratory muscle strength, gas exchange, or exercise endurance. IPPV also may have a role in the management of acute exacerbations of COPD. A prospective randomized clinical trial reported lower $Paco_2$ levels, improved respiratory acidosis, and a significant reduction in mortality in 30 COPD patients with acute exacerbation treated with IPPV when compared to conventional treatment.[13] Patients with hypercapnia who do not improve with IPPV may be rebreathing $CO_2$ within the mask, which may improve with use of a nonrebreathing device. IPPV requires a significant amount of patient motivation and education. Mask discomfort, nasal congestion, dry mouth, and interference with sleep and bed partners are frequent limiting factors. IPPV should not be used in patients with excessive secretions, reduced gag reflex, or altered sensorium.

## Intermittent negative-pressure ventilation

The application of negative pressure to the chest wall acts to augment expansion of the chest cavity, decreasing the work of breathing performed by the patient. This method applies cyclic negative pressures to the chest wall using a vacuum apparatus attached to a shell cuirass, body wrap, or iron lung. Significant improvements in inspiratory muscle strength, arterial blood gases, and vital capacity were reported in 18 patients who received negative-pressure ventilation 4 to 10 hours daily for several months. However, a large controlled study of 184 patients with COPD randomized to either negative-pressure ventilation or sham therapy did not show any statistically significant differences in exercise capacity, daytime arterial blood gases, respiratory muscle strength, severity of dyspnea, or quality of life.[14] Home intermittent negative-pressure ventilation results in little benefit to most patients with COPD. Certain highly motivated patients may have subjective improvement, however.

# INVASIVE METHODS OF VENTILATION

Some patients can be managed using chronic positive-pressure ventilation delivered through a cuffed tracheostomy tube, either for part of the day or continuously. For patients requiring partial support, a fenestrated tracheostomy tube can be used, whereby removal of the inner cannula permits airflow across the vocal cords and vocalization. Portable or semiportable ventilators are available for use in wheelchairs, home, or subacute-care institutions. Use of these ventilators over a long term requires a high degree of patient (and family or caregiver) motivation and effort. However, in the appropriate setting, an adequate quality of life can be achieved.

# PULMONARY REHABILITATION

The most disturbing symptom to patients with COPD is dyspnea, resulting in limitation of activity. Dyspnea is related to multiple factors including abnormal pulmonary mechanics, impairment in pulmonary gas exchange, an abnormal perception of breathlessness and ventilatory control, the presence of impaired cardiac performance caused by cor pulmonale or ischemic heart disease, poor nutritional status, and the development of respiratory muscle dysfunction. When dyspnea persists and activities are limited despite optimal medical control, a rehabilitation program can increase exercise capacity, reduce anxiety, and improve quality of life and functional status. Several studies show decreased inpatient hospital days in patients undergoing rehabilitation programs. It is unclear, however, whether pulmonary rehabilitation programs improve survival.[15]

Patients should be considered for pulmonary rehabilitation when they are medically stable on maximal medical therapy. Initial screening includes spirometry, arterial blood gases, and exercise evaluation by a standard 12-minute walk, cycle ergometry, or treadmill testing. Psychosocial evaluation is an essential part of the screening process because well-motivated patients are more likely to benefit from the rehabilitation program.

Rehabilitation programs usually are supervised by a pulmonologist and are staffed by a multidisciplinary team composed of a respiratory nurse, respiratory therapist, occupational therapist, dietitian, social worker, and psychologist. Most patients participate in outpatient programs; however, severely disabled patients may require an inpatient program for evaluation and initial care until functional capacity has improved. The program structure should provide the following[2]: (1) exercise reconditioning by stair climbing, treadmill walking, or cycle ergometry; (2) upper extremity strength training to improve accessory respiratory muscle function; (3) breathing retraining, including pursed-lip breathing, expiratory muscle augmentation, synchronized movement of the abdomen and thorax, and relaxation techniques directed at accessory respiratory muscles; (4) instruction in work simplification and the use of energy conservation devices that allow improved ability to perform independent activities; (5) psychosocial rehabilitation, employing education, counseling, biofeedback, relaxation, and group supportive therapies; (6) smoking cessation programs; and (7) nutritional support. For patients unwilling or unable to participate in an extensive program, significant benefit can still be derived from an unstructured program using a treadmill, free-range walking, or cycling, for 1 to 2 hours per week.

## NUTRITIONAL SUPPORT

The exact incidence of undernutrition in patients with COPD is not known but ranges from 24% of stable outpatients to 47% of hospitalized patients.[16] Undernutrition has been associated with decreased survival in patients with severe COPD because of reduced respiratory muscle strength and impaired immune function manifested by lymphopenia, anergy, and susceptibility to infection.

Nutritional assessment should include clinical history of anorexia, difficulty in chewing or swallowing, degree of breathlessness on eating, and assessment of caloric intake and energy requirements. Body weight should be compared to ideal body weight and to weight history. Anthropometric measurements, including triceps-skinfold thickness (a reflection of total body fat) and forearm muscle circumference (a marker of protein content), also are useful. Patients with COPD often display reduced fat stores but preservation of protein content. Several small studies indicate that improvement in muscle strength, endurance, and pulmonary function occurs only when there is a net gain in weight. However, survival is not increased in successfully nourished patients for unclear reasons. A conservative approach to nutrition in these patients therefore is to start with dietary counseling if weight loss is mild. If this approach is unsuccessful or if there is severe weight loss, a trial of food supplements can be attempted. For patients with hypercapnia or elevated minute ventilation or both, adding high fat-content supplements to the diet may be beneficial, though this is not proved. Many patients will not gain weight despite adequate caloric intake and therefore do not benefit from aggressive nutritional supplementation.

## SURGICAL THERAPY

The role of surgery in the management of advanced COPD is very limited and in general should be avoided. There are, however, special situations where a surgical approach may be helpful. Patients considered for such an approach should be carefully evaluated and the risks and benefits meticulously weighed and explained to the patient.

### Lung transplantation
The International Lung Transplant Registry lists over 2000 patients as lung-transplant recipients since 1983, two thirds over the past 2 years. Long-term results on large populations of patients therefore are not

**Table 38-3.** *Recipient criteria for lung transplantation in advanced COPD*

| Indications | Contraindications |
|---|---|
| End-stage disease resulting in: | **ABSOLUTE** |
|   Frequent hospitalizations | Serious psychiatric illness, that is, |
|   Progressive deterioration of |   functional psychosis, organic |
|     pulmonary function |   brain disease, history of self- |
|   Inability to perform normal |   destructive acts, history of |
|     daily activities |   noncompliance with therapy |
|   Life expectancy of less than | Refractory right ventricular failure |
|     18 months | Irreversible hepatic or renal disease |
| Conditions included: | Active systemic infection, HIV |
|   Severe COPD (emphysema, | Presence of systemic disease |
|     chronic bronchitis, |   affected by immunosuppression |
|     bronchiectasis, asthma) | Active neoplastic disease |
|   Bronchiolitis obliterans | **RELATIVE** |
|   Congenital lobar emphysema | Active coronary artery disease |
|   Alpha$_1$-antitrypsin deficiency | Age over 55 years |
|   Bronchopulmonary dysplasia | Drug, alcohol, tobacco abuse |
|   Cystic fibrosis | Chronic use of oral steroids |
|   Pulmonary agenesis | |

yet available. Currently, obstructive lung disease, including COPD and alpha$_1$-antitrypsin deficiency, is the most common indication for lung transplantation. In the St. Louis series, the 2-year survival rate is 94% for patients with COPD and 73% for all alpha$_1$-antitrypsin deficiency.[17] Preliminary long term results indicate that 5 year survival rates may be significantly less than this, in the 50% to 60% range. The most common causes of early postoperative death are sepsis and cardiac failure, whereas chronic rejection is the primary cause of late posttransplant death. On average, COPD patients can double the distance they can walk in 6 minutes after a single lung transplant and can triple this distance after a bilateral lung transplant. Single lung transplantation is the most common procedure for patients with severe COPD because bilateral transplants result in greater short-term mortality. Waiting periods are often 200 to 500 days, and 20% to 40% of lung transplant candidates die while waiting for a donor.

The guidelines for selecting patients for lung transplantation vary among transplant centers, but in general the patient should have severe COPD and poor short-term prognosis using medical therapy alone. Table 38-3 describes the guidelines for lung transplantation used by the Massachusetts Consortium for Lung Transplantation. Although prior cardiothoracic surgery or pleurodesis increases the technical difficulty and complications of the operation, these conditions are not considered an absolute contraindication to lung transplantation. In addition, chronic use of low-dose steroids (less than 10 mg of prednisone per day) is not an absolute contraindication. Patients who fulfill the criteria for lung transplantation are referred to specialized centers for further evaluation and participation in a structured rehabilitation and nutritional program. During and after transplantation, patients receive an immunosuppressive regimen of antilymphocyte antibodies, corticosteroids, azathioprine, and cyclosporin A. Despite this, about 25% of patients develop some degree of bronchiolitis obliterans syndrome (BOS), believed to be attributable to persistent, low-level rejection. The presence of BOS often causes severe impairment in allograft function. The increased immunosuppression required to suppress the underlying rejection leads to a greater incidence of opportunistic infections. Although some episodes of BOS are reversible with therapy, BOS remains the most important impediment to the long-term success of transplanted lungs.

## Bullectomy

Bullae are large air-containing spaces in the lung without functional lung tissue. They usually occur congenitally, or in severe emphysema, and radiographically present as large areas of hyperlucency. Specific intervention is not usually indicated; however, large subpleural bullae occasionally may enlarge to such a massive degree that compression of adjacent functional lung tissue causes incapacitating dyspnea. Chest CT scanning is often useful in differentiating functional lung from scar tissue abutting the bullae. If a bullae occupies more than one third of the hemithorax, surgical excision or laser ablation of the bullae can result in significant functional improvement.

## Volume reduction surgery

This technique recently has led to dramatic improvement in a few, selected patients. The patient undergoes sequential thoracotomies, with resection of multiple areas of emphysematous lung tissue. The result is a smaller lung with less air-trapping, allowing areas of functional lung to expand with improved ventilation-perfusion relationships. The decreased lung volume also enables the diaphragm, respiratory muscles, and chest wall to undergo remodeling, thereby improving their force-tension relationships and chest-wall mechanics. As of this writing, only short-term results have been published.[18,19] The mean $FEV_1$ was doubled from 0.77 to 1.4 L, and the distance walked in 6 minutes was substantially improved. Some patients could discontinue the use of supplemental oxygen, and most reported subjective improvements in dyspnea, functional abilities, and a sense of well-being. These results are preliminary, however, and are highly dependent on proper patient selection, the use of vigorous preoperative and postoperative rehabilitation programs, and a highly experienced thoracic surgical team.

## References

1. Feinleib M, Rosenberg RM, Collins JG, et al: Trends in COPD morbidity and mortality in the United States, *Am Rev Respir Dis* 140:S9, 1989.

2. Anthonisen NR: Prognosis in chronic obstructive pulmonary disease: results from multicenter clinical trials, *Am Rev Respir Dis* 140:S95, 1989.

3. American Thoracic Society: Lung function testing: selection of reference values and interpretative strategies, *Am Rev Respir Dis* 144:1202, 1991.

4. American Thoracic Society: Standards for the diagnosis and care of patients with chronic obstructive pulmonary disease (COPD) and asthma, *Am Rev Respir Dis* 136:225, 1987.

5. Callahan CM, Dittus RS, Katz BP: Oral corticosteroid therapy for patients with stable chronic obstructive pulmonary disease: a meta-analysis, *Ann Intern Med* 114:216, 1991.

6. Dallari R, Barozzi G, Pinelli G, et al: Predictors of survival in subjects with chronic obstructive pulmonary disease treated with long term oxygen therapy, *Respiration* 61:8, 1994.

7. Nocturnal Oxygen Therapy Group: Continuous or nocturnal oxygen therapy in hypoxemic chronic obstructive lung disease: a clinical trial, *Ann Intern Med* 93:391, 1980.

8. Report of the Medical Research Council Working Party: Long term domiciliary oxygen therapy in chronic hypoxic cor pulmonale complicating chronic bronchitis and emphysema, *Lancet* 1:681, 1981.

9. Goldstein RS, Ramcharan V, Bowes G, et al: Effect of supplemental nocturnal oxygen on gas exchange in patients with severe obstructive lung disease, *N Engl J Med* 310:425, 1984.

10. American Thoracic Society: Guidelines for the approach to the patient with severe hereditary alpha$_1$-antitrypsin deficiency, *Am Rev Respir Dis* 140:1494, 1989.

11. Fuchs HJ, Borowitz DS, Christiansen DH, et al: Effect of aerosolized recombinant human DNase on exacerbations of respiratory symptoms and on pulmonary function in patients with cystic fibrosis, *N Engl J Med* 331:637, 1994.

12. Elliot M, Moxham J: Noninvasive mechanical ventilation by nasal or face mask. In Tobin MJ, editor: *Principles and practice of mechanical ventilation,* New York, 1994, McGraw-Hill.

13. Bott J, Carroll MP, Conway JH, et al: A randomised controlled study of nasal ventilation in acute ventilatory failure due to chronic obstructive airways disease, *Lancet* 341:1555, 1993.

14. Shapiro SH, Ernst P, Gray-Donald K, et al: Effect of negative pressure ventilation in severe chronic obstructive pulmonary disease, *Lancet* 2:1425, 1992 (with comment on pp 1440–1441).

15. Sahn SA, Nett LM, Petty TL: Ten year follow-up of a comprehensive rehabilitation program for severe COPD, *Chest* 77(suppl):311, 1980.

16. Donahoe M, Rogers RM: Nutritional assessment and support in chronic obstructive pulmonary disease, *Clin Chest Med* 11:487, 1990.

17. Cooper JD, Patterson A, Trulock EP: Results of single and bilateral lung transplantation in 131 consecutive recipients, *J Thorac Cardiovasc Surg* 107:460, 1994.

18. Cooper JD, Truelock EP, Triantafillou GA: et al: Bilateral pneumectomy (volume reduction) for chronic obstructive pulmonary disease, *J Thorac Cardiovasc Surg* 109:106, 1995.

19. Sciurba FC, Rogers RM, Keenan RJ, et al: Improvement in pulmonary function and elastic recoil after lung-reduction surgery for diffuse emphysema, *N Engl J Med* 334:1095, 1996.

## Chapter 39

# *Perioperative Evaluation of Pulmonary Risk*

Scott K. Epstein

Pulmonary complications constitute the most frequent cause of postoperative disease and death. The incidence of pulmonary complications ranges from 5% to 40% depending on how complications are defined, the percentage of patients with lung disease, and the type of operations performed. As a general rule, the closer the surgical incision is to the diaphragm, the higher the pulmonary risk. For thoracic and upper abdominal surgery, the incidence of complications ranges from 20% to 80%, for lower abdominal surgery from 0 to 20%, and for nonthoracic and nonabdominal operations less than 5%.[1,2] For patients with obstructive lung disease the risk is substantially increased, often exceeding 50% for cardiac or upper abdominal surgery.[3] Nevertheless, except for lung resection, it is rare for surgery to be absolutely contraindicated on the basis of pulmonary risk. When surgery is elective and the assessed pulmonary risk is high, a relative contraindication may exist. Under most circumstances, however, the goal of perioperative pulmonary risk assessment is to design a strategy that reduces the likelihood of complications while maintaining the benefits derived from surgery.

The physician who evaluates a patient's perioperative pulmonary risk must answer a series of critical questions. The remainder of this discussion is a proposal of answers to these questions.

## WHAT ARE PERIOPERATIVE PULMONARY COMPLICATIONS AND HOW DO THEY OCCUR?

The box on p. 415 lists the commonly identified pulmonary complications. The effect of less severe complications derives from the resulting prolongation of hospitalization and delay in postoperative rehabilitation. Some complications such as "microatelectasis" or asymptomatic mild hypoxemia are of little clinical relevance.

The genesis of most pulmonary complications can be found in the disruption of pulmonary defense mechanisms and, most significantly,

## Pulmonary Complications

Respiratory death
Respiratory failure
Hypoxemia
Hypercapnia
Prolonged mechanical ventilation
Atelectasis
Lobar atelectasis
"Macroatelectasis" (abnormal chest roentgenogram)
"Microatelectasis" (normal chest roentgenogram, hypoxemia, crackles)
Pneumonia (fever, cough, change in sputum, leukocytosis, radiographic infiltrate)
Tracheobronchitis
Increase respiratory secretions
Exacerbation of disease of the airways
Respiratory muscle weakness
Hypoventilation
Pulmonary embolism

the alterations of the pulmonary physiologic characteristics that occur in the perioperative period. The former abnormalities occur principally from mucus hypersecretion with reduced cough and decreased mucociliary clearance. The physiologic abnormalities occur because of the effects of both anesthesia and surgery. General anesthesia (inhalational, intravenous) causes atelectasis by reducing resting lung volume (functional residual capacity, FRC), by cephalad repositioning of the diaphragm, and by inhibition of sigh.[1] The resulting intrapulmonary shunt, together with ventilation-perfusion mismatch and increased dead space, produce gas exchange abnormalities that are further exacerbated by a blunted response to hypercapnia and hypoxemia. For the most part, these changes reverse rapidly and are of little importance in the postoperative period. Spinal and epidural anesthesia also lead to a reduced FRC while also decreasing expiratory muscle function and cough effectiveness. Regional nerve blockade (brachial plexus, supraclavicular, and so on), though intuitively safer, may be associated with some pulmonary risk because of the possibility of pneumothorax or paralyzed phrenic nerves through local anesthetic spread.

Significant pulmonary risk principally complicates surgery on the thorax (such as lung resection, sternotomy for cardiac surgery, or esophagectomy), upper abdomen, thoracoabdominal aorta, or the lower abdomen. These surgeries substantially diminish lung function, permanently in the obvious case of lung resection and transiently for both nonresection thoracic and upper abdominal operations. Extrathoracic and extra-abdominal procedures, such as neurologic procedures or amputations, are not characterized by reduced lung function and are associated with minimal if any perioperative pulmonary morbidity.

Thoracic surgery (without lung resection) and upper abdominal surgery lead to a restrictive pulmonary physiologic condition with reductions in forced vital capacity (FVC), forced expired volume in one second (FEV$_1$), and FRC that typically persists for up to 2 weeks postoperatively.[1,2] Although minute ventilation does not change, alveolar ventilation falls because a pattern of rapid and shallow breathing is assumed. These changes predispose to atelectasis and consequent hypoxemia because tidal breathing occurs at a lung volume below that at which alveolar units are collapsed (closing volume). Although postoperative pain and its treatment, through reduction of cough and sigh, may contribute to these alterations, other physiologic mechanisms appear to be more important. With cardiac surgery, pulmonary restriction results from altered chest-wall mechanics and from left lower lobe atelectasis that occurs with retraction during surgery and related pleural injury. The phrenic nerve or nerves may be injured because of freezing with cold cardioplegia or disruption of its blood supply with dissection of the internal mammary artery.[1] With upper abdominal surgery, the supine position and the effects of the abdominal incision surprisingly are not the principal contributors to the observed pulmonary restriction. The primary mechanism for the decreased lung function is diaphragmatic dysfunction resulting from reflex phrenic nerve inhibition that occurs with surgical manipulation of the viscera. This dysfunction can be overcome by voluntary efforts at diaphragmatic breathing, by electrical stimulation of the phrenic nerves, or by thoracic extradural anesthetic blockade. Laparoscopic abdominal surgery leads to a smaller reduction in FEV$_1$, FVC, and peak flow rate and less oxygen desaturation than laparotomy does, perhaps because of the smaller incision required, less pain, and a reduced need for analgesics.[4] Because of the arguments made earlier, less inhibition of the phrenic nerve also may occur with laparoscopic surgery. Lower abdominal surgery, which is not associated with diaphragmatic dysfunction, produces a smaller decrease in VC and less significant hypoxemia. These changes typically resolve rapidly (in 24 hours), and significant pulmonary complications are not common.

# WHO IS AT RISK FOR PULMONARY COMPLICATIONS? HOW CAN THE RISK BE QUANTITATED?

When one is evaluating a patient for surgery, it is useful to go through a checklist of factors that are known to be linked with an increased risk for pulmonary complications (see box on p. 417). Simultaneously, one should consider which factors can be modified to reduce the risk.

**1. Does the patient have known lung disease?** The most crucial factor in the assessment of pulmonary risk is the presence of chronic obstructive pulmonary disease (COPD). Although the abnormal pulmonary function seen with anesthesia and surgery may have a minimal effect when there is little or no underlying pulmonary disease, the patient with significant lung disease may be severely affected. Pulmonary risk

## Risk Factors for Pulmonary Complications

Obstructive lung disease (COPD, asthma)
Restrictive lung disease
Respiratory muscle weakness
Abnormal pulmonary function (reduced $FEV_1$, DLCO)
Hypercapnia
Hypoxemia
Hypoventilation syndrome (obstructive sleep apnea)

Type of surgery (lung resection, other thoracic surgery, upper abdominal surgery, lower abdominal surgery, major abdominal vascular surgery, laparoscopy)
Type of anesthesia and anesthesia time

Smoking
Productive cough
Wheezing
Dyspnea

Age
Bodyweight (obesity or underweight)
Malnutrition

*COPD*, Chronic obstructive pulmonary disease; *DLCO*, single-breath diffusing capacity in the lungs; $FEV_1$, forced expiratory volume in 1 second.

increases as the $FEV_1$ falls, but the correlation between this value and the risk for nonlung resection surgery is not always strong. Significantly, no $FEV_1$ has been found to be absolutely prohibitive for nonlung resection surgery. Those patients with severe COPD ($FEV_1$ <50% predicted) can successfully undergo surgery, though the risk for serious pulmonary complications is increased, especially for upper abdominal and cardiac surgery.[3] The reported risk for cardiac surgery is substantial, with respiratory mortality as high as 20% for those with an $FEV_1$ <50% predicted.[3] An additional consideration is an elevated $Paco_2$ (greater than a range of 45 to 50 mm Hg), one of the strongest pulmonary risk factors identified. Hypercapnia may reflect severe ventilation-perfusion mismatch, respiratory muscle weakness, or an abnormal control of breathing. Although these mechanisms probably significantly increase risk, one recent study could not find a difference in pulmonary complications after lung resection between normocapnic and hypercapnic patients.[5] Although hypoxemia may also predispose to pulmonary complications, the magnitude is much less than that with hypercapnia. Hypoxemia does not generally reflect respiratory muscle weakness or hypoventilation. Hypoxemia, usually a result of ventilation-perfusion mismatch, is readily corrected with supplemental oxygen.

Although much less dramatic than COPD, patients with asthma are at elevated risk, with up to 20% suffering a pulmonary complication. Placement of an endotracheal tube and manipulation of viscera may precipitate bronchospasm and complicate the perioperative period. Importantly, the pulmonary risk for asthmatics falls significantly when wheezing is absent at the time of surgery.[6] The risk for patients with restrictive lung disease, though elevated, appears to be significantly lower than for those with obstructive lung disease. These patients usually have preserved respiratory muscle function and capacity for effective cough, and the airways are typically free of secretions. In the setting of significant chest-wall restriction (such as ankylosing spondylitis) and unusual dependence on the diaphragm, upper abdominal surgery may be particularly treacherous.

**2. What type of surgery and anesthesia is the patient to undergo?** The surgical procedure undertaken is a crucial determinant of pulmonary risk. Those operations associated with the greatest pulmonary risk are thoracic (with or without lung resection), upper abdominal, aortic, lower abdominal, and head and neck (given the increased risk of COPD). For upper abdominal surgery, subcostal (horizontal) and smaller incisions are associated with fewer pulmonary complications than midline (vertical) or larger ones. Further reduction in the complication rate is seen when laparoscopic abdominal surgery is substituted for laparotomy.

Procedures lasting more than 3 to 4 hours are associated with a greatly increased pulmonary risk. In all likelihood this finding has more to do with the procedure being performed than the duration of anesthesia. Although they produce very different effects on respiratory function, there is no clear-cut difference in the rate of pulmonary complications between general and spinal epidural anesthesia. Nevertheless, under some circumstances one method may have advantages over the other. Although the mechanism is unclear, high thoracic spinal-epidural (above T6) anesthesia has been associated with severe bronchospasm in patients with asthma. In contrast, general volatile agents such as enflurane and halothane and the dissociative agent ketamine are bronchodilators and may be favored in asthma. On the other hand, histamine-releasing agents, such as some of the paralytic agents, should probably be avoided in these patients.

**3. What is the smoking history?** Studies in patients undergoing cardiac surgery indicate a greatly elevated risk for those who have smoked more than 20 pack-years or 1 pack/day.[7] This adverse risk occurs because smoking leads to increased closing volumes (the volume at which alveoli at the lung bases are collapsed), decreased small-airway function, and impaired ciliary function and tracheobronchial clearance, which predispose to atelectasis and pneumonia. Once smoking is discontinued it takes 6 to 8 weeks for these abnormalities to resolve. Not surprisingly, tobacco must be discontinued 8 weeks before cardiac surgery to reduce the risk of postoperative pulmonary complications.[7]

**4. Does the patient have productive cough?** Several studies have noted that increased respiratory secretions preoperatively predispose to postoperative pulmonary complications after cardiac surgery or lung resection.[8] In the perioperative period, additional mucus hypersecretion, together with reduced capacity for secretion clearance, will increase the likelihood of obstructive atelectasis and consequent pneumonia.

**5. Is the patient wheezing?** Increased expiratory airflow obstruction, often manifested as wheezing, increases pulmonary risk by decreasing secretion clearance and reducing the effectiveness of cough. In addition, worsening air-trapping and consequent hyperinflation may occur, leading to diminished mechanical diaphragmatic function. Patients with COPD undergoing lung resection and those with asthma are at increased pulmonary risk if wheezing is detected on physical exam before surgery.[6,8]

**6. Is there obesity or significant weight loss?** Obesity, especially in the supine position, reduces FRC, predisposing to atelectasis and thus may accentuate many of the problems associated with upper abdominal surgery. Early studies suggested that slight increases in body weight increased the risk of postoperative atelectasis. Recent work indicates that only the morbidly obese (>250 lb or 100% over ideal body weight) are at increased risk for significant pulmonary complications.[2] Additionally, patients who are obese may have the obstructive sleep apnea syndrome. Pulmonary risk may increase when these patients inadvertently or injudiciously receive benzodiazepines or narcotics perioperatively. In contrast to the above, substantial weight loss and associated malnutrition predispose to pulmonary complications by decreasing immune function and reducing respiratory muscle strength. Although a reduced serum albumin has been a good predictor in some studies, more comprehensive nutritional assessment, including anthropomorphic measures, usually is required for accurate assessment of nutritional status.

**7. How old is the patient?** Early studies had suggested that older patients were at elevated risk for surgery. Recent analyses, using multivariate statistical methods, indicate that, once the preceding factors are controlled for, age is not an independent risk factor.[2] Although age alone should rarely be taken into account when one is assessing the risk for a pulmonary complication, it does signal the need to look carefully for the presence of other risk factors.

# HOW SHOULD THE PATIENT BE EVALUATED?

History and physical examination, directed at the questions posed above, are the mainstay of intelligent and effective preoperative evaluation. In addition, quantification of dyspnea using a scale such as how far the patient can walk before resting or which activities induce breathlessness (dressing or talking) may provide additional prognostic information. Anesthesiologists' assessment, using the American Society of Anesthesiologists (ASA) classification, has been useful in predicting postoperative complications. In essence, this system divides patients into five groups based on severity of underlying disease: class 1 (healthy); class 2 (mild to moderate systemic disease); class 3 (severe); class 4 (severe and life threatening); and class 5 (moribund). An ASA class >2 predicts increased pulmonary complications for major thoracic and abdominal surgery.[9] Although hyperinflation or the presence of infiltrates on the preoperative chest roentgenogram (CXR) may signal increased pulmonary risk, it is not clear whether the CXR adds useful additional information to standard history and physical and pulmonary function testing.[9] Nevertheless, I routinely obtain a preoperative CXR to serve as a base-line view for comparison to that of postoperative films.

## What is the role for pulmonary function testing (PFT)?

There has been great debate about the role of preoperative PFT for nonlung resection surgery, but its effect on postoperative outcome has not been demonstrated conclusively. The logic behind obtaining PFT in all patients undergoing high-risk surgery is that abnormalities may be found in patients without other evidence of pulmonary disease. Although this "occult" abnormality in lung function may place them at increased risk compared to those with clinically detectable lung disease, the increase in risk may be minor. The majority of studies clearly indicate an increased risk for pulmonary complications when the spirometric values are reduced. When the FVC is <70% of the predicted value, the $FEV_1/FVC$ is <50%, or the maximal voluntary ventilation (MVV) is <50%, the risk for postoperative complications increases.[1,2] Unfortunately there appears to be no good "cutoff" value to separate those who will from those who will not suffer a pulmonary complication. This is the case for upper abdominal surgery, where a wide range in positive and negative predictive values for various PFTs in estimating postoperative pulmonary complications has been reported.[10] Similarly for cardiac surgery, those with reduced FVC and $FEV_1$ are at increased risk for prolonged intensive-care-unit stay and death, but overall, PFT appears not to be an accurate predictor of outcome.

Given the role of diaphragmatic dysfunction in upper abdominal surgery, one would predict that the presence of respiratory muscle weakness would indicate a substantially increased pulmonary risk. This appears to be the case because measurement of either the maximal inspiratory (MIP) or expiratory (MEP) pressure allows prediction of increased complications for upper abdominal surgery.[1]

Although accurate threshold values for spirometry may not exist, combining these data into a multivariate analysis, including clinical information such as smoking, dyspnea, exercise capacity, productive cough, wheezing, and tests of respiratory muscle strength may allow for improved prediction of outcome. Recommendations for pulmonary function testing are outlined in the box on p. 421.

Several studies have utilized exercise testing to assess pulmonary fitness for nonthoracic surgery. The best of these showed that elderly patients (>65 years) undergoing major abdominal or noncardiac thoracic surgery had a fivefold reduction in major pulmonary complications if they could do supine bicycle exercise for ≥2 minutes achieving a heart rate of ≥99 beats/min.[11]

---

## Indications for Preoperative Pulmonary Function Testing

A. Patients scheduled for pulmonary resection
B. Patients scheduled for all other procedures who are considered at high risk: those with two in category A, one in category A and either one in category B or one in category C, two in category B, one in category B and one in category C, or three or more in category C.

**Category A**
1. High-risk surgery (thoracic, upper abdominal, abdominal vascular)
2. History or physical examination compatible with COPD

**Category B**
1. Intermediate-risk surgery (lower abdomen or pelvic, head, and neck)
2. History or physical examination compatible with asthma or restrictive lung disease

**Category C**
1. Smoking within 8 weeks of surgery
2. Age >70
3. Dyspnea
4. Wheezing on physical examination
5. Productive cough
6. Morbid obesity

---

If spirometry results are abnormal, obtain arterial blood gas and make plans for preoperative and postoperative therapy.

## How should the patient be evaluated before pulmonary resection?

The preoperative evaluation for pulmonary resection differs substantially from that with other surgeries. The risk is increased because the incidence of COPD is high and surgery will result in a permanent reduction in lung function. The benefit is clear because surgical therapy for lung cancer offers the best chance for cure. In general, the more lung to be removed, the higher the risk of surgery. Although the mortalities range from 1% for segmentectomy to 3% for lobectomy to 6% for pneumonectomy; overall complication rates are similar for these procedures. This comparable morbidity is attributable to patients with more severe underlying lung disease undergoing less extensive procedures. Although the correlation between abnormal pulmonary function and pulmonary risk may be stronger for lung resection than for other procedures, the predictive accuracy is similarly suboptimal. Various studies have indicated that the pulmonary risk of lung resection is increased when the preoperative FVC is less than a range of 50% to 70% predicted, $FEV_1$ is less than a range of 1.2 to 2 liters or <50% predicted, maximum voluntary ventilation (MVV) is <50% predicted, residual volume/total lung capacity (RV/TLC) is >50%, or diffusion capacity (DLCO) is <50% predicted.[1,2] As with upper abdominal surgery, the positive and negative predictive values of spirometry for pulmonary complications or cardiopulmonary death are wide ranging.[10] In contrast, the amount of functional lung remaining after resection has a more predictable influence on postoperative outcome. With lung resection, one can estimate the remaining lung function by combining the preoperative $FEV_1$ or DLCO and the results of a split perfusion nuclear scan that directly quantifies the amount of lung to be removed (as a percentage of all of the functioning lung). In the absence of nuclear scanning, one can obtain a reasonable estimate by multiplying the $FEV_1$ by the number of segments to be removed divided by the total number of segments. For patients undergoing resection, a predicted postoperative $FEV_1$ ($ppoFEV_1$) <800 mL or <40% predicted or a ppoD-LCO <40% is associated with greatly increased morbidity and mortality.[12]

Even after calculation of the predicted postoperative lung function, perioperative pulmonary risk is still only imperfectly assessed. Some patients estimated to be at high risk experience no complications, whereas others believed to be at low risk suffer significant morbidity and mortality. In addition, although perioperative pulmonary morbidity is important, the majority of studies also demonstrate that cardiac complications represent the major aspect of perioperative outcome. To some degree, pulmonary complications predispose to cardiac ones and vice versa, and most authorities lump these together as "cardiopulmonary" complications. Based on this logic, physiologic (exercise) testing methods, which simultaneously stress both the cardiac and pulmonary systems, have been explored as tools for risk stratification. It is commonly believed that a patient who can successfully walk up one or two flights of stairs without stopping to rest will have sufficient physiologic reserve to withstand lung resection. Unfortunately some patients who climb more than two flights still suffer serious postoperative cardiopulmonary complications. Furthermore, it has been shown that most patients with an $FEV_1$ <1 liter can climb more than three flights of stairs.[1]

Although some studies have focused on the predictive capacity of stair climbing or distance walked (the 6- or 12-minute walk), cardiopulmonary exercise testing using a bicycle ergometer and a metabolic cart to measure oxygen uptake has been the most extensively studied tool. The majority of studies, but not all, demonstrate increased cardiopulmonary risk when the peak oxygen uptake (peak $\dot{V}O_2$) during maximal symptom-limited exercise is reduced. The risk for cardiopulmonary complications is greatest when the peak $\dot{V}O_2$ is <10 mL/kg/min (or <500 mL/m$^2$ of body surface area), moderate when 10 to 19 mL/kg/min, and minimal when ≥20 mL/kg/min.[13] Not surprisingly, the peak $\dot{V}O_2$ correlates with the number of stairs climbed, with 4.6 flights correlating with $\dot{V}O_2$ >20 mL/kg/min.[1] It has been further noted that patients incapable of performing an exercise test because of musculoskeletal, neurologic, psychologic, or peripheral vascular disease are at considerably elevated risk for cardiopulmonary disease and death. Although these patients may have more significant underlying cardiopulmonary disease than those who can exercise, the inability to exercise appears to be an independent predictor of risk.[14] I believe the role for cardiopulmonary exercise testing is in selecting patients believed to be at high risk by traditional testing who actually are capable of withstanding curative lung resection.

## How are these risk factors combined to yield an overall assessment?

Unlike for cardiac risk, multivariate assessment of pulmonary risk is less well developed. In a study of 42 patients for lung resection for cancer, a multifactorial risk index (CPRI) combining a cardiac risk index and a pulmonary risk index was highly predictive of postoperative cardiopulmonary complications (Table 39-1). When the CPRI was $\geq$ 4, the risk of cardiopulmonary complications was 22 times that for those with a score less than 4.[8] Although this study suggested no additional prognostic information when the peak $\dot{V}O_2$ from exercise testing was added to the CPRI, only a third of the patients had an $FEV_1$ <2 liters. Based on this, the best overall approach to risk assessment, especially for patients with severe reduction in preoperative lung function, is probably a multifactorial one. In Fig. 39-1, I have outlined my method for evaluating patients who are scheduled for lung resection.

# HOW SHOULD THE PATIENT BE PREPARED FOR SURGERY?

Except for lung resection, an absolute contraindication to surgery because of pulmonary risk is rare. The utility of risk assessment is principally to identify the high-risk patient who requires preoperative preparation to reduce perioperative risk or who requires a change in surgical or anesthetic approach. Several older studies have demonstrated that inpatient preoperative preparation in those identified to be at increased risk could have reduced pulmonary complications and possibly improved survival in abdominal and thoracic procedures.[15] In general, these preoperative regimens are based on some combination of chest physiotherapy (breathing exercises, encouraged cough, postural drainage, incentive spirometry, intermittent positive-pressure breathing [IPPB], bronchodilators, antibiotics, smoking cessation, and theophylline. One recent study suggests that similar benefits can occur if breathing exercises are started as an outpatient, 1 week before surgery.[1] As yet, there is no evidence that preoperative preparation benefits the low-risk patient. Based on these and other reports, I favor the following preoperative strategy for patients considered to be at high risk for postoperative pulmonary complications.

**Smoking cessation.** Although conclusive benefits have been demonstrated only after 8 weeks of cessation in those undergoing cardiac surgery, I still recommend even short-term smoking cessation for all surgical procedures based on the early studies of successful preoperative preparation.

**Table 39-1.** *Multifactorial risk index for cancer lung resection*

| CARDIAC RISK INDEX | | PULMONARY RISK INDEX | |
| --- | --- | --- | --- |
| Parameter | Points | Parameter | Points |
| Congestive heart failure | 11 | Obesity (body mass index $\geq$27 kg/m$^2$) | 1 |
| ($S_3$, jugular venous distension, LVEF $\leq$40%) | | Cigarette smoking within 8 weeks of surgery | 1 |
| Myocardial infarction during the previous 6 months | 10 | Productive cough within 5 days of surgery | 1 |
| Greater than 5 PVCs/min (noted anytime preoperatively) | 7 | Diffuse wheezing or rhonchi noted within 5 days of surgery | 1 |
| Rhythm other than NSR or PACs (on preoperative ECG) | 7 | | |
| Age >70 years | 5 | $FEV_1/FVC$ <70% | 1 |
| Important valvular aortic stenosis | 3 | $Paco_2$ >45 mm Hg | 1 |
| Poor general medical condition | 3 | | |
| Cardiac risk index (CRI) points = 3 to 47 | | Pulmonary Risk Index score (PRI) = 0 to 6 | |

CRI score: 1 (0–5 points), 2 (6–12 points), 3 (12–25 points), 4 (>25 points)

Cardiac risk index score (CRI) = 1 to 4

Cardiopulmonary risk index score (CPRI) = CRI + PRI = 1 to 10

*Left,* Cardiac indices (modified from Goldman L, Caldera DL, Nussbaum SR, et al: *N Engl J Med* 297:845, 1977) and, *right,* pulmonary indices. Cardiopulmonary risk index score (CPRI) is derived when CRI score and PRI score are added together. *LVEF,* Left ventricular ejection fraction; *NSR,* normal sinus rhythm; *PAC,* premature atrial contraction; *PVC,* premature ventricular contraction; $S_3$, third heart sound. (Modified from Epstein SK, Faling LJ, Daly BDT, et al: *Chest* 104(3):695, 1993.)

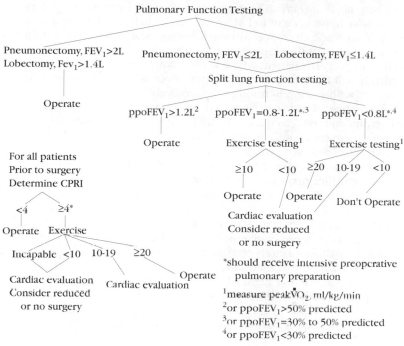

**Figure 39-1.** *Strategy for evaluating patients before thoracotomy with lung resection for lung cancer. For pneumonectomy, split lung function testing is indicated when the FEV₁ percentage predicted is less than 60% predicted, and for lobectomy, it is less than 50% predicted. Exercise testing should be performed (and the algorithm for ppoFEV₁ <0.8 L followed) when the ppoFEV₁ is less than 40% predicted. Diffusion capacity percentage predicted (DLCO percentage predicted) may be used instead of FEV₁ percentage predicted. Patients with hypercapnia (Pa$CO_2$ >44 mm Hg) should undergo exercise testing. FEV₁, Preoperative forced expiratory volume in I second; ppoFEV₁, predicted postoperative FEV₁; peak $\dot{V}O_2$, peak oxygen uptake during symptom-limited maximal exercise test; exercise testing, cardiopulmonary stress test; CPRI, cardiopulmonary risk index.*

**Bronchodilators.** For stable patients, I continue the same agents used preoperatively, changing from metered-dose inhalers to nebulizer therapy for the perioperative period. If a COPD patient is not taking ipratropium bromide, I start it empirically, at a dose of 2 to 4 puffs qid, because of the benign side-effect profile. The safety of empiric beta-adrenergic agonists has not been demonstrated and because of adverse effects, I neither start it nor empirically increase the dose in an otherwise stable patient. Beta-agonists should be used immediately if symptoms or signs of bronchospasm arise in the perioperative period. In general, nonemergent surgery should be delayed until an attempt at correcting and resolving preoperative wheezing is made.

**Chest physiotherapy.** The basic goal of these maneuvers is lung expansion, improvement in FRC, reduction in atelectasis, and improvement in secretion clearance. Although it is not clearly proved beneficial, I recommend that the respiratory therapist see and instruct the patient before surgery. The patient who is familiar with these manuevers preoperatively will likely be more cooperative even when pain or narcotics interfere with comprehension postoperatively.

**Antibiotics.** When there is productive cough or an unexplained radiographic infiltrate, a course of antibiotics should be administered. If possible, surgery should be delayed for a minimum of 7 to 10 days or until the patient's symptoms have resolved.

**Theophylline and other respiratory stimulants.** Several studies suggest that theophylline may improve the respiratory muscle dysfunction seen with upper abdominal surgery. This area remains controversial, and the clinical relevance of these observations is unclear. For patients receiving these preparations chronically, intravenous therapy can be used during the perioperative period. Because of the real potential for cardiac arrhythmias, I rarely recommend instituting this drug in a patient not already taking this medication. When it is used, the goal level is 8 to 10 $\mu$g/dL because higher levels are associated with toxicity and little additional benefit. Other respiratory stimulants, such as doxapram, seem to reduce postoperative pulmonary complications in patients undergoing abdominal surgery, perhaps by countering the reflex inhibition of the phrenic nerve.

**Steroids.** Preoperative (outpatient) and perioperative use of steroids in asthmatics decreases the rate of complications to that seen in a nonasthmatic population.[6] For mild asthmatics with a normal $FEV_1$, requiring only as-needed bronchodilators and not using systemic or inhaled steroids, perioperative steroid therapy is not clearly beneficial. For patients taking regular or intermittent systemic or inhaled steroids, I routinely recommend administering these during the perioperative period at a dose of 0.5 to 1.0 mg/kg of methylprednisolone every 6 to 8 hours beginning 6 hours preoperatively and continuing for a minimum of 24 hours. For symptomatic patients, steroids should be started up to a week beforehand, and the patient should be free of wheezing, if possible, before surgery. Importantly, such a perioperative course of steroids does not increase the risk of wound infection or abnormal wound healing.[6]

# WHAT SHOULD THE POSTOPERATIVE TREATMENT BE?

Preoperative and perioperative therapy with bronchodilators, theophylline, and steroids should be continued in the postoperative period until patients approach their base-line pulmonary function. Although not of proved benefit, it seems prudent to remove nasogastric tubes and to mobilize the patient as early as feasible. Postoperative narcotics and

---

## Lung-Expansion Maneuvers
..................................................................

1. **Incentive spirometry:** slow maximal inspiration to 50% to 100% of vital capacity with breath hold, performed every hour while awake
2. **Continuous positive airway pressure (CPAP):** settings 5 to 15 cm $H_2O$ every 4 hours while awake
3. **Intermittent positive-pressure breathing (IPPB):** infrequently used
4. **Deep breathing:** sequential breathing to achieve total lung capacity, followed by a breath hold and forced cough
5. **Diaphragmatic breathing**

---

sedatives may predispose to atelectasis by reducing sigh and should be minimized if possible. Some but not all studies suggest that epidural anesthesia or intercostal nerve blocks may reduce postoperative pulmonary complications. Much of postoperative care centers on lung-expansion methods designed to counteract the pulmonary pathophysiologic changes produced by surgery (see box above). Chest physiotherapy, such as percussion and postural drainage, is indicated only when abundant pulmonary secretions are present. For upper abdominal surgery, continuous positive airway pressure (CPAP), incentive spirometry, and deep breathing (especially diaphragmatic breathing) appear to be equally effective in reducing pulmonary complications.[1] Incentive spirometry has the advantage that it can be performed unsupervised, and the cost of the device is reasonable. The duration and number of treatments for optimal efficacy is unknown, but I recommend 5 minutes every hour while awake. Patients who have no additional pulmonary risk factors do not clearly benefit from these postoperative maneuvers. Similarly, lung-expansion maneuvers are not clearly beneficial in unselected patients undergoing routine cardiac surgery. Although there are fewer studies available for lung resection, the benefits of lung expansion seem to extend to these patients as well.

## References

1. Celli BR: What is the value of preoperative pulmonary function testing? *Med Clin North Am* 77:309-325, 1993.
2. Mohr DN, Jett JR: Preoperative evaluation of pulmonary risk factors, *J Gen Intern Med* 3:277-287, 1988.
3. Kroenke K, Lawrence VA, Theroux JF, Tuley MR: Operative risk in patients with severe obstructive pulmonary disease, *Arch Intern Med* 152:967-971, 1992.
4. McMahon AJ, Russell IT, Ramsay G, et al: Laparoscopic and minilaparotomy cholecystectomy: a randomized trial comparing postoperative pain and pulmonary function, *Surgery* 115:533-539, 1994.
5. Kearney DJ, Lee TH, Reilly JJ, et al: Assessment of operative risk in patients undergoing lung resection: importance of predicted pulmonary function, *Chest* 105:753-759, 1994.

6. Pien LC, Grammer LC, Patterson R: Minimal complications in a surgical population with severe asthma receiving prophylactic corticosteriods, *J Allergy Clin Immunol* 82:696-700, 1988.
7. Warner MA, Divertie MB, Tinker JH: Preoperative cessation of smoking and pulmonary complications in coronary artery bypass patients, *Anesthesiology* 60:380-383, 1984.
8. Epstein SK, Faling LJ, Daly BDT, Celli BR: Predicting complications after pulmonary resection: preoperative exercise testing vs a multifactorial cardiopulmonary risk index, *Chest* 104:694-700, 1993.
9. Kroenke K, Lawrence VA, Theroux JF, et al: Postoperative complications after thoracic and major abdominal surgery in patients with and without obstructive lung disease, *Chest* 104:1445-1451, 1993.
10. Zibrak JD, O'Donnell CR, Marton K: Indications for pulmonary function testing, *Ann Intern Med* 112:763-771, 1990.
11. Gerson MC, Hurst JM, Hertzberg VS, et al: Prediction of cardiac and pulmonary complications related to elective abdominal and noncardiac thoracic surgery in geriatric patients, *Am J Med* 88:101-107, 1990.
12. Markos J, Mullan BP, Hillman DR, et al: Preoperative assessment as a predictor of mortality and morbidity after lung resection, *Am Rev Respir Dis* 139:902-910, 1989.
13. Gass GD, Olsen GN: Preoperative pulmonary function testing to predict postoperative morbidity and mortality, *Chest* 89:127-135, 1986.
14. Epstein SK, Faling LJ, Daly BDT, Celli BR: Inability to perform bicycle ergometry predicts increased morbidity and mortality after lung resection, *Chest* 107:311-316, 1995.
15. Gracey DR, Divertie MB, Didier EP: Preoperative pulmonary preparation of patients with chronic obstructive pulmonary disease, *Chest* 76:123-129, 1979.

# Part 6

# Hematologic Disease and Cancer

## Chapter 40

## *Anemia*

Kenneth B. Miller

Anemia results from a wide variety of disorders and nearly always requires further evaluation because it provides an objective sign of an underlying disease. Early diagnostic evaluation in many cases may have a major salutory effect on clinical outcome. For example, carcinoma of the colon may initially present with iron deficiency anemia. A National Health and Nutrition Examination Survey estimated that approximately 3.8% of all noninstitutionalized Americans are anemic, and other studies indicate that approximately one in four medical inpatients is anemic.[1] An orderly approach to the etiology of the anemia is essential if the clinician is to avoid either inadequate or excessive evaluation and treatment. Evaluation of the anemic patient relies on clinical and laboratory information to narrow the scope of the differential diagnosis and to aid in management.

# INITIAL CONSIDERATIONS

## Is the patient anemic?

Anemia represents a reduction of the body's red cell mass, a quantity that under normal conditions is maintained within narrow limits by the regulatory hormone erythropoietin. Erythropoietin is released from the renal peritubular cells in response to a fall in the tissue oxygen content. In response to erythropoietin, red cell precursors in the bone marrow undergo proliferation and accelerated maturation and are released into the blood. Red blood cells circulate in the blood for approximately 120 days. Therefore the bone marrow must replace approximately 0.8% of the red blood cells lost each day to senescence. The erythropoietic feedback loop ensures that the hemoglobin mass available for oxygen delivery matches the body's needs and that production equals destruction. Anemia results when the normal balance of destruction and production is disturbed. Anemia may result from a primary disorder within the bone marrow, increased loss or destruction of red blood cells, or as a manifestation of several systemic disorders.

The evaluation of anemia begins with a laboratory measurement that indicates an abnormally low concentration of hemoglobin or an abnormally low packed red blood cell volume (hematocrit). Before proceeding with additional diagnostic studies, the clinician must first determine whether the abnormal laboratory result correctly indicates that the patient is anemic. Aside from acute blood loss, a reduction in red blood cells is usually accompanied by an increase in plasma volume such that the blood volume remains constant. A reduction in the mass of circulating red blood cells, that is, anemia, therefore is most readily detected as a decrease in the concentration of hemoglobin or red cells in the blood.

The hemoglobin and hematocrit, however, also decrease when the plasma volume expands. This phenomenon occurs routinely during the third trimester of pregnancy, in marathon runners and other endurance athletes, in patients with massive splenomegaly,[2] and in some patients with an IgM paraprotein. In these instances it is difficult to equate the concentration of hemoglobin or red cells with the total red cell mass. Direct measurement of the red cell mass by use of radiolabeled red cells therefore may be necessary to differentiate between simple expansion of plasma volume and actual anemia.

## The definition of normal

A second aspect of determining whether a patient is anemic relates to the definition of the normal range of the hemoglobin and of the hematocrit. Normal values are derived from the distribution of these measurements in a healthy reference population of men and women. Androgens enhance both the renal erythropoietin secretion and the bone marrow response and explain in part the gender differences in hemoglobin and hematocrit. Geographic differences also exist and reflect ambient oxygen tensions, such that the lower oxygen tensions at higher altitudes are associated with a compensatory increase in the hemoglobin and hematocrit.

The red blood cell number, hemoglobin, and hematocrit are routinely generated by accurate electronic counters. The electronic counters directly measure the red blood cell number and the mean corpuscular volume (MCV).[3] The hemoglobin concentration is determined by chromatographic quantitation of the hemoglobin present in a defined volume of red blood cells. These values are then used to calculate the hematocrit, the mean corpuscular hemoglobin (MCH), and the mean corpuscular hemoglobin concentration (MCHC). Many electronic counters also generate a red blood cell size index, the RDW, which is a measurement of the distribution of the red cell size.

# CLINICAL EVALUATION

The evaluation of anemia begins with the history and physical examination and then proceeds with selected laboratory testing. The evaluation of anemia all too often begins with a barrage of laboratory testing, perhaps because anemia is usually first recognized when laboratory test results are found to be abnormal. Although such an approach may be considered expeditious, more often than not it leads to confusion and frustration when the results fail to indicate the diagnosis. As with most complex clinical problems, laboratory results are most informative when considered in the context of information obtained from the history and physical examination.

## History
The evaluation of the anemic patient begins with an attempt to answer the five questions listed in the box below. The history provides key information regarding the nature, duration, and severity of the patient's symptoms.

## Inherited disorders
The history is useful in approaching the question of whether anemia is congenital or acquired. This issue should not be overlooked because the differential diagnosis of the inherited disorders that result in anemia is quite different from that of the disorders that result in acquired

---

**Evaluating Anemia**

1. Is there a family history of anemia or other blood disorders?
2. Is the patient complaining of fatigue, weight loss, fevers, night sweats, or other systemic complaints?
3. Is the patient taking any medications, even over-the-counter medications, and has the patient ever been exposed to hematotoxins?
4. Is there evidence of blood loss or hemolysis? In women a detailed menstrual and childbirth history should be obtained.
5. Is there a history of systemic or chronic inflammatory disease?

anemia. A past or family history of anemia, splenectomy, or refusal as a blood donor should be sought and, when present, indicates the possibility that the disorder is congenital. Furthermore, because the frequency of several of the inheritable anemias varies greatly in different ethnic groups, a brief exploration of the patient's ancestry is often helpful. Sickle cell disease, the thalassemias, glucose-6-phosphate dehydrogenase deficiency, and hereditary spherocytosis and elliptocytosis account for most of the inherited anemias.[4] When anemia is caused by one of these disorders, the primary mechanism is either chronic or episodic hemolysis, and there are prominent red cell morphologic abnormalities, which usually are present on the routine blood smear preparation.

## Drugs and toxins

A history of exposure to certain drugs or toxins provides important clues to the cause of anemia. Special care must be given to detecting these exposures because over-the-counter medications and environmental toxins are frequently overlooked by patients. Drugs may result in anemia when they suppress bone marrow function or provoke either immune or oxidative hemolysis, or when they cause or promote blood loss. Prominent examples are listed in the box on p. 433. Drug-induced oxidative hemolysis occurs almost exclusively in individuals with glucose-6-phosphate dehydrogenase deficiency.

Aspirin and nonsteroidal anti-inflammatory drugs are readily available over the counter and are associated with gastrointestinal bleeding. Many patients may not consider these agents as drugs and therefore should be specifically questioned about their use. Alcohol and its metabolites can directly suppress erythropoiesis and antagonize the action of folate.[5] Furthermore, excessive alcohol consumption frequently is associated with a diet poor in folates and with both chronic and acute gastrointestinal blood loss.

Although it rarely presents with isolated anemia, lead intoxication interferes with a variety of red blood cell enzyme systems required for hemoglobin synthesis and results in either a microcytic or normocytic anemia with prominent basophilic stippling of the red cells in the peripheral blood and ringed sideroblasts in the bone marrow. A blood lead level should be obtained whenever lead intoxication is suspected.

## Blood loss and hemolysis

Bleeding and hemolysis often occur episodically and may not be active at the time of evaluation. Therefore the history is particularly important when one is considering whether these processes are contributing to the development of anemia. A detailed menstrual and pregnancy history should be obtained on all women. Recent surgery and possible autologous blood donations should not be overlooked as potential sources of blood loss. Symptoms such as pica (craving to eat dirt, clay, ice, or laundry starch) or sore tongue and signs such as koilonychia (spooned nails), glossitis, or angular stomatitis are suggestive of iron deficiency. A history of jaundice or change in the color of the urine may indicate intravascular hemolysis.

## Drugs That May Result in Anemia

DRUGS THAT MAY INTERFERE WITH RED CELL PRODUCTION BY INDUCING MARROW SUPPRESSION OR APLASIA

Alcohol
Antineoplastic drugs
Antithyroid drugs
Antibiotics
Oral hypoglycemic agents
Phenylbutazone
Azidothymidine (AZT)

DRUGS THAT INTERFERE WITH $B_{12}$, FOLATE, OR IRON ABSORPTION OR UTILIZATION

Nitrous oxide
Anticonvulsant drugs
Antineoplastic drugs
Isoniazid, cycloserin A

DRUGS CAPABLE OF PROMOTING HEMOLYSIS

**Immune-mediated**

Penicillins
Quinine
Alpha-methyldopa
Procainamide
Mitomycin C

**Oxidative stress**

Antimalarials
Sulfonamide drugs
Nalidixic acid

DRUGS THAT MAY PRODUCE OR PROMOTE BLOOD LOSS

Aspirin
Alcohol
Nonsteroidal anti-inflammatory agents
Corticosteroids
Anticoagulants

## Chronic or systemic disease

An attempt to identify the various chronic or systemic disorders that may result in anemia begins with a history and physical examination. The major disease categories to be considered are neoplasia, chronic renal disease, chronic liver disease, endocrine disorders, chronic infection, and chronic inflammatory disorders such as rheumatoid arthritis, ulcerative colitis, and Crohn's disease.[6,7] In addition, a history of ulcer disease or bowel surgery may provide an important clue to identifying the source of iron, $B_{12}$, or folate deficiency. A personal or family history of gallstones or a cholecystectomy, splenectomy, or episodes of dark or cola-colored urine should prompt consideration of the various hemolytic disorders outlined in the box on p. 435.

## Physical examination

Many findings on physical examination help to direct the clinician's attention to the cause of anemia. A rectal and pelvic examination must not be overlooked in the evaluation of the anemic patient. Particular attention should be paid to the findings listed in Table 40-1.

# LABORATORY INVESTIGATION

The list of laboratory tests that may be indicated during the evaluation of the anemic patient is as diverse as the various underlying disorders that result in anemia.

## Initial studies

Red blood cell size is used to classify anemia. Electronic counters determine the size of the cell and therefore the mean corpuscular volume (MCV), which provides an important means of categorizing the type and causes of anemia. The normal MCV is 80 to 95 femtoliter (fL), and cells with a larger or smaller value are characterized as "macrocytic" and "microcytic" respectively. Therefore, anemia can be broadly grouped as microcytic (MCV <80 fL), normocytic (MCV 80 to 99 fL), or macrocytic (MCV >100 fL). The box on p. 437 characterizes the approach to anemias according to their MCV.[8]

The microcytic anemias generally result from deficient hemoglobin synthesis and represent the most common types of anemias in adults and children. This group includes iron deficiency, the anemias of chronic disease (inflammation), and the inherited defects in globin chain synthesis, that is, thalassemias. The anemias resulting from abnormalities of heme synthesis such as sideroblastic anemia and lead poisoning result in hemoglobin-deficient microcytic anemia.

The macrocytic anemias usually are associated with vitamin deficiencies or drugs that interfere with DNA synthesis. Folate and $B_{12}$ deficiency are the most common causes of macrocytic anemia. Liver disease, hypothyroidism, and abnormalities in purine metabolism also may result in a macrocytic anemia. The myelodysplastic syndromes and preleukemic states can present with a refractory and unexplained macrocytic anemia. Chemotherapeutic drugs such as hydroxyurea and the antimetabolites that interfere with DNA synthesis can cause a macrocytic anemia.

An elevated MCV may also be a manifestation of a reticulocytosis. because reticulocytes are larger than the more mature red cells. Clump-

# Classification of the Hemolytic Disorders

## INTRINSIC TO RED BLOOD CELL

**Hemoglobinopathy**

Sickle-cell disease
Thalassemia

**Membrane abnormality**

Hereditary spherocytosis
Hereditary elliptocytosis
Bur cell anemia associated with severe liver disease
Bur cell anemia associated with renal disease

**Enzymopathy**

Glucose-6-phosphate dehydrogenase deficiency
Pyruvate kinase deficiency

**Paroxysmal nocturnal hemoglobinuria**

## EXTRINSIC TO RED BLOOD CELL

Immune-mediated (microspherocytosis)

**Warm-reactive antibodies (Coombs' positive)**

Autoimmune drug-induced lymphoproliferative disease

**Cold-reactive antibodies**

Paroxysmal cold hemoglobinuria
Chronic idiopathic
Acute transient (after viral illness)
Syphilis
Cold agglutinin syndrome
Mycoplasmosis
Epstein-Barr virus causing mononucleosis
Lymphoproliferative disease

**Traumatic (schistocytes)**

Microangiopathy
Valvular heart disease
Marching
Trauma

**Table 40-1.** *Physical examination findings associated with anemia*

| Findings | Associated anemia |
|---|---|
| Pallor, tachypnea, tachycardia, orthostatic hypotension | Blood loss |
| Green-tinged pallor, koilonychia, glossitis, angular stomatitis, blood in stool | Iron deficiency |
| Fever, cachexia, chronic infection, rheumatoid arthritis, Crohn's disease, or other inflammatory disorders | Chronic disease |
| Diminished vibration and position sense, dementia | $B_{12}$ deficiency |
| Pallor, glossitis, signs of malabsorption, alcohol abuse, pregnancy | Folate deficiency |
| Bradycardia, hypothermia, cool coarse dry skin, sallow pallor, reduced scalp and body hair, nonpitting edema, goiter, husky voice, slow speech, poor hearing, poor memory, peripheral neuropathy, "hung-up" reflexes, hyperpigmentation, acne, excess hair growth | Endocrine disorders |
| Jaundice, icterus, spider angiomas, gynecomastia | Liver disease |
| Gingival lead line, abdominal tenderness, peripheral neuropathy | Lead poisoning |
| Ecchymoses, bone tenderness, recent fractures | Multiple myeloma |
| Fever, pallor, petechiae, ecchymoses | Aplastic anemia |
| Fever, pallor, petechiae, ecchymoses, adenopathy, sternal tenderness, splenomegaly | Leukemia, myelodysplasia |

ing or agglutination of red cells may cause a pseudomacrocytosis resulting in a false elevation of the MCV. The factitious macrocytosis caused by the agglutination of red cells attributable to a cold agglutinin or cryoglobulin can be corrected by warming the specimen before one determines the MCV.

Normocytic anemias generally reflect anemias because of underproduction of red cells as reflected by a low reticulocyte count. The anemias of chronic disease, aplastic anemia, and some of the anemias associated with thyroid dysfunction and other endocrine disorders usually result in normocytic anemias. The anemia of renal insufficiency

## Classification of the Causes of Anemia Based on Mean Corpuscular Volume (MCV)

### MICROCYTIC ANEMIA (MCV LESS THAN 80 FL)

Iron deficiency
Thalassemia trait
Anemia of chronic disease
Sideroblastic anemia
Lead poisoning

### NORMOCYTIC (MCV 81 TO 100 FL)

Anemia of chronic disease
Sickle cell disease
Recent blood loss
Hemolysis
Liver disease
Renal disease
Hypothyroidism
Adrenal insufficiency
HIV infection
Aplastic anemia
Myelophthisis
Leukemia
Lymphoma
Myeloma
Metastatic cancer

### MACROCYTIC (MCV GREATER THAN 100 FL)

**Megaloblastic**

Vitamin $B_{12}$ deficiency
Folate deficiency
Antineoplastic drugs

**Nonmegaloblastic**

Reticulocytosis
Alcohol
Liver disease
Hypothyroidism

and other disorders associated with impaired erythropoietin synthesis and secretion also are normochromic.

The MCV is an average value representing the arithmetic mean volume of red cells, and therefore combined abnormalities or partially treated anemias can result in a normal MCV. The red blood cell distribution width index (RDW) gives the distribution of the size of the red cells and reflects the heterogeneity of the RBC population. The RDW is elevated in patients with combined or partially treated anemias and in patients with a prominent reticulocytosis.

The mean corpuscular hemoglobin (MCH) and the mean corpuscular hemoglobin concentration (MCHC) generally reflect the findings of the MCV. Both values are low in iron deficiency but occur later than a decrease in the MCV. In hereditary spherocytosis the MCHC is elevated because it is associated with a population of smaller denser red cells. The finding of an elevated MCHC is very suggestive of the diagnosis of hereditary spherocytosis.

The electonically generated hematocrit (Hct) is generally three times the measured hemoglobin. A departure from this ratio occurs when there is brisk intravascular hemolysis or agglutination of red cells. The total and differential white cell count and the platelet count also must be reviewed when investigating anemia. Leukopenia or thrombocytopenia in conjunction with anemia (pancytopenia) is strongly suggestive of the presence of either a primary or a secondary disorder of the bone marrow, megaloblastic anemia, or hypersplenism.

## Examination of peripheral blood smear

The initial laboratory evaluation of the anemic patient should always include a review of the peripheral blood smear and a determination of the reticulocyte count.[9] The examination of the peripheral blood smear permits the recognition of many variations in the size and shape of the red blood cells. Oval macrocytes and hypersegmented neutrophils are suggestive of megaloblastic anemia. Circulating nucleated red blood cells and immature white cells (leukoerythroblastic picture) are suggestive of an infiltrative disorder involving the bone marrow. Abnormal WBCs can confirm the diagnosis of one of the leukemias.

The red cell shape is useful in the differential diagnosis of hemolytic anemias. Fragmented red cells are suggestive of a traumatic hemolysis often associated with a mechanical heart valve; spherocytes are a marker of hereditary spherocytosis; target cells are suggestive of liver disease, thalassemia, or hemoglobin C disease. Microspherocytes are suggestive of an immune-mediated hemolytic anemia. Table 40-2 reviews the common peripheral blood smear findings.

## The reticulocyte count

As noted earlier, each day approximately 0.8% of the RBC mass needs to be replaced by young erythrocytes released from the bone marrow. Reticulocytes are larger than mature RBCs, and they still contain portions of polyribosomal RNA material. Supravital stains (reticulocyte stain) of the peripheral blood smear detect these reticulated cells, and their number permits an assessment of the bone marrow's response to anemia. The corrected reticulocyte count provides an insight into the mechanism of the anemia. When the cause of the anemia is blood loss or destruction, the bone marrow normally responds by making more red blood cells resulting in an elevation of the reticulocyte count (reticulocytosis). An absence of an appropriate reticulocytosis indicates

**Table 40-2.** *Peripheral blood smear findings in the diagnosis of anemia*

| Findings | Associated anemia |
| --- | --- |
| Oval macrocytes, hypersegmented neutrophils | Megaloblastic anemia |
| Schistocytes (fragmented red cells) | Traumatic hemolysis, disseminated intravascular coagulation |
| Microspherocytes | Immune-mediated hemolysis |
| Elliptocytes (more than 25%) | Hereditary elliptosis |
| Spherocytes | Hereditary spherocytosis |
| Target cells | Liver disease, thalassemia |
| Basophilic stippling | Thalassemia, lead poisoning, myelodysplasia |
| Sickle cells | Sickle cell disease and variants |
| Microcytic, hypochromic red cells | Iron deficiency, chronic disease, sideroblastic anemia |
| Nucleated red cells | Marrow infiltration, infections, granuloma |
| Teardrop-shaped red cells | Myelofibrosis |
| Rouleau formation | Myeloma, macrolobulinemia, HIV |
| Agglutinated red cells | Cold agglutinin disease |
| Intracellular parasites | Babesiosis, malaria |
| Polychromasia | Reticulocytosis |

that the anemia results from impaired RBC production. The reticulocyte count is usually expressed as "percentage of RBCs examined." In the presence of anemia, when the red cell count is decreased, the percentage of reticulocytes is proportionally increased because the denominator, the number of red cells, in this fraction is decreased. The reticulocyte count therefore must be corrected for the degree of anemia according to the following formula:

$$\text{Corrected reticulocyte count} = \% \text{ reticulocytes} \times \frac{\text{Patient's Hct}}{45}$$

The normal reticulocyte count is 1% to 2%. A corrected reticulocyte count of greater than 5% implies that the erythroid marrow compartment is responding appropriately to the anemia. The absence of an appropriate reticulocytosis does not exclude peripheral destruction or blood loss but indicates that an additional disorder that interferes with a normal marrow response to the anemia also may be present. Corrected values of less than 0.5% in association with anemia are strongly suggestive of a primary bone marrow disorder that should be evaluated with a bone marrow aspiration or biopsy.

Testing of stool for the presence of occult blood should be part of the evaluation of the anemic patient, especially if the anemia is microcytic. Because gastrointestinal bleeding often occurs episodically, multiple samples should be obtained over 1 to 2 weeks.

## Additional laboratory testing

After a history and physical examination have been completed and the initial test results have been reviewed, further laboratory investigations usually are required to establish the cause or causes of anemia. Each component of this phase of the evaluation is directed to test a specific hypothesis generated during the initial evaluation.

Iron studies should be performed early in the evaluation of most patients with anemia because iron deficiency anemia is common and its presence indicates the need to identify a possible source of the blood loss. The interpretation of iron studies can be confusing in a patient with intercurrent medical problems. Tests used to assess an individual's iron stores are altered during the acute phase response and therefore may not accurately reflect the patient's iron stores in the presence of fever or of acute infection[10] (see the box).

The tests used to evaluate iron stores include the serum ferritin, serum iron, total iron-binding capacity (transferrin), transferrin saturation, free erythrocyte protoporphyrin, and bone marrow iron stores. The serum ferritin reflects the total body iron stores. The serum ferritin

---

### Causes of Iron Deficiency

Gastrointestinal blood loss
Pregnancy, lactation, and delivery
Blood donation
Medical phlebotomy
Dietary insufficiency in infants, adolescents, menstruating women, and strict vegetarians
*Genitourinary losses:* menstrual bleeding; uterine, cervical, or vaginal lesions; renal, ureteral, or bladder lesions; chronic intravascular hemolysis; hemodialysis
*Malabsorption:* after gastric or small bowel surgery or in malabsorption syndromes (celiac disease, nontropical sprue)
*Pulmonary losses:* idiopathic pulmonary hemosiderosis
Self-induced phlebotomy

falls in iron deficiency and rises in iron overload. In the "uncomplicated" patient, the serum ferritin accurately reflects iron stores and is a useful test to determine if the patient is iron deficient. The serum ferritin, however, also rises in response to inflammation. In the patient with fever and inflammation the serum ferritin may be normal even in the context of iron deficiency. The total iron-binding capacity (TIBC) rises as iron stores are depleted. In the context of inflammation the TIBC falls even in the presence of iron deficiency. The serum iron falls in both iron deficiency and acute inflammation. The transferrin saturation reflects the total iron-binding capacity and the serum iron. The ratio is decreased in iron deficiency and in inflammation. Free erythrocyte protoporphyrin (FEP) rises in iron deficiency and is not affected by recently administered iron therapy. FEP is most useful in recognizing iron deficiency in infants and differentiating the microcytosis of iron deficiency from the anemia associated with lead poisoning.

Tests of thyroid, renal, and liver function may be helpful in the evaluation of many patients with anemia. The creatinine clearance should be estimated in the evaluation of normocytic anemia of uncertain cause. Anemia caused by chronic renal disease is usually proportional to the degree of renal insufficiency. Because other causes of anemia occur frequently in patients with chronic renal failure, their presence should be carefully excluded before one attributes the anemia to renal disease.

When chronic liver disease is suspected, the serum albumin concentration and the prothrombin time should be determined along with the direct and indirect bilirubin, the lactate dehydogenase (LDH), the alkaline phosphatase, and the transaminases. It is unlikely that anemia is a result of liver disease if all these tests are normal. In addition to detection of liver disease, elevations of the indirect bilirubin and the LDH are useful indicators of hemolysis and ineffective erythropoiesis. When liver disease is present, mild to moderate anemia may develop as a consequence of shortened red cell survival. In these cases, examination of the blood smear usually reveals target cells or burr cells. Other potentially correctable causes of anemia, such as folate deficiency, blood loss, or hypersplenism, should be sought before attributing anemia to liver disease alone.

## Tests for hemolysis

Anemia caused by decreased red cell survival (hemolysis) may be suspected on the basis of the history, physical examination, or initial laboratory evaluation. Before attempting to establish a diagnosis of one of the disorders listed in the box on p. 435, evidence of hemolysis should be sought by determination of the levels of the indirect serum bilirubin, LDH, and haptoglobin. Although the presence of reticulocytosis indicates that hemolysis (or blood loss) may be present, the absence of reticulocytosis cannot be considered as evidence against hemolysis because other processes may prevent a normal marrow response to anemia. Both intravascular and, to a lesser degree, extravascular (reticuloendothelial) destruction of red cells result in increases in the levels of the indirect bilirubin and the LDH and decreases in the haptoglobin level. Recent transfusions also may alter the haptoglobin and the bilirubin, making the evaluation of hemolysis more difficult. In cases where an episode of hemolysis is believed to have occurred and resolved before an evaluation could begin, the presence of hemosiderin-containing renal tubular cells may be helpful. In contrast to the aforementioned blood tests, these cells may be observed in the urine sediment for up to 14 days after episodes of intravascular hemolysis. The urinary hemosiderin is also a useful test to detect intermittent and chronic hemolysis.

Once the presence of hemolysis has been established, further evaluation to determine the cause of hemolysis should be sought (see box p. 435). For example, Coombs' test should be used to establish the presence of warm antibody-mediated hemolysis, hemoglobin electrophoresis should be performed if the presence of an abnormal hemoglobin is suspected, and osmotic fragility should be evaluated when hereditary spherocytosis is suspect.

### Tests for vitamin $B_{12}$ deficiency and folate deficiency

The presence of vitamin $B_{12}$ (cyanocobalamin) deficiency or folate deficiency should be confirmed by direct level measurement. Vitamin $B_{12}$ deficiency or folic acid deficiency results in a megaloblastic anemia that is almost always accompanied by the characteristic presence of hypersegmented neutrophils and oval macrocytes on the peripheral blood smear. Macrocytosis may be absent in the presence of megaloblastic hematopoiesis as a result of other concomitant medical and nutritional deficiencies.

When megaloblastic hematopoiesis is recognized, however, $B_{12}$ and folate levels should be measured to define which deficiency is present.[11] The serum folate level, however, may not accurately reflect folate deficiency because the serum folate level may rapidly normalize as a consequence of improved diet soon after hospital admission. In the absence of transfusions, the red cell folate level is the test of choice in hospitalized patients because it is not subject to rapid alterations. A low folate level may occur in combination with $B_{12}$ deficiency. Replacement of the folic acid without $B_{12}$ may correct the hematologic manifestation of the $B_{12}$ deficiency but allow irreversible neurologic damage attributable to untreated $B_{12}$ deficiency to progress. Some measure of caution is therefore appropriate in the interpretation of the results of either of these tests for folate deficiency. The serum $B_{12}$ level is generally not affected by changes in diet and therefore is useful to detect $B_{12}$ deficiency. However, falsely low levels of $B_{12}$ are also occasionally reported.[12] This occurs primarily in the presence of folate deficiency, transcobalamin I deficiency, multiple myeloma, pregnancy, or oral contraceptive use. In the presence of $B_{12}$ deficiency there is reduced activity of intracellular $B_{12}$-dependent enzyme levels resulting in increased urinary excretion of methylmalonic acid (MMA). MMA excretion is increased in $B_{12}$ deficiency but not in folate deficiency and other causes of macrocytosis.[13] The serum cobalamin levels fall as people age. The incidence of low serum level is between 5% and 20%

in the elderly population.[14] The meaning of these low levels is unclear, but they indicate that the metabolic deficiency of $B_{12}$ may be underestimated in the elderly population. The cause of low $B_{12}$ levels in the elderly is multifactorial. In some patients it represents classical pernicious anemia, whereas in others malabsorption limited to food-bound cobalamine may be responsible.

## Bone marrow examination

The presence of bicytopenia or pancytopenia, reticulocytopenia, or leukoerythroblastosis (circulating immature myeloid and erythroid precursors) should be evaluated with bone marrow evaluation. The bone marrow examination is useful in the evaluation of anemia to determine the status of iron stores, to confirm the presence of megaloblastosis, to evaluate combined nutritional deficiency states, and to recognize abnormal marrow function or maturation.

# SELECTED CAUSES OF ANEMIA

The two most common causes of anemia, chronic disease, and iron deficiency, as well as the anemia of chronic renal disease and of megaloblastic anemia are of sufficient importance to the clinician to merit additional brief discussion in this chapter.

## The anemia of chronic disease

The anemia of chronic disease (ACD) is the anemia that accompanies chronic inflammation, infections, or neoplasms.[15] Although the name is suggestive that this syndrome occurs in any one of a vast array of chronic diseases, this diagnosis should be considered only in association with an inflammatory, infectious, or neoplastic process. The anemia of chronic disease is one of the most frequently encountered anemias. Furthermore, because other causes of anemia are frequently present in these settings, the anemia of chronic disease should be considered as a diagnosis of exclusion to avoid missing other less readily apparent causes of anemia.

The ACD syndrome is characterized by a moderate anemia (hematocrit rarely less than 25%), with normocytic or microcytic red blood cells. ACD is primarily an anemia caused by underproduction of red cells with a low reticulocyte production. Although ACD is generally considered a normochromic anemia, in 30% to 50% of patients the red cells are microcytic. The concentrations of serum iron, iron-binding capacity, and transferrin saturation are reduced with adequate iron stores. The serum ferritin is increased. The latter two features are helpful in distinguishing the anemia of chronic disease from that of iron deficiency. In iron deficiency, the serum transferrin increases and the ferritin decreases. The mechanism responsible for ACD is not clear but may in part be mediated by the endogenous release of cytokines associated with the underlying disease, which in turn inhibits erythropoiesis.[16] In the absence of intercurrent pulmonary or cardiac disease the anemia of chronic disease rarely is symptomatic, and transfusions generally are not needed.

## Iron-deficiency anemia

A lack of iron is the most common nutritional deficiency affecting humans. It has been estimated that one billion people in the world are anemic, and over half have iron deficiency as the cause (see box, p. 440). Iron deficiency can have profound effects on the mental and motor development in infants and children.[17] Iron-deficiency anemia typically presents with hypochromic and microcytic red blood cells, decreased serum iron, ferritin levels, transferrin saturation, and increased serum transferrin levels (iron-binding capacity). Not infrequently, however, one or several of these features are absent, and establishing the diagnosis is more challenging. A low serum ferritin level, less than 10 $\mu$g/L, is generally considered diagnostic of iron deficiency, and values less than 20 $\mu$g/L are suggestive of an iron-deficiency state.[18] However, a plasma ferritin in the normal range does not necessarily rule out iron deficiency. Infections, inflammation, liver disease, and malignant disorders can increase the ferritin level. In patients with chronic inflammation, a ferritin level of greater than 100 $\mu$g/L makes iron deficiency unlikely (Table 40-3). When iron deficiency is suspected and blood iron studies are inconclusive, the status of the patient's iron stores should be evaluated, either with an examination of the marrow for stainable iron or with a therapeutic trial of oral iron supplements (such as 325 mg of ferrous sulfate tid for 2 months).

Once recognized, the proper management of iron-deficiency anemia includes not only treatment with iron supplements, but also a search for the source of the deficiency (blood loss). In developed countries, iron deficiency in adults usually occurs as a consequence of gastrointestinal blood loss. Other causes of iron deficiency are listed in the box on p. 440. Oral iron supplements should be administered for at least 6 months to correct both the anemia and the depleted body iron stores. Failure of the anemia to respond completely to iron therapy within 2 months after starting therapy implies either continued blood loss, noncompliance with therapy, impaired ability to absorb iron as a consequence of a gastric or small bowel pathologic condition, or an incorrect or incomplete initial diagnosis.

**Table 40-3.** *Laboratory measurements of iron status*

| Test | Iron deficiency | Hemolysis | Inflammation |
|------|-----------------|-----------|--------------|
| Serum ferritin ($\mu$g/L) | <12 | Normal | >100 |
| Serum iron ($\mu$g/L) | <15 | >100 | <20 |
| Transferrin ($\mu$g/L) | >250 | Normal | <200 |
| Transferrin saturation | <16% | >25% | 15%–40% |

## The anemia of chronic renal disease

Anemia is a common effect of acute and chronic renal failure. The anemia, though multifactorial in origin, is primarily attributable to erythropoietin deficiency.[19] Other factors may contribute to the development of anemia in this setting. These include iron deficiency attributable to both hemodialysis-associated and gastrointestinal blood loss, dietary or dialysis-induced folate deficiency, aluminum toxicity, hyperparathyroidism, decreased red blood cell survival, and perhaps nondialyzable uremic inhibitors of erythropoiesis. In addition, hemolysis may occur in these patients as a consequence of the uremia or improper hemodialysis if blood is exposed to formaldehyde, heat, or hypotonic media. In renal failure, erythropoietin (rhEPO) can induce a dose-dependent increase in erythropoiesis. Most patients require a dose of 50 to 125 IU/kg intravenously or subcutaneously three times per week to maintain a hematocrit in the 30% to 35% range. Patients who fail to respond to rhEPO may have intercurrent iron deficiency. As in other settings, patients who do not respond to rhEPO should be investigated in an attempt to identify and correct other reversible causes of anemia.

## Megaloblastic anemia

Once megaloblastic anemia has been recognized and the results of serum $B_{12}$ and folate tests indicate that deficiency is present, treatment should be instituted, and a cause of the deficiency identified. When $B_{12}$ deficiency is present, pernicious anemia is the most likely cause and can be documented when one performs a Schilling test that corrects with exogenously administered intrinsic factor. The Schilling test assesses the ability of the gut to absorb $B_{12}$. The Schilling test has three parts: the first part administers radiolabeled $B_{12}$ and requires the secretion of endogenous intrinsic factor; the second part administers $B_{12}$ with intrinsic factor and tests the ability of the terminal ileum to absorb the $B_{12}$–intrinsic factor complex. If there is evidence of a possible blind-loop disease or bacterial overgrowth, part two should be repeated after a trial of oral antibiotics (part three). The presence of anti-intrinsic factor antibodies supports the diagnosis of pernicious anemia.

Folate deficiency occurs as a consequence of any one of the following associated disorders: dietary insufficiency; nutritional malabsorption caused by drugs, enteritis, enteropathy, or gastric or jejunal resection; or the increased nutritional requirements of infancy, pregnancy, chronic hemolytic disease, malignancy (also attributable to poor diet), or chronic exfoliative dermatitis. In patients who drink alcoholic beverages on a regular basis, poor diet, ethanol-induced interruption of the enterohepatic circulation of folates, and a direct antifolate action of ethanol frequently lead to folate deficiency. Folate deficiency can occur within 3 weeks of stopping of the folic acid. When features of megaloblastic hematopoiesis are identified but $B_{12}$ and folate levels are not decreased, a primary bone marrow disorder such as myelodysplasia or marrow dysfunction caused by drug or toxic exposure should be considered.

Many patients with low $B_{12}$ levels do not have megaloblastic anemia or neurologic disease. Patients with AIDS have abnormal serum $B_{12}$

levels. In a majority of AIDS patients, the low $B_{12}$ level is not a physiologic deficiency of $B_{12}$ but rather results from impaired transcobalamin transport, and replacement therapy does not improve the anemia.[20] The meaning of a low serum $B_{12}$ in the asymptomatic patient is controversial. For example, about 20% of healthy elderly individuals have low serum cobalamin levels without evidence of anemia or neurologic disease. The box below lists the common causes of a low serum $B_{12}$ level. A Schilling test should be performed on patients with an unexplained low $B_{12}$ level. Do all patients require treatment with $B_{12}$ in the absence of symptoms? At present it is advisable to institute therapy in patients with low cobalamin levels of uncertain cause, especially if there is evidence of possible malabsorption. However, in patients in whom it is clear that cobalamin deficiency does not exist, that is, early in pregnancy, treatment may not be needed.

# MANAGEMENT

The optimal management of the anemic patient must include efforts directed, not only at treating the symptoms attributable to anemia itself,

---

## Common Causes of Low Serum Cobalamin Levels

### DISORDERS INVOLVING COBALAMIN DEFICIENCY

**Malabsorption of free cobalamin**

Pernicious anemia
Postgastrectomy
Small bowel disease

**Malabsorption of food cobalamin**

Atrophic gastritis
Postgastrectomy
Chronic gastritis

### DISORDERS IN WHICH COBALAMIN STATUS IS UNCLEAR

**Deficiency in some but not all cases**

Elderly
Vegans (strict vegetarians)
AIDS
Idiopathic

**Deficiency uncommon**

Pregnancy
Folate deficiency
Multiple myeloma

but also at correcting the cause or causes of the anemia insofar as that may be possible.

## Transfusion

The transfusion of packed red cells to correct anemia is indicated if the patient is symptomatic or if anemia threatens damage to the brain, heart, or other vital organs. Common symptoms attributable to severe anemia include exertional dyspnea and other forms of exercise intolerance, headache, dizziness, faintness, profound fatigue, angina pectoris, and claudication. A great deal of individual variation exists with regard to which symptoms predominate. When anemia develops over a prolonged period, as is often the case, these problems generally do not develop until the hemoglobin falls below 7 g/dL unless there is coexisting pulmonary or cardiovascular disease.

## Hormonal therapy

The effects of pharmacologic doses of androgens on erythropoiesis may be useful in the treatment of anemia in selected clinical settings. Androgens such as oxymetholone and fluoxymesterone have been used for many years to stimulate erythropoiesis in patients with anemia caused by diminished production of red cells. These compounds sometimes are able to induce clinically significant increases in red blood cell production both by increasing the production of erythropoietin and by enhancing the effects of erythropoietin on the marrow. The androgens have been used with variable results in patients with idiopathic myelofibrosis, myelodysplasia, aplastic anemia, paroxysmal nocturnal hemoglobinuria, and the anemia of chronic renal disease. Their clinical use is frequently limited by the development of unacceptable side effects such as cholestatic hepatitis, virilization, or salt-and-water retention, and the lack of a durable response.

The recent cloning and expression of the human gene for erythropoietin has had important clinical implications for the management of anemia. Recombinantly produced human erythropoietin (rhEPO) has resulted in the elimination of transfusion dependency for patients with renal insufficiency without meaningful side effects.[21] The role of rhEPO in the management of other causes of anemias remains controversial. In patients with nonrenal causes of anemias, the measurement of endogenous erythropoietin levels may help in identifying those patients most likely to benefit from rhEPO therapy. A low endogenous level of less than 100 U is generally associated with a more favorable response to treatment.

## References

1. Self KG, Conrady MM, Eichner ER: Failure to diagnose anemia in medical inpatients: Is the traditional diagnosis of anemia a dying art? *Am J Med* 81:786-790, 1986.
2. Hess CE, Ayers CR, Sandusky WR, et al: Mechanism of dilutional anemia in massive splenomegaly, *Blood* 47:629-644, 1976.
3. Gulati GL, Bong HH: The automated CBC: a current perspective, *Hematol Oncol Clin North Am* 8:593-603, 1994.

4. Lux SE, Palek J: Disorders of red cell membrane. In Handin RI, Lux SE, Stossel TP, editors: Blood: principles and practice of hematology, Philadelphia, 1995, Lippincott.

5. Larkin EC, Watson-Williams EJ: Alcohol and the blood, *Med Clin North Am* 68:105-120, 1984.

6. Eschbach JW, Adamson JW: Anemia of end-stage renal disease (ESRD), *Kidney Int* 28:1-5, 1985.

7. Baer AN, Dessypris EN, Goldwasser E, Krantz SB: Blunted erythropoietin response to anaemia in rheumatoid arthritis, *Br J Haematol* 66:559-564, 1987.

8. Bessman JD, Gilmer PR. Gardner FH: Improved classification of anemias by MCV and RDW, *Am J Clin Pathol* 80:322, 1983.

9. Gulati GL, Hyun BH: Blood smear examination, *Hematol Oncol Clin North Am* 8:631-650, 1994.

10. Cook JD: Clinical evaluation of iron deficiency, *Semin Hematol* 19:6-18, 1982.

11. Herbert V: Megaloblastic anemias, *Lab Invest* 52:3-19, 1985.

12. Blundell EL, Matthews JH, Allen SM, et al: Importance of low serum vitamin $B_{12}$ and red cell folate concentrations in elderly hospitalized inpatients, *J Clin Pathol* 38:1179-1184, 1985.

13. Joosten E, Pelemans W, Devos P, et al: Cobalamin absorption and serum homocysteine and methylmalonic acid in elderly subjects with low serum cobalamin, *Eur J Haematol* 51:25-30, 1993.

14. Pennypacker LC, Allen RH, Kelly JP, et al: High prevalence of cobalamin deficiency in elderly outpatients, *J Am Geriatr Soc* 40:1197-1204, 1992.

15. Lee GR: The anemia of chronic disease, *Semin Hematol* 20:60-69, 1983.

16. Means RT, Krantz SB: Inhibition of human erythroid colony forming units by gamma interferon can be corrected by recombinant human erythropoietin, *Blood* 78:2564-2576, 1991.

17. Oski FA: Iron deficiency in infancy and childhood, *N Engl J Med* 329:190-193, 1993.

18. Guyatt GH, Patterson C, Ali M, et al: Diagnosis of iron deficiency in the elderly, *Am J Med* 88:205, 1990.

19. Eschbach JW, Egrie JC, Downing MR, et al: Correction of the anemia of end-stage renal disease with recombinant human erythropoietin: results of a combined phase I and II clinical trial, *N Engl J Med* 316:73-78, 1987.

20. Burkes RL, Cohen H, Krailo M, et al: Low serum cobalamin levels occur frequently in the acquired immune deficiency syndrome and related disorders, *Eur J Haematol* 38:141-152, 1987.

21. Erslev AJ: Erythropoietin, *N Engl J Med* 324:1339-1344, 1991, with comment in 324:1360-1362, 1991.

# Chapter 41

# An Approach to the Bleeding Patient

Kenneth B. Miller

## EVALUATION

The evaluation of a patient with a bleeding disorder must take into account the physiology of blood vessels, platelets, and coagulation proteins. The evaluation of the bleeding patient should start with the following questions:

### Where is the location of the bleeding?

Spontaneous hemarthroses and muscle hemorrhages are highly suggestive of severe hemophilia or other congenital bleeding disorders, whereas epistaxis, gingival bleeding, and menorrhagia are more commonly found in patients with thrombocytopenia, platelet disorders, or von Willebrand's Disease (vWD).

### What is the timing of the bleeding event? Did it occur after a procedure, biopsy, or surgery, or did it occur spontaneously?

Bleeding after a surgical experience may be related to the surgery or an underlying bleeding disorder. Patients without a history of bleeding who bleed in excess after a procedure suggest a more subtle defect of coagulation such as von Willebrand's disease or defects of platelet dysfunction or thrombocytopenia.

### Is there a personal history of bleeding or bruising?

Most patients with profound coagulation disorders have a history of abnormal bleeding. Specifically, questions about prolonged bleeding after a minor surgical experience such as a tooth extraction or a biopsy should be asked. A prior history of a transfusion after surgery or history of metrorrhagia and recurrent nose bleeds may indicate a prior bleeding disorder. A menstrual and obstetrical history should be obtained in all women.

### Is there a family history of bleeding?

A detailed family history is critical for evaluating a possible bleeding disorder. Many of the coagulation disorders are inherited; for example, hemophilia is a sex-linked disorder, whereas von Willebrand's disease is autosomally transmitted.

## What medications is the patient taking?

Many medications interfere with platelet function. The recent addition of an oral antibiotic and poor oral intake or malnutrition may place the patient at risk for vitamin K deficiency. The use of anticoagulants should be noted. Even a small dose of heparin, used to flush intravenous lines, may be associated with thrombocytopenia. Idiosyncratic reactions to drugs may produce profound thrombocytopenia. Recent medications may also interfere with coagulation studies. ASA (arylsulfatase-A) and nonsteroidal anti-inflammatory drugs (NSAIDs) affect platelet function and prolong the bleeding time (Table 41-1). A detailed medication history may also provide insight into underlying illnesses that can be associated with bleeding such as systemic lupus erythematosus or renal insufficiency.

# SCREENING TESTS

In the laboratory, screening tests are a useful start in the investigation of the bleeding patient and may be followed by more specialized and diagnostic tests. Before describing the clinical manifestations and laboratory perturbations of the different bleeding disorders, I briefly review normal hemostasis.

## Normal hemostasis

Hemostasis is divided into two separate but related phases: (1) primary hemostasis, in which there is rapid occlusion of a vascular lesion by a

**Table 41-1.** *Medications commonly associated with platelet dysfunction*

| Agent | Mechanism and effect |
|-------|----------------------|
| Aspirin | Irreversible acetylation of platelet, increases BT, blocks cyclo-oxygenase (for full life of platelet) <br> Abnormal platelet aggregation |
| Dipyridamole | Inhibits platelet phosphodiesterase, no change in BT |
| NSAID | Reversible inhibitor of platelet cyclo-oxygenase, alters platelet aggregation <br> Reversible within 24 to 48 hours of stopping medication, can prolong BT |
| Ticlopidine | Inhibits platelet aggregation, prolongs BT; platelet dysfunction lasts 4 to 10 days |

*BT,* Bleeding time; *NSAID,* nonsteroidal anti-inflammatory drug.

platelet plug, and (2) secondary hemostasis, which results in the formation of a stable fibrin clot. Disruption of vascular endothelium results in immediate vasoconstriction, which is both intrinsic to the vessel and secondary to the release of humoral factors. These factors also modulate platelet adherence and promote platelet aggregation and foster formation of the platelet plug. Once this plug forms, the secondary phase of hemostasis begins by factor activation through the coagulation cascade, ultimately resulting in a stable fibrin clot overlying and strengthening the initial platelet plug. Factor activation by the coagulation cascade requires a series of enzymatic reactions depicted in Fig. 41-1. Central to the coagulation cascade is the activation of factor X, which converts prothrombin to thrombin; thrombin, in turn, cleaves fibrinogen to fibrin. The result is the formation of an interlinked, insoluble fibrin. Factor X can be activated by either the intrinsic pathway, generally measured by the partial thromboplastin time (PTT), or by the extrinsic pathway, measured by the prothrombin time (PT).

This scheme of blood coagulation is important for our understanding of clot formation in vitro and the laboratory monitoring of anticoagulation and the diagnosis of coagulation disorders. However, the cascade does not accurately reflect hemostasis in vivo. For instance patients with hereditary factor XII deficiency have a greatly prolonged PTT but

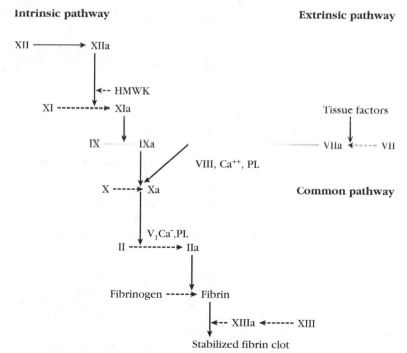

**Figure 41-1.** *The clotting cascade. IIMWK, High-molecular-weight kininogen; Ca<sup>++</sup>, calcium; PL, phospholipids; a, active factor.*

have no bleeding problems, whereas patients deficient in factor VII bleed abnormaliy.[1] The in vivo events are suggestive that the key to initiation of blood coagulation is the exposure of cell surfaces expressing tissue factor that bind to factor VII.

Clotting factors are made predominantly in the liver. Factor VIII is also made by endothelial cells. In the hepatocyte, vitamin K is required for the synthesis of prothrombin (II) and factors VII, IX, and X. These "vitamin K–dependent" clotting factors contain a unique amino acid residue called gamma-carboxyglutamic acid.

The fibrinolytic system, which is mediated by the proteolytic enzyme plasmin, is responsible for the dissolution and remodeling of the fibrin clot. The regulation and control of the fibrinolytic system are mediated by specific molecular interactions among its main components and by controlled synthesis and release of plasminogen activators and plasminogen-activator inhibitors from endothelial cells. Disorders of the fibrinolytic system may result either from impaired activation, which results in thrombotic events, or from excessive activation, which results in bleeding complications. The proteolysis of fibrin by plasmin produces debris designated "fibrin split products" (FSP); these low-molecular-weight proteins inhibit the action of thrombin on fibrinogen and interfere with platelet activation.

Patients with an abnormality of one coagulation factor (such as hemophilia) form a normal platelet plug and therefore have normal primary hemostasis. Individuals with vascular or platelet abnormalities (such as vasculitis or thrombocytopathy) have a defect in primary hemostasis but are able to form a normal fibrin clot. Coagulation studies help to determine whether a primary or a secondary hemostatic abnormality is present.

Four readily available tests are useful in the initial evaluation of the bleeding patient (Table 41-2):

1. Bleeding time (BT)
2. Platelet count
3. Prothrombin time (PT) and partial thromboplastin time (PTT)

A platelet count of less than $50,000/mm^3$ is associated with an increased risk of posttraumatic bleeding, whereas a platelet count of less than $20,000 \ mm/^3$ is associated with spontaneous bruising and petechiae. There is a linear correlation between the platelet count and the risk of spontaneous bleeding, provided that there is not a concomitant platelet dysfunction.

The bleeding time reflects platelet adherence and intrinsic platelet function and is not, as the name implies, a global test of the hemostatic system. The bleeding time is prolonged in disorders that affect platelet function or number. The bleeding time is normal in most disorders that affect the soluble coagulation cascade and prolong the PT and PTT. The bleeding time is prolonged in patients with a platelet count below $100,000/mm^3$, disorders associated with platelet dysfunction including the recent administration of aspirin, and deficiencies or func-

**Table 41–2.** *Tests used in evaluation of bleeding patient*

| Test | Normal | Pathway | Prolonged in |
|------|--------|---------|--------------|
| Partial thromboplastin time (PTT) | 25–40 seconds | Intrinsic | Hemophilia, von Willebrand's disease, factor deficiency (VIII, IX, XII, X, fibrinogen), circulating anticoagulant, DIC, heparin therapy |
| Prothrombin time (PT) | 8–12 seconds INR = 1 | Extrinsic | Warfarin therapy, vitamin K deficiency, liver disease, DIC, Factor deficiency (X, V, prothrombin, fibrinogen) |
| Bleeding time (BT) | 4–9 minutes | Primary hemostasis | Platelet disorders, von Willebrand's disease, intrinsic platelet dysfunction, thrombocytopenia |
| Thrombin time (TT) | 10–15 seconds | Fibrinogen → fibrin | Dysfibrinogenemia, DIC with FSP, hypofibrinogenemia, heparin |

*DIC,* disseminated intravascular coagulopathy; *FSP,* fibrin split products; *INR,* international normalized ratio.

tional abnormalities of plasma proteins required for normal interaction of platelets and the vessel wall such as von Willebrand's disease. The bleeding time may also be prolonged in patients with defects of vascular structure, vasculitis, or defects of collagen synthesis. The bleeding time is influenced by many factors, including the depth, location, skin thickness, and skill of the technologist performing the test.[2] The bleeding time is prolonged in a linear fashion as the platelet count falls from 100,000 to 10,000/mm$^3$ and therefore is not a useful test in patients with thrombocytopenia.[3]

The use of the bleeding time to evaluate the primary phase of coagulation is controversial. Analysis of the performance of the bleeding time indicates that the test functions poorly as a screening test for bleeding disorders.[4] However, in selected patients the bleeding time, carefully performed, may be helpful in defining an underlying disorder of primary hemostasis.[5] I recommend the bleeding time test for patients with a normal platelet count and unexplained bleeding to evaluate a possible defect of platelet interaction with the vessel wall. Many disorders and medications can affect platelet function and the bleeding time (see box). The bleeding time therefore must be interpreted with caution.

## Common Drugs That Inhibit Platelet Function

NONSTEROIDAL ANTI-INFLAMMATORY AGENTS

Aspirin
Indomethacin
Ibuprofen, naproxen, etc.

BETA-LACTAM ANTIBIOTICS

Ticarcillin
Methicillin
Piperacillin
Carbenicillin
Cephalosporins

CARDIOVASCULAR DRUGS

Nitroglycerin
Nitroprusside
Calcium channel blockers (nifedipine, verapamil, etc.)

PSYCHOTROPIC DRUGS

Tricyclic antidepressants
Phenothiazines

OTHER DRUGS

Dextrans
Furosemide
Phentolamine
Dypridamole
Ticlopidine

## The platelet count

The platelet count should be a routine part of the evaluation of all bleeding patients. The platelet count can rapidly fall and be associated with increased destruction or impaired production. The finding of thrombocytopenia should be confirmed by a review of the peripheral blood smear. Abnormalities of platelet size and the presence of red blood cell fragments that are suggestive of disseminated intravascular coagulation or other microangiopathies may provide important clues to direct the further evaluation of the bleeding patient.

## The prothrombin time

The prothrombin time (PT) measures the extrinsic and common pathways and is prolonged with abnormalities of factors VII, V, and X and prothrombin and fibrinogen. The PT may be prolonged because of a deficiency of one of the clotting factors or because of the presence of an inhibitor or circulating anticoagulant.

## Partial thromboplastin time

The partial thromboplastin time (PTT) measures the intrinsic and common pathways. The PTT may be prolonged because of a deficiency of one or more of the clotting factors or because of the presence of inhibitors that affect their function. A clotting factor level of less than 30% is needed before the PTT is prolonged.

To further define the cause of bleeding or a prolonged PTT/PT, specialized clotting tests are often required to further define the hemostatic abnormality, including thrombin time (TT), reptilase time, Stypven (Russell's viper venom) time, fibrinogen and fibrin split product measurement, intrinsic platelet function tests, and the ristocetin cofactor assay. The thrombin time is prolonged in the presence of heparin, fibrin split products, or abnormal or low serum fibrinogen. If the thrombin time is prolonged, a reptilase time should be performed. The reptilase time is not prolonged in the presence of heparin and is therefore helpful in evaluating a patient with a prolonged PTT when a heparin effect is questioned. The Stypven time directly measures the activation of factor X and is independent of factor VII activation. The ristocetin cofactor assay is most useful in the evaluation of von Willebrand's disease.

# COAGULATION AND PLATELET DISORDERS

## Hereditary coagulation disorders

The most commonly inherited disorders of coagulation are hemophilia A, hemophilia B, and von Willebrand's disease. Although inherited hypofibrinogenemias and quantitative and qualitative abnormalities of factors V, VII, XII, and XIII have been described, these are rare disorders.

The diagnosis of hemophilia A (factor VIII deficiency) should be suspected in any man with a hemarthrosis or in men with abnormal PTTs and family histories of bleeding. Hemophilia A is a sex-linked recessive disease that affects more than 15,000 males in the United States.[6] The defect in hemophilia A is a mutation in the q28 region of the X chromosome that results in failure to make functional factor VIII. Laboratory tests reveal a prolonged PTT and a low factor VIII level and activity. The PT and bleeding time are normal. The frequency and severity of the bleeding are directly related to the factor VIII level. Severe hemophiliacs have a factor VIII activity of less than 1% and often bleed in infancy; moderate hemophiliacs have activities between 1% and 5%; individuals with levels greater than 5% generally have mild disease and seldom spontaneously bleed.

Patients with moderate to severe hemophilia have a variety of lifelong bleeding problems related to soft-tissue and intra-articular bleeding, and yet mucosal bleeding are rare. The most notable problem is hemarthrosis, which commonly involves the knees and other large joints. A hemarthrosis is a painful, tender, and swollen joint with blood in the intracapsular space.

In general, patients with mild hemophilia have little serious bleeding. Spontaneous bleeding is rare. These patients may be asymptomatic and may only be diagnosed during adulthood. The mild hemophiliac, however, can develop serious bleeding after trauma or surgery and may require treatment before surgical or dental procedures.

Therapy for hemophilia A historically required the infusion of cryoprecipitate and, later, factor VIII concentrates. This practice, however, was complicated by the transmission of infectious hepatitis and human immunodeficiency virus (HIV). Monoclonal-purified, virus-inactivated factor VIII has become available. Recombinant factor VIII products are also available.[7] These agents are not associated with the transmission of infections. Factor VIII products should be administered at the first sign of a bleeding event. Restoration of normal hemostasis after serious bleeding usually requires a factor VIII level of 30% to 50%. Therapy should be continued for several days after cessation of bleeding and for at least 10 days after surgery. The use of epsilon-aminocaproic acid (EACA, Amicar) decreases the amount of factor VIII required after dental surgery.

In patients with mild to moderate hemophilia A, DDAVP, the synthetic vasopressin analog, is an important therapeutic alternative. DDAVP administered intravenously causes an increase in circulating factor VIII by releasing endothelial stores. An intravenous dose of 0.3 $\mu$g/kg often raises the level of factor VIII fourfold for 6 to 24 hours. This may be adequate in patients with mild disease, but it is rarely sufficient to prevent bleeding during minor surgery or trauma in those patients with severe disease. As many as 10% to 15% of hemophilia patients do not have a rise in factor VIII level after adequate factor administration. This is attributable to the presence or development of an antibody to factor VIII, which inhibits its action. Two groups of patients have inhibitors: patients with a low, constant level of antibody that is not affected by antigenic stimulation (noninducible) and patients whose antibody titer rises dramatically after administration of factor XIII (inducible). Patients with a noninducible inhibitor generally require a substantial increase in factor VIII dosage. Patients with an inducible inhibitor may require extremely high doses of factor VIII, or alternative forms of treatment to stop the bleeding.

Hemophilia B, a sex-linked recessive disorder, is clinically identical to hemophilia A, though attributable to factor IX deficiency.[8] The pattern of standard coagulation test abnormalities is identical to hemophilia A, but the factor IX activity is low. Treatment of hemophilia B requires the infusion of factor IX concentrate.

Von Willebrand's disease is a heterogenous collection of inherited disorders associated with bleeding into the skin and mucous membranes associated with the deficiency or abnormality of von Willebrand factor (vWF).[9] It is an autosomally transmitted defect that affects males and females equally. As with the clotting factor disorders, the defect may be qualitative or quantitative. vWF, a high-molecular-weight multimeric protein, circulates as the factor VIII carrier protein. vWF is important for platelet adherence to the damaged endothelial surface. vWF binds both to the endothelial surface at the site of vessel injury and to the platelet surface membrane. In the absence of a normal vWF, platelets cannot bind to ruptured vascular endothelium, and bleeding ensues.

The clinical manifestations of von Willebrand's disease are variable but usually include some form of mucous membrane bleeding. Patients may have a long history of recurrent nose bleeds, easy bruising, or menorrhagia. Spontaneous hemarthroses are extremely rare. Because the history in patients with von Willebrand's disease is difficult to interpret, all patients with prolonged postsurgical bleeding or with a history of excessive bruising after mild trauma should be evaluated for this disorder.

Three major subtypes of von Willebrand's disease have been described, depending on the specific vWF abnormality. Type I patients have a quantitative decrease in vWF. Type II patients have qualitative abnormalities, including abnormal assembly of multimeric vWF or abnormalities that lead to rapid vWF clearance. Type III is the absolute absence of vWF, and patients present with severe bleeding at a young age. An acquired form of vWD has been described in a small number of patients with no family history of bleeding disorders. These patients have antibodies that interfere with vWF function or may adsorb vWF onto malignant cells. These forms of acquired vWF have been described in lymphoma, in multiple myeloma, and in other cancers. These patients respond poorly to DDAVP.

Laboratory tests obtained in patients with suspected von Willebrand's disease are listed in Table 41-3. Because von Willebrand's factor is required for platelet adherence, patients have a prolonged BT, and since vWF is the factor VIII carrier protein, affected patients have reduced levels of factor VIII, and thus the PTT is prolonged. Platelet-adhesion studies and the ristocetin agglutination tests are abnormal,

**Table 41-3.** *Coagulation tests in von Willebrand's disease*

| Abnormal | Normal |
| --- | --- |
| Bleeding time (BT) | Prothombin time (PT), thrombin time (TT) |
| Partial thromoplastin time (PTT) | Platelet aggregation |
| Platelet adhesion | |
| Ristocetin cofactor assay | |
| Ristocetin agglutination | |
| Von Willebrand's factor antigen | |
| Factor VIII activity and antigen | |

whereas intrinsic platelet aggregation (platelet-platelet binding) tests are normal.

Treatment of von Willebrand's disease requires the replacement of the missing or abnormal vWF. DDAVP may raise the level of vWF by releasing endothelial stores and is best used in mild, type I, disease after a test dose ensures an adequate response. A rare subtype of type II is associated with DDAVP-induced thrombocytopenia. Tachyphylaxis to DDAVP occurs over time. Furthermore, the response to DDAVP is quite variable. Emergency replacement of vWF is most easily accomplished by the twice-daily infusion of cryoprecipitate, a plasma fraction rich in both factor VIII and vWF. Factor VIII concentrates have no role in the therapy of von Willebrand's disease. See the box on p. 459 for guidelines for the use of widely used blood products.

## Acquired coagulation disorders

Acquired coagulation disorders may be divided into four groups: (1) disorders of decreased factor production, (2) disorders of increased factor destruction, (3) circulating factor inhibitors, and (4) factor dilution secondary to massive transfusion. Any one of these defects can cause severe bleeding. The PT or PTT, or both, are prolonged in each of these disorders.

Vitamin K deficiency, the most common of the acquired coagulation disorders, results in decreased factor production because factors II, VII, IX, and X require vitamin K for their terminal activation.

Decreased vitamin K levels are found in patients receiving warfarin. Vitamin K synthesis and absorption from the gastrointestinal tract are interfered with by broad-spectrum antibiotics, by poor oral intake, and in patients with intestinal malabsorption. The antibiotics interfere with vitamin K metabolism and reduce gut flora that synthesizes vitamin K. Acute and chronically ill patients with poor oral intake, especially those taking antibiotics, are at highest risk for the development of vitamin K deficiency and subsequent severe bleeding.

Therapy is aimed at replacing vitamin K. Patients suspected of vitamin K deficiency generally have a prolonged PT and are at risk for serious bleeding and should receive vitamin K replacement (10 mg subcutaneously daily for 3 days) while the PT is monitored. Most deficiencies become corrected in 12 to 18 hours. In the bleeding patient administration of fresh frozen plasma (FFP) immediately replaces the needed clotting factors. Patients requiring warfarin are of special concern because administration of vitamin K to correct an excessively prolonged PT may make reinitiation of orally administered anticoagulation difficult. These patients are best treated with FFP to transiently treat the bleeding problem while holding the oral anticoagulation.

Acquired coagulation defects secondary to increased factor destruction include disseminated intravascular coagulopathy (DIC), liver disease, uremia, and postcardiopulmonary bypass.

In severe liver disease, vitamin K–dependent factors are not synthesized. Because most clotting proteins are made in the liver, both the PT and the PTT are prolonged. In addition, patients with severe liver disease may have thrombocytopenia from accompanying hypersple-

## Guidelines for the Use of Blood Products
........................................................................

### FRESH FROZEN PLASMA

1. Multiple coagulation factor deficiencies with prothrombin time >16 seconds or PTT >55 seconds and either active bleeding or planned surgical procedure
2. Previously documented deficiency of factor V or factor XI and either active bleeding or planned surgical procedure
3. Correction of warfarin anticoagulation with active bleeding or surgery planned within 6 to 12 hours
4. Thrombotic thrombocytopenic purpura (TTP) with plasmapheresis

### CRYOPRECIPITATE

1. Documented deficiency of fibrinogen (<100 mg/dL) and either active bleeding or planned surgical procedure
2. Documented deficiency of factor XIII and either active bleeding or planned surgical procedure
3. Active bleeding or a planned procedure in a patient with von Willebrand's disease not responsive to DDAVP; treatment of type II von Willebrand's disease
4. Disseminated intravascular coagulation

### PLATELETS

1. Prophylactic for a platelet count <15,000 to 20,000/mm$^3$
2. Active bleeding or planned major surgical procedure and a platelet count <100,000/mm$^3$
3. Documented platelet function disorder and active bleeding or planned surgical procedure
4. Active bleeding in a patient with uremia, recent aspirin ingestion, or after cardiopulmonary bypass or massive transfusion (>1 blood volume transfused within 24 hours)

nism. Patients with severe liver disease may also have increased fibrinolysis and dysfibrinogenemia. Although vitamin K is an important initial treatment, few patients with severe liver disease will respond. During episodes of bleeding, attempts to correct the clotting factor deficiency in severe liver disease require large quantities of FFP.[10] In cirrhosis of the liver fibrinogen levels fall, and cryoprecipitate may be required to replace the fibrinogen and control bleeding.

The hemostatic disorder in DIC is multifactorial.[11] DIC is suggested by a pattern of laboratory results that includes an elevation in PT, PTT, and thrombin time, thrombocytopenia, and the presence of fibrin split products (FSP). DIC results from the activation of the coagulation and fibrinolytic system in response to an illness or injury. The generation of thrombin and plasmin predisposes to both thrombotic and hemorrhagic complications. The peripheral blood smear allows documentation of the microangiopathic hemolytic changes, including fragmented erythrocytes and thrombocytopenia. The PT and PTT are prolonged in DIC because of the consumption of fibrinogen and other coagulation factors as well as the presence of FSPs that interfere with fibrin polymerization. The fibrinogen concentration is usually depressed but may remain in the normal range in low grade but clinically significant DIC. DIC usually results from several systemic diseases, and treatment must be aimed at the underlying disorder (see box below).

---

## Common Disorders Associated with Disseminated Intravascular Coagulopathy (DIC)

Infection
   Meningococcus
   Sepsis (gram positive and gram negative)
   Fungal sepsis
Malignancy
Vascular disease
   Aortic aneurysm
   Giant hemagioma (Kassabach-Merrit syndrome)
   Aortic balloon pump
   Vasculitis
Liver disease
   Fulminant hepatic failure
   Cirrhosis
Surgery
   Vascular surgery
   Liver transplantation
   Cardiac bypass
Obstetric complications
   Amniotic fluid embolism
   Abruptio placentae
   Retained dead fetus
   Toxemia
Heat stroke
Burns
Trauma
Promyelocytic leukemia
Acute intravascular hemolysis
Systemic lupus erythematosus
Fibrinolytic therapy
Pancreatitis
Snake bites

Acute treatment of the bleeding patient with DIC is aimed at replacement of the consumed clotting factors. Patients should receive platelets, FFP, and cryoprecipitate with measurement of coagulation parameters and fibrinogen levels. Most importantly, therapy must be directed at the underlying disease to interrupt the cause for consumptive coagulopathy. The use of heparin to inhibit coagulation remains controversial and is currently recommended only when thrombosis complicates the DIC.

Circulating inhibitors of specific coagulation factors also may cause severe bleeding. Factor inhibition is secondary to an antibody directed against a specific factor, most often factor VIII or X. These antibodies may occur with autoimmune diseases such as systemic lupus erythematosus or rheumatoid arthritis. Inhibitors are measured in Bethesda units (BU), a measure of concentration. In nonhemophiliacs, an inhibitor level greater than 15 BU is associated with major hemorrhage, whereas bleeding with an inhibitor level less than 10 BU is usually minor. Acute therapy may be ineffective and expensive and includes very high factor VIII dosing, porcine factor VIII, exchange transfusion, therapeutic plasmapheresis, or activated procoagulant complex.

In 5% to 10% of patients with active systemic lupus erythematosus (SLE), the PTT often is prolonged in vitro because of an antibody toward the test-dependent phospholipid.[12] These "lupus anticoagulants," often seen in patients with SLE, represent an important cause of a prolonged PTT in asymptomatic individuals. A one-to-one mixture of FFP with patient plasma fails to correct the abnormality. Lupus anticoagulants do not selectively inactivate any of the clotting factors and rarely interfere with hemostasis in vivo. Paradoxically, these patients have a 30% incidence of thrombosis.

Transfusions of large quantities of blood and colloid can result in a dilutional coagulopathy because these replacement products do not contain significant amounts of coagulation factors. Generally, 2 units of FFP are required for every 10 units of packed red cells administered, and cryoprecipitate is given to correct a measured fibrinogen deficiency. Close monitoring of the PT, PTT, and platelet count is required to avoid overlooking a concomitant consumptive coagulopathy. In addition, most patients will develop dilutional thrombocytopenia after 10 to 20 units of banked blood have been transfused. It is difficult to distinguish the role of dilutional coagulopathy from that of platelet consumption either during bleeding or clotting or secondary to consumption. Patients with pure dilutional thrombocytopenia require platelet infusion to prevent bleeding (see box on p. 459).

## Quantitative platelet disorders

Bleeding may result from either low platelet numbers or poor platelet function. There are many rare platelet disorders that cause significant bleeding.

Abnormalities in platelet production can be attributable to congenital megakaryocytic hypoplasia, marrow infiltration caused by granuloma or tumor, aplastic anemia, or toxic or immunologic bone marrow damage. Drug-induced thrombocytopenia can occur from either bone marrow toxicity or peripheral platelet destruction. Heparin-induced thrombocytopenia occurs in approximately 5% of patients receiving bovine heparin. Heparin-induced thrombocytopenia can occur even in patients who are receiving heparin only in line-flush solutions.[14] Heparin-induced thrombocytopenia in many cases is a diagnosis of exclusion; however, it should be suspected whenever a patient becomes thrombocytopenic while receiving any form of heparin. Patients who develop heparin-associated thrombocytopenia are also at risk for arterial and venous thrombosis. Moreover, patients who develop heparin-induced thrombocytopenia frequently demonstrate increased resistance to heparin therapy. In patients with heparin-induced thrombocytopenia the heparin should be discontinued and an alternative anticoagulant should be used.

Alcohol abuse often is implicated in bone marrow suppression, and it may be accompanied by folate deficiency and hypersplenism; severe bleeding rarely is seen without coexisting liver disease. The platelet count usually returns to normal within 1 to 2 weeks after cessation of alcohol use.

Drug-induced thrombocytopenia is often paroxysmal, and severe bleeding may ensue. In life-threatening cases, we recommend the administration of platelets even though the infused platelets have a short half-life. The use of steroids is controversial. Bone marrow recovery usually occurs within 4 to 10 days after cessation of the medication.

Idiopathic thrombocytopenic purpura (ITP), an immune-mediated thrombocytopenia purpura unrelated to drugs, occurs in acute and chronic forms and is a relatively common disorder. Antiplatelet antibodies often are implicated, though they may not be detected.

Acute ITP may be seen in any age group but is more common in children, especially after a viral infection. Except for petechiae and purpura, the children appear well, and hepatosplenomegaly is rare. The platelet count is low, and additional clotting tests are normal. Acute ITP in children generally has a favorable outcome, and over 80% of patients recover spontaneously. The remainder develop chronic ITP and require long-term corticosteroids, maintenance immunoglobulin, or splenectomy. Of concern are the 1% to 2% of acute ITP patients at risk for intracranial bleeding. Recent data indicate that 500 to 1000 mg/kg per day of intravenously administered immunoglobulin may be a reliable means of rapidly raising the platelet count. Adults presenting with acute ITP are usually initially treated with steroids. If clinical bleeding develops, intravenous immunoglobulin (400 mg/kg daily for 4 days) will often raise the platelet count rapidly.

Thrombocytopenia associated with infection with the human immunodeficiency virus is the most common hematologic manifestation of early HIV infection.[15] The majority of patients have mild thrombocytopenia, with less than 5% of patients having severe thrombocytopenia ($<50,000/mm^3$). The clinical course of HIV-associated thrombocytopenia shares many features with classical ITP. Bleeding manifestations are unusual in patients with platelet counts greater than $50,000/mm^3$. Most patients will not require treatment. In severe thrombocytopenia treatment with antiretroviral agents, steroids, IgG, and splenectomy are options.

Chronic ITP, predominantly an adult disease, may present acutely but often is insidious and has no relation to a viral illness. Patients are usually treated with steroids, and those patients who are refractory require splenectomy. Occasionally, patients respond to anabolic steroids such as danazol or to long-term immunosuppressive therapy. Chronic ITP may occur in a primary form or may be seen in association with chronic lymphocytic leukemia, lymphoma, or SLE.

Thrombotic thrombocytopenic purpura (TTP), a rare syndrome, is associated with low platelet counts, purpura, anemia, atypical neurologic findings, fever, and renal insufficiency. The anemia is a microangiopathic hemolytic anemia with schistocytes and reticulocytes seen on peripheral blood smear. Arteriolar occlusion may be responsible for renal dysfunction. Neurologic signs include headache, psychosis, and coma. TTP remains a severe disease with a mortality exceeding 60%. Therapy must include plasma infusion with plasma exchange (with plasma as the replacement fluid).

## Qualitative platelet disorders

Despite an adequate number of platelets, abnormalities in platelet function can result in bleeding. Abnormal laboratory tests include abnormal agglutination with ristocetin, epinephrine, or adenosine diphosphate (ADP). These disorders occur in both hereditary and acquired forms. Platelet dysfunction frequently occurs after aspirin consumption resulting in the acetylation of platelet cyclo-oxygenase that lasts for the life of the platelet (10 days). Platelet administration thus may be required if there is severe bleeding and a prolonged BT.

Uremia is associated with bleeding of the mucous membrane, gastrointestinal tract, and skin. The cause of this bleeding is primarily attributable to extrinsic platelet dysfunction that increases as uncleared metabolites accumulate. The BT is often greatly abnormal as are specialized platelet-function tests. Dialysis will partially correct the abnormal platelet function. DDAVP has been shown to sometimes correct the coagulopathy of uremia. The mechanism of action of DDAVP in these patients is unclear but may relate to the release of vWF from the vascular endothelium. The use of cryoprecipitate is controversial.

## References

1. Broze GJ Jr: The role of tissue factor pathway inhibitor in a revised coagulation cascade, *Semin Hematol* 29:159-169, 1992.
2. Roger RPC, Levin J: A critical reappraisal of the bleeding time, *Semin Thromb Hemost* 16:1, 1990.
3. Harker LA, Slichter SJ: The bleeding time as a screening test evaluation of platelet function, *N Engl J Med* 287:155-159, 1972.
4. Lind SE: The bleeding time does not predict surgical bleeding, *Blood* 12:2547-2552, 1991.
5. Triplet DA: The bleeding time—neither pariah nor panacea, *Arch Pathol Lab Med* 113:1207-1208, 1989.

6. Furie B, Limantain SA, Rosenfield CG: A practical guide to the evaluation and treatment of hemophilia, *Blood* 84:3-9, 1994.

7. Lusher JM: Transfusion therapy in congenital coagulopathies, *Hematol Oncol Clin North Am* 8:1167-1180, 1994.

8. Aledof LM: Safe approach to treatment of factor IX-deficient patients, *Semin Hematol* 28:21-29, 1991.

9. Triplett DA: Laboratory evaluation of von Willebrand's disease, *Mayo Clin Proc* 66:832-845, 1991.

10. NIH Consensus Conference: Fresh frozen plasma: indications and risks, *JAMA* 253:201-203, 1985.

11. Blick RL: Disseminated intravascular coagulation, *Hematol Oncol Clin North Am* 6:1259, 1992.

12. Khamashto MA, Cuadrado JE, Mujic F, et al: The management of thrombosis in the antiphospholipid-antibody syndrome, *N Engl J Med* 332:993-997, 1995.

13. Burstein SA: Thrombocytopenia due to decreased platelet production. In *Hematology: basic principles and practice,* Hoffman, Benz, Shantil, Furie, Cohen, Silberstein editors: New York, 1995, Churchill Livingstone.

14. Boshkov LK, Warkentin LE, Hayward CP, et al: Heparin-induced thromocytopenia and thrombosis: clinical and laboratory studies, *Br J Haematol* 84:322-328, 1993.

15. Mientjes GHC, van Ameijden EJC, Mulder JW, et al: Prevalence of thromocytopenia in HIV-infected and non-HIV infected drug users and homosexual men, *Br J Hematol* 82:615-619, 1992.

# Chapter 42

## *Leukocytosis*

Kenneth B. Miller

Leukocytosis, an elevation of the white blood cell count (WBC), is one of the most common problems in clinical medicine. Leukocytosis can reflect an acute infection, inflammation, exposure to a noxious agent, malignant disease, or even a benign physiologic response. The normal ranges for the absolute leukocyte and differential counts are presented in Table 42-1. In the normal adult, approximately 55% to 70% of the circulating leukocytes are neutrophilic granulocytes, 20% to 40% are lymphocytes, and the remaining 1% to 8% are monocytes and eosinophils.[1] Basophils are not usually seen during a 100-cell differential count. Lymphocytes are divided based on their functional and phenotypic markers, that is, T cell, B cell, NK cell, and so on.

Approximately 100 billion granulocytes and monocytes are produced in the bone marrow and released into the peripheral circulation each day. In the peripheral circulation, neutrophils are evenly divided into a circulating and a marginal pool. The peripheral WBC reflects the cells in circulating pools, whereas cells adherent to the vascular endothelium of the microcirculation are part of the marginal pool. The average neutrophilic leukocyte circulates in the blood for approximately 3 to 12 hours and can move freely between these two pools. However, once the neutrophil leaves the marginal pool to enter the tissues it cannot return. In contrast, lymphocytes can recirculate between the blood and the peripheral lymphoid tissues. Granulocytes leave the marginal pool (demarginate) and enter the circulating pool in response to stimuli that alter blood flow through the microcirculation or that affect cell adhesion to the vascular endothelium. Demargination results in a shift in the normal equilibrium between the circulating and the marginal pools and can result in a transient but sometimes pronounced leukocytosis.

In the bone marrow, granulocytic precursors are divided into two compartments: the mitotic compartment contains the cells capable of cell division including myeloblasts, promyelocytes, and myelocytes; the postmitotic (or maturation) compartment contains the metamyelocytes, bands, and segmented neutrophils, which cannot undergo cell division. The postmitotic compartment, containing twice the number of cells as the mitotic compartment, is a reservoir for the rapid release of mature granulocytes into the circulation. To provide a sustained

**Table 42-1.** *Normal adult leukocyte and leukocyte differential counts*
................................................................

| Type | Number (cells/mm³) | Percentage |
|------|------|------|
| Total leukocytes | 4100-10,900 | — |
| Neutrophils | 2266-7670 | 55-70 |
| Eosinophils | 0-492 | 0-1 |
| Monocytes | 123-804 | 1-8 |
| Basophils | 0-156 | 0 |
| Lymphocytes | 832-3140 | 20-40 |

granulocytosis, the bone marrow increases the rate and number of cells undergoing mitosis at each stage in the mitotic compartment. In the postmitotic compartment, the transit time can be accelerated and neutrophils can be released into the peripheral blood at an earlier stage, the metamyelocyte stage or the band stage. Neutrophil production, maturation, and release are under the control of several different growth and colony-stimulating factors.[2]

Although granulocytes have a short life span, lymphocytes may survive as immunocompetent cells for the life of the individual. When exposed to the appropriate antigen or stimuli, lymphocytes transform, undergo activation, and divide. Lymphocyte proliferation and activation are also under the control of several growth factors that are important in the immunoregulatory process.[2]

## IS THE WBC COUNT ELEVATED?

Leukocytosis refers to the elevation of the total white blood cell (WBC) count. In most laboratories the WBC count is determined by an electronic cell counter.[3] These automated hematology instruments report the relative percentage and absolute number of various cell types. Although these counters generally provide reliable, reproducible, and accurate measurements of cell concentrations, there are possible sources for error.[4] The WBC count can be falsely elevated in the presence of circulating nucleated red blood cells (RBCs) or large abnormal platelets. Therefore the review of the peripheral blood smear should be the first step in the evaluation of all patients with an elevated total WBC count. The differential count obtained from the peripheral smear is important in the evaluation of the leukocytosis. An elevated WBC count should be designated by the name of the prinicpal cell type, that is, neutrophilic, eosinophilic, basophilic, lymphocytic, or monocytic leukocytosis.

# CLINICAL EVALUATION

In a patient with an elevated WBC it is critical to determine whether the circulating leukocytes or lymphocytes are normal, mature cells typically found in the peripheral blood, or abnormal and suggestive of an underlying leukemia or malignant disease. Moreover, on review of the peripheral smear several distinctive morphologic features in the granulocytes may provide important clues to the cause of the leukocytosis. For example, the finding of Döhle's bodies, toxic granules, or vacuoles in the granulocytes is suggestive of an ongoing infection. Auer rods, malformed granules containing lysosomal enzymes, when present in immature granulocytes, are diagnostic of acute myelogenous leukemia or one of the myelodysplastic syndromes.

Reviewing the peripheral smear also provides information on the other cellular elements. For example, teardrop-shaped red blood cells are suggestive of myelofibrosis. The finding of circulating nucleated red blood cells and immature granulocytes, termed *leukoerythroblastosis*, is strongly suggestive of a metastatic or infiltrative disease that involves the bone marrow. Atypical "activated" lymphocytes are suggestive of a recent viral infection. Epstein-Barr virus infections result in transformed lymphocytes that are atypical and may resemble lymphoblasts with irregular nuclei.

The most common cause of an elevated total WBC is an increase in the absolute and relative neutrophil count (Table 42-2). A *bacterial infection* is the most frequent reason for a neutrophilic leukocytosis. The neutrophilia that accompanies a bacterial infection is usually associated with a "shift to the left" of the circulating granulocytes. A shift to the left refers to a relative increase in bands and metamyelocytes in the peripheral blood smear. Occasionally, neutrophilia may be the presenting or only sign of an occult infection. Chronic bacterial endocarditis, or partially treated abscesses, and chronic fungal infections

**Table 42-2.** *Causes of neutrophilic leukocytosis*

| | |
|---|---|
| Physiologic conditions | Exercise, pregnancy, ovulation, stress, cigarette smoking, nausea, vomiting, chronic idiopathic neutrophilia, asplenia |
| Infections | Bacterial, fungal, viral, parasitic |
| Hematologic disorders | Leukemia, myeloproliferative disorders, hemolytic anemias, hemorrhage |
| Inflammatory disorders | Rheumatoid arthritis, vasculitis, gout |
| Metabolic disorders | Uremia, diabetic acidosis, eclampsia |
| Tissue breakdown | Myocardial infarction, carcinoma |
| Cell necrosis | Lymphomas, Hodgkin's disease, brain tumors |
| Drugs | Steroids, epinephrine, lithium carbonate, tegretol |

should be considered in the differential diagnosis of an unexplained neutrophilia associated with a persistently left-shifted differential count. As noted, the presence of Döhle's bodies or toxic granules in the granulocytes is further evidence of an ongoing infection. Qualitative disorders in neutrophil function do not usually result in an elevation of the peripheral neutrophil count.

*Noninfectious causes* of neutrophilia can reflect (1) a physiologic response, (2) a response to metabolic disorders or tissue necrosis, (3) part of an underlying hematologic disease, or (4) a response to the administration of many different drugs or chemicals.[5] Physiologic causes of neutrophilia reflect changes in the distribution of the neutrophils between the circulating and marginal pools. Neutrophils demarginate in response to stress, strenuous exercise, epinephrine, and corticosteroids. The demargination results in an increase in the total neutrophil count and generally does not cause a shift to the left. Transient neutrophil counts as high as 22,000 per cubic millimeter can occur after a brief period of strenuous exercise. The magnitude of the leukocytosis with exercise appears to depend primarily on the intensity of the activity, rather than on its duration. Pain, nausea, vomiting, and intense anxiety also may cause a transient neutrophilic leukocytosis in the absence of infection. A neutrophilia can occur during ovulation, reflecting an increase in the level of circulating 17-hydroxycorticosteroids. A normal pregnancy may be associated with a neutrophilic leukocytosis in the range of 15,000 to 20,000/mm³; the neutrophilia increases as term approaches. The onset of labor rarely may be accompanied by a neutrophilic leukocytosis as high as 34,000/mm³ in the absence of an infection. However, the neutrophilia occurring during pregnancy also may signify a serious complication such as eclampsia, bleeding, or fetal distress. Neutrophilia in the absence of an infection may be seen in cigarette smokers. Idiopathic neutrophilia, a sporadic familial disorder, is characterized by a chronic mild elevation of the neutrophil count (12,000 to 20,000/mm³) without evidence of any underlying disorder. The elevated WBC count is presumed to represent the normal range for these individuals.[6] Chronic neutrophilia, 11,000 to 14,000/mm³, may occur in patients who have no underlying disorders.[6] These patients have chronic idiopathic neutrophilia.[7]

Although neutrophilia may be a physiologic response to a variety of stimuli, it is more commonly encountered as a reaction to an underlying disease process. Inflammation or tissue damage and necrosis can produce a greatly elevated leukocyte count. The finding of a leukocytosis may help differentiate a myocardial infarction with tissue necrosis from angina pectoris. Neutrophilia may occur with many collagen-vascular diseases such as acute glomerulonephritis, serum sickness, and rheumatic fever. Metabolic disorders such as ketoacidosis, uremia, and eclampsia may produce prominent neutrophilia. A neutrophilic leukocytosis may accompany poisoning by a variety of chemicals and drugs including lead, mercury, digitalis, and benzene derivatives. Patients taking therapeutic doses of lithium carbonate or carbamazepine (Tegretol) may develop a chronic neutrophilia without evidence of toxicity or infection. In malignant diseases the neutrophilia may reflect tissue injury or inflammation. Metastatic cancer to the liver or bone marrow may present with a elevated leukocyte count that, in some cases, may mimic a leukemia.

## LEUKEMOID REACTION

A WBC count of greater than $50,000/mm^3$, with circulating immature myeloid cells mimicking a leukemia, is called a *leukemoid reaction.* The leukemoid reaction is characterized by a leukocytosis of a greater degree than would be expected with the underlying diseases and immature myeloid cells in the peripheral smear. The leukemoid reaction must be differentiated from chronic myeloid leukemia (CML) and other myeloproliferative disorders (Table 42-3). The leukocyte alkaline phosphatase (LAP) score and cytogenetic testing are particularly helpful studies to differentiate CML from a leukemoid reaction.

The LAP is a cytochemical stain that is scored from 0 to +4 based on the intensity of the staining. One hundred leukocytes are counted, and the score of each of the cells is totaled. Therefore an LAP score may vary from 0 (no cells staining) to 400 (all cells staining). In stable-phase CML, the LAP score is very low (0 to 5), whereas, in the leukemoid reaction, the LAP score is high (100 to 400). However, the interpretation of an LAP score is difficult in certain clinical settings. In some patients with CML, the LAP score in fact may be elevated, thereby reflecting an intercurrent infection, pregnancy, or an inflammatory reaction. Therefore, although a 0 LAP score is diagnostic of CML, a mildly elevated LAP score does not exclude the diagnosis. In these settings it is necessary to confirm the diagnosis of chronic myelogenous leukemia by cytogenetic or molecular markers. A bone marrow should be performed to search for the diagnostic cytogenetic marker of CML, the Philadelphia chromosome. The Philadelphia chromosome, a balanced cytogenetic translocation involving chromosomes 9 and 22 (t 9;22), reflects the rearrangement of a defined area on chromosome 22 (*bcr* region). The

**Table 42-3.** *Evaluation of a leukemoid reaction*

| Test | Leukemoid reaction | Chronic myeloid leukemia |
|---|---|---|
| White blood cells | $20,000-50,000/mm^3$ | $20,000-150,000/mm^3$ |
| Basophils | Normal | Increased |
| Platelets | Normal | Normal or increased |
| Uric acid | Normal | Increased |
| LAP score | High (100-400) | Low (0-5) |
| Cytogenetics | Normal | Philadelphia chromosome |
| Spleen size | Normal | Enlarged |

*LAP,* Leukocyte alkaline phosphatase.

molecular marker for CML reflects the rearrangement of the *bcr* region which codes for an abnormal protein.[8]

# LEUKEMIA

Patients with leukemia may present with a very high WBC count. Although a WBC count of greater than 100,000/mm³ generally requires treatment, it is the absolute blast count that is most important. A circulating blast count of greater than 50,000/mm³ predisposes the patient to the signs and symptoms of leukostasis and requires urgent treatment. However, an elevated WBC count composed mainly of mature neutrophils and rare myeloblasts (chronic phase CML) or mature lymphocytes (chronic lymphocytic leukemia) does not require emergency intervention. The treatment and prevention of leukostasis is aimed at rapidly lowering the WBC count. Leukapheresis, hydroxyurea, allopurinol, and adequate hydration are important components of the therapy of leukostasis.

# MYELOPROLIFERATIVE DISORDERS

When all other causes of neutrophilia have been excluded, consideration should be given to one of myeloproliferative disorders. Polycythemia vera is associated with an elevation of the RBC mass, thrombocytosis, and splenomegaly. The leukocytosis in polycythemia vera is often modest in contrast to the elevated hematocrit. In myelofibrosis and myeloid metaplasia, spenomegaly is prominent, and the peripheral smear usually reveals teardrop-shaped RBCs and nucleated RBCs. However, early in the course of myelofibrosis or polycythemia vera, leukocytosis may be the presenting finding.

The therapy of neutrophilia depends on the underlying disease; an infection must be treated with the appropriate antibiotics; the specific inflammatory disease, acute injury, or tissue necrosis should be identified and treated. In the myeloproliferative disorders, therapy should be directed toward the primary disease. In polycythemia vera, periodic phlebotomy may be required, followed by cytotoxic chemotherapy if necessary to control the symptoms. In chronic myelogenous leukemia, there are several therapeutic options, depending on the age of the patient, the extent of the disease, and the presenting symptoms. Bone marrow transplantation, interferon, and chemotherapy represent possible therapies for patients with CML.

# EOSINOPHILIA

Eosinophils are derived from a separate bone marrow progenitor cell and make up 3% of the circulating leukocytes. Eosinophils are increased in certain allergic conditions and parasitic infections, thereby reflecting the release of material chemotactic for eosinophils from activated local tissue mast cells. Like the neutrophil, the eosinophil moves freely between a circulating and a marginal pool. Eosinophilia is diagnosed when the absolute blood eosinophil count is in excess of $500/mm^3$. Eosinophils are increased in atopic and parasitic diseases, drug reactions, neoplastic conditions, and collagen vascular disorders. Table 42-4 lists the major causes of eosinophilia. The most common cause for eosinophilia in hospitalized patients is a drug reaction. Allergic disorders and hypersensitivity states associated with parasitic infections are also common causes of eosinophilia. However, the mere presence of a parasitic infestation is not necessarily associated with an eosinophilia. The parasite must actually invade the host to cause an eosinophilia. *Strongyloides, Schistosoma,* filarial worms of many species, *Toxocara,* and other tissue-invasive helminths are most commonly associated with an eosinophilia. Trichinosis should be suspected in cases with muscle tenderness and weakness, prominent eosinophilia (20% to 70%), elevated muscle enzymes, and a normal sedimentation rate. Serologic testing, skin tests, or a muscle biopsy may be necessary to confirm this diagnosis. Stool examination for ova and parasites should be part of the evaluation of all patients with an unexplained eosinophilia. Eosinophilia is seen in most types of allergic or hypersensitivity respiratory diseases including asthma, hay fever, and occupational lung disease. Allergic rhinitis and nasal polyps are common causes of eosinophilia.

An extreme and persistent elevation of the eosinophilic count without a detectable cause is referred to as the *hypereosinophilic syndrome*.[9] This disorder is defined by three criteria: (1) a persistent eosinophilia above $1500/mm^3$ for more than 6 months, (2) organ dysfunction secondary to infiltration with mature eosinophils, and (3) the absence of a known cause for the eosinophilia. The hypereosinophilic syndrome

## Table 42-4. *Causes of eosinophilic leukocytosis*

| Condition | Cause |
|---|---|
| Allergic conditions | Asthma, hay fever, insect bites, urticaria, drug reactions, allergic rhinitis |
| Neoplastic disease | Hodgkin's disease, polycythemia vera, metastatic carcinoma, leukemia |
| Collagen vascular disease | Polyarteritis nodosa, systemic lupus erythematosus |
| Parasitic disease | Trichinosis, visceral larva migrans, strongyloidiasis, filariasis |
| Pulmonary disease | Löffler's syndrome, occupational lung disease |
| Infections | Aspergillosis, coccidioidomycosis |
| Endocrine disorders | Adrenal insufficiency, hypothyroidism |
| Miscellaneous | Hypereosinophilic syndrome, graft-versus-host disease, Wiskott-Aldrich syndrome |

is a heterogeneous disorder with a range of organ involvement from minor skin changes to life-threatening cardiovascular and neurologic complications. Patients may present with only cardiac symptoms secondary to endocardial fibrosis and a restrictive endomyocardiopathy. An endomyocardial biopsy may be required to demonstrate damage to the endothelium and the eosinophilic infiltrate. Patients with the hypereosinophilic syndrome are at risk for thrombotic events related to the endomyocardial disease and the development of mural thrombi.

The evaluation of eosinophilia should start with a personal and family history, including details of all recent travel. Physical examination should focus on skin, pulmonary, and cardiac findings. Laboratory evaluation should include liver and renal functions studies, immunoglobulin E (IgE) levels, stools for ova and parasites, chest roentgenograms, and pulmonary function studies where appropriate. If these studies do not reveal the cause of the eosinophilia, markers for a possible myeloproliferative disorder, including an LAP score, and a bone marrow aspirate with chromosome analysis may be helpful. If all tests fail to define an underlying cause of the eosinophilia, the diagnosis of the hypereosinophilic syndrome should be considered. Treatment of the eosinophilia depends on the underlying disease. Therapy of the hypereosinophilic syndrome is aimed at preventing the complications of progressive organ involvement and thromboembolic complications and includes the use of corticosteroids, cytotoxic chemotherapy, and anticoagulation.

# BASOPHILIA

The basophil, the least numerous of the circulating leukocytes, is a rare cause of leukocytosis.[10] The basophil matures in the bone marrow through stages similar to the other granulocytes. However, the fate of the basophil in the peripheral blood remains poorly understood. Basophilia is defined as a basophilic leukocyte count greater than 50 cells/mm$^3$ or persistently greater than 1% of the circulating leukocytes. Table 42-5 lists the most common causes of basophilia. Basophilia is associated with hypersensitivity states and myeloproliferative disorders.

**Table 42-5.** *Causes of basophilic leukocytosis*

| Condition | Cause |
|---|---|
| Hematologic disorders | Myeloproliferative disorders, chronic myelogenous leukemia, polycythemia vera, pernicious anemia |
| Inflammatory disorders | Ulcerative colitis |
| Miscellaneous disorders | Hypersensitivity drug eruptions, myxedema |

The finding of a persistent basophilia should alert one to the possibility of an evolving myeloproliferative disorder. In chronic myelogenous leukemia, for example, basophilia is a common presenting finding. However, a persistent basophilia of greater than 15% is an ominous sign and often heralds the onset of the terminal, blastic stage. Basophilia is seen in the other myeloproliferative disorders, including polycythemia vera and myelofibrosis, but does not have the same adverse prognostic significance in these disorders.

# MONOCYTOSIS

The monocyte spends only a short time in the peripheral circulation but, unlike the neutrophil, continues to differentiate in the tissues to form a variety of mononuclear phagocytic cells that can survive for weeks to years. Monocytes have a ubiquitous role in inflammation and host defense.[11] Monocytosis is defined as greater than 750 monocytes/mm$^3$. Neoplastic, immune, and chronic inflammatory or infectious diseases are the leading causes of monocytosis (Table 42-6). This condition is associated with several primary hematologic disorders, including hemolytic anemias, myelodysplastic syndromes, Hodgkin's disease, lymphomas, and acute leukemias.

Because the monocyte plays a pivotal role in immunologic reactions and the host response to neoplasia, a monocytosis may be one of the early signs of a malignant disease. An unexplained, persistent monocytosis with either a macrocytosis or low-grade anemia is suggestive of a myelodysplastic or myeloproliferative disorder. Monocytosis is also seen in many chronic infections, including tuberculosis, subacute bacterial endocarditis, secondary syphilis, and brucellosis. Cirrhosis of

**Table 42-6.** Causes of monocytosis

| Condition | Cause |
|---|---|
| Infections | Tuberculosis, syphilis, brucellosis, leprosy, rickettsial disease, typhoid fever, subacute bacterial endocarditis |
| Neoplastic diseases | Hodgkin's disease, myelodysplastic syndrome, monocytic leukemias, histiocytic medullary reticulosis |
| Collagen vascular diseases | Rheumatoid arthritis, systemic lupus erythematosus, periarteritis nodosa |
| Chronic inflammation | Cirrhosis, ulcerative colitis, regional enteritis |
| Miscellaneous disorders | Sarcoidosis, drug reactions, lipid storage disorders, hemolytic anemia, recovery from myelosuppression and agranulocytosis |

the liver from multiple causes may be associated with a relative but persistent monocytosis. The primary malignant monocytic disorders include acute monocytic leukemia and chronic myelomonocytic leukemia. These disorders may be associated with prominent gum and skin infiltrates with atypical monocytes.

Monocytosis often appears during the recovery phase of viral or bacterial infections. Monocytes also are the first cells to reappear after agranulocytosis or chemotherapy-induced myelosuppression. Monocytosis may occur in the context of lipid storage diseases, including Gaucher's and Niemann-Pick disease. Collagen-vascular disorders such as rheumatoid arthritis, systemic lupus erythematosus, and periarteritis nodosa rarely may present with a mild monocytosis.

As noted, monocytosis is usually associated with a chronic inflammatory disease. Tuberculosis, chronic liver disease, and partially treated subacute bacterial endocarditis are often overlooked causes for a persistent monocytosis. The combination of a monocytosis and a macrocytic anemia is suggestive of a myelodysplastic or myeloproliferative disorder. Moreover, the peripheral smear may reveal basophilic stippling of the RBCs and atypical neutrophils. A history of chemotherapy for a prior malignancy or of an occupational exposure to a known or possible carcinogen is important in planning the work up.

All patients with an unexplained monocytosis and anemia should be evaluated for a possible myelodysplastic syndrome. A bone marrow aspirate and biopsy may reveal ringed sideroblasts and dysplastic changes in the myeloid, erythroid, and megakaryocytic precursors. A myelodysplastic syndrome developing in a patient exposed to a known hematotoxin is a poor prognostic sign. These patients typically rapidly progress to an acute myeloblastic leukemia that responds poorly to standard chemotherapy.

## LYMPHOCYTOSIS

Lymphocytes make up 20% to 40% of peripheral blood leukocytes. A lymphocytosis is defined as greater than 4000 cells/mm$^3$. The causes of a lymphocytosis are listed in Table 42-7. Viral infections are the most

**Table 42-7.** *Causes of lymphocytosis*

| Condition | Cause |
|---|---|
| Acute infections | Infectious mononucleosis, pertussis, mumps, rubella, infectious hepatitis, CMV |
| Chronic infections | Brucellosis, tuberculosis, secondary syphilis |
| Hematopoietic disorders | Acute lymphocytic leukemia, chronic lymphocytic leukemia, lymphoma, T-cell disorders |
| Metabolic disorders | Thyrotoxicosis |

common causes of a transient lymphocytosis. Mumps, varicella, and cytomegalovirus (CMV) are associated with a prominent lymphocytosis. Infectious mononucleosis typically produces a pronounced lymphocytosis in association with splenomegaly and lymphadenopathy. The lymphocytosis is characterized by many atypical and large reactive cells. Lymphocytosis is rare during acute bacterial infections, except for pertussis in which the total WBC count is usually between 20,000 to 50,000/mm$^3$ with 60% or more lymphocytes. Most of the lymphocytes are of the small mature type with rare atypical reactive cells. Other infections associated with a lymphocytosis include brucellosis and chronic tuberculosis. A relative lymphocytosis, usually in the presence of neutropenia, is seen in hyperthyroidism and in many drug reactions.[12]

An increase in the number of mature lymphocytes in the absence of an intercurrent viral infection is one of the earliest signs of chronic lymphocytic leukemia. Chronic lymphocytic leukemia (CLL), one of the most common hematologic neoplasms in adults, is characterized by the proliferation and accumulation of mature-appearing lymphocytes. In most cases the cells are of B-cell origin and, by definition, are derived from a single clone. When an elderly patient presents with a total WBC count of greater than 20,000/mm$^3$ with 80% small lymphocytes, generalized lymphadenopathy, and splenomegaly, the diagnosis of CLL is obvious. However, a modest elevation of the lymphocyte count with a normal total WBC in a middle-aged patient may be difficult to interpret. The diagnosis of CLL in the early stages relies on the demonstration of an expansion of a monoclonal population of cells. In B-CLL the normal T-cell/B-cell ratio is reversed with the B cells accounting for greater than 80% of all circulating lymphocytes. Immuno-phenotyping of the peripheral blood lymphocytes is necessary to diagnos CLL in the early stages. In CLL the malignant cell expresses a low surface density of immunoglobulins, usually IgM or IgM and IgD, which are monoclonal, as revealed by the expression of single light chains, either kappa or lambda, and are simultaneously marked with the CD5 antibody.[13] Although B-cell CLL is the most common cause of an unexplained lymphocytosis in an adult, the other lymphocytic neoplasms can cause a lymphocytosis. The leukemic phase of indolent lymphomas, prolymphocytic leukemia, Sézary syndrome, and, rarely, hairy-cell leukemia may resemble CLL. The leukemias of differentiated T cells can also present with a lymphocytosis. Adult T-cell leukemia, an endemic disorder in certain regions in southwest Japan and in the Caribbean, can present with a lymphocytosis. This type of leukemia is associated with a unique human retrovirus, the human T-cell lymphotrophic virus (HTLV-1).[14] After a several-year incubation period, infection with the HTLV-I virus can result in an acute, rapidly progressive, fatal T-cell lymphoproliferative disorder. The disease is characterized by large numbers of atypical-appearing circulating T lymphocytes, prominent skin lesions, hypercalcemia with lytic bone lesions, and lymphadenopathy. Other T-cell disorders that can present with a lymphocytosis include Sézary syndrome and T-cell chronic lymphocytic leukemia.[15]

The evaluation of lymphocytosis should start with a review of the peripheral smear. As noted, the appearance of many atypical "reactive"

**Table 42-8.** *Surface markers in lymphocytosis*

| Disorder | Surface immunoglobulin | CD5+ | CD19/CD20 |
|---|---|---|---|
| B-CLL | + | +++ | +++ |
| T-CLL | − | +++ | − |
| Prolymphocytic leukemia | +++ | ± | +++ |
| Hairy cell leukemia | +++ | − | +++ |
| Sézary syndrome | − | − | − |
| Lymphoma-leukemic phase | +++ | − | +++ |
| Reactive lymphocytosis | ± | − | + |

*B-CLL,* B-cell chronic lymphocytic leukemia; *T-CLL,* T-cell chronic lymphocytic leukemia.

  + Marker positive in 20% to 40% of cells.
 ++ Marker positive in 40% to 80% of cells.
+++ Marker positive in >80% of cells.
 ± Marker positive in 10% to 20% of cells.
 − Marker positive in <10% of cells.

lymphocytes is suggestive of an ongoing viral illness. The presence of many circulating large granular lymphocytes is suggestive of a T-cell disorder, and small mature-appearing lymphocytes are suggestive of chronic lymphocytic leukemia. The use of surface markers or T-cell receptor studies are helpful in defining the clonal nature of the lymphocytes in selected cases. In the evaluation of an unexplained lymphocytosis, immunophenotyping of the lymphocyte population will define if the population is monoclonal and determine if the lymphocytosis is reactive, associated with a transient viral illness or related to an underlying malignant disorder[16] (Table 42-8). Serologic studies may help in the diagnosis of an active or resolving viral illness. Many of the special viral titers are now available at selected laboratories or regional centers.

Therapy of a lymphocytic disorder clearly depends on the underlying cell population. In CLL or one of its variants, the choice of therapy depends on the stage of the disease, the age of the patient, the symptoms, and other associated medical conditions.[17]

## References

1. Shapiro MF, Greenfield S: The complete blood count, *Ann Intern Med* 106:65-74, 1987.
2. Garnick MB: Hematopoietic growth factors, *Semin Oncol,* vol 19, 1992.
3. Gulati GL, Bong HH: The automated CBC: a current perspective, *Hematol Oncol Clin North Am* 8:593-603, 1994.
4. Krause JR: The automated white blood cell differential, *Hematol Oncol Clin North Am* 8:605-616, 1994.
5. Malech HL, Gallin JI: Neutrophils in human diseases, *N Engl J Med* 317:687-694, 1987.

6. Herring WB, Smith LG, Walke RJ, Herion JC: Hereditary neutrophilia, *Am J Med* 56:729-738, 1974.

7. Ward H, Reinhard E: Chronic idiopathic leukocytosis, *Ann Intern Med* 75:193-199, 1971.

8. Kantarjian HM, Deisseroth A, Kurzock R, et al: Chronic myelogenous leukemia: a concise review, *Blood* 82:691-703, 1993.

9. Fauci AS, Harley JB, Roberts WC, et al: The idiopathic hypereosinophilic syndrome: clinical, pathophysiologic, and therapeutic considerations. *Ann Intern Med* 97:78-92, 1982.

10. Dvorak HF, Dvorak AM: Basophilic leukocytes: structure, function and role in disease, *Clin Haematol* 4:651-684, 1974.

11. Johnston RB: Monocytes and macrophages, *N Engl J Med* 318:747-752, 1988.

12. Miller KB: Reactive lymphocyte disorders and lymphadenopathy. In Handin RI, Lux S, Stossel TP, editors: *Blood: principles and practice of hematology,* Philadelphia, 1994, Lippincott.

13. Chesson BD, Bennett JM, Rai KR, et al: Guidelines for clinical protocols for chronic lymphocytic leukemia (CLL): recommendations of the NCI-Sponsored Working Group, *Am J Hematol* 29:152-164, 1988.

14. Franchini G: Review: molecular mechanisms of human T-cell leukemia/lymphotropic virus type I infection, *Blood* 86:3619-3639, 1995.

15. Newland AC, Catousky D, Linch D, et al: Chronic T-cell lymphocytosis: a review of 21 cases, *Br J Haematol* 58:433-446, 1984.

16. Knapp W, editor: Leukocyte typing. IV: White cell differentiation antigens, Oxford, 1989, Oxford University Press

17. Champlin R, Gale RP, Foon KA, Golde DW: Chronic leukemias: oncogenes, chromosomes, and advances in therapy, *Ann Intern Med* 104:671-688, 1986.

# Chapter 43

# *Lymphadenopathy*

Richard A. Rudders

Enlarged lymph nodes are a common clinical sign that requires further evaluation. The potentially malignant nature of adenopathy necessitates that the diagnostic work up be selective and proceed in an expeditious manner. As a general rule the older the patient and the larger the lymph node, the greater is the likelihood that a neoplasm is present. The definitive diagnostic test in many cases is a lymph node biopsy. It is important that a pathologist experienced in lymph node pathology participate in the evaluation. Incorrect diagnosis that results from inadequately prepared or processed biopsy material or from inexperience is unfortunately all too common in this difficult area of pathology.

## NORMAL LYMPH NODE ANATOMY

Organized lymphoid tissue consists of a network of lymph nodes, liver, spleen, bone marrow, Waldeyer's ring (referring to lymphatic tissue in the oropharynx), and Peyer's patches in the gut. Blood and lymph are vehicles that allow traffic between these way stations. There are numerous other deposits of lymphoid tissue scattered in almost every organ, but they are not termed lymph nodes because of their lack of strict anatomic organization and structure. Lymph nodes are distributed peripherally and centrally, with the largest bulk of nodal tissue being found in the midline in the thorax and abdomen. The amount of nodal tissue declines as one moves peripherally. This is an important point because the patient usually detects enlargement of peripheral nodes, as in the neck, axilla, or groin, and often the great bulk of node enlargement is hidden and not obvious clinically.

## HOW BIG IS BIG?

The most important initial clinical decision to be made is whether to call lymph nodes enlarged. Lymph nodes less than 0.5 cm in diameter (barely palpable) are not a cause of concern. This is particularly true in the younger patient who is likely to have enlarged neck nodes related to respiratory infections. There is, however, no guarantee that small nodes are benign, and they must be viewed in the context of the entire picture. For example, an individual with multiple small nodes and abnormal blood counts may have a serious underlying disease, whereas a child with multiple small nodes may be entirely normal. Another potentially confusing problem relates to groin nodes. Individuals of all ages are likely to have palpable groin nodes. If the nodes are small, they are likely to be normal. The larger the nodes, the greater is the cause for concern. Lymph nodes greater than 2 to 3 cm in diameter, particularly when multiple, have a high risk of malignancy in any age group and in any location and should be evaluated promptly. One cannot emphasize too strongly that there is a fine line between the urgent needs to evaluate significantly enlarged nodes and the inadvisability of needlessly subjecting individuals to expensive and morbid diagnostic procedures.

# WHY DO LYMPH NODES ENLARGE?

Lymph nodes are organized collections of lymphoid tissue and consist of several types of immunocompetent cells such as lymphocytes and macrophages. There are three major causes of lymph node enlargement: lymphadenitis, lymphadenopathy, and neoplasia (see box on p. 480). Lymphadenitis is the normal physiologic response to an inflammatory (infectious) stimulus that can be either regional or systemic. In some cases the inflammatory agent is not readily identified (such as benign reactive hyperplasia), but in many cases a clear relationship to a viral or bacterial agent can be defined. Prominent generalized adenopathy may be a feature of mononucleosis, cytomegalovirus, and toxoplasmosis infections.

Lymphadenopathies consist of a diverse group of diseases. Many, such as systemic lupus erythematosus and other collagen diseases, are associated with immunologic hyperfunction, which leads to node enlargement. Any systemic disorder associated with hyperfunction or abnormal function of the lymphoid system can be associated with adenopathy. Lymphadenopathy may be prominent in the case of drug reactions, such as those related to phenytoin. The adenopathy in such cases waxes and wanes with the activity of the underlying disease.

The most important cause of adenopathy from the therapeutic standpoint is neoplasia.[1] This is particularly the case in recent years, since a great many of the primary neoplasms of lymph nodes, namely, lymphoma and leukemia, are potentially curable. It is essential to identify as quickly as possible individuals with neoplasms that are curable to ensure the highest likelihood of therapeutic success. Non-Hodgkin's lymphoma and Hodgkin's disease are two such examples (Fig. 43-1). Metastatic tumors also may cause lymph node enlargement. Although this may be a less favorable situation, regional metastases from an occult primary cancer such as breast, oropharynx, or melanoma are important to identify, since in many cases cure or extended remission with appropriate treatment is possible.

## Selected Causes of Adenopathy

### LYMPHADENITIS

**Benign reactive hyperplasia**

**Viral diseases**
Infectious mononucleosis
Varicella zoster
Cytomegalovirus
German measles

**Bacterial diseases**

Gram-positive and negative bacteria
Tuberculosis
Leprosy
Syphilis

**Other**

Toxoplasmosis
Cat-scratch disease
Lymphogranuloma venereum

### LYMPHADENOPATHY

Systemic lupus erythematosus
Rheumatoid arthritis
Sjögren's syndrome
Drug reactions
Reactions to chemicals and tumor products
Sarcoidosis

### NEOPLASIA

**Hematopoietic**

Non-Hodgkin's lymphoma
Hodgkin's disease
Chronic leukemia
Acute leukemia

**Nonhematopoietic**

Lung cancer
Breast cancer
Melanoma
Nasopharyngeal carcinoma
Soft-tissue sarcoma
Seminoma

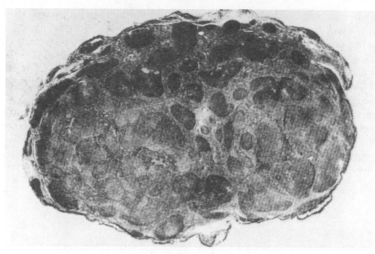

**Figure 43-1.** *Low-power microscopic view of lymph node from patient with follicular (nodular) non-Hodgkin's lymphoma. The lymphoma nodules can be seen clearly at this magnification.*

## CLINICAL CLUES TO THE CAUSES OF ADENOPATHY

In the clinical evaluation several important clues help decide whether further evaluation is mandatory. As stated, age is an important variable that influences our level of concern. The older the patient with significant adenopathy, the more likely is the presence of serious illness. The distribution of nodes is an important clue. Abnormal nodes in a single area indicate the possibility of a local cause, whereas generalized abnormal nodes are suggestive of a systemic process. In either case distribution does not distinguish benign from malignant enlargement. Another important characteristic to appreciate is the consistency of the nodes. If the nodes are extremely firm and matted, a neoplastic process is suggested. If they are discrete and painful, and particularly if they are regional, an infectious cause is more likely. Again, this is not an absolute sign, since more than one neck node from a suspected abscessed tooth has proved to be a metastasis from an oropharyngeal carcinoma. Since it is common for tumors to infarct, pain may be produced in the node, thereby mimicking inflammation.

One cannot overemphasize the value of the clinical history in this type of evaluation. The rate of progression of the adenopathy, the presence of pain, and the association with another illness, either chronic or acute, are vitally important clues. One should also pay particular attention to drug ingestion and to exposure to animals to rule out infections such as toxoplasmosis and cat-scratch disease.

Based on these considerations, one must make an initial decision regarding further evaluation. If the adenopathy appears to be the result of a benign self-limited problem, no further studies are indicated. However, I would urge that all patients have at least one follow-up examination to confirm that the adenopathy is benign and is not progressive. If an infectious agent, particularly a virus, is suspected, further evaluation should include appropriate cultures and serum viral antibody titers. No further evaluation is necessary if the suspected infection is proved, though again a follow-up examination is advisable. Most individuals seen in the office, particularly younger individuals with a definable infectious illness, require no further evaluation other than careful follow-up. But what of the patient with significant adenopathy that is progressive and not infectious in origin? In such cases the next step is biopsy.

# LYMPH NODE BIOPSY

There are several types of biopsy techniques that are useful.[2] Needle aspiration biopsies with or without ultrasound guidance may be done with a fine needle, or a sizable core of tissue can be obtained with a variety of larger bone instruments. Needle biopsies in general have the advantage of ease and speed, but the amount of material obtained may be sufficient only for culture and cytologic exam. Core biopsies provide more tissue but do not usually suffice for flow cytometric or special studies. Needle biopsies are most useful in distinguishing neoplastic from nonneoplastic diagnosis such as infection but are inadequate for subclassification of malignancies such as lymphoma. For this reason if malignancy is highly suspected, an excisional or incisional node biopsy is preferred. The surgeon should be advised to remove as large a node as is feasible, preferably intact.

In certain circumstances enlarged nodes may be present in the thorax or abdomen, thus making biopsy more problematic. Although computerized tomography or ultrasonography can be helpful in guiding a needle biopsy, more often than not an excisional biopsy is necessary. It is a matter of clinical judgment as to when a thoracotomy or laparotomy should be done to establish a diagnosis. Often other more accessible areas, such as the bone marrow, are biopsied first in order to avoid surgery to diagnose leukemia or lymphoma. Many patients with central adenopathy require an excisional biopsy even after exhausting noninvasive maneuvers.

One cannot overemphasize the importance of proper handling of the biopsy material. Material should be sent to the pathology laboratory fresh in sterile saline, not fixed in formalin. This ensures that lymphocyte-marker studies, immunocytochemistry, and cultures can be done on the material. These tests are not possible with formalin-fixed material. Close collaboration with the pathologist is needed to ensure that maximum information is obtained from each biopsy and that an accurate diagnosis can be made. Lymph node disorder diagnosis can be extremely difficult, and good preparation of material is vitally important to improve diagnostic accuracy[3] (Table 43-1).

**Table 43-1.** *Studies performed on lymph node biopsy specimens*

| Study | Comment |
|---|---|
| Light microscopy | Hematoxylin and eosin stain |
| Immunocytochemistry | Fluorescent 1-labeled antibodies |
| Surface marker studies | Flow cytometry |
| Electron microscopy | In selected cases |
| Culture and special stains | In selected cases |
| Cytogenetic studies | To detect genetic markers |

# OTHER DIAGNOSTIC TESTS

## CT and MRI scanning

Computerized tomography (CT) and magnetic resonance imaging (MRI) scanning are the best studies to evaluate the size of lymph nodes, since they can detect nodes as small as 0.5 to 1.0 cm in diameter with reasonable accuracy and are noninvasive.[4] CT scans of the chest and abdomen have become a routine part of the evaluation of all patients with neoplastic adenopathy (Fig. 43-2). Based on these findings, patients with lymphoma, for example, can be placed into a stage and the correct treatment modality can be chosen. Patients with nonneoplastic adenopathy documented by biopsy rarely require further evaluation.

## Pedal lymphangiography

Pedal lymphangiography delineates the size and characteristics of pelvic and low retroperitoneal nodes. The use of this diagnostic study has declined with the widespread availability of CT and MRI scanning. However, there are selected situations where lymphangiography may be useful (Fig. 43-3). This is particularly the case in patients with lymphomas or pelvic cancers that have equivocal CT scan findings. The disadvantage of this type of study is that it is invasive and potentially morbid, particularly in older persons. Dye allergy and pulmonary disease are contraindications to this type of study.[5]

## Gallium scanning

Gallium scanning is a noninvasive study that can provide information about the presence of disease in multiple anatomic sites. Gallium is taken up by neoplastic lymphoid tissue and by certain solid tumors, such as a melanoma. Gallium also localizes in abscesses. If lymph nodes are enlarged and also take up gallium, they are likely to be neoplastic. The opposite is not true, however, since many tumors do not avidly bind gallium. Therefore a normal gallium scan does not necessarily rule out neoplastic lymphadenopathy. Numerous studies have shown a significant false-positive and false-negative rate in hematologic malig-

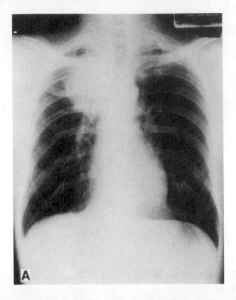

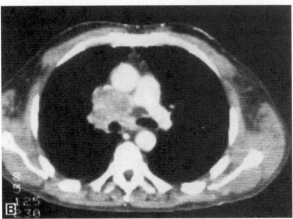

**Figure 43–2.** *A, Chest roentgenogram of patient with large right-sided mediastinal and paratracheal mass. B, CT scan of the chest of the same patient with delineation of the mass, which is composed of lymph nodes subsequently shown to be lung cancer.*

nancies; thus gallium scans are performed now only in selected situations.

## DIFFICULT PREMALIGNANT LESIONS

There are several instances where the cause of adenopathy is obscure or its biologic significance is not clear. Many such lesions fall into the category of premalignancy. Many cases of lymphadenopathy in this

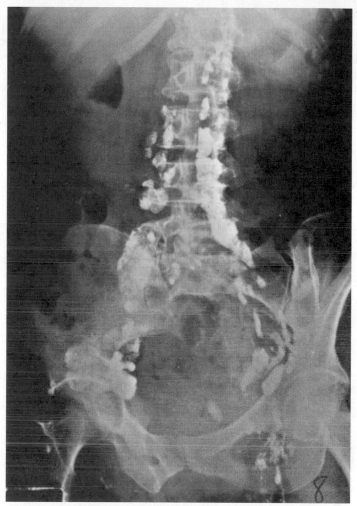

**Figure 43–3.** *Lymphangiogram from patient with Hodgkin's disease. Lymph nodes on the right are enlarged and have a foamy appearance. For comparison, lymph nodes on the left are normal.*

group regress spontaneously or remain stable for long periods of time. Many, however, evolve into frank malignancy, usually a non-Hodgkin's lymphoma.

## Atypical lymphoid hyperplasia

Individuals with atypical lymphoid hyperplasia present with adenopathy that is often generalized and that may either persist or wax and wane. When a node is biopsied, the pathologist is unable to state that it is benign or malignant, since atypical features that are disturbing are present in the node. Such changes may be cellular atypia, capsular spillage, or architectural distortion. In our experience many such individuals progress to frank malignant lymphoma over a period of time. It is not clear whether the original biopsy could have represented a sampling error in some of these cases, but in other cases a clear evolution to lymphoma can be documented. Lymphoctye phenotype or

**Table 43-2.** *Cell-surface marker and cytogenetic studies of lymph node tissue*

| Type of study | Specificity | Cell lineage or tumor |
|---|---|---|
| ANTIBODY | | |
| Ig | Heavy and light immunoglobulin chains | B cell |
| CD3 | T-cell receptor | T cell |
| CD4 | HIV receptor | T helper |
| CD5 | gp 67 | T cell |
| CD8 | Class I receptor | T suppressor |
| CD10 | CALLA | Leukemia/lymphoma |
| CD11 | Integrin receptor | Monocyte, granulocyte |
| CD15 | — | Granulocyte, R scale |
| CD16 | IgG Fc receptor | Granulocyte, NK cell |
| CD19 | gp 95 | B cell |
| CD20 | — | B cell |
| CD21 | C'/EBV receptor | B cell |
| CD25 | IL-2 receptor | B and T cells |
| CD30 | Ki-1 | R-S cells |
| CD34 | gp 105–120 | Precursor cell |
| CD45 | Leukocyte common antigen | Leukocytes |
| CD56 | N-CAM | NK cells |
| CYTOGENETIC | | |
| $t$ (14; 18) | bcl-2 | Follicular lymphoma |
| $t$ (8; 14) | c-myc | Burkitt's lymphoma |
| $t$ (11; 14) | bcl-1 | Mantle zone lymphoma |
| $t$ (2; 5) | p80 | Anaplastic large cell lymphoma |

*bcl*, B cell leukemia; *C'*, complement; *CALLA*, common acute lymphocytic leukemia antigen; *EBV*, Epstein-Barr virus; *Fc*, fragment c; *gp*, glycoprotein; *HIV*, human immunodeficiency virus; *Ig*, immunoglobulin; *IL-2*, interleukin-2; *Ki*, Kiel; *N-CAM*, nerve cell adhesion molecule; *NK*, natural killer; *p*, protein; *R-S*, Reed-Sternberg; *t( )*, translocation and rearranged chromosomes.

cytogenetic analysis of the nodal tissue has been illuminating, since such studies often define a malignant clone of lymphocytes.[6,7] Restricted expression of surface-membrane immunoglobulin or a cytogenetic marker have been most useful in defining malignant proliferations of B lymphocytes (Table 43-2).

## Angioimmunoblastic lymphadenopathy

Some patients present with lymphadenopathy and a host of associated immunologic abnormalities and thus have angioimmunoblastic lymphadenopathy. The cause of the syndrome is not clear, but it most likely represents an abnormal immune response to an undefined antigen and associated faulty immunoregulation. Although one-third of these patients remit spontaneously, one-third die of progressive disease, and the remainder progress to frank malignant lymphoma. The lymph node biopsy is characteristic and displays a pleomorphic lymphoid infiltrate, extensive necrosis, and neovascularization (Fig. 43-4). A definitive diagnosis of lymphoma usually cannot be made at this stage. Because of the varied outcome, most patients are not treated aggressively with chemotherapy unless they progress to frank lymphoma.

## Abnormal immune responses

Some patients present with adenopathy that is neither atypical hyperplasia nor classic immunoblastic lymphadenopathy. Such cases have been lumped into a separate category termed *abnormal immune response.*[8] Again, in my experience this may be considered a potentially premalignant lesion, since many patients progress to frank lymphoma or have

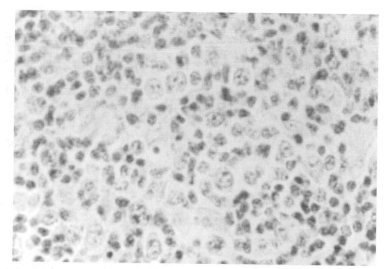

**Figure 43-4.** *High-power microscopic view of cervical lymph node biopsy from patient with angioimmunoblastic lymphadenopathy. Notice large immunoblasts with prominent nuclei.*

a progressive and fatal disease. This is an extremely difficult group of patients to evaluate, since no definite malignancy is present. As with atypical hyperplasia, lymphocyte phenotyping has been helpful in defining malignant subpopulations of lymphocytes.

## Acquired immunodeficiency syndrome

The retrovirus-related disease acquired immunodeficiency syndrome (AIDS) often presents with generalized adenopathy in its early stages.[9] This lymphadenopathic phase is a precursor to full-blown AIDS and to the potential development of frank malignant lymphoma. HIV may be cultured from the lymph nodes in these cases. Initially the histologic picture in the lymph node is that of an abnormal immune response and is not frankly neoplastic. It is not known what proportion of patients with lymphadenopathy will progress to full-blown AIDS or how many have reversible findings. Again, lymphocyte phenotyping of the lymph nodes has been helpful in defining the abnormality, since there is usually total T-cell depression and a reduction in helper T cells, thereby causing a reversed helper T: suppressor T ratio. See Chapter 47 for a more detailed discussion of AIDS-related lymphoma.

## References

1. Rosenberg SA: Lymphosarcoma: a review of 1269 cases, *Medicine* 40:31-84, 1961.
2. Ioachim HL, editor: *Lymph node biopsy,* Philadelphia, 1982, Lippincott.
3. Knowles DM, editor: *Neoplastic hematopathology,* Baltimore, 1992, Williams & Wilkins.
4. Mass AA, editor: *Computed tomography of the body,* Philadelphia, 1983, Saunders.
5. Cabanillas F: Comparison of lymphangiograms and gallium scans in the non-Hodgkin's lymphomas, *Cancer* 39:85-88, 1977.
6. Rabbitts TH: Chromosomal translocations in human cancer, *Nature* 372:143-149, 1994.
7. Aisenberg AC: Coherent view of non-Hodgkin's lymphoma, *J Clin Oncol* 13:2656-2675, 1995.
8. Lukes RJ: Immunologic approach to non-Hodgkin's lymphomas and related leukemias: analysis of the results of multiparameter studies of 425 cases, *Semin Hematol* 15:322-351, 1978.
9. NIH Conference. Acquired immunodeficiency syndrome: epidemiologic, clinical, immunologic and therapeutic considerations. Ann Intern Med 100:92-106, 1984.

# Chapter 44

# *Cancer Screening*

Kenneth B. Miller
Roger Platt

Cancer screening and cancer-related checkups, including the tests, procedures, and counseling related to the prevention and early detection of cancer, have enormous medical, social, and economic implications. To be accepted by physicians and patients, cancer screening should adhere to the following five basic principles:

1. The cancer being screened for should be an important health problem for the individual or the community.
2. A screening test should be reliable, acceptable to patients, ideally risk free, and inexpensive.
3. The natural history of the disease should be well understood and should have a recognizable early or asymptomatic stage.
4. There should be an acceptable, practical, and effective form of therapy available for patients found to have an early cancer. Screening for a disease with no effective therapy offers only a diagnosis and is of questionable value.
5. Screening and early treatment of the cancer should be proved to favorably influence the survival time or quality of life for the patient.

There are several kinds of bias that characterize early detection programs and that may affect the interpretation of screening results. "Lead-time bias" refers to the fact that a disease found by screening has a longer course, or natural history, simply because of its earlier discovery. The longer survival of the screened patient therefore may be independent of any benefit resulting from having discovered the cancer early. "Length bias" refers to the fact that cancers with an inherently slower growth rate and thus a relatively more favorable outlook are disproportionately detected. The longer the preclinical duration of the disease, the stronger is this length bias. Patient self-selection bias is obvious; people who select or seek out screening programs may be more concerned about their health and take better care of themselves and may be healthier than those who do not participate in such programs. Finally, overdiagnosis or erroneous diagnosis can affect the interpretation of results of screening. When is a cancer a cancer? When dealing with very early, limited disease, some patients who are diagnosed as having a cancer may in fact not have a malignancy. Patients without a true cancer obviously will have a more improved outcome than patients with cancer.

Screening tests must also address the issues of sensitivity, specificity, and predictive value. Sensitivity is the likelihood of the test being positive when the disease is present; specificity is the likelihood of the test being negative when the disease is absent. The reciprocal of specificity is referred to as the false-positive rate. Predictive value is the proportion of patients with positive tests who have the disease in question. The predictive value of a test is what most concerns the physician.

The predictive value of a test is critically dependent on not only the specificity of the test but also the prevalence of the disease in the population being screened. For example, if a population of 100,000 were screened for a disease with a 2% prevalence (which would make the disease very common), and if sensitivity and specificity of the test were 95%, there would be a total of 6800 positive tests (Fig. 44-1). However, only 1900 would be true positive, that is, positive tests in patients who have the disease. In this example the positive predictive value is only 28%, defined as:

$$\frac{\text{True positives}}{\text{True positives + False positives}}$$

Therefore in this example:

$$\frac{1900}{1900 + 4900} = 28\%$$

Therefore, when one screens large numbers of patients even for a common disease with a very specific test, the positive predictive value is still low. This problem is further magnified when the disease is less common and the population is very large.

Cancer screening needs to be routinely repeated at intervals that detect a high proportion of cancers in the early, presymptomatic stage.

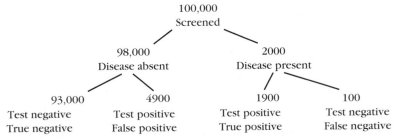

**Figure 44-1.** *Screening test: the predictive value is dependent on the prevalence of the disease and the sensitivity of the test.*

The interval between routinely repeated tests is determined by the rate at which detectable but presymptomatic disease progresses to the symptomatic stage when it would normally be present. In addition, the interval between tests must be acceptable to the target population.

The financial and resource costs associated with a screening program include those of identifying the target population, the screening procedure itself, the diagnostic workup of test-positive people, and the treatment of cancers diagnosed. The cost of screening can be expressed as cost per person, cost per case detected, or cost per unit of benefit. Health economists express benefit in terms of quality-adjusted life-years (QALYs). The extra years of life gained are adjusted for any effects of the program on the quality of life.

Cancer detection in the asymptomatic patient has focused on a number of cancers including those of the breast, colon, cervix, uterus, prostate, skin (melanoma), and lung. The evaluation of cancer-screening tests is such a lengthy and costly research undertaking that there are only a few cancers for which public health authorities have sufficient evidence to recommend or not recommend cancer screening. The American Cancer Society has recently updated its recommendations regarding screening for cancers (Table 44-1).

# BREAST CANCER

Breast cancer is the most common cancer in American women and the second most common cause of cancer deaths. Breast cancer occurred in more than 180,000 women in 1995 and accounted for greater than 46,000 deaths.[1] One in 8 women will be affected sometime during her lifetime with breast cancer. The risk factors for breast cancer include a positive family history, particularly in the mother or sisters, previous breast cancer, increasing age, obesity, not having children, having children late, and early menarche. Exercise and a diet low in saturated and animal-derived fat may possibly lower the risk of breast cancer. Mutations of the tumor-suppressor gene p53, and the BRCA1 gene have been noted in familial breast cancer and are associated with a significantly increased risk for breast cancer.[2] The ability to identify carriers of these mutated genes may someday allow for screening of breast cancer on a molecular level.

There are three established ways of finding breast cancer at an early stage: (1) breast self-examination, (2) physical examination of the breast by a trained clinician, and (3) mammography. In clinical practice, however, only about half of all cancers of the breast are detected at a stage in which the cancer is small and has not spread to regional lymph nodes. The prognosis is dependent on the extent of the disease at the time of diagnosis.

Breast self-examination has been recommended for many years. Self-examination has been the subject of review by the World Health Organization and the U.S. Preventive Services Task Force. The task force concluded that the sensitivity of self-examination is quite low (20% to 30%) compared with mammography and physical examination of the

**Table 44-1.** *Summary of American Cancer Society Recommendations for the early detection of cancer in asymptomatic people*

| Test or procedure | Population Sex | Age | Frequency |
|---|---|---|---|
| Sigmoidoscopy | M, F | Over 50 | Every 3-5 years |
| Stool guaiac slide test | M, F | Over 50 | Every year |
| Digital rectal examination | M, F | Over 40 | Every year |
| Papanicolaou test | F | 20-65 | All sexually active women over 18 years, annually. After 3 negative exams 1 year apart, perform at discretion of her physician. |
| Pelvic examination | F | At menopause | At menopause |
| Breast self-examination | F | Over 20 | Every month |
| Breast physical examination | F | 20-40 | Every 3 years |
| | F | Over 40 | Every year |
| Mammography | F | 40-49 | Every 1 or 2 years yearly |
| | | Over 50 | |
| Chest roentgenogram | | | Not recommended |
| Sputum cytology | | | Not recommended |
| Health counseling* and cancer checkup. | M, F | Over 20 | Every 3 years |
| | M, F | Over 40 | Every year |

* Includes examination of skin, thyroid, ovaries, lymph nodes, and oral region. Data from Shingleton HM, Patrick RL, Johnston WW, Smith RA: *CA Cancer J Clin* 45:305-320, 1995; Slawin KM, Ohori M, Dillioglugil O, Scardno PT: *CA Cancer J Clin* 45:134-147, 1995; and Mettlin C, Jones G, Averett H, et al: *CA Cancer J Clin* 43:42-46, 1993.

breast by a physician. Although the task force did not recommend abandoning self-examination, serious questions were raised about its usefulness. The World Health Organization concluded that "there is insufficient evidence that breast self-examination as applied to date is effective in reducing mortality from breast cancer . . . although there is equally insufficient evidence to change them [guidelines] where they exist."[3] In calling for additional research on breast self-examination, both organizations noted that the problem with self-examination, was not evidence for the lack of effect of breast self-examination but lack of evidence. We agree with these findings, but continue to recommend breast self-examination for all female patients.

We suggest to our patients that the breast self-examination should be performed at the same time each month, preferably after each menstrual period, and any new masses should be reported to their physicians.

Screening for breast cancer with mammography has been the principal focus of many studies over the last decade. The sensitivity of the mammogram is about 80% to 90% and is age dependent because in young women with dense breasts, lesions are more difficult to locate and define. Specificity is approximately 15% to 25%; that is, about one of every four to five mammographic lesions found prove to be malignant. Radiation exposure is low with newer mammographic technology, averaging six one-hundredths of a rad (0.06 rad), which is about the same as two chest roentgenograms.

Studies of breast cancer screening by mammography began in the late 1960s. The Health Insurance Plan (HIP) of New York enrolled some 31,000 women 40 to 64 years of age in a prospective breast cancer screening study.[4] These women were screened by a combination of yearly physical examinations of the breast and mammograms. The control group consisted of a matched group of 31,000 women from the same prepaid medical group plan who received their usual medical care. Ten years after this study was initiated, the mortality in the screened group was 30% less than that of the nonscreened group. At age 18 years, the difference between screened and nonscreened women was 21%. A significant difference applied only to women over 50 years of age. There was no significant reduction in breast cancer deaths in the HIP study for women under 50 years of age at the time of diagnosis in the first 5 years of the study. However, after 6 years, analysis revealed a beneficial effect in the screened group 40 to 49 years of age.[5] However, the effect observed in this younger population has been questioned and may have been attributable to improved survival within each stage of breast cancer and not a direct result of the screening.[6]

The HIP study was not designed to assess a possible differential effect of screening at various ages, and the differences observed could be attributable to chance alone. The HIP study raised questions on the differential effect of age on screening for breast cancer.

The American Cancer Society and the National Cancer Institute jointly sponsored a large study known as the Breast Cancer Detection Demonstration Project (BCDDP).[7] The project started in 1974 and ended in 1981. Twenty-nine sites around the country were selected and a total of 283,000 women were enrolled. The age range was between 35 and 74 years, with a median age of 50. The woman were younger than those screened in the HIP study. All women were screened with a combination of physical examination and mammography. The BCDDP was organized as a demonstration project and not as a research study. There was no control population, and the asymptomatic women were self-selected. Moreover, in this study there was an overrepresentation of women at higher risks for breast cancer as compared with the general population, a bias also found in the HIP study. Because of a concern over possible radiation-induced breast cancer in younger women, the BCDDP study recommended mammography for women under 50 years of age only if there was a family history of breast cancer.[8]

After 10 years, 4485 breast cancers were found; 3507 (80%) were discovered by the screening process. Fifty-nine percent of the noninfiltrating tumors and 53% of the small (<1.0 cm) cancers were found only by mammography. Forty-two percent of all cancers were found only by mammography; of note, 20% of patients with breast cancer were found to have abnormal nodes at surgery in this study. This low percentage of nodal involvement compares with approximately 53% of patients in studies of breast cancer not detected by screening programs. The BCDDP study confirmed the improved detection ability of mammography in women over 50 years of age with an overall reduction in mortality of 40% in women over 50 years of age. For women 35 to 49 years, however, there was little overall survival benefit.[9]

There has been a great deal of controversy regarding the BCDDP data base; the study was not controlled and the women were self-selected. However, despite these limitations, the data demonstrated the effectiveness of mammography in detecting breast cancer at its early stage. These data, along with similar studies that were done in Sweden and in Utrecht, the Netherlands, demonstrated that yearly screening with mammography results in finding more breast cancers that are smaller and at a more favorable stage for surgical intervention.[10] Mortality, though not an end point in both studies, was favorably affected in the women over 50 years of age. Both studies, however, showed no significant reduction in breast cancer mortality for women 40 to 49 years of age.[6,11] The Canadian National Breast Screening Study, designed to investigate the effects on mortality from screening mammograms in women 40 to 49 years of age, also did not demonstrate a decrease in breast cancer mortality.[12] The study did, however, demonstrate a significant increase in the detection of smaller, node-normal tumors. The results of this study continue to be criticized because of flaws in the study's methodology, staff expertise, and quality of the mammograms.[13]

Given the findings of these studies, the American Cancer Society developed very strong recommendations regarding breast cancer screening with mammography. The recommendations have been revised a number of times and presently include the following points:[14,15]

1. Monthly breast self-examination for all women 20 years of age or more.

2. A clinical breast examination every 3 years for women 20 to 40 years of age. Yearly breast examination for women 40 years or over.
3. Mammography for all women 40 to 49 years of age every 1 to 2 years.
4. Mammography yearly on all women 50 years of age or over.

Nevertheless, there has been controversy about routine mammograms for women under 50 years of age. The benefits of mammography after 50 years of age are well documented, but for the younger age group the evidence is still inconclusive. The incidence of breast cancer is considerably lower below 50 years of age, and, as noted, mammograms are more difficult to interpret in this age group. At present there is simply no consensus among experts whether mammograms should be done as a screening test in this age group.[6] Performing mammograms on asymptomatic women between 40 and 49 years of age at 1- to 2-year intervals as recommended by the American Cancer Society is not cost effective and has not yet been proved in long-running studies to result in lower mortality. In the HIP study at 18 years there was a difference of only six deaths in screened versus nonscreened patients under 50 years of age. Moreover, the American College of Physicians, the Canadian Task Force on the Periodic Health Examination, the American College of Obstetricians and Gynecologists, and the screening committee of the International Union Against Cancer do not recommend mammography for women under 50 years of age. Recently the National Cancer Institute (NCI) altered its guidelines, omitting recommendations for mammography and clinical breast examination for women in the 40 to 49 years of age bracket. Unsure of what to recommend, the NCI stopped issuing guidelines for breast cancer screening altogether and replaced guidelines with a statement of evidence.[16] The American Cancer Society continues to recommend mammography for women 40 to 49 years of age. The American Cancer Society does not dispute the lack of evidence supporting the use of routine screening mammography for younger women. However, they note that the clinical but not significant trends in younger women cannot be ignored.[14] Given the lack of consensus, our approach is to provide patients with the evidence and let them make up their own minds. We tell patients under 50 years of age that the mammogram carries a very low risk for harm but the chance of finding a lesion is likewise low. We believe this is the best approach at this time. On the other hand, we strongly recommend annual mammograms for patients in this age group with one of the known risk factors for breast cancer.

For women over 50 years of age, we agree with the recommendations of the American Cancer Society and recommend yearly mammography.

## COLON CANCER

Colon cancer affects 150,000 people each year and accounts for 56,000 deaths annually. Risk factors include previous colon cancer, familial polyposis, villous or adenomatous polyps, and ulcerative colitis. Favorable influences may include low dietary fat and a high-fiber diet. Epidemiologic studies indicate that low doses of aspirin may be useful in preventing colorectal cancers.[17] The polyp-neoplasia sequence for the genesis of carcinoma of the colon is now well accepted. This refers to the concept that most colon cancer arises from preexisting villous or adenomatous polyps. Malignant transformation of these polyps occurs over a prolonged period of time, thus providing an opportunity for early diagnosis at the time when the disease is localized. The screening tests available for colon cancer include digital rectal examination, stool blood testing, sigmoidoscopy, and colonoscopy.

Digital rectal examination remains a recommended part of the routine comprehensive physical exam. Its value as a method for early detection of polyps or colon cancer is unknown. Current data indicate that only 10% of colon cancers are within the reach of an examining finger. Cancer of the colon has seemingly migrated away from the rectum and toward the cecum. However, we believe that this examination should continue to be performed.

Fecal occult blood testing (FOBT) is usually guaiac based and detects the peroxidase-like activity of hemoglobin. The test can detect blood loss that is about three times the normal level. False-positive results may be attributable to dietary sources of peroxidase, myoglobin, or hemoglobin (see box below). Consumption of drugs such as aspirin may cause enough bleeding to create a positive test. High doses of vitamin C increase the false-negative rate. One recently published clinical trial using rehydrated slides demonstrated a 33% reduction in colon cancer mortality. However, 10% of the screening tests were positive with a positive predictive value for colon cancer at about 2% and for cancer and adenomas combined at 30%. The high false-positive rate resulted in 38% of the screened population undergoing colonoscopy at some point during the study. A recent case control study suggested that yearly FOBT screening could reduce colon cancer mortality by 25%.[19] Although FOBT testing appears to lead to lower colon cancer mortality, its specificity in actual practice is low, and its sensitivity is

---

## Substances That Interfere with the Stool Guaiac Test

MAY PRODUCE A FALSE-POSITIVE TEST

Rare red meat, broccoli, cantaloupe, cauliflower, red radish, horseradish, parsnips, artichoke, zucchini, iron medication

MAY PRODUCE A FALSE-NEGATIVE TEST

Vitamin C, prolonged storage of sample

also limited. Studies suggest that most polyps and even the majority of invasive cancers do not consistently bleed.

Since approximately half the patients with positive stool guaiac tests have no demonstrable disorder, many persons without disease undergo the cost, discomfort, and anxiety of endoscopy or barium contrast studies to evaluate the positive Hemoccult test. Using a combination of fecal occult blood tests improves the specificity and sensitivity of testing program.[19,20]

The American Cancer Society and the Canadian Task Force on the Periodic Health Examination have endorsed the use of screening by means of the stool guaiac test on a yearly basis after 50 years of age. The U.S. Preventive Services Task Force has recently changed its view that there is insufficient evidence for or against colon-cancer screening but endorses occult blood screening or sigmoidoscopy, or both, starting at age 50.[19]

We agree with these findings and accept the limitations of the stool guaiac test but continue to recommend the stool guaiac test on a yearly basis after 50 years of age.

The issue of routine sigmoidoscopy is more controversial. Adenomatous and villous polyps are the precursors for cancer of the colon, but the rate of malignant degeneration is low, on the order of less than 1%. When flexible sigmoidoscopy to 60 cm is performed, approximately 8% to 10% of asymptomatic people over 50 years of age are found to have adenomatous polyps. These polyps are frequently multiple, and on colonoscopy, up to 50% have synchronous lesions beyond 60 cm. These observations have given rise to the recommendation that the discovery of one polyp on a screening sigmoidoscopy must be followed by colonoscopic examination of the entire colon.[21] The benefit of proctosigmoidoscopic screening is suggested by several studies including the Preventive Medicine Institute–Strang Clinic study in New York City, the Kaiser Permanente Study in Oakland, California, and the one at St. Marks hospital in London, England.[22,23] These studies, though not prospective and uncontrolled, did demonstrate a reduced risk for fatal colorectal cancers in the population screened with a sigmoidoscopy.

The American Cancer Society, the National Cancer Institute, and others recommend a digital rectal examination to detect colorectal cancer for all persons 40 years and over. Up to now, only the American Cancer Society from those major advisory groups has recommended that sigmoidoscopy be done on a regular screening program. They recommend that all persons over 50 years of age have a sigmoidoscopy performed every 3 to 5 years.[24]

The U.S. Preventive Services Task Force acknowledged that evidence from controlled trials to either recommend or not recommend the use of sigmoidoscopy as a screening test in populations with no known risk is unclear. However, they recommended colonoscopy for high-risk patients so as to evaluate the entire colon.

We agree with the American Cancer Society recommendation of a routine flexible sigmoidoscopy to 60 cm every 3 to 5 years for patients over 50 years. In patients with adenomas found on sigmoidoscopy we recommend colonoscopy every 3 to 5 years for an indefinite period after adenoma removal. We explain to our low-risk patients that there are insufficient data to support the routine screening of all patients with colonoscopy. All patients with a strong family history, two or more affected first-degree relatives, or a single first-degree relative developing colorectal cancer before age 55, or familial polyposis coli, are encouraged to have periodic colonoscopy.[24]

# CANCER OF THE CERVIX

In the United States, invasive cancer of the cervix occurs in about 15,000 women annually and is responsible for 5000 cancer-related deaths. Sexual activity is the most important risk factor, with intercourse before 18 years of age, multiple sexual partners, and a high number of sexual partners associated with an increased cancer risk. Sex as a risk factor is now believed to be related to infection with a human papillomavirus. Other known risk factors are in utero exposure to diethylstilbestrol and smoking.

The rationale for screening is based on a long average presymptomatic period for cervical cancer (5 years) and an even longer period of asymptomatic cervical intraepithelial neoplasia (CIN) that is believed to precede invasive cervical cancer in most patients. CIN encompasses cervical dysplasia and carcinoma in situ (CIS) and is believed to last, on average, 10 years or longer. Dysplasia frequently reverts to normal without treatment, but CIS is more likely to progress to invasive cancer.

The Papanicolaou smear has been used to detect cervical abnormalities for over 50 years. Problems with specimen collection and cytologic interpretation reduce test sensitivity. Endocervical and cervical cells are best collected with newer instruments designed for this purpose. Lack of endocervical cells on the slide (especially in premenopausal women) indicates that specimen collection may have been inadequate.

If the Pap smear shows dysplasia, a woman's risk of developing invasive cervical cancer increases manyfold. With mild dysplasia, two repeat pap smears should be done at 3-month intervals, and if either is abnormal, the patient should be referred to a gynecologist. If both are normal, the patient should be counseled that she should have an annual pap smear indefinitely. Patients with smears demonstrating higher grade dysplasia, CIS, or invasive cancer should be referred immediately to a gynecologist.

The Pap test for screening for cancer of the cervix is accepted by most women and their physicians. Epidemiologic studies have shown that in populations in which use of the Pap smear is high, the rate of decline of death from cervical cancer has been above average. No randomized trial to evaluate the efficacy of Pap smears has ever been done. All evidence supporting the use of this test is indirect and is based on projections from what is known of the natural history of the disease. However, this concept has been questioned in some studies.[25]

The Pap test has many real and potential technical problems. The Pap test interpretation can vary greatly among different laboratories. The Pap test is easy to perform but difficult to read. In one representative study the diagnosis was questioned in a third of the specimens referred to a panel of expert pathologists. Moreover, abnormal cells may not appear on the slide. In a study evaluating dysplasia of the cervix, 50% of the slides showed a discrepancy on two slides taken at the same time from the same woman.[25]

Despite the limitations of the Pap test, it remains an important and widely used screening test. Several large epidemiologic studies have demonstrated that the use of the Pap test has contributed to the reduction of mortality from cervical cancer. In August 1987 the American Cancer Society held a workshop to reexamine the scientific data about Pap smears and cervical cancer. That report recommended that all women who are or have been sexually active or are over 18 years of age have an annual Pap test and pelvic examination. After a woman has had three or more consecutive normal annual examinations, the Pap test may be performed "less frequently at the discretion of her physician." This recommendation attempts to address the uncertainty about the optimal frequency of screening and the likelihood that cervical cancer may be related to a sexually transmitted agent, one of the human papillomavirus (HPV) group. The new guidelines do not place an upper age limit of testing for cervical cancer. Other groups now have similar recommendations including the National Cancer Institute, the American Medical Association, and the American College of Obstetricians and Gynecologists. In contrast, programs in England and Canada still recommend a Pap smear every 3 years from 18 to 35 years of age in sexually active women, and then every 5 years until 60 years.

The cytologic nomenclature for the classification of the Pap smear has resulted in confusion among clinicians and pathologists. Originally, Papanicolaou described five classes: class I, absence of atypical or abnormal cells, to class 5, cytologic evidence conclusive for malignancy. Others have used terms to define it from the preinvasive continuum of the cervical dysplasia to cervical intraepithelial neoplasia (CIN) and to invasive carcinoma. The National Cancer Institute workshop developed the Bethesda System to classify cervical and vaginal cytologic features[26] (Table 44-2).

Despite the difficulties associated with the Pap Smear, we agree with the recommendations of the American Cancer Society.

## CANCER OF THE UTERUS

Over 95% of uterine cancers are adenocarcinomas of the endometrium. In the United States, there are about 40,000 new cases and 4000 deaths each year. Risk factors include nulliparity, obesity, diabetes mellitus, a mother or sister with endometrial cancer, and previous breast or colon cancer. A major risk factor is the postmenopausal use of estrogen without progesterone, and the risk is dose related. The Pap smear is not a sensitive test for endometrial cancer.

The prevalence of carcinoma of the endometrium has increased steadily over the last 90 years, an increase thus reflecting the increased life span of women and perhaps the decreased likelihood of cervical

**Table 44-2.** Relationship of the Bethesda System to Papanicolaou classification

Bethesda System*

| Within normal limits | Benign cellular changes | | LGSIL HPV | HGSIL | | Invasive carcinoma |
|---|---|---|---|---|---|---|
| | Infection Reactive repair | ASCUS AGUS | Mild dysplasia[†] | Moderate dysplasia[†] | Severe dysplasia[†] CIS[†] | |
| | | | | Epithelial cell abnormalities | | |
| | | | CIN1[‡] | CIN2[‡] | CIN3[‡] | |

The Papanicolaou Classification

| Class I No abnormal cells | Class II Atypical cytology but no evidence of malignancy | Class III Cytology suggestive of, but not diagnostic of malignancy | Class IV Cytology strongly suggestive malignancy | Class V Cytology conclusive for malignancy |
|---|---|---|---|---|

ASCUS, Atypical squamous cells of unknown significance; AGUS, atypical glandular cells of unknown significance; HGSIL, high-grade squamous intraepithelial lesion; HPV, human papillomavirus; LGSIL, low-grade squamous intraepithelial lesion.

*The Betheseda Terminology.[26]

[†]CIN1, CIN2, CIN3, cervical intraepithelial neoplasia; terminology from Reagan, et al.[25]

[‡]CIS, carcinoma in situ; terminology from Richard.[25]

cancer. Endometrial cancer is most common in postmenopausal women.

Endometrial aspiration and biopsy has been recommended as a screening test. In a screening study of endometrial carcinoma in asymptomatic women using endometrial aspiration, eight cancers were found in 1280 women.[27] Seven of the eight had one or more risk factors for endometrial cancer. The role of endometrial aspiration or biopsy in asymptomatic patients without one of the previously noted risk factors remains unclear. Endometrial sampling appears to be a more sensitive test, but the test is probably too uncomfortable to use on a routine basis. The American Cancer Society recommends that every woman at the time of menopause have a pelvic examination and that high-risk women have an endometrial tissue sample examined. Despite these recommendations, less than 2% of all women have undergone this screening test. At this time we recommend that only high-risk women should consider an endometrial aspiration. We do not recommend the routine use of this screening test. However, women should be informed about the importance of promptly reporting any postmenopausal bleeding to their physician.

## CANCER OF THE LUNG

Lung cancer is the most common cause of cancer death in the United States; over 170,000 new cases are diagnosed annually with 160,000 cancer-related deaths. Five-year survival rates remain below 10%. Survival rates are low even when an asymptomatic tumor is discovered.

Several randomized trials have evaluated chest roentgenograms and sputum cytologic findings as screening tests for lung cancer. In the Philadelphia Pulmonary Neoplasm Research Project, over 6000 smokers were offered semiannual chest roentgenograms.[28] Over a 10-year period, 121 cancers were detected with a 5-year survival of 8%. A British trial of semiannual chest roentgenograms in 29,000 men found 101 cancers in 3 years. In 25,000 controls, 76 tumors were found. Five-year survival rates were 15% in the intervention group and 6% in controls. Cancer death rates in the two groups were almost identical.

An additional problem with chest roentgenographic screening is that the predictive value of a positive test is low, from 5% to 20% in different studies.

Trials at Johns Hopkins, Memorial Sloan-Kettering and the Mayo Clinic, each enrolled more than 10,000 male smokers and examined the value of annual chest roentgenograms (every 4 months at Mayo) combined with sputum cytology every 4 months. Mortalities in the control and intervention groups were not significantly different in any of the trials.

These trials also demonstrated that a sputum cytology test is less sensitive than previously believed. Only 10% to 13% of tumors were initially detected by cytology testing alone. Although false-positive tests were rare, they required extensive bronchoscopic evaluation to rule out the presence of cancer. In sum, large-scale screening programs using chest roentgenograms and sputum cytology have not reduced the death rate from lung cancer.

Given the data, we believe that at this time there is no proved benefit of routine screening of patients for lung cancer with chest roentgenograms or sputum cytology. The physician's primary role in preventing lung cancer is to educate patients regarding the many risks associated with smoking and to strongly encourage patients who do smoke to stop. The American Cancer Society does not recommend screening roentgenograms or sputum cytology tests.

# MELANOMA

The incidence of melanoma is rising rapidly. Currently, over 30,000 new cases are identified annually, and there are over 6000 deaths each year. Risk factors include extensive sun exposure (especially when associated with sunburn), presence of congenital nevi (especially ones over 1.5 cm in diameter), and history of melanoma in a first-degree relative.

Although no randomized trial of screening has been done, there is strong evidence that early detection and removal of abnormal nevi reduces the death rate from melanoma. Case death rates have declined since physicians and others have become more aware of the appearance of melanoma and its precursor, the dysplastic nevus.

Examination of the skin, especially all sun-exposed areas, should be part of every routine physical exam. The ABCD criteria should be utilized to detect suspicious lesions:

**A** - Asymmetry of lesion shape
**B** - Border irregularity
**C** - Multiple colors
**D** - Diameter greater than 6 millimeters

The presence of one or more of these findings should lead to biopsy or to dermatology referral.

Patients should be counseled to seek immediate evaluation for a change in size or color of any pigmented lesion. Bleeding or itching also requires immediate evaluation. Any individual with a previous dysplastic nevus or melanoma is at higher risk for a second lesion and should have annual skin screening throughout life.

# PROSTATE CANCER

In the United States, about 250,000 men will be diagnosed with prostate cancer each year, and there will be 40,000 deaths. Currently about 40% of newly diagnosed men already have metastases. The incidence is two to three times higher in black Americans and twice as high when a father or brother has prostate cancer. Prevalence of histologic prostate cancer at autopsy is about 20% for men in their sixties and 40% for those over 70 years.

A problem in considering a screening program is that definitive treatment of prostate cancer carries considerable morbidity. Radical prostatectomy has been associated with a 30% incidence of incontinence and a 60% risk for impotence. Newer nerve-sparing techniques have reduced these numbers somewhat. For radiotherapy, the numbers are about 5% and 35%, respectively.[29]

The two currently used screening techniques are digital rectal exam (DRE) and prostate-specific antigen test (PSA). Randomized trials demonstrating the effects of these tests on prostate cancer mortality are not available.

In screening studies using both DRE and PSA, DRE detected 50% to 60% of cancers, and PSA found 75% to 80%.[30] Both techniques detected about the same percentage of localized cancer. In population studies, DRE is abnormal in 10% to 20% of men (higher with advancing age). When patients with an abnormal DRE are subject to biopsy, 15% to 25% will have cancer.

The PSA test measures a glycoprotein produced by prostate epithelial cells. Normal values are related to gland volume and therefore rise somewhat with age. A value of 5 ng/mL is usually considered elevated in a 50 year old but normal in a 70 year old. The PSA level can also be elevated for weeks after prostatitis, acute urinary retention, or an invasive procedure. DRE does not elevate PSA. The likelihood of cancer is related to the degree of PSA elevation. In one study, 22% of biopsies in men with PSAs between 4 and 10 were positive, whereas 67% of PSAs over 10 were associated with a positive biopsy.[31]

The PSA test is associated with a sensitivity of up to 80% in detecting prostate cancer but is associated with a high false-positive rate. False-positive results in benign prostatic hypertrophy and prostatitis range from 25% to 40%. The reported predictive value of PSA in screening studies is 28% to 35%, reflecting that one third of men with elevated PSA levels (>4 mg/mL) will be found to have prostate cancer whereas two thirds will not.[31] The use of the PSA as a screening test for prostate cancer therefore remains controversial. Several prospective studies are underway to evaluate the role of PSA, but these studies are at least a decade away from completion. In 1993 the American Cancer Society recommended that all men over 50 years of age have an annual prostate examination and a PSA level.[32] The American Urological Association issued a similar recommendation. Support for PSA screening is not, however, universal. The U.S. Preventive Services Task Force, the Canadian Task Force on the Periodic Health Examination, and the Canadian Urologic Association have not recommended periodic screening with PSA.

In summary, we believe that clinical trials have demonstrated that screening for prostate cancer lowers cancer mortality. DRE is a part of the routine examination in patients over 40 years of age and the presence of a prostatic nodule should lead to referral to a urologist. Many urologists recommend use of the PSA test annually beginning at 50 years, provided that the patient's life expectancy exceeds 10 years.

The benefit and risks (including the complications of definitive therapy) of PSA screening should be discussed with men over 50. Given existing data, the routine use of the PSA test cannot be recommended.

# OVARIAN CANCER

Advances in the medical and surgical treatment of ovarian cancer have improved the outcome for early-stage disease. However, early diagnosis remains an uncommon event. At present, physical examination, or the use of CA-125 tests and pelvic ultrasound lack the necessary specificity for population-based screening.[33]

# ROLE OF TUMOR MARKERS

Several "tumor" markers that are useful in the management of patients with known cancer have been developed in the last decade. These markers include carcinoembryonic antigen (CEA) for patients with colon, breast, pancreatic, and ovarian cancer; alpha-fetoprotein (AFP) for liver and germ cell tumors; CA 125 for ovarian cancer; and mammary serum antigen (MSA) for patients with breast cancer. None of these markers is specific enough to be used as a screening test for cancer, and we do not recommend their use in screening tests.[34]

## References

1. Wingo PA, Tong T, Bolden S: Cancer statistics, *CA Cancer J Clin* 45:8-30, 1995.
2. King MC, Rowell S, Love SM: Inherited breast and ovarian cancer: What are the risks? What are the choices? *JAMA* 269:1975-1980, 1993.
3. Self-examination in the early detection of breast cancer, Geneva, 1983, World Health Organization.
4. Habbeman JDF, van Oortmarssen GJ, van Pucten DJ, et al: Age-specific reduction in breast cancer mortality by screening: an analysis of the results of the Health Insurance Plan of Greater New York, *J Natl Cancer Inst* 7:277-317, 1986.
5. Chu KC, Connor RJ: Analysis of the temporal patterns of benefits in the Health Insurance Plan of Greater New York trial by stage and age, *Am J Epidemiol* 133:1039-1049, 1991.
6. Miller AB: Mammography in women under 50, *Hematol Oncol Clin North Am* 8:165-177, 1994.
7. Baker LH: Breast Cancer Detection Demonstration Project: five year summary report, *Cancer* 32:194, 1982.
8. Breslow L, Thomas LB, Upton AC: Final reports of the National Cancer Institute Ad Hoc Working Groups on Mammography in Screening for Breast Cancer and summary report of their joint findings and recommendations, *J Natl Cancer Inst* 59:467-541, 1977.
9. Morrison AS, Brisson J, Khalid N: Breast cancer incidence and mortality in the Breast Cancer Detection Demonstration Project, *J Natl Cancer Inst* 80:1540-1547, 1988.

10. Tabár L, Fagerberg CJG, Gad A, et al: Reduction in mortality from breast cancer after mass screening with mammography, *Lancet* 1:829-832, 1985.

11. Verbeek ALM, Hendricks JHCL, Holland R, et al: Mammographic screening and breast cancer mortality: age-specific effects in Nijmegen Project, 1975-1982, *Lancet* 1:865-866, 1985.

12. Mettlin CJ, Smart CR: The Canadian National Breast Screening Study: an appraisal and implications for early detection policy, *Cancer* 72(suppl): 1461-1465, 1993.

13. Kopans DB: The Canadian screening program: a different perspective, *AJR* 155:448-479, 1990.

14. Mettlin CJ, Smart CR: Breast cancer detection guidelines for women aged 40 to 49 years: rationale for the American Cancer Society reaffirmation of recommendations, *CA* 44:248-255, 1994.

15. Dodd GM: American Cancer Society guidelines from the past to present, *Cancer* 79(suppl):1429-1432, 1993.

16. Volkers N: NCI replaces guidelines with statement of evidence, *J Natl Cancer Inst* 86:14-15, 1994.

17. Garewall HS: Aspirin in the prevention of colorectal cancer, *Ann Intern Med* 121:303-303, 1994.

18. Allison JE, Twkawa IS, Ranson LJ, Adrian AL: A comparison of fecal occult-blood tests for colorectal-cancer screening, *N Engl J Med* 334:155-159, 1996.

19. Ransohoff DF, Lang CA: Improving the fecal occult-blood test, *N Engl J Med* 334:189-190, 1996.

20. Toribara NW, Sleisenger MH: Current concepts: screening for colorectal cancer, *N Engl J Med* 332:861-867, 1995.

21. Ransohoff DF, Lang CA: Sigmoidoscopic screening in the 1990s, *JAMA* 269:1278-1281, 1993.

22. Selby JV, Friedman GD, Quesenberry CPJ, Weiss NS: A case control study of screening sigmoidoscopy and mortality from colorectal cancer, *N Engl J Med* 326:653-657, 1992.

23. Atkin WS, Morson BC, Cuzick J: Long term risk of colorectal cancer after excision of rectosigmoid adenomas, *N Engl J Med* 326:658-662, 1992.

24. Levin B, Murphy GP: Revisions in American Cancer Society recommendations for the early detection of colorectal cancer, *CA Cancer J Clin* 42:296-299, 1992.

25. Shingleton HM, Patrick RL, Johnston WW, Smith RA: The current status of the Papanicolaou smear, *CA Cancer J Clin* 45:305-320, 1995.

26. National Cancer Institute Workshop: The 1988 Bethesda System for reporting cervical/vaginal cytological diagnosis, *JAMA* 262:931-934, 1989.

27. Koss LG, Schreiberk, Oberlander SG, et al: Screening of asymptomatic women for endometrial cancer, *CA Cancer J Clin* 31(6):301-317, 1981.

28. Weiss W, Boucot KE, Cooper DA: The Philadelphia pulmonary neoplasm research project: survival factors in bronchogenic carcinoma, *JAMA* 216:2119-2123, 1973.

29. Chodak GW, Thisted RA, Gerber GS, et al: Results of conservative management of clinically localized prostate cancer, *N Engl J Med* 330:242-248, 1994.

30. Slawin KM, Ohori M, Dillioglugil O, Scardno PT: Screening for prostate cancer: an analysis of the early experience, *CA Cancer J Clin* 45:134-147, 1995.

31. Woolf SH: Screening for prostate cancer with prostate specific antigen, *N Engl J Med* 333:1401-1405, 1995.
32. Mettlin C, Jones G, Averett H, et al: Defining and updating the American Cancer Society guidelines for cancer-related checkup: prostate and endometrial cancers, *CA Cancer J Clin* 43:42-46, 1993.
33. Teneriello MG, Park RC: Early detection of ovarian cancer, *CA Cancer J Clin* 45:71-87, 1995.
34. Hayes DF, editor: Tumor markers in adult solid malignancies, *Hematol Oncol Clin North Am* 8(3), 1994.

## Chapter 45
# *Adjuvant Treatment of Cancer*

Richard A. Rudders

As new cancer treatments are developed, strategies to optimize the results of these treatments follow. Predicated on persuasive theoretical and practical arguments, so-called adjuvant treatment is such a strategy. In oncologic practice we now are usually able to remove the bulk of a given tumor with one of several modalities. The residual disease (both metastatic and microscopic), however, is a major cause of treatment failure leading to overt recurrence of cancer and death. Since the total tumor burden is often quite small after an initial attempt at curative treatment, there is an opportunity to eradicate successfully any residual tumor, even though there is distant spread. Use of a variety of treatment modalities to eradicate residual disease is a guiding principle of adjuvant treatment. Before discussing some specific examples of adjuvant therapy, I review some fundamental concepts regarding adjuvant therapy. This background information will aid the clinician in analyzing newly published data on adjuvant cancer therapy and in answering a common question: Should I have additional treatment either before or after my operation?

## ADJUVANT TREATMENT — A DEFINITION

Broadly speaking, the term "adjuvant" signifies 'something in addition to or added.' With respect to cancer treatment, adjuvant therapy is any form of therapy given in addition to a primary mode of treatment, again, with the intent of improving outcome. Such a definition has no restriction in terms of type, mode of administration, or duration, as long as the intent is to improve results without jeopardizing the result of the primary therapy. Thus adjuvant cancer treatment may be chemotherapy, radiation therapy, surgery, or any other modality deemed suitable. In contrast, the use of a second mode of treatment that is directed at bulk tumor as part of primary therapy, strictly speaking, should be classified as "combined modality" treatment, rather than adjuvant treatment.

# BASIC PRINCIPLES

Historically the rationale for adjuvant treatment was closely tied to prevailing concepts of tumor cell kinetics. From animal and in vitro model systems, early investigators recognized that anticancer interventions were more successful when tumor burdens were small and when treatments were given in maximum doses.[1] It then was reasoned that treatment would more likely be successful in situations where a minimal tumor burden existed. We now know that, with increasing tumor size and proliferation, the degree of tumor heterogeneity also increases (through mutational events), thereby setting the stage for resistance to treatment.[2] Both of these factors, sheer tumor bulk and cellular resistance, tend to defeat therapeutic maneuvers. Ideally, then, to optimize outcome, treatment should be given as early as possible in the course of the disease when tumor bulk is small and cellular resistance is minimal. This concept remains the basis for adjuvant therapy.

Given this foundation, what remains is to define the proper setting in which to use adjuvant therapy. Historically, adjuvant therapy was employed after surgical removal of a tumor in situations where there remained a high rate of recurrence or relapse. In such instances, tumor progression was primarily attributable to growth of occult micrometastases at distant sites that were present before surgery. It was argued and demonstrated that postoperative chemotherapy could eradicate these microscopic foci of disease. One classic adjuvant treatment protocol therefore would be systemic treatment, such as chemotherapy, after primary resection of a tumor. This concept logically can be extended to include any situation where primary therapy may not suffice and additional treatment may add benefit.

Adjuvant treatment need not be chemotherapy but may be radiation therapy, a so-called biologic response modifier (see subsequently), or surgery. Furthermore, a regional approach may be warranted, rather than a systemic approach, if a specific site of micrometastases constitutes the greatest liability in terms of future recurrence and morbidity. An example of such a regional approach is regional infusion of the liver with 5-fluorouracil after primary resection for colon cancer in patients at high risk for hepatic recurrence.

So-called neoadjuvant treatment has recently become popular and offers certain advantages. This strategy employs the adjuvant treatment as the initial treatment to improve the result of the primary curative modality; in most cases this modality is surgery. Not only may cure rates be improved, but also the surgery itself may be technically easier (see later discussion of esophageal and rectal cancer).

It seems obvious that to choose a form of adjuvant therapy that is not likely to be successful is counterproductive. Unfortunately this is often done with the best of intentions. In an effort to spare the patient morbidity from an additional treatment, a drug regimen that is ineffective is employed. A basic principle of adjuvant chemotherapy is: If the drug is not an effective treatment in a nonadjuvant setting, don't use it in an adjuvant setting. This argument does not apply, however, to substances classified as biologic response modifiers. Biologic response modifiers are geared to work optimally in patients with low tumor burdens and may have little or no demonstrable activity when tumor burdens are high.

Cancer treatment to a considerable extent remains empiric, and certain aspects of strategies such as adjuvant treatment remain hard to define. One such dilemma relates to the duration of treatment. Since very often no visible tumor exists, how does one gauge the adequacy of adjuvant chemotherapy? Empiric observations, long-term follow-up, and occasionally the use of tumor markers are the only methods. Anything less assures no likelihood of obtaining useful information. Clearly, careful planning in implementing adjuvant treatment is necessary.

# THE DESIGN OF AN ADJUVANT TREATMENT

Except in certain specific settings (see subsequently), adjuvant therapy remains largely experimental. Adjuvant therapy therefore is ideally given in the context of a clinical trial using a well-defined protocol. I believe that ad hoc or random treatment of patients with unproved adjuvant therapy should not be carried out without a protocol. In general, an adjuvant therapy study requires a sizable number of patients and a long follow-up study to be statistically valid. The foundation of a well-designed study of adjuvant therapy is the principle of randomization. Patients are assigned randomly to one of several treatment options. A simple adjuvant study randomizes patients between a primary treatment option only and a primary treatment along with an adjuvant treatment option. In this way, the single variable in the system is the adjuvant therapy. When a large enough patient sample is entered and sufficient time has elapsed, the effect of the adjuvant treatment can be quantified when one compares the responses in the experimental group to the relapses in the control group. More complicated studies that ask several questions at once can be designed. Although this approach may be appealing because it appears quicker and more cost effective, more complicated studies are more difficult to analyze, and the results are more difficult to interpret.

The goal of all adjuvant treatment is to increase disease-free survival and ultimately to cure. This means that, for a given cohort of patients, the number of patients that remain free of any evidence of tumor after therapy is statistically significantly increased compared to a control population (Fig. 45-1, curve A). If such a cohort is followed long enough, disease-free survival of sufficient duration becomes equivalent to cure. The accuracy of judging cure varies with the natural history of each tumor. Certain tumors recur early, and survival without relapse for more than 2 years allows one to predict a high cure rate. Other tumors may recur late, and many years must elapse before a cure is assured. The usual presentation of cure rates as 5-year survivals is therefore arbitrary, and cure rates must be evaluated in the context of individual tumors.

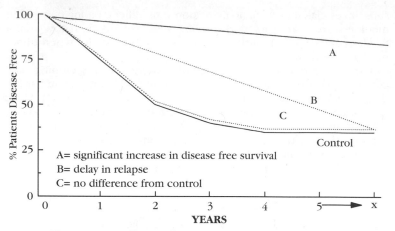

**Figure 45-1.** *Three different results of adjuvant treatment.*

Although less desirable, an increase in total patient survival or in delay of relapse (Fig. 45-1, curve *B*), even if cure is not achieved, may be the most a given adjuvant treatment can accomplish. This effect, although less than hoped for, may be highly desirable, depending on the magnitude of the increase in survival relative to the case; the latter must be measured both in true cost and in terms of toxicity of the treatment and of side effects suffered by the patient. The more successful the treatment, the higher is the therapeutic index. The lower the therapeutic index is, the more the toxicity and the less the benefit, and survival curves with and without adjuvant therapy will be comparable (Fig. 45-1, curve *C*).

The clinician should know the common pitfalls in interpreting the results of adjuvant therapy trials. The most common error is to draw a hasty conclusion from preliminary data, that is, after too little time has elapsed. Early prolongation of disease-free survival may be meaningless in terms of cure if relapse is merely delayed. Projecting a considerable increase in disease-free survival or in cure rate based on preliminary data is a common practice in studies of adjuvant treatment and should be discouraged. More often than not, a totally different picture emerges when the data mature. If the cure rate is not increased, a new approach may be necessary. However, if a lesser but still desirable effect occurs, such as prolongation of total survival or delay of relapse, modification of the original treatment may be indicated as the next step.

Judging the benefit of any treatment is difficult but particularly so when toxic treatments with low therapeutic indices are used. The benefits of adjuvant treatment must be carefully weighed against the cost in terms of both acute and delayed side effects.

## SPECIFIC EXAMPLES OF ADJUVANT THERAPIES

Several specific examples of current adjuvant therapies are listed in Tables 45-1 and 45-2. The list is in no way intended to be comprehensive

**Table 45–1.** *Adjuvant treatment of common cancers*

| Cancer | Patient characteristics | Therapy | Outcome |
|---|---|---|---|
| Breast | Postsurgical resection | | |
| | Node negative* | | |
| | *Premenopausal* | | |
| | Receptor positive | Hormonal therapy | Unknown |
| | Receptor negative | Chemotherapy | Unknown |
| | *Postmenopausal* | | |
| | Receptor positive | Hormonal therapy | Unkown |
| | Receptor negative | Chemotherapy | Unknown |
| | Node positive | | |
| | *Premenopausal* | | |
| | Receptor positive | Chemotherapy | Increase DFS |
| | Receptor negative | Chemotherapy | Increase DFS |
| | *Postmenopausal* | | |
| | Receptor positive | Hormonal therapy and chemotherapy | Increase DFS |
| | Receptor negative | Chemotherapy and hormonal therapy | Increase DFS |
| Colon | Postsurgical resection | | |
| | Dukes stage C | Chemotherapy | Increase DFS |
| | Dukes stage B2* | Various | Unknown |
| Rectum | Postsurgical resection | | |
| | Dukes stages B and C | Chemoradiotherapy | Increase DFS |
| | Preoperative | | |
| | Bulky, locally advanced | Chemoradiotherapy | Sphincter Preservation |
| Esophagus | Preoperative* | | |
| | Bulky, locally advanced | Chemotherapy | Unknown |
| Lung | | | |
| Small cell | Postchemotherapy induction | Radiation to CNS or primary site, or both | Decrease local recurrence |
| Non–small cell* | Postsurgical resection | Chemoradiation | Unknown |
| | Stage II B | | |
| | Preoperative | Chemoradiation | Unknown |
| Prostate* | Postsurgical positive margins or extracapsular extension | Radiotherapy | Unknown |

*CNS,* Central nervous system; *DFS,* disease-free survival.
* Treatment on clinical trial strongly recommended.

**Table 45-2.** *Adjuvant treatment of less common cancers*

| Cancer | Patient characteristics | Therapy | Outcome |
|---|---|---|---|
| Melanoma* | Postsurgical resection of primary site | Chemotherapy BRM | Unknown |
| Osteogenic sarcoma | Preoperative | Chemotherapy | Limb salvage Increase DFS |
| Testicular | Postsurgical stage II retroperitoneal node dissection, no choriocarcinoma | Chemotherapy | Increase in DFS |
| Lymphoma | Large cell, stages I and II | Chemoradiotherapy | Increase DFS |
| | Burkitt's and lymphoblastic | CNS radiation with or without chemotherapy | Unknown |
| | All types,* advanced disease, postinductional | High-dose chemoradiation stem-cell rescue | Unknown |
| Leukemia | All | CNS radiation with or without chemotherapy | Increase DFS |

*BRM,* Biologic response modifier; *DFS,* disease-free survival.
* Treatment on clinical trial strongly recommended.

but serves to illustrate several common tumor types considered amenable to adjuvant treatment. The competent consultant must be aware of these examples and of the various approaches to adjuvant treatment they exemplify.

## Breast cancer—an adjuvant success story

More has been written about the adjuvant therapy of surgically resectable breast cancer than perhaps any other cancer.[3-5] Breast cancer is an important tumor for several reasons. First, it is extremely common and is one of the leading causes of cancer death in women. Second, adjuvant therapy in breast cancer clearly works! The studies of adjuvant therapy have been numerous, international, well controlled, and carefully done. Adjuvant treatment with either tamoxifen or various different combination chemotherapy regimens, usually given for 6 months in the postoperative period, clearly prolongs disease-free and total survival for certain well-defined subsets of patients (see Fig. 45-1, curve *A*). This effect has been demonstrated in patients who fall into two broad categories: premenopausal patients treated with chemotherapy and postmenopausal patients treated with hormonal therapy (tamoxifen). Patients with cancerous axillary lymph nodes derive the most benefit from adjuvant therapy (see Table 45-1). The challenge of the future is to define subgroups of node-negative patients who may also benefit. This is best done in the context of a clinical trial. Node-negative patients with risk factors for recurrence are likely to benefit the most. These factors include a large primary tumor (more than about 1 to 2 cm), tumor aneuploidy with or without a high S (synthesis)-phase fraction, and a high content of the HER-2 marker.

As with any therapy, the potential benefits of adjuvant chemotherapy for breast cancer must be weighed against the risks of treatment. The short-term effects of chemotherapy are well defined and vary with the type of drugs used and the duration of treatment. Tolerance of drug therapy for 6 months (the usual duration of treatment) is highly variable, potentially morbid, but rarely fatal. We are just now in a position to evaluate the potential long-term effects. I believe that the greatest concern is the development of second malignancies, particularly leukemia with myelodysplasia, though sterilization is also an important issue. The incidence of leukemia is definitely increased, particularly in patients treated with the alkylating agent melphalan. The incidence, however, is in the range of only 1.7% at 10 years. An increase in leukemia in patients treated with cyclophosphamide, the other alkylating agent in common use, is very low, in the range of 5 cases per 10,000 at 10 years.

Fortunately the acute toxic adverse effects of hormonal therapy with tamoxifen, the agent most commonly used, have been few. Little is known about the potential long-term carcinogenic effect of chronic tamoxifen use (greater than 5 years). The possible effect on endocrine-sensitive tumors, such as endometrial cancer, is of concern.

Overall, the adjuvant story in breast cancer has been a successful one. This experience serves as a model for the development of similar strategies in other tumors.

## Gastrointestinal cancer

Cancers of the gastrointestinal tract are very common, causing approximately one out of four cancer deaths in the United States.[6] Clinical trials of postoperative adjuvant therapy for upper gastrointestinal (GI) cancers such as those of the stomach and pancreas have failed to show a benefit and are not considered the standard of care outside of a clinical trial. The situation with esophageal cancer is different. So-called neoadjuvant therapy, defined in this case as treatment given before definitive surgery, appears to be a promising approach. A platinum-containing chemotherapy regimen along with radiotherapy when given preoperatively has produced exciting results in patients with locally advanced disease who would be at high risk for recurrence with surgery alone. Again, such patients should be treated in the context of a clinical trial.

The situation with lower GI malignancies is much clearer. Adjuvant postoperative chemotherapy for Dukes stage C colon cancer is the standard of care and provides a modest but clear-cut survival advantage. Standard regimens include 5-fluorouracil with either levamisole or leukovorin given for 1 year. Less-advanced Dukes stage B2 cancers have not benefited from this therapy, and if adjuvant therapy is contemplated, it should be done in the context of a clinical trial.

Rectal cancer presents additional unique issues in the adjuvant setting. An NIH consensus conference in 1990 clearly endorsed the concept that postoperative adjuvant therapy for Dukes stages B and C rectal cancer patients is advantageous and should be the standard of care.[7] Therapy is by the use of 5-fluorouracil combined with radiotherapy initiated 1 to 2 months after surgery. This concept has recently been extended in phase II and phase III clinical trials to treating bulkier more locally advanced rectal tumors with preoperative chemoradiotherapy (neoadjuvant). This strategy may have considerable advantages in terms of anal sphincter preservation and better tolerance of treatment but should be approached in the context of a clinical study.

## Other tumors—clear-cut or potential success stories

Adjuvant therapy has had a clear-cut effect on either survival or cure in patients with other types of cancer (see Tables 45-1 and 45-2). Although some of these tumors are relatively uncommon, some results have been so exciting that the potential to apply these principles to other more common tumors is an important spin-off from these experimental studies. Certain subsets of patients with testicular cancer, non-Hodgkin's lymphoma, sarcomas, and acute leukemia benefit from adjuvant treatment.[8] For example, aggressive treatment of testicular cancer has resulted in a substantial increase in cure rate. In the case of osteogenic sarcoma, chemotherapy treatment may alleviate the need for radical amputation of a limb.

# PROSPECTS FOR THE FUTURE

As previously stated, I believe the adjuvant treatment of cancer is an exciting, but to a great extent, experimental approach. However, as noted above, for many tumors it may be considered standard treatment. For tumors where it is not standard treatment, patients should be encouraged to enter into clinical trials, obviously after giving consent. The future of adjuvant therapy looks bright. As newer treatments are developed, the patient with a small body burden of tumor is a favorable testing ground for this approach. A partially effective treatment in patients with "bulk disease" may be highly effective in the patient with only microscopic disease. The recent development of a host of exciting new classes of compounds referred to as biologic response modifiers (antibodies, vaccines, cytokines, immunomodulators) is an extremely interesting and promising approach with applicability especially to patients with low tumor burden. In future years, these compounds may prove to be invaluable in salvaging patients at high risk for recurrence of cancer.

## References

1. Skipper HE, Schnabel FM Jr, Wilcox WS: Experimental evaluation of potential anticancer agents. XII. On the criteria and kinetics associated with the

"curability" of experimental leukemia, *Cancer Chemother Rep* 54:431-450, 1950.

2. Goldie JH, Coldman AJ: Quantitative model for multiple levels of drug resistance in clinical tumors, *Cancer Treat Rep* 67(10):923-931, 1983.

3. Shapiro CL, Henderson IC: Adjuvant therapy of breast cancer, *Hematol Oncol Clin North Am* 8:213-231, 1994.

4. Early Breast Cancer Trialists' Collaborative Group: Effects of adjuvant tamoxifen and of a cytotoxic therapy on mortality in early breast cancer: an overview of 61 randomized trials among 28,896 women, *N Engl J Med* 319:1681-1692, 1988.

5. Gasparini G, Pozza F, Harris AL: Evaluating the potential usefulness of new prognostic and predictive indicators in node negative breast cancer patients, *J Natl Cancer Inst* 85:1206-1219, 1993.

6. Kelsen D: Neoadjuvant therapy for gastrointestinal tumors, *Oncology* 7(9):25-32, 1993.

7. Adjuvant therapy for patients with colon and rectum cancer: NIH consensus Development Conference Consensus Statement, 8(4):1-21, 1991.

8. Abeloff MD, editor: Clinical oncology, New York, 1995, Churchill Livingstone.

# Chapter 46

# *Pigmented Skin Lesions*

Francis Renna

Pigmented skin lesions are important because they are suggestive of a melanocytic neoplasm, the most worrisome being cutaneous melanoma. They derive their color from the melanocytic pigment, melanin, which, depending on its amount and location within the skin, may produce the colors brown, black, tan, or their shades—tan, dark brown, blue-black, and gray. Melanoma can spread internally and cause death after arising from a seemingly external, superficial, and usually friendly outpost of our bodies, our skin. The appearance of a single death from melanoma, especially in a young, productive, and otherwise healthy person, can cause widespread concern, even panic, in a community. Many individuals will then call their own physicians asking if they have to worry about their own pigmented lesions. By knowing the early signs of melanoma and its precursors and by teaching them to our patients, we can help allay their fears and reduce the risk of fatal disease when these lesions do appear.

The incidence of melanoma is increasing faster than any other human cancer.[1] In 1991, there were 32,000 melanomas diagnosed, almost triple the number that were diagnosed in 1979[2]; the lifetime risk of a white child developing melanoma has increased from about 1 in 150 in 1985 to a predicted risk of 1 in 90 by year 2000.[3] In the United States, melanoma is the second leading cause of death in women 15 to 35 years of age[2] and the seventh most common cancer in the United States.[4] This increase in melanoma is largely attributable to increased, unprotected sun exposure, especially among fair-skinned people who sunburn easily.[2] Blistering sunburns during adolescence double the risk of later melanoma,[2] underscoring the need for sun protection, especially given the thinning of the earth's ozone layer. A personal history of melanoma increases the risk of having another melanoma by about 5% compared to the 1% lifetime risk of melanoma in whites.[5] It now appears that pregnancy and the use of oral contraceptives do not increase the risk of melanoma, but the risk of pregnancy in someone who has melanoma is less clear.[6,7] I agree with those who recommend postponing pregnancy for 2 to 3 years after melanoma removal, a time when melanoma is most likely to recur.

Fortunately the prognosis for patients with melanoma is improving. In the 1940s, the 5-year survival from melanoma was 40%, whereas in the 1980s it rose to 85% for clinical stage I (localized, primary skin tumor).[1] Credit for this improved outlook is attributable to the earlier recognition of melanoma when it is thinner and less likely to have metastasized. No effective treatment for metastatic melanoma currently exists. Further reduction in the incidence and mortality from melanoma has come from the recognition of its precursor lesions: congenital melanocytic nevi, lentigo maligna (melanoma in situ), acral and mucosal lesions, and the atypical mole (dysplastic nevus)—the most important precursor and marker for melanoma based on its incidence and tendency for malignant change.[8]

Given these facts, our ability to diagnose melanoma early and to recognize its precursors becomes of paramount importance. Use of this knowledge by physicians, other health care workers, and patients should result in a reduction of the overall death rate from melanoma to less than 5%.[9] My emphasis in this chapter is to review the early signs of worrisome pigmented lesions (melanoma and its precursors) and to distinguish them from benign pigmented growths.

Potentially dangerous pigmented growths can be diagnosed only if we look for them and educate and encourage our patients to perform self-examinations. Examination of the entire skin for pigmented lesions, including hidden sites (scalp, genital, perineal, perianal, and mucous membranes), should be part of every physical examination. Such examination requires the naked eye aided by the use of a hand magnifier (5 to 10 power) and oblique (side) lighting, the latter to distinguish slightly elevated (possibly early melanoma) from macular (flat) benign or precancerous pigmented growths.

## CLINICAL GUIDELINES

Microscopic cellular atypia and malignant changes in melanocytes translate into the macroscopic "disorderly" change that can be detected with the naked eye. The most important observation for early detection of a dangerous lesion is its disorderly appearance. Clinical observation of the degree of disorderliness within a pigmented lesion, reflected in four physical features (in order of their importance: color, border, surface topography, and size, abbreviated CBSS), will reliably alert the clinician and patient to the need for further diagnostic confirmation by surgical excision and histologic examination.[4] The clinical danger signs for pigmented lesions are also referred to by the mnemonic *ABCD* (*A*, asymmetry, *B*, border irregularity, *C*, color variegation, *D*, diameter greater than 6 mm).[5]

I educate patients about the danger signs for pigmented lesions during their examination by showing them photographs from two pamphlets, *The ABC's of Moles and Melanoma* and *Dysplastic nevi and malignant melanoma* (available from the Skin Cancer Foundation, Box 561, New York, NY 10156). I review the dangerous features (color variegation, border irregularity, surface irregularity, and size) in detail and compare the photographs with the patient's pigmented lesions if any are present. If the patient has a recent or past history of a dangerous pigmented lesion (such as a melanoma, atypical moles), I provide pamphlets for all first-degree relatives and encourage patients to have their relatives examined by their own physician or dermatologist to check for a familial pattern of melanoma or one of its precursors, especially atypical moles.

The removal of any suspicious pigmented lesion should include excision of the entire lesion, size and location permitting, so that dangerous foci will not be missed. If the lesion is a melanoma, microscopic thickness can be determined because it directly relates to prognosis. The 10-year survival for clinical stage I melanoma (local disease without node involvement) based on tumor thickness less than or equal to 0.85 mm is 95.7%; 0.85 to 1.69 mm, 87.1%; 1.70 to 3.59 mm, 66.5%; and greater than or equal to 3.60 mm, 46%.[5]

Once the diagnosis and thickness of a melanoma are determined, a wider reexcision carried down to the muscle fascia is indicated. The reexcision margins required are narrower than in the past, and in stage I melanoma, elective lymph node dissection is not recommended, except for melanoma thickness between 1.50 and 4.0 mm, when it is optional. The reexcision margins for thicknesses less than 1.0 mm, 1.0 to 1.5 mm, 1.5 to 4.0 mm, and greater than 4.0 mm are 1.0, 1.5, 2 to 3, and 3.0 cm, respectively.[4] A more detailed description of the four physical features that define a pigmented lesion's potential for melanoma follows.

**Color.** Color is the most important of the four features. Benign pigmented lesions have a uniform brown or tan color or a regular pattern or colors (stippled). Early melanoma, especially superficial spreading and lentigo maligna melanoma, has haphazard or variegated shades of brown (tan, medium, and dark brown) mixed with red (representing focal sites of inflammation and secondary vasodilatation), white (focal regressed or amelanocytic melanocytes), blue (caused by the scattering of incident light), and black or shades of black, that is, blue-black, blue-gray, and purple. Black, or its shades, is the most ominous color and is an important exception to the requirement for variegated color. When black occurs uniformly as the only color, it signals the potential presence of nodular melanoma, which invades early in its biologic life and carries the worst prognosis of all melanomas. Hence the dictum that any uniformly black or shades-of-black lesion, unless diagnosable by some other objective criterion (such as a small traumatic hematoma that can be evacuated by needle aspiration) demands removal for definitive histologic diagnosis. Although many black lesions turn out to be benign, such as seborrheic keratoses, small hemangiomas, and the blue nevus (a benign nevus whose deep dermal component appears blue because of reflected and scattered light), the possibility of missing a nodular melanoma at a more curable stage justifies their removal.

**Border.** Benign pigmented lesions are symmetric and have a uniformly round or oval shape. Early melanoma, especially superficial spreading and lentigo maligna melanoma, has irregular borders. Superficial spreading melanoma has a horizontal, noninvasive growth phase, providing an opportunity for cure by early diagnosis. Lentigo maligna melanoma also has a delayed invasive phase and arises within a precursor lesion, lentigo maligna (melanoma in situ), which may be present for up to 25 years as a mottled-brown macule on sun-exposed skin before the emergence of melanoma. Superficial spreading melanoma, the most common and easily recognizable form, has the most dramatic irregularity to the border, often appearing jaggedly irregular and asymmetric, with one or more notches or protrusions along its edge. Nodular melanoma is an exception in that it usually has a uniform round or oval margin and sometimes appears large and polypoid in shape. Polypoid melanoma may be pink with small islands of brown or black at the periphery; it often is the most rapidly growing melanoma, arising over a period of months.

**Surface.** Benign pigmented nevi have a uniformly elevated surface. If multiple elevations are present, they are similar in size and shape and are symmetrically placed (cobblestone-like pattern). Early melanoma demonstrates an asymmetrically placed elevation, often with darker color within the elevation or an irregular arrangement of multiple elevations. Nodular melanoma presents as a solitary elevation from its onset.

**Size.** Size alone is the least reliable indicator for melanoma. Remember that most early melanomas are greater than 6 mm, whereas most benign nevi are less than 6 mm in diameter. Lentigo maligna melanoma may be quite large, 3 to 6 cm, whereas superficial spreading melanoma is usually 2.5 cm or less in diameter. Of course, melanomas can be less than 6 mm. Hence reliance on size alone will cause the missing of smaller melanomas that demonstrate other suspicious features. Relative size is important because any pigmented lesion that is clearly larger than the surrounding majority catches the physician or patient's eye as marching out of step compared to the others. If other diagnostic features are present, the lesion should be removed.

The absence of definitely worrisome physical, chronologic, or subjective features allows the lesion to be monitored for the development of such changes. Alternatively the lesion could be removed if the patient or physician continues to worry about it, especially if there is a personal or family history of atypical moles or melanoma (Table 46-1).

The diagnosis of dangerous pigmented lesions also is aided by the history and symptoms. The most telling historical early warning signs are a change in color or size in a preexisting melanocytic nevus or the appearance of a new pigmented lesion, often noted by the patient, spouse, or friend. Other risk factors for worrisome pigmented lesions include a light complexion that sunburns easily, a history of blistering sunburns during childhood or adolescence, blue eyes, blond or red hair, a personal or family history of melanoma or atypical moles, and an increased number of normal moles.[9] The presence of symptoms without obvious cause, such as friction, trauma, or sunburn, especially within one of many pigmented lesions in the absence of other physical signs, could reflect an early malignant change.

Features that may deceive physicians into discounting the presence of melanoma include the absence of symptoms. The physical changes described so far usually occur in the absence of symptoms. Likewise,

**Table 46-1.** *Clinical features of several pigmented skin lesions*

| | Common nevi | Atypical moles | Cutaneous melanoma |
|---|---|---|---|
| Overview | Orderly, regular, and symmetric | Orderly or disorderly, symmetric or asymmetric | Disorderly, irregular, asymmetric |
| Color | Uniform shades of brown | Regular or mixture of browns, often pink, rarely black | Haphazard pattern of any mixture of brown, black, blue, gray, white, pink, or red Uniform black, blue, or blue-black is suggestive of nodular melanoma |
| Border | Regular, well demarcated, round, or oval | Regular, round, oval, or irregular with less severe notching Edge may fade into surrounding skin | Jaggedly irregular; may have a large notch |
| Surface | Uniform; if multiple, elevations of similar size and shape and symmetrically placed (cobblestone-like) | Regular, symmetric or irregularly asymmetric, single or multiple | Asymmetrically placed single or multiple, different-sized elevations |
| Size | Usually less than 6 mm | Usually greater than 6 mm Can be diagnosed when smaller | Usually greater than 6 mm Can be diagnosed when smaller |

the presence or absence of hair within the lesion has no bearing on its being benign or malignant. The duration of a pigmented lesion is helpful only if it has recently appeared. A long duration does not exclude a dangerous lesion because often patients are not aware of subtle, gradual changes in lesions they have come to take for granted.

Although less commonly, children may also develop dangerous pigmented lesions, including congenital melanoma and prepubertal atypical moles and melanoma.[10] We should weigh the danger signs for pigmented lesions just as heavily for newborns and children as for teenagers and adults.

To summarize, disorderliness or any change in color, border, surface, or size (CBSS) or a uniform black or blue-black color within a pigmented lesion, especially a change in color toward black, warrants definitive diagnosis by surgical removal and histologic studies. Less reliable but often important is the appearance of unprovoked and unremitting symptoms within a pigmented lesion or a patient's unremitting worry over such a lesion.

# COMMON BENIGN PIGMENTED LESIONS

## Seborrheic keratosis

Seborrheic keratosis, a common flat-topped plaque ranging in size from a few millimeters to several centimeters, often is uniformly colored with shades of brown or even black. It represents a benign proliferation of epidermal cells (keratinocytes) that retain the ability to form keratin (scale). The pattern of growth is outward, above the plane of the surrounding skin, providing their "stuck-on" appearance and their ability to be flicked or scraped off without penetration of the dermis. Seborrheic keratoses have a cobblestone or wartlike surface of many uniform, small-sized, closely set symmetric elevations. Older lesions are obviously covered by flat scales (hyperkeratotic) that may not be readily visible in early lesions unless the edge is scraped. The border is well demarcated and slightly pedunculated or square-shouldered on cross section. They appear anywhere but are most common on the trunk, chest, and neck.[3]

Seborrheic keratoses are the most common "look-alike" for melanoma. The pattern of color may be asymmetric and irregular and may be associated with irregular, well-demarcated margins. A round or oval seborrheic keratosis with uniform black or blue-black color may be confused with nodular melanoma. The presence of hyperkeratotic scales throughout the lesion and the stuck-on appearance are important clinical signs, arguing against melanoma, which normally is not a keratinizing tumor. It may be difficult to detect scales, and, moreover, the color and pattern as well as the irregular margins may be so suggestive of melanoma that histologic examination is necessary.

## Lentigines

Lentigo ('freckle', from Latin) refers to any small brown macule (flush with the surrounding skin) composed of an increased number of normal melanocytes. Three types of lentigines are recognized: simple lentigo, solar lentigo, and lentigo maligna (melanoma in situ). Freckles are probably a variant of the solar lentigo. A simple lentigo is small, about 1.5 mm, may be the first stage of the common acquired mole beginning in childhood, and is well demarcated and round with a uniform brown or dark brown color. Occasionally a simple lentigo is a dark brown color with smooth or regular, finely jagged edges.

A solar lentigo, a benign melanocytic hyperplasia present on sun-exposed skin especially of the face, chest, and dorsum of the hands, is erroneously referred to as a "liver spot" instead of a "sun spot." A solar lentigo often is larger than a simple lentigo and ranges from a few millimeters to several centimeters. It often has an irregular border, but as long as it is not black, lacks islands of darker and lighter shades of brown, white, or gray, and has no component elevated (oblique lighting often is required), then lentigo maligna (a macule with shades of brown or black; see subsequently) and lentigo malignant melanoma (elevated darkly pigmented islands appearing against a macular, mottled brown background) need not be considered.

# COMMON ACQUIRED NEVOMELANOCYTIC NEVI (COMMON NEVI)

Common nevi are round or oval, well demarcated with a smooth border, tan to dark brown and occasionally black, with varying degrees of elevation from macular to dome-shaped papules, and most often up to 5 mm in size. Common nevi represent accumulations of nevus cells (immature melanocytes that have not completed their migration from the neural crest to the epidermis as mature melanocytes) at different anatomic levels within the skin. Accumulations at the dermoepidermal junction appear as flat or slightly raised brown to dark brown lesions called *junctional nevi.* If the nevus cells are within both the superficial dermis and the dermoepidermal junction, the lesion is more raised, may include hair, and is called a *compound nevus.* If the nevus cells are only in the deeper dermis, the lesion is called a *dermal nevus* and may have a smooth or rough surface and contain coarse hairs.

All these nevi are easily recognized as benign pigmented lesions because of their overall orderly appearance, regular borders and surfaces, and regular shades of brown.

Junctional nevi usually arise in childhood or around puberty but occasionally appear later in life. Since their appearance after 40 years of age is uncommon, their appearance beyond this age demands that they be followed closely for possible evolution into atypical moles or melanoma.[4] Before 40 years of age, junctional nevi also may evolve into compound or intradermal nevi, becoming more raised and larger but retaining their orderly appearance. If these changes arouse physician or patient concern, especially if they appear disorderly, removal is in order. Normal changes in common nevi are likely to occur during growth spurts in toddlers, just before or during puberty, or during pregnancy; however, all nevi should change together. Any one nevus marching out of step, changing in color, border, surface, or size at any time in life, warrants removal.[11]

Several other criteria in addition to visible changes argue for removal. A nevus that is continually irritated may assume symptoms, size, and color changes that can be confused with an early melanoma. Nevi in hidden sites, especially if darkly colored or if there is a personal or family history of atypical moles or melanoma, should be removed, since they are difficult to monitor.

I urge clinicians to make special note of darkly pigmented or irregularly marginated lesions on acral sites, especially palms, soles, and toewebs, because these pigmented lesions are often not appreciated by patients and, if they are not identified and checked by their physician, could develop into a more advanced and dangerous melanoma. Delayed diagnosis of such pigmented lesions has led in the past to their worse prognosis. Although the more darkly pigmented races normally have darkly pigmented nevi, their occurrence on the palms and soles carries the same hazard. In a white person, pigmented lesions involving the nail folds, which manifest as a longitudinal brown pigmented streak within the nail plate, as well as pigmented conjunctival lesions, warrant biopsy; these lesions are uncommon and carry a greater malignant potential. Darkly pigmented people have a higher incidence of benign nail-associated and conjunctiva-pigmented lesions, so their lesions are biopsied or removed on an individual basis, according to whether there has been a recent change in a long-standing lesion, the appearance of a new lesion, or a personal or family history of melanoma or its precursors.[11]

## Melanoma precursors lentigo maligna

Lentigo maligna, also called *melanoma in situ,*[12] is a macular hyperplasia of atypical melanocytes along the epidermal basement membrane. The color is variegated with shades of brown to black occurring together with an irregular border. Often there are colors that are suggestive of focal regression: white, blue-gray, pink, or, more rarely, no color (amelanosis). Size varies from a few millimeters to a few centimeters, and these lesions appear mostly on sun-damaged skin on the head, neck, and upper extremities usually around 50 to 60 years of age.[11] Lentigo maligna grows slowly; about 30% eventually develop focal invasive melanoma (lentigo maligna melanoma) after a long latent period (5 to 50 years).[4] Invasion manifests as a small, slightly or obviously raised segment, usually of darker color, within the macular background. Any macular, mottled brown to dark brown lesion, even in the absence of black, on the face, neck, or upper extremity in an elderly patient should be biopsied either by complete excision with 2 to 3 mm margins for a smaller lesion or, if the lesion is larger, by a punch biopsy from the darkest or most raised portion. If it is a lentigo maligna, the entire lesion should be excised with a 5 mm margin when possible. Lentigo maligna seldom causes symptoms and, because of its long duration and slow change, may not worry or be noticed by the patient. Thus, although the patient may not bring it to my attention, I always look for lentigo maligna when examining an elderly patient.

## Congenital melanocytic nevi (congenital nevi)

Congenital melanocytic nevi are present at birth or appear within the first 12 months and consist of nevus cells that are present deeper in the dermis than common acquired nevi penetrate. In the absence of a reliable history, a congenital nevus should be suspected in a pigmented lesion greater than 1.5 cm[11]; at the same time the lesion will have none of the features of an atypical mole (see later discussion of atypical moles). They appear as round or oval raised lesions with a uniform brown or dark brown color and smooth regular borders. Frequently the surface is covered by papillomatous elevations that become more raised and irregular with time. Coarse long hairs are often present and may become darker and coarser in late childhood. More atypical congenital nevi have haphazard shades of brown, dark brown, black, and blue-black and may be poorly demarcated with or without irregular margins. Clearly these latter are worrisome and require removal when feasible.

Congenital nevi are arbitrarily subclassified as small if less than or equal to 1.5 cm in diameter, medium if 1.5 to 19.9 cm, and large if greater than or equal to 20 cm in diameter.[5] When large congenital nevi cover a major portion of the body, they are referred to as giant, garment, or great hairy nevi. The lifetime risk for melanoma in giant congenital nevi is estimated at 6%.[13] Melanomas appear within giant congenital nevi early, often within the first 3 years of life, and are difficult to detect because of their dark color and rough surface as well as the often deep origin of the melanoma within these lesions. Hence, full-thickness excision is recommended after the first 6 months of life; before 6 months the risk of general anesthesia is too great.

There is controversy over the management of small and medium-sized congenital nevi because there is no agreement over the degree of risk for melanoma in these lesions. However, it is known that small and medium-sized congenital nevi are responsible for up to 15% of melanomas.[11] Any congenital nevus that displays irregular size, shape, or color is best removed without delay. For nonworrisome-appearing small and medium-sized congenital nevi, the increased risk for melanoma begins just before puberty, increases through the teen-age years, and then decreases. Since most parents, physicians, and children are uneasy about monitoring such lesions during these higher-risk years, I examine them yearly until the child is 8 to 10 years of age (patients and parents check them every 2 to 3 months), at which time I suggest that these congenital nevi be excised, barring problems with cosmetics and functional deficits. This is also a time when children are better able to tolerate local anesthesia and minor surgery.

## Atypical mole (dysplastic nevus)

The dysplastic nevus has been renamed the *atypical mole* because of past confusion regarding histologic diagnostic criteria. The revised histologic description is "nevus with architectural disorder" followed by a comment regarding the presence and degree of melanocytic atypia.[12] The atypical mole is the most frequently occurring melanoma precursor, appearing in about 5% of white people,[13] and it occurs in both a familial and sporadic (nonfamilial) pattern.[14] Since it can be confused clinically with common nevi and melanoma, definitive diagnosis depends on the histologic characteristics of the excised lesion.

There is varying risk for melanoma among people with atypical moles. The risk is most related to a personal or family history of melanoma. Those at lowest risk (a relative risk of from 2 to 8 compared with the general population) are people with atypical moles and no personal or family history of melanoma. Those at highest risk (lifetime risk approaching 100%) have a hereditary syndrome, the familial atypical multiple-mole melanoma (FAMMM) syndrome, defined by (1) melanoma in one or more first- or second-degree relatives, (2) large numbers of moles (often greater than 50) some of which are atypical, and (3) moles that have the histologic changes associated with atypical moles.[15] Atypical moles begin around puberty and continue to appear throughout life, hence the need for lifelong surveillance.

Often the family history regarding atypical moles is not known, or if there is a family history of atypical moles, melanoma may not yet have developed. Therefore the risk for melanoma in a person or family cannot be accurately known at the outset. Thus it is best that all first-degree relatives of people with atypical moles be examined for their presence. In the setting of atypical moles, melanoma most often arises within an atypical mole but may also arise in normal-appearing skin; hence, the entire skin, not just the atypical moles, needs to be watched.

Clinically, atypical moles appear on any mucocutaneous surface and usually are larger than common nevi, 6 to 12 mm in diameter. The surface is often macular with slightly to moderately elevated components. The border is often irregular and may be ill defined, fading into the surrounding skin. The color is often variegated, tan to dark brown, often with a prominent pink component. Atypical moles are common on the sun-exposed trunk and extremities but also on the sun-protected scalp, buttocks, breasts, and genital skin.[15] Unlike melanoma, there is usually the absence of black or its shades and an overall milder degree of disorderliness. The atypical mole can be thought of as a "watered-down melanoma," intermediate in appearance between common nevi and melanoma.

Current knowledge regarding the atypical mole dictates a prudent stepwise plan for the management of patients with these melanoma precursors as well as of their blood relatives. First, after examination of the entire skin, the diagnosis should be confirmed by excision of one to three of the most atypical-appearing moles. The pathologist will also grade the degree of cellular atypia, aiding the decision for future removals based on clinical correlation with the degree of histologic atypia. Also, atypical-appearing nevi should be removed if located in hidden sites, if they are changing or have an extremely atypical appearance, or if the patient is on immunosuppressive medications or has Hodgkin's disease. Second, remaining atypical moles can be mapped or photographed to detect changes or new lesions. Third, the patient should perform self-examinations every 4 to 6 weeks looking for changes in one of the four features or for new lesions. Fourth, patients should have physician examinations at a frequency that reflects the degree of risk for melanoma. If there is a positive personal or family history of melanoma, examinations are done every 3 to 6 months, whereas, if the personal and family history are negative for melanoma, examinations can be 6 months to a year. Fifth, blood relatives of people with atypical moles or melanoma also need to be examined based on the following considerations. Children within the kindred who have multiple common acquired nevi should be checked carefully just before and during puberty and yearly throughout the teen-age years for the evolution of atypical moles.

If there have been two or more people with melanomas within the family, *all* blood relatives should be examined once and then the children by 10 years of age and then yearly to 20 years of age if no atypical moles are found. For people with one or more atypical moles and no personal or family history of melanoma, only *first-degree* relatives beyond puberty need to be checked once and then followed only if atypical moles are found. Sixth, all patients with atypical moles should minimize ultraviolet-ray exposure and use high-potency sun protection, preferably a broad-spectrum UVB and UVA sunscreen with at least a no. 15 sun protection factor along with the use of protective clothing when outdoors.[11] Sunglasses are also recommended to protect the eyes from the hazardous effects of ultraviolet exposure. For patients and physicians alike, it is encouraging to remember that melanomas detected as part of an atypical mole surveillance program have been removed at a nearly 100% curable stage (see box on p. 527).[16,17]

# SUMMARY

Any pigmented lesion that appears disorderly; that is manifested by an *irregular color* pattern, consisting of shades of brown mixed with red, white, or blue or by the presence of black or its shades; or that has an *irregular border* or *surface* topography is a suspect for melanoma and should be removed for definitive diagnosis. Other warning signs for melanoma are as follows:

1. Size greater than 6 mm
2. Any change in color or shape
3. Unprovoked nonremitting symptoms
4. New pigmented lesions after 40 years of age
5. Any precursor lesions, lentigo maligna, congenital nevus, acral or mucosal lesions, and atypical moles
6. Pigmented lesions in hidden sites

Since early melanoma is often curable and later melanoma often is not, patients should be instructed to perform regular self-examinations, and physicians should check the skin during routine examinations, more often if there is a personal or family history of melanoma or one

## Management of Patients with Atypical Moles

1. Examine the entire skin, including hidden areas.
2. Review the family history for the presence of atypical moles.
3. Excise 1 to 3 of the most atypical-appearing moles for definitive histologic diagnosis and grading of atypia.
4. Examine all first-degree relatives for the presence of atypical moles or melanoma.
5. Instruct all affected individuals how to recognize atypical moles and melanoma and in the technique of self-examination, to be done at 4- to 6-week intervals.*
6. Map or photograph the patient's lesions.
7. Regular physician examinations for life. If there is a personal or family history of melanoma, examinations are done every 3 to 6 months. If there is no personal or family history of melanoma, examinations are done 6 months to yearly. Children who are first-degree relatives of people with dysplastic nevi or melanoma should be checked just before and during puberty and throughout the teen years for the evolution of atypical moles and melanoma.
8. Regular eye examinations.
9. Avoid unprotected ultraviolet-radiation exposure. Use sunscreens, protective clothing, and sunglasses.
10. Excise any moles undergoing suspicious changes.

* Slade J et al: *J Am Acad Dermatol* 32:479, 1995.

of its precursors, especially atypical moles. Examination should include the entire skin including hidden sites. With greater awareness and detection of early dangerous pigmented lesions, the death rate from melanoma should decrease to less than 5%.

## References

1. Boring CC, Squires TS, Tong T: Cancer statistics *CA* 41:19, 1991.
2. Sober AJ: Cutaneous melanoma: opportunity for cure, *CA Cancer J Clin* 41:197, 1991.
3. Koh HK: Cutaneous melanoma, *N Engl J Med* 325:171, 1991.
4. Barnhill RL, Mihm MC, Fitpatrick RB, et al: Neoplasms: malignant melanoma. In Fitzpatrick TB, Eisen AZ, Wolff K, et al, editors: *Dermatology in general medicine,* ed 4, New York, 1993, McGraw-Hill.
5. Friedman RJ, Rigel DS, Silverman MK, et al: Malignant melanoma in the 1990's: the continued importance of early detection and the role of physician examination and self-examination of the skin, *CA Cancer J Clin* 41:201, 1991.
6. Driscol MS, Grin-Jorgenson CM, Grant-Kels JM: Does pregnancy influence the prognosis of malignant melanoma? *J Am Acad Dermatol* 29:619, 1993.
7. Palmer JR, Rosenberg L, Strom BL, et al: Oral contraceptive use and risk of cutaneous malignant melanoma, *Cancer Causes Control* 3:547, 1992.

8. Rhodes AR, Weinstock MA, Fitzpatrick TB, et al: Risk factors for cutaneous melanoma: a practical method of recognizing predisposed individuals, *JAMA* 258:3146, 1987.

9. Rigel DS: Epidemiology and prognostic factors in malignant melanoma, *Ann Plast Surg* 28:7, 1992.

10. Ceballos PI, Ruiz-Maldonado R, Mihm MC: Melanoma in children, *N Engl J Med* 332:656, 1995.

11. Rhodes AR: Neoplasms: benign neoplasias, hyperplasias, and dysplasias of melanocytes. In Fitzpatrick TB, Eisen AZ, Wolff K, et al, editors: *Dermatology in general medicine,* ed 4, New York, 1993, McGraw-Hill.

12. Consensus development panel on early melanoma: Diagnosis and treatment of early melanoma, *JAMA* 268:1314, 1992.

13. Walton RG: Recognition and importance of precursor lesions in the diagnosis of early cutaneous malignant melanoma, *Int J Dermatol* 33:302, 1994.

14. Rivers JK: Management of precursors and primary lesions of melanoma, *Curr Opin Oncol* 5:377, 1993.

15. Slade J, Marghoob AA, Salopek TG, et al: Atypical mole syndrome: risk factors for cutaneous malignant melanoma and implications for management, *J Am Acad Dermatol* 32:479, 1995.

16. Clark WH: The dysplastic nevus syndrome, *Arch Dermatol* 124:1207, 1988.

17. Parker T, Zitelli J: Malignant melanoma, *Dermatol Surg* 22:234, 1996.

# Chapter 47

# *AIDS-Related Cancer*

Richard A. Rudders

Traditionally, infectious diseases have complicated the course of many malignant diseases. For example, years ago tuberculosis was the bane of patients with Hodgkin's disease until effective therapy was discovered. Also, aggressive cancer treatments potentially produce immunodeficiency that results in infectious complications. This relationship between neoplasia and its treatment and infection has a new twist in the setting of the current AIDS epidemic. Chronic HIV infection now leads to the development of a variety of cancers! Ironically what has been learned in the past decade is that these cancers appear to arise in this setting as the result of coinfection with several other viral agents. If you believe in the viral cause of cancer, AIDS provides considerable food for thought.

## THE MAGNITUDE OF THE PROBLEM

AIDS-related cancer is not a trivial issue and is likely to worsen. Currently, approximately 1 million patients in the United States are infected with HIV. Of these, approximately 20% to 25% will develop a serious often fatal malignancy.[1] In view of these figures there will be 200,000 to 250,000 new cases of cancer in the current pool of HIV-infected patients. These numbers are likely to increase as the number of infected persons increases and patients with AIDS live longer. Furthermore, the rate of HIV infection is probably underestimated and thus the pool of patients at risk is considerably larger than current estimates. Most of the increase in cancer risk is attributed to three malignancies: non-Hodgkin's lymphoma,[2] Kaposi's sarcoma,[3] and anogenital cancer (Table 47-1). A fourth malignancy, invasive cancer of the cervix, may be increased as well. The latter suspicion is based on an observed increase in preinvasive cervical lesions. Recent reports also indicate that two other rare malignancies may be increased in patients with HIV infection. Reported increases in testicular cancer and leiomyosarcoma[4] appear to be real and are currently under investigation. There is no doubt that the recognition and treatment of malignancy have become a significant part of the care of HIV-infected individuals.

**Table 47-1.** *AIDS-associated cancer*

| Cancer | Incidence (%) | Associated virus | Treatment |
|---|---|---|---|
| Non-Hodgkin's lymphoma | | | |
| Systemic | 10 | EBV | Combination therapy, Colony-stimulating factors, antiretroviral, PCP prophylaxis |
| CNS | 2 | EBV | Radiotherapy with or without chemotherapy |
| Kaposi's sarcoma | 10 | HPV CMV ?HSV | Surgery and radiotherapy, single-agent chemotherapy, biologic response modifier, antivirals |
| Anogenital | <1 | HPV HSV-2 | Surgery and radiotherapy |
| Cervical | ? | HPV | Surgery and radiotherapy |
| Leiomyosarcomas | ? | EBV | Surgery |
| Testicular | ? | ? | Surgery and chemotherapy |

*CMV,* Cytomegalovirus; *EBV,* Epstein-Barr virus, *HPV,* human papillomavirus; *HSV,* herpesvirus; *PCP, Pneumocystis carinii* pneumonia.

## NON-HODGKIN'S LYMPHOMA

In the early 1980s the association between non-Hodgkin's lymphoma and the AIDS epidemic was first noted. It was rapidly appreciated that these observations were extremely important. Since then the incidence of lymphoma has increased to approximately 10%, and in 5% of HIV-infected patients, lymphoma is the AIDS-defining illness. Many clinical features of AIDS-associated lymphoma are distinct and noteworthy. Systemic lymphomas are predominantly of high grade and are disseminated and extranodal in distribution. Furthermore, primary CNS lymphoma, which is a rare disease in the general population, is seen frequently in this disease (Fig. 47-1) in the setting of progressive immunodeficiency (CD4 counts <200).[5] Virtually all CNS lymphoma is associated with the presence of EBV,[6] and a large proportion (30% to 60%) of systemic lymphoma express the EBV genome. In this setting it is not surprising that most lymphomas are derived from B cells and are generally monoclonal.

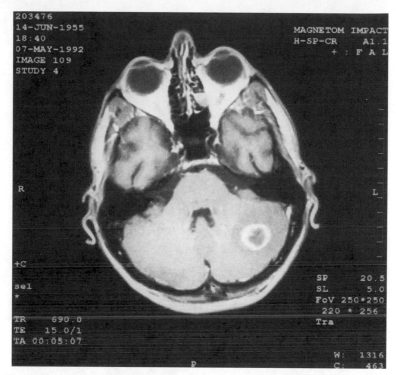

**Figure 47–1.** *CT scan of head in primary central nervous system lymphoma. There is a discrete ring-enhancing lesion in the left hemisphere.*

High-grade lymphoma, usually immunoblastic or small noncleaved cell (Burkitt's) lymphoma, predominate particularly in the primary CNS variety (Fig. 47-2). Less aggressive variants or Hodgkin's disease are seen occasionally with systemic lymphoma but even these tumors behave in an aggressive manner. Another striking clinical feature is the advanced stage of systemic disease at presentation. Bone marrow and CNS involvement are very common (65% to 90%), and there is a predilection for extranodal sites, such as the gastrointestinal tract, Waldeyer's ring, and nasal sinuses, to be involved.

Treatment is less than satisfactory and if possible should be conducted in the setting of a clinical trial. Prognosis is better in patients with less profound underlying immunodeficiency, a good performance status, and no prior AIDS-defining illnesses. The results of trials with standard CHOP (cytoxan, doxorubicin, vincristine, prednisone) indicate remission rates that may vary widely (20% to 60%), and median survivals are between 4 and 7 months. Aggressive therapy is often complicated by severe myelosuppression and infections. The role of antiretrovirals, cytokines, and CNS prophylaxis has not been proved. The concurrent administration of zidovudine is contraindicated because of its myelosuppression. This is a difficult group of patients to treat

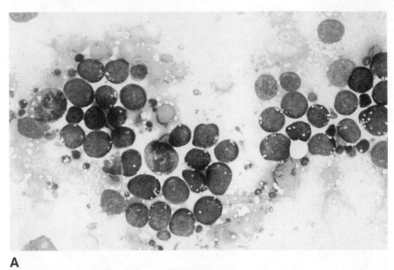

**Figure 47–2.** *A, Small noncleaved cell lymphoma. Touch preparation of lymph node. (Wright's stain.) B, Immunoblastic sarcoma lymph node. (Hematoxylin and eosin stain.)*

because of the underlying immunodeficiency. In general, good-risk patients are treated with combination chemotherapy (CHOP or a clinical trial), and poor-risk patients are treated with various regimens at reduced doses. In addition, all patients should receive PCP prophylaxis and antiretroviral therapy. CNS prophylaxis is routinely given only to patients with small non-cleaved cell lymphoma or those with bone marrows positive for the disease.

The treatment of primary CNS lymphoma is even more problematic. Once a definite diagnosis is established by biopsy, radiotherapy is the treatment of choice. Whether adding systemic chemotherapy will improve results is the subject of ongoing study. With radiotherapy alone good-risk patients survive up to 6 months, and an occasional patient may survive a year. Poor-risk patients have a median survival of only a few months.

Despite these dismal results, there is reason to believe that as our knowledge of lymphomagenesis expands, new approaches perhaps involving cytokines or other immunomodulators may improve the outlook for these patients.

## KAPOSI'S SARCOMA

The mysterious tumor Kaposi's sarcoma occurred sporadically in older individuals long before the current AIDS epidemic. Typically, Ashkenazi Jews, usually of eastern European origin, Mediterraneans, particularly Italians, and certain groups of African blacks were afflicted. In its original form it is usually an indolent disorder characterized by the appearance of flat or raised brown purplish lesions on the skin of the lower extremities. Over a period of time lesions progressed locally, and in a small percentage of patients, frank sarcomatous change and visceral dissemination ensued. The gastrointestinal and respiratory tracts were the most frequent sites of extracutaneous spread. The exact origin of this tumor was never clear because early lesions consisted of vascular endothelial and lymphoreticular proliferation that was not frankly neoplastic. Progression to sarcoma or leukemia-lymphoma did occur with time in a subset of patients, a characteristic confirming the premalignant nature of this lesion.

The AIDS epidemic has changed the face of this disease. Early in the epidemic, lesions of Kaposi's sarcoma were recognized with increasing frequency, predominantly in homosexual men. What was notable was the very aggressive, often explosive, nature of the disease in this new setting.[7] Today approximately 10% of HIV-infected individuals will develop this cancer. A larger proportion of HIV-infected homosexuals, predominantly male, will develop Kaposi's sarcoma. This is in contrast to the much lower prevalence in other high-risk groups such as intravenous drug abusers and transfusion-related AIDS. The presence of known or as yet uncharacterized viral agents in the homosexual group may explain this difference in prevalence.[8] The disease usually begins in the skin with a predilection for the head and neck area (Fig. 47-3), but skin lesions in any location are suspect and should be biopsied. The most striking difference compared to the endemic variety of Kaposi's sarcoma is the highly aggressive biologic behavior in the AIDS patient. Rapid progression with early visceral dissemination is the rule rather than the exception. In a large series, skin involvement occurs in greater than 90% of patients, and lymph nodes, the lungs, and the gastrointesti-

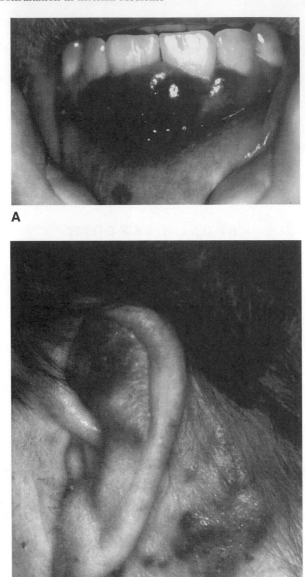

**Figure 47–3.** *A, Kaposi's sarcoma presenting in the gumline of a homosexual male. B, Kaposi's sarcoma involving the skin of the ear and the scalp.*

nal tract are involved in 50% to 60%. Approximately 5% of patients have visceral involvement without skin lesions. Complications result mainly from bleeding, ulceration of lesions, and compression of vital adjacent structures.

Management of Kaposi's syndrome in AIDS patients represents a challenge and is summarized in Table 47-2. If lesions are small and asymptomatic, they are best left alone. When lesions enlarge to the point that they ulcerate, hemorrhage, or compress local structures, radiotherapy can be an effective and rapid treatment. The instillation of chemotherapeutic agents such as vinblastine sulfate (Velban) directly into accessible lesions has been tried, and the results may be dramatic. If all else fails, systemic therapy may be given. Generalized disease with visceral involvement may require systemic therapy. Single-agent or combination chemotherapy will work but is highly toxic in this group of patients and is poorly tolerated because of pancytopenia and systemic toxicity. Biologic agents such as interferon-$\alpha$ have activity at doses of 6 to $10 \times 10^6$ U given 2 or 3 times weekly, but again toxicity is often prohibitive. As is so often the case in AIDS, treatment is poorly tolerated, the dose is compromised, and results are suboptimal, particularly in advanced stages of the disease.

## ANOGENITAL CANCER

Although the incidence of anogenital cancer in the AIDS population is low (<1%), management can be a challenge. The human papillomavirus and perhaps other viruses play a pathogenetic role. There is a transition

---

**Table 47-2.** *Treatment of Kaposi's sarcoma*

| Modality | Indication |
|---|---|
| Radiotherapy | Localized hemorrhage, compression, or ulceration |
| Chemotherapy | Refractory local disease Systemic disease |
| Regimens with Velban, Oncovin, and Adriamycin* | Injected directly into individual lesions |
| Biological drugs such as interferon-$\alpha$ | Refractory local disease Systemic disease |
| Surgery | Selected local problems, such as gastrointestinal obstruction or perforation |

*Adriamycin (doxorubicin HCl); Velban (vinblastine sulfate); Oncovin (vincristine sulfate).

from the premalignant anal intraepithelial neoplasia to frank squamous cell carcinoma with time. This cancer is highly aggressive, invades adjacent structures, and metastasizes systemically to regional nodes.

Surgery and radiotherapy are the mainstays of management. Radiotherapy has the advantage of anal-sphincter preservation but does not achieve local control in many patients. A local surgical excision may suffice for small tumors, but more extensive lesions may require sacrifice of the anal sphincter.

## OTHER CANCERS

Three other cancers are likely to be associated in higher frequency with AIDS than in the general population, but definitive proof is lacking at this time. These cancers are invasive cervical cancer, leiomyosarcoma, and testicular cancer. In each instance management parallels the management in the non-AIDS setting. As with all cancers in AIDS patients the therapeutic plan often requires modification because of debility of the patient and increased toxicity of the proposed treatment.

## FUTURE INSIGHTS

Cancers associated with AIDS provide a unique opportunity to learn about the role of viruses in the pathogenesis of specific cancers. Translation of advances in our understanding of their etiology must ultimately lead to the development of new and improved therapeutic approaches. One would hope that advances in molecular genetics will lead to entirely new treatments for these devastating illnesses.

### References

1. Levine HM: AIDS related malignancies: the emerging epidemic, *J Natl Cancer Inst* 85:1382-1397, 1993.
2. Ziegler JL, Drew WL, Miner RC, et al: Outbreak of Burkitt's-like lymphoma in homosexual men, *Lancet* 2:631-633, 1982.
3. Hymes KB, Cheung T, Greene JB, et al: Kaposi's sarcoma in homosexual men—a report of eight cases, *Lancet* 2:598-600, 1981.
4. McClain KL, Leach CT, Jenson HB, et al: Association of Epstein-Barr virus with leiomyosarcomas in children with AIDS, *N Engl J Med* 332:12-18, 1995.
5. Snider WD, Simpson DM, Aronyk KE, Nielsen SL: Primary lymphoma of the nervous system associated with acquired immunodeficiency syndrome, *N Engl J Med* 308:45, 1983.
6. MacMahon EM, Glass JD, Hayward SD, et al: Epstein-Barr virus in AIDS-related primary central nervous system lymphoma, *Lancet* 338:969-973, 1991.
7. Safai B, Johnson KG, Myskowski PL, et al: The natural history of Kaposi's sarcoma in the acquired immunodeficiency syndrome, *Ann Intern Med* 103:744-750, 1985.
8. Monini P, De Lelli SL, Fabris M, et al: Kaposi's sarcoma-associated herpes virus DNA sequences in prostate tissue and human semen, *N Engl J Med* 334: 1168-1177, 1996.

# Chapter 48

# *Splenomegaly*

Richard A. Rudders
Frederick R. Aronson

Splenomegaly occurs in association with a wide range of underlying disorders. Some are benign and self-limited; others are malignant and may be fatal despite treatment. The cause of splenomegaly can be difficult to determine; however, common causes of splenic enlargement vary significantly in different age groups as well as in different parts of the world. Knowledge of these factors can therefore help narrow the list of likely causes in a particular patient. In conjunction with the history, a careful physical examination and selected laboratory tests focus the differential diagnosis and indicate appropriate areas for additional investigation. Management of the patient with splenomegaly depends primarily on the underlying disease. In some cases, simple observation is appropriate; in others, exploratory laparotomy or cytotoxic chemotherapy is indicated. Clearly, no one management strategy is best in all cases.

This chapter provides a brief description of the characteristics of normal and enlarged spleens and of some of the diagnostic tests used to evaluate suspected splenomegaly. The differential diagnosis and the principles of management of splenomegaly are then reviewed.

## THE ENLARGED SPLEEN

Normal spleen size averages 150 g, with a range of 100 to 250 g. Spleen size varies to a greater extent between individuals than in the same individual over time. Although the size of the spleen often decreases to as little as 50 g after 70 years of age, the cause of this change is uncertain, and splenic function is generally preserved.

Splenomegaly more often than not represents an important clue to potentially serious underlying disease, particularly in older patients, and indicates the need for additional diagnostic evaluation. Occasionally, however, a clearly palpable spleen is detected in the absence of any demonstrable underlying disease. The majority of such cases occur in infants and in children and are believed to be caused by the generalized lymphatic hypertrophy that accompanies the immune response to the viral infections that are prevalent in this age group. Most cases of

537

splenomegaly of undetermined cause in young adults are also probably attributable to unrecognized viral infection because modest splenic enlargement may persist for weeks after viral infection. In one study, 58 (2.6%) of 2200 freshmen entering Dartmouth College in the 1960s had palpable spleens that could not be attributed to body habitus or to associated disease. Although splenomegaly persisted in many of these students for several years, they had no greater prevalence of illness after 10 years of follow-up examination than students without splenomegaly.

**Symptoms.** Rapid enlargement or parenchymal infarction of the spleen usually results in left upper quadrant pain or tenderness. Parenchymal infarction caused by local thrombosis is an important cause of splenic pain that occurs periodically in children with sickle cell disease and occasionally in patients with myeloproliferative disorders, Hodgkin's disease, acute leukemia, or vasculitis. Painful splenic infarcts occur, perhaps even more frequently, because of thromboemboli or septic emboli of cardiac origin.[2] Rapid splenic enlargement with capsular stretching and pain, a relatively uncommon problem, occurs primarily in patients with acute infection, aggressive lymphoma, or traumatic subcapsular or intraparenchymal hemorrhage. In these and other clinical settings when rapid enlargement does occur, the patient is at risk for splenic rupture, a potentially life-threatening event.[3] Pain and signs of an acute abdomen are usually but not invariably present if rupture occurs. Pain referred to the left shoulder occurs when the diaphragmatic surface of the spleen becomes inflamed. This is an ominous symptom that should not be ignored because it indicates that the patient is at risk for splenic rupture.

Splenic enlargement more often proceeds slowly and produces few if any symptoms. The likelihood of experiencing ill-defined symptoms, such as early satiety, bloating, fullness, and swelling or asymmetry of the abdomen, increases as spleen size increases, though patients with chronically enlarged spleens often experience none of these symptoms. The disorders most frequently associated with massive splenomegaly but minimal if any symptoms are vascular congestion,[4] the myeloproliferative diseases,[5-7] the indolent lymphoproliferative diseases,[8-9] sarcoidosis,[10] Gaucher's disease,[11] and cystic lesions of the spleen.[12-14]

**Physical findings.** Palpation is the most sensitive technique for demonstrating splenic enlargement by physical examination.[15] Increases of as little as 40% above normal size can be detected by use of this technique. The enlarged spleen is first palpable beneath the left lateral costal margin as a tip that descends with inspiration. As the spleen enlarges, its tip descends inferiorly and to the right just beneath the anterior abdominal wall. With progressive enlargement, the spleen becomes palpable as a mass that extends along a diagonal from the left upper quadrant toward and, in cases of massive enlargement, into the right lower quadrant.

Not all enlarged spleens are palpable, however. Obesity, ascites, or surgical scars of the abdomen decrease the sensitivity of the physical examination for the detection of splenomegaly. Local tenderness and other causes of limited patient cooperation also tend to interfere with the abdominal examination. Even with the patient in the right lateral decubitus position and with careful bimanual palpation, the spleen may be up to twice its normal size yet remain undetectable. Extremely large spleens may also be missed if the examiner fails to search the entire path of enlargement, from the extreme right lower quadrant to the left costal margin, for the characteristic lower edge.

In addition, not all left upper quadrant masses are attributable to enlarged spleens. When a structure adjacent to the spleen becomes palpable, it may simulate splenomegaly.[16] The most common example of this is enlargement of the left lobe of the liver. However, gastric or colonic tumors, cysts or tumors of the pancreas, left ovary, left kidney, or adrenal gland, metastatic carcinoma, or hematomas or tumors of the structures of the anterior abdominal wall also may be misinterpreted as splenomegaly. In addition, a noticeable flattening of the left hemidiaphragm, a subphrenic abscess, or other processes that produce a mass effect occasionally displace a normal spleen to within reach of the examiner's hand.

Several findings on physical examination are useful in distinguishing splenomegaly from other left upper quadrant masses. Movement of the inferior margin, or tip, of the spleen downward with inspiration is probably the best known of these findings. The presence of an inferior edge, but no palpable superior edge, is another characteristic finding when the mass in question is caused by splenomegaly. In addition, a single indentation in the lower medial margin—the splenic notch—is often apparent on gentle palpation in patients with moderately enlarged spleens. Care must be taken, however, not to confuse the splenic notch with a polycystic left kidney, which may produce a left upper quadrant mass with a "notch." In these cases, the presence of a superior margin and the relative lack of movement with respiration suggest that the mass in question is not an enlarged spleen.

## IMAGING TECHNIQUES

Given the frequent clinical use of plain chest and abdominal roentgenograms, it is not surprising that unsuspected splenomegaly is sometimes first detected by these studies.[17] When there is a question about the nature of a left upper quadrant mass or when splenomegaly is suspected but not clearly present on examination, one or more of several radiologic imaging techniques should be used to confirm the examiner's impressions and to search for associated findings. Computerized axial tomographic (CAT) and magnetic resonance imaging (MRI) scans, radionuclide scintigraphic scanning, ultrasound imaging, and plain roentgenography may all be of use in the initial or the serial evaluation of patients with suspected splenomegaly.

**Ultrasonography.** Ultrasound imaging is essentially without risk to the patient and is usually accurate in measuring spleen size and detecting the presence of cystic structures. This modality is particularly useful to assess the parenchymal texture of an enlarged spleen and to guide needle aspiration in the rare case where this procedure is indicated.[18] However, high-quality studies are difficult to obtain in some patients for technical reasons, and these problems occasionally limit the usefulness of this technique in the evaluation of patients with splenomegaly.

**Scintigraphic scans.** The [99mtechnetium]-sulfur colloid liver-spleen scan, widely used to image functional splenic tissue, is most useful in the evaluation of spleen size and function and in the detection of accessory splenic tissue.[19,20] In addition, the liver-spleen scan is sometimes useful diagnostically, as when increased marrow uptake of isotope is seen in patients with hepatic cirrhosis and congestive splenomegaly. Scintigraphic scans performed after the infusion of blood cells that are labeled with various radioisotopes are sometimes used in cytopenic patients with suspected hypersplenism in an effort to predict patient response to splenectomy. Although this approach is theoretically attractive and has research applications, it is not sufficiently accurate to be recommended for routine clinical use at present.[21,22] As with all noninvasive tests, the liver-spleen scan cannot be used reliably either to document or exclude splenic involvement by tumors, particularly infiltrative lesions, since both false-positive and false-negative results are fairly common.

**Computerized tomographic (CT) and magnetic resonance imaging (MRI) scans.** CT and MRI offer some advantages in the evaluation of patients with a newly discovered left upper quadrant mass. They are the most accurate of the noninvasive techniques in the assessment of the size and parenchymal consistency of the spleen and other abdominal viscera and are the only noninvasive methods capable of evaluating intra-abdominal lymph nodes above the level of the renal bed.[23,24] Furthermore, a single scan is often preferable to a series of other noninvasive tests because it provides information about most of the abdominal viscera and spaces. Limitations of MRI and CT scans include the production of artifacts by patient movement, by surgical clips, or by other metallic foreign bodies, and the relative disadvantages of greater patient radiation exposure and higher cost than that of other techniques. In general, MRI scans are preferred over CT scans to evaluate soft tissues or if the individual has very little abdominal fat. Figure 48-1 illustrates the utility of scanning in the evaluation of splenic disease. In this instance an enlarged asymptomatic spleen was found accidentally and all work-up results were normal. A CT scan of the spleen without contrast was inconclusive. A scan with contrast clearly demonstrated a space-occupying lesion. At splenectomy this lesion proved to be a primary splenic lymphoma.

# DIFFERENTIAL DIAGNOSIS

The box on pp. 542 and 543 lists the wide variety of disorders that may be associated with splenomegaly. As with other clinical findings caused by a wide range of underlying disorders, establishment of the correct diagnosis is the critical first step in determining the optimal management of the patient with splenomegaly. To accomplish this, the clinician first prepares a differential diagnosis based on the patient's history, the findings on physical examination, and the results of prelimi-

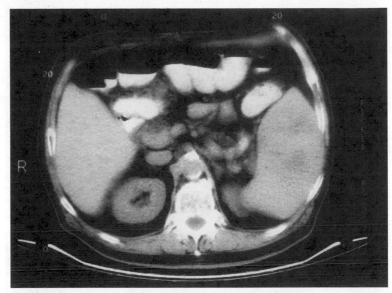

**A**

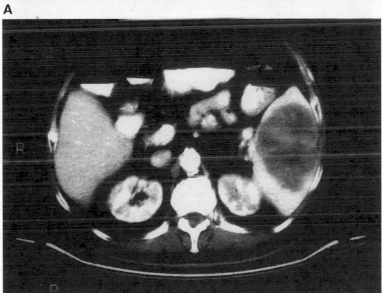

**B**

**Figure 48–1.** *A, CT scan of spleen without contrast. B, Same study with intravenously administered contrast agent disclosing large space-occupying lesion.*

## Causes of Splenomegaly

### INFECTIOUS CAUSES

Infectious mononucleosis
Endocarditis
Human immunodeficiency virus (HIV) infection
Abscess
*Salmonella* infection
Brucellosis
Mycobacterial infection
Spirochetal infection
Rickettsial infection
Psittacosis
Histoplasmosis
Tularemia
Listeriosis
Toxocariasis
Malaria and other tropical diseases

### HEMATOLOGIC CAUSES

Lymphoproliferative disroders
Chronic lymphocytic leukemia
Hodgkin's disease
Non-Hodgkin's lymphoma
Waldenström's macroglobulinemia
Heavy-chain disease
Angioimmunoblastic lymphadenopathy
Acute lymphocytic leukemia
Myeloproliferative disorders
Chronic myelogenous leukemia
Polycythemia vera
Myeloid metaplasia
Essential thrombocythemia
Chronic myelomonocytic leukemia
Acute myelogenous leukemia
Red blood cell disorders
Hereditary spherocytosis
Thalassemia
Hemoglobin SC
Other hemoglobinopathy or hemolytic syndrome
Histiocytosis
Systemic mastocytosis
Malignant hypereosinophilic syndrome

*continued*

*continued*

## IMMUNE CAUSES

Collagen-vascular diseases
Rheumatoid arthritis
Systemic lupus erythematosus
Behçet's syndrome
Granulomatous diseases
Sarcoidosis
Crohn's disease
Berylliosis
Hypersensitivity reaction
Phenytoin

## ENDOCRINE CAUSES

Hyperthyroidism

## INFILTRATIVE CAUSES

Lipoidosis
Gaucher's disease
Niemann-Pick disease
Hyperlipidemias
Amyloidosis

## CONGESTIVE CAUSES

Hepatic cirrhosis (Banti's syndrome)
Splenic or portal venous thrombosis
Congestive heart failure (rarely)

## TUMORS OR CYSTS, OR BOTH

Tumors
Metastatic (melanoma, carcinoma of the lung, breast, pancreas)
Locally invasive (carcinoma of the pancreas, left kidney, stomach)
Primary (see Hematologic causes)
Cysts
Epithelial
Lymphangiomatous
Posttraumatic

## UNKNOWN ETIOLOGY

Idiopathic nontropical (Dacie's syndrome)
Chronic renal failure patients on hemodialysis
Idiopathic portal hypertension

nary laboratory tests and then uses additional tests both to establish the correct diagnosis and to exclude the incorrect diagnoses in the differential.[17,25,26] The ability to construct a differential diagnosis and to select the tests necessary to establish a diagnosis requires a knowledge of the epidemiology and the clinical features of the various disorders listed in the box. Although a detailed discussion of all these disorders is beyond the scope of this chapter, the following comments should be helpful in most cases encountered in practice today.

**Splenic biopsy.** Unlike most other organs the spleen is very hazardous as a site to be biopsied. Ultrasound-guided needle biopsies should be contemplated only in the most extreme situations. Any type of needle biopsy has a prohibitive incidence of capsular tear leading to subcapsular hemorrhage, splenic rupture, and intraperitoneal hemorrhage. Emergency splenectomy often follows splenic needle biopsy. If a biopsy is absolutely required to make a diagnosis, the entire spleen usually has to be removed and examined. This is not a trivial procedure and should not be done casually, particularly in young individuals, because of the subsequent increased risk of serious infection with encapsulated organisms such as pneumococci (*Streptococcus pneumoniae*) and certain rare rickettsial diseases such as babesiosis. Splenectomy in adults seems to present less of a long-term problem with infection but pneumococcal and *Haemophilus influenzae* vaccines are recommended. The wisdom of performing a splenic biopsy and if so what type is performed is a matter of careful clinical judgment that weighs the potential benefits versus the risks.

**Infectious diseases.** Splenomegaly occurs in a large number of infectious diseases (Table 48-1). Many of these diseases, however, are uncommon in the United States. For example, malaria,[27] the tropical splenomegaly syndromes,[28,29] schistosomiasis,[30] and various other tropical infections can usually be excluded from the differential diagnosis in the absence of an appropriate history of exposure. However, it is important to recall that malaria can be acquired abroad and imported to the United States, since infection may be inapparent for up to 12 months. Intravenous drug abuse and exposure to blood or blood products are also risk factors for acquiring malaria, but these exposures are even more important as risk factors for other causes of splenomegaly such as bacterial endocarditis[31,32] and the acquired immunodeficiency syndrome (AIDS).[33-35] In addition, several of the other infections listed in Table 48-1 that do occur in the United States are found almost exclusively in patients who are infected as a consequence of a well-defined exposure. Splenic abscess occurs almost exclusively in patients with congenital or acquired immunodeficiency, including that caused by treatment with chemotherapy or steroids, and in patients with disseminated infections or with various other serious illnesses. Splenic abscess is notably uncommon in patients with AIDS.[36] Other examples include tularemia after contact with infected rabbit meat or brucellosis in patients employed as meat packers. Thus, in most cases, these disorders can be excluded from further consideration on the basis of the history.

**Table 48-1.** *Infectious diseases associated with splenomegaly*

| Disease | Comments |
|---|---|
| Infectious mononucleosis | Heterophil-positive Epstein-Barr virus, heterophil-negative Epstein-Barr virus, cytomegalovirus |
| Endocarditis | Splenomegaly occurs more often in the subacute form; may simulate mononucleosis |
| Human immunodeficiency virus infection | Splenomegaly occurs as a part of the AIDS-related complex (ARC), during acute infection, and when involved by lymphoma or metastatic tumor in patients with AIDS |
| Mycobacterial infection | Splenomegaly occurs primarily in the elderly with subacute disseminated tuberculosis that resembles mononucleosis |
| Rickettsial infections | Rocky Mountain spotted fever and typhus; Colorado tick fever (a viral infection) resembles spotted fever without rash |
| *Salmonella* infections | Typhoid and paratyphoid; the spleen is rarely palpable in shigellosis |
| Brucellosis | Meat packers or handlers with chronic fever |
| Tularemia | Infected wild rabbit meat; typhoidal form resembles mononucleosis; other forms include ulceroglandular, glandular, and gastrointestinal |
| Spirochetal infections | Congenital syphilis, occasionally secondary or late syphilis, and pretibial (Fort Bragg) fever, a form of leptospirosis |
| Psittacosis | Splenomegaly occurs in 10 percent to 70 percent of cases |
| Abscess | Splenomegaly frequently absent |
| Histoplasmosis | Splenomegaly occurs primarily in patients with the infrequent disseminated form of infection |
| Listeriosis | Splenomegaly occurs in severe infection of the newborn |
| Toxocariasis | Visceral larva migrans; splenomegaly occurs primarily in patients with severe infection |
| Tropical | Malaria, tropical splenomegaly syndrome, schistosomiasis, kala-azar, trypanosomiasis, filarial tropical eosinophilia, borreliosis, and others |

The mononucleosis syndrome of malaise, fever, adenopathy, and splenomegaly with circulating atypical lymphocytes occurs in patients of all ages and is caused by a variety of infectious, immune, and neoplastic disorders. This syndrome occurs most commonly in adolescents as a consequence of infection by the Epstein-Barr virus.[37] In the elderly, splenomegaly may be a prominent feature of the chronic subacute form of disseminated tuberculosis that occurs with recrudescent infection and may present with a mononucleosis-like syndrome.[38] Cytomegalovirus infection may resemble infectious mononucleosis; however, splenomegaly is uncommon in this syndrome, in toxoplasmosis, in other leptospiral diseases with the rare exception of pretibial (Fort Bragg) fever, and in the mononucleosis-like syndromes that occasionally accompany infection by adenovirus, herpes simplex type II, rubella, varicella-zoster, and other unidentified agents. In cases where the clinical course or the results of serologic tests are not consistent with a viral cause of infectious mononucleosis, the clinician should give careful consideration to other diseases that may resemble mononucleosis, such as bacterial endocarditis, lymphoproliferative disease, collagen vascular disease, or an atypical form of one of the infections listed in the box on p. 547.

Some disorders that may result in splenomegaly typically present with other, more prominent, features. The differential diagnosis in these patients, therefore, is not based solely on the isolated finding of an enlarged spleen but, rather, is suggested by the presence of the characteristic associated features. For example, fever, rash, headache, and myalgia coupled with an recent history of a tick bite should lead to the consideration of Rocky Mountain spotted fever,[39] typhus, or Colorado tick fever. Fever, gastrointestinal symptoms, rash, and splenomegaly are typical of the typhoid and paratyphoid forms of *Salmonella* infection. Disseminated infection with obvious multisystem disease is present in most patients who have splenomegaly caused by histoplasmosis or toxicariasis and in neonates with listeriosis, toxoplasmosis, rubella, syphilis, or cytomegalovirus disease. Lymphadenopathy is present in many patients with infection or neoplastic disease, and thus there is a great deal of overlap in the differential diagnosis of patients with these findings. Patients with several noninfectious causes of splenomegaly, such as lupus, rheumatoid arthritis,[40] thalassemia major,[41] amyloidosis,[42,43] Behcet's syndrome,[44] the histiocytoses,[45] systemic mastocytosis,[46] the hypereosinophilic syndromes,[47,48] and the granulomatous disorders, generally present with other more prominent clinical features that should be suggestive of the correct diagnosis.

In contrast, infectious mononucleosis, subacute bacterial endocarditis, the lymphoproliferative and myeloproliferative disorders, some red blood cell disorders, brucellosis, early rickettsial infection, disseminated tuberculosis, the lipoidoses, and others sometimes present with splenomegaly and either nonspecific or absent associated features.[49] Blood cultures, careful examination of the peripheral blood and bone marrow, and serologic tests are often required in these cases to establish a diagnosis.

**Hematologic disorders.** Abnormalities of the blood counts, blood smear, bone marrow, lymph nodes, or serum proteins typically are present in patients with splenomegaly caused by hematologic disease.

## Common Causes of Splenomegaly in the United States (by Age)

### INFANTS AND CHILDREN

Red blood cell disorder, including sickle cell disease
Infection, especially in the newborn as part of the TORCH (*T*oxoplasmosis, *R*ubella, *C*ytomegalovirus, *H*erpes simplex) syndrome
Trauma
Hematologic or neoplastic disease
Lipoidosis
Congestive disorder

### ADOLESCENTS

Infectious mononucleosis, usually attributable to Epstein-Barr virus
Other infection
Hodgkin's disease, non-Hodgkin's lymphoma, leukemia
Other hematologic disorders
Collagen-vascular or other immune disorders
Lipoidosis

### ADULTS

Congestive disorder
Myeloproliferative disorder
Lymphoproliferative disorder
Infection
Red blood cell disorder
Immune disorder
Amyloidosis
Lipoidosis

Patients with chronic hemolysis usually develop mild to moderate splenomegaly. Hemolysis may be caused by either a congenital red blood cell disorder, such as hereditary spherocytosis[50] or thalassemia,[41] or any of a variety of acquired disorders. Establishment of a diagnosis of one of these disorders begins by demonstrating active hemolysis and then depends on a systematic search for a specific cause of hemolysis.

The myeloproliferative disorders are usually discovered in older patients and may present with asymptomatic splenomegaly. Polycythemia vera, myelofibrosis with myeloid metaphasia, essential thrombocythemia, and chronic myelogenous leukemia are generally easily recognized by their characteristic clinical and peripheral blood features.[5-7] Bone marrow examination is usually necessary, however, to establish the diagnosis of either acute leukemia[51] or chronic myelomonocytic leukemia,[52] a myelodysplastic or preleukemic disease that is associated with splenomegaly.

Splenomegaly is often present in patients with chronic lymphocytic leukemia, Waldenström's macroglobulinemia, or heavy-chain disease.[8] In contrast, splenomegaly is only rarely a prominent feature or a diagnostic clue in patients with acute lymphocytic leukemia, Hodgkin's disease, or one of the non-Hodgkin's lymphomas.[53] Hairy-cell leukemia, though relatively uncommon, should be considered in elderly patients with mild pancytopenia, splenomegaly, and recurrent infections.[9] The finding of tartrate-resistant, acid phosphatase–positive lymphocytes in peripheral blood or bone marrow is strongly suggestive of a diagnosis of hairy-cell leukemia. Establishing the diagnosis of any of the lymphoproliferative diseases nearly always requires careful examination of the peripheral blood, the bone marrow, and lymph node biopsy and may require electrophoresis of serum or urine proteins.

**Congestive disorders.** Vascular congestion is frequently the cause of chronic splenomegaly in adults. Hepatic cirrhosis, primarily caused by alcohol abuse, chronic hepatitis, or both, is the most common cause of portal hypertension in the United States that results in splenic congestion and enlargement.[4] Disorders that result in portal or splenic vein thrombosis, such as pancreatitis, local tumor, or aneurysm, and, occasionally, severe congestive heart failure, may also result in this syndrome.[54] Most patients with congestive splenomegaly have variable cytopenias (hypersplenism) attributable to splenic sequestration of blood cells and show signs of either chronic liver disease or portal hypertension. Splenectomy may be indicated in the management of variceal bleeding in these patients but is rarely required to manage hypersplenism.[21,22]

**Lipid storage diseases.** Although severe forms of the lipoidoses often present in childhood, variant forms may present with splenomegaly in any age group. Gaucher's and Niemann-Pick disease are autosomal recessive disorders characterized by the accumulation in macrophages of glucocerebroside or of sphingomyelin and ceroid, respectively.[12,55] Examination of marrow or other biopsy material in these cases usually reveals Gaucher's cells or the foam cells typical of Niemann-Pick disease. Assays of white blood cells or cultured fibroblasts for glucocerebrosidase or sphingomyelinase activity can be used to confirm these diagnoses.

# MANAGEMENT

Since splenomegaly is most often associated with another disease, usually systemic, it is not surprising that management is directed primarily at the underlying disorder. The splenomegaly that occurs secondary to most infectious, congestive, hyperimmune, and infiltrative disorders does not require treatment as such. Treatment of the underlying disease or observation usually suffices.

On the other hand, interventions directed at the spleen may be required in patients with splenomegaly caused by neoplastic diseases, particularly if symptoms are severe. Systemic chemotherapy or local radiotherapy may be useful in alleviating symptoms. More often, however, splenomegaly is seen in the context of widespread disease; in these cases treatment is and should be systemic, rather than directed solely at the spleen.

The acute splenomegaly associated with infectious disease, particularly infectious mononucleosis, may lead to splenic rupture. Patients who develop this catastrophic life-threatening event should be evaluated promptly for exploratory laparotomy.[3,49] Early splenectomy is also indicated in the rare patient with a splenic abscess.[36]

The clinician may need to consider surgical removal of the spleen because of peripheral blood cytopenias attributable to hypersplenism.[21] For example, splenectomy may be necessary if blood counts are severely depressed because of congestive splenomegaly or if blood cytopenias accompany infiltrative diseases of the spleen. In such cases, the blood counts often improve, and bleeding and infectious complications resolve after surgery. The decision to remove a spleen for hypersplenism must be weighed carefully, however, since the splenectomy may fail if bone marrow compromise is also contributing to the peripheral cytopenias.[22] In addition, the surgical risk of splenectomy and the risk of postoperative infection are often relatively high in these patients.[22,56] Splenectomy is occasionally required to manage hemolytic anemia when other treatments fail. Splenic irradiation may also be effective when splenectomy is indicated but cannot be performed safely.[57] Finally, splenectomy is indicated in the management of some patients with congenital defects of the red blood cell membrane, such as hereditary spherocytosis or elliptocytosis, and in some patients with Gaucher's disease.[58,59]

# CONCLUSION

Splenomegaly is associated with a host of diseases. Attention to certain clues, however, frequently narrows the differential diagnosis to the more likely causes. When evaluating any patient with suspected splenomegaly, the clinician should ask the following questions:

1. Is the spleen really enlarged?
2. What is the age (see box, p. 547) and geographic background of the patient?
3. Is the enlargement acute or chronic?
4. What are the pertinent findings from the history, physical examination, blood smear, and routine laboratory tests?

Additional diagnostic tests should then be selected to investigate the most likely diagnoses based on this information. In most cases a diagnosis can be established on the basis of a careful history and physical examination combined with appropriate laboratory and imaging studies. Although bone marrow or lymph node biopsy may be required to diagnose hematologic or neoplastic disease, laparatomy and splenectomy are rarely necessary. Likewise, splenic biopsy is indicated to establish a diagnosis only rarely, particularly in view of the potential hazards of splenic aspiration. The management of patients with spleno-megaly is based, to a large extent, on the underlying disease. The therapeutic approach varies from observation alone to treatment of the underlying condition. Occasionally, enlarged spleens are so symptomatic that they have to be surgically removed or irradiated, but this is not often necessary.

## References

1. Ebaugh FG, McIntyre OR: Palpable spleens: ten-year follow-up, *Ann Intern Med* 90:130-131, 1979.
2. O'Keefe JH Jr, Holmes DR Jr, Schaff HV, et al: Thromboembolic splenic infarction, *Mayo Clin Proc* 61:967-972, 1986.
3. Peters RM, Gordon LA: Nonsurgical treatment of splenic hemorrhage in an adult with infectious mononucleosis, *Am J Med* 80:123-125, 1986.
4. Okuda K, Kono K, Ohnishi K, et al: Clinical study of eighty-six cases of idiopathic portal hypertension and comparison with cirrhosis with spleno-megaly, *Gastroenterology* 86:600-610, 1984.
5. Koeffler HP, Golde DW: Chronic myelogenous leukemia—new concepts, *N Engl J Med* 304:1201-1209, 1269-1274, 1981.
6. Laszlo J: Myeloproliferative disorders: myelofibrosis, myelosclerosis, extra-medullary hematopoiesis, undifferentiated, and hemorrhagic thrombocy-themia, *Semin Hematol* 12:409-432, 1975.
7. Adamson JW, Fialkow PJ, Murphy S, et al: Polycythemia vera: stem-cell and probable clonal origin of the disease, *N Engl J Med* 295:913-916, 1976.
8. Gale RP, Foon KA: Chronic lymphocytic leukemia: recent advances in biology and treatment, *Ann Intern Med* 103:101-120, 1985.
9. Cheson BD, Martin A: Clinical trials in hairy cell leukemia: current status and future directions, *Ann Intern Med* 106:871-878, 1987.
10. Peter SA: Massive splenomegaly as the presenting manifestation of sarcoido-sis, *J Natl Med Assoc* 78:243-244, 1986.
11. Beaudet AL: Gaucher's disease, *N Engl J Med* 316:619-621, 1987.
12. Dawes LG, Malangoni MA: Cystic masses of the spleen, *Am Surg* 52:333-336, 1986.
13. Pistoia F, Markowitz SK: Splenic lymphangiomatosis: CT diagnosis, *AJR* 150:121-122, 1988.
14. Tada T, Wakabayashi T, Kishimoto H: Peliosis of the spleen, *Am J Clin Pathol* 79:708-713, 1983.
15. Sullivan S, Williams R: Reliability of clinical techniques for detecting splenic enlargement, *Br Med J* 2:1043-1044, 1976.
16. Noseda A, Bellens R, Gansbeke DV, et al: Rectus sheath hematoma mimick-ing acute splenic disease, *Am J Gastroenterol* 78:566-568, 1983.
17. Rosenthal DS, Harris NL: Case records of the Massachusetts General Hospital (Case 48-1985), *N Engl J Med* 313:1405-1412, 1985.
18. Solbiati L, Bossi MC, Bellotti E, et al: Focal lesions in the spleen: sonographic patterns and guided biopsy, *AJR* 140:59-65, 1983.
19. Larson SM, Tuell SH, Moores KD, et al: Dimensions of the normal adult spleen scan and prediction of spleen weight, *J Nucl Med* 12:123-126, 1971.
20. Zhang B, Lewis SM: Use of radionuclide scanning to estimate spleen size in vivo, *J Clin Pathol* 40:508-511, 1987.
21. Coon WW: Splenectomy for splenomegaly and secondary hypersplenism, *World J Surg* 9:437-443, 1985.

22. Wilson RE, Rosenthal DS, Moloney WC, et al: Splenectomy for myeloproliferative disorders, *World J Surg* 9:431-436, 1985.

23. Heymsfield SB, Fulenwider T, Nordlinger B, et al: Accurate measurement of liver, kidney, and spleen volume and mass by computerized axial tomography, *Ann Intern Med* 90:185-187, 1979.

24. Gilbert T, Castellino RA: Critical review: the spleen in Hodgkin's disease: diagnostic value of CT, *Invest Radiol* 21:437-439, 1986.

25. Eichner ER, Whitfield CL: Splenomegaly: an algorithmic approach to diagnosis, *JAMA* 246:2858-2861, 1981.

26. Schnipper LE, Harris NL: Case records of the Massachusetts General Hospital (Case 15-1982), *N Engl J Med* 306:918-925, 1982.

27. Rosse WF: The spleen as a filter, *N Engl J Med* 317:704-706, 1987.

28. Hoffmann SL, Piessens WF, Ratiwayanto S, et al: Reduction of suppressor T lymphocytes in the tropical splenomegaly syndrome, *N Engl J Med* 310:337-341, 1984.

29. DeCook KM, Lucas SB, Rees PH, et al: Obscure splenomegaly in the tropics that is not the tropical splenomegaly syndrome, *Br Med J* 287:1347-1348, 1983.

30. DeCook KM: Hepatosplenic schistosomiasis: a clinical review, *Gut* 27:734-745, 1986.

31. Von Reyn CF, Levy BS, Arbeit D, et al: Infective endocarditis: an analysis based on strict case definitions, *Ann Intern Med* 94:505-518, 1981.

32. Laufer D, Lew PD, Oberhansli I, et al: Chronic Q fever endocarditis with massive splenomegaly in childhood, *J Pediatr* 108:535-539, 1986.

33. Abrams DI, Lewis BJ, Beckstead JH, et al: Persistent diffuse lymphadenopathy in homosexual men: endpoint or prodrome? *Ann Intern Med* 100:801-808, 1984.

34. Cooper DA, Gold J, Maclean P, et al: Acute AIDS retrovirus infection: definition of a clinical illness associated with scroconversion, *Lancet* 1:537-540, 1985.

35. Smith R: Liver-spleen scintigraphy in patients with acquired immunodeficiency syndrome, *AJR* 145:1201-1204, 1985.

36. Nelken N, Ignatius J, Skinner M, et al: Changing clinical spectrum of splenic abscess: a multicenter study and review of the literature, *Am J Surg* 154:27-34, 1987.

37. Evans AS, Niederman JC, McCollum RW: Seroepidemiologic studies of infectious mononucleosis with EB virus, *N Engl J Med* 279:1121-1127, 1968.

38. Glassroth J, Robins AG, Snider DE: Tuberculosis in the 1980s, *N Engl J Med* 302:1441-1450, 1980.

39. Turner RC, Chaplinski TJ, Adams HG: Rocky Mountain spotted fever presenting as thrombotic thrombocytopenic purpura, *Am J Med* 81:153-157, 1986.

40. Thorne C, Urowitz MB: Long-term outcome in Felty's syndrome, *Ann Rheum Dis* 41:486-489, 1982.

41. Orkin SH, Nathan DG: The thalassemias, *N Engl J Med* 295:710-714, 1976.

42. Kyle RA, Greipp PR: Amyloidosis (AL): clinical and laboratory features in 229 cases, *Mayo Clin Proc* 58:665-673, 1983.

43. Gertz MA, Kyle RA, Greipp PR: Hyposplenism in primary systemic amyloidosis, *Ann Intern Med* 98:475-477, 1983.

44. Chajek T, Fainaru M: Behcet's disease: report of 41 cases and a review of the literature, *Medicine* 54:179-188, 1975.

45. Deuel T, Pikul F: Clinicopathologic conference: fever, pancytopenia, renal insufficiency, and death in a 22-year-old man, *Am J Med* 82:787-795, 1987.

46. Roth J, Brudler O, Henze E: Functional asplenia in malignant mastocytosis, *J Nucl Med* 26:1149-1152, 1985.

47. Alfaham MA, Ferguson SD, Sihra B, et al: The idiopathic hypereosinophilic syndrome, *Arch Dis Child* 62:601-613, 1987.

48. Wynn SR, Sachs MI, Keating MU, et al: Idiopathic hypereosinophilic syndrome in a 5½-month-old infant, *J Pediatr* 111:94-97, 1987.

49. Patel JM, Rizzolo E, Hinshaw JR: Spontaneous subscapular splenic hematoma as the only clinical manifestation of infectious mononucleosis, *JAMA* 247:3243-3244, 1982.

50. Croom RD, McMillan CW, Orringer EP, et al: Hereditary spherocytosis: recent experience and current concepts of pathophysiology, *Ann Surg* 203:34-39, 1986.

51. Bennet JM, Catovsky D, Daniel MT, et al: Proposals for the classification of the acute leukemias, *Br J Haematol* 33:451-458, 1976.

52. Bennett JM, Catovsky D, Daniel MT, et al: Proposals for the classification of the myelodysplastic syndromes, *Br J Haematol* 51:189-199, 1982.

53. Spier CM, Kjeldsberg CR, Eyre HJ, et al: Malignant lymphoma with primary presentation in the spleen, *Arch Pathol Lab Med* 109:1076-1080, 1985.

54. Moossa AR, Gadd MA: Isolated splenic vein thrombosis, *World J Surg* 9:384-390, 1985.

55. Dawson PJ, Dawson G: Adult Niemann-Pick disease with sea-blue histocytes in the spleen, *Hum Pathol* 13:1115-1120, 1982.

56. Gelfand JA, Grabbe JP: Case records of the Massachusetts General Hospital (Case 20-1983), *N Engl J Med* 308:1212-1218, 1983.

57. Markus H, Forfar JC: Splenic iradiation in treating warm autoimmune haemolytic anaemia, *Br Med J* 29:839-840, 1986.

58. Agre P, Asimos A, Casella JF, et al: Inheritance pattern and clinical response to splenectomy as a reflection of erythrocyte spectrin deficiency in hereditary spherocytosis, *N Engl J Med* 315:1579-1583, 1986.

59. Hobbs JR, Jones KH, Shaw PJ, et al: Beneficial effect of pretransplant splenectomy of displacement bone marrow transplantation for Gaucher's syndrome, *Lancet* 1:1111-1115, 1987.

# Part 7

# Chronic Disease

## Chapter 49

## The Patient with Pain

Jennifer Daley
John T. Harrington

Pain is one of the most common reasons why patients seek a physician.[1] Difficult to define, promethean in its guises, and challenging to treat, pain has two major components. First, pain is the perception in the central nervous system (CNS) of a pathophysiologic stimulus often severe enough to cause tissue injury. The objective signal is transmitted through complex neural paths from the site of injury through the spinal column to the brain. The second crucial component of pain is the emotional and affective response of the injured person to the injury and pain. It is this second component (denoted as suffering in this chapter), influenced by the severity, significance, and course of the injury, that makes the definition, diagnosis, and treatment of pain difficult in many instances.[2]

On a temporal basis, pain can be considered either acute (minutes to several days) or chronic (months to years). Although it is not difficult to define and distinguish the classic syndromes of acute pain, it is less easy to define the syndrome of chronic pain. Patients experiencing acute pain can usually describe the characteristics of the pain accurately; that is, they can relate the onset, character, radiation, and timing of the pain. If patients are in acute pain, they show signs of autonomic discharge with diaphoresis, tachycardia, and pallor. The psychologic reaction of the patient to acute pain is usually appropriate. Both pain (the first component) and suffering (the second component) can be relieved by identification and treatment of the underlying cause of the acute pain and by the provision of adequate analgesia. For example, patients with the severe pain of renal colic, an acute myocardial infarction, or an acute fracture are usually diagnosed readily, and adequate analgesic therapy can be instituted in a short time.

The syndromes of chronic pain are more difficult to define; on a temporal basis, patients with chronic pain may have intermittent or unremitting complaints for months to years.[3,4] The longer the patient has suffered with the pain, the more difficult it becomes to characterize the pain accurately and reliably. The patient's report of the character, timing, and quality of chronic pain is often contradictory, vague, and uncertain. The patient's report of the pain usually does not conform to the classic acute pain syndromes. In addition, chronic pain is poorly relieved by the therapies used in acute pain. Thus the physician is often led to the conclusion that the patient is consciously manufacturing the symptom of pain or exaggerating the severity of both the pain and the resulting disability. All too often, the physician and the patient end their professional relationship on an unpleasant note—the patient angry and frustrated, feeling that the physician has been insensitive to his or her pain; the physician skeptical about the authenticity and the magnitude of the patient's pain and suffering.

This chapter describes our approach to patients with both acute and chronic pain. The first section discusses the general diagnostic approach to any patient with pain. In the subsequent sections, we describe the approach to the treatment of acute pain and the evaluation and management of the patient with chronic pain.

# DIAGNOSIS OF THE PATIENT WITH PAIN

Diagnosis of the patient with pain begins with a meticulous medical history and careful physical examination. The importance of a detailed review of the patient's medical records cannot be overemphasized. The patient should be asked to bring medical records from other physicians to the first visit. In patients who have had chronic pain syndromes for many years, have seen numerous physicians, and have had extensive previous diagnostic evaluations, review of the medical record can seem like a burdensome and unnecessary task. The record, however, almost always reveals critical information about the extent of prior evaluations and the patient's physical and emotional response to attempts to diagnose and relieve the pain. Careful review of prior evaluations can also save both the patient and the physician from unnecessarily repeating previous studies.

The history should focus on a detailed and accurate description of the pain. What is the nature of the pain? Where does the pain arise and where is it distributed? When does the pain occur and in relation to what events? What are the factors that make the pain worse? What are the factors that make the pain better? What diagnostic efforts have been made to determine the cause of the pain? What therapies have been attempted and with what degree of success? A complete medical history is critical, and special emphasis should be placed on ascertaining if the patient has any chronic illnesses that are strongly associated with pain (such as rheumatoid arthritis or metastatic cancer with bony involvement).

An equally important and often neglected part of the medical history of the patient with pain is a careful psychiatric history. The psychiatric history should focus on any signs or symptoms of depression. Particular attention should be paid to the presence of any vegetative signs of depression and the presence of sleep disorders. The patient should be questioned carefully about the extent to which pain inhibits or interferes with the patient's home, work, and sexual life. In patients with long-standing chronic pain, some symptoms of depression are appropriate reactions to the long-standing and debilitating nature of the problem. The physician should specifically inquire how the patient's behavior during pain affects his relationships with his family, friends, and co-workers and how those around him respond to the patient's pain and suffering.

The physical examination should be complete and thorough and should include a detailed neurologic examination. First the physician should direct his or her attention to the site of pain, thereby assessing any abnormality or inflammation. Second, if the patient has reported any radiation of pain, the areas of radiation should be inspected. Regardless of whether the patient has reported radiation of pain, the physician should then thoroughly inspect the segmental dermatomes associated with the area of pain. For example, a patient complaining of persistent arm or shoulder pain may have involvement of the neural plexus by a Pancoast tumor, even in the absence of other neurologic signs. Finally, the physician should be aware of the common patterns of referred pain. Referred pain is pain perceived at a site distant from the actual source of injury, usually in some visceral organ. Commonly, referred pain is experienced by the patient in the cutaneous distribution of the segmental dermatome from which the visceral organ arises. Familiar examples of referred pain are the pain of an acute myocardial infarction experienced as pain radiating down the left arm or into the jaw, or the pain of renal colic experienced as groin or testicular pain.

Laboratory examination should be directed to the local area of pain as well as to the related areas of dermatome distribution, or referred pain. In the patient with acute pain, appropriate studies should be instituted immediately. In the patient with chronic pain who does not present with an acute emergency, it is mandatory to review the extent and quality of previous evaluations before one embarks on extensive additional and perhaps repetitive laboratory testing.

## TREATMENT OF THE PATIENT WITH ACUTE PAIN

Appropriate treatment of the patient with acute pain requires identification of the cause of the pain and treatment of that underlying cause.

Space precludes the description of the causes and treatments of all the acute pain syndromes here. The general management of the patient with acute pain is outlined here with special attention to the management of the pain of the terminally ill.

An informed patient and a compassionate physician who takes time to explain the course of the patient's illness to the patient and his family and friends can significantly reduce the agitation, turmoil, and confusion that often accompany the patient in acute pain. Too often an afterthought in the evaluation of the patient with acute pain, communication and empathy can often prevent further acceleration of cycles of pain. However, in the patient with severe acute pain, patient education, reassurance, and the institution of appropriate therapy for the underlying disorder are usually insufficient to alleviate the pain. Many physicians are reluctant to prescribe narcotic analgesics for fear of addicting the patient to narcotics.[5] This fear is unfounded in patients who have acute pain.[6,7,8]

Several general principles should be remembered in treating acute pain. Analgesic therapy should be instituted promptly unless cardinal manifestations of the underlying disorder would be obscured by analgesic therapy (such as acute right lower quadrant pain in which appendicitis or visceral perforation is suspected). Analgesic therapy should be prescribed at frequent, regular intervals around the clock; the patient should have the right to refuse analgesic medication but should be encouraged to accept prescribed medication for minor pain rather than waiting until pain becomes severe. Solid evidence demonstrates that relying on a patient's request for pain medication results in larger total doses of analgesic medication to control wide swings in intensity of pain and burdens the patient with deciding "when the pain is too much to bear." For these reasons, dosing schedules for "when-necessary (PRN)" pain medications in patients with severe acute pain should be avoided. Narcotic analgesics should never be given in combination with each other. Frequently, a combination of a nonnarcotic analgesic such as phenothiazine (chlorpromazine 25 to 50 mg four times a day) and a narcotic analgesic achieves greater pain control and reduces the overall amount of narcotic administered, since the effects of these two separate classes of drugs are synergistic.

Analgesic agents, drugs that diminish pain without causing loss of consciousness, fall into three main categories: nonnarcotic analgesics used in the treatment of mild pain, narcotic analgesics used for moderate pain, and narcotic analgesics used both parenterally and orally for severe pain (Table 49-1).

The physician should be intimately familiar with the dosing schedules, side effects, and drug interactions of two or three drugs of the hundreds available in each category. In patients with mild to moderate pain, drugs should be combined and rapidly added in a stepwise fashion until satisfactory pain control has been achieved. Aspirin (600 mg PO every 3 to 4 hours), acetaminophen (650 mg PO every 3 to 4 hours), or a nonsteroidal anti-inflammatory agent such as ibuprofen (400 mg every 6 hours) are good agents to initiate the treatment of mild pain. Both aspirin and nonsteroidal anti-inflammatory agents cause gastroin-

**Table 49–1.** *Some commonly prescribed analgesic medications used in patients with acute pain*

| Drug | Usual starting dose | |
| --- | --- | --- |
| | Oral | Subcutaneous or intramuscular |
| NONNARCOTIC ANALGESICS FOR MILD TO MODERATE PAIN | | |
| Aspirin | 600 mg q3 to 4h | |
| Ibuprofen | 200 to 600 mg q6h | |
| Acetaminophen | 650 mg q6h | |
| NARCOTIC AND NARCOTIC ANTAGONISTS FOR MODERATE TO SEVERE PAIN | | |
| Codeine | 15 to 30 mg q4 to 6h | |
| Oxycodone | 5 mg q4 to 6h | |
| Meperidine | 50 to 100 mg q3 to 4h | 75 mg q3 to 4h |
| NARCOTIC AND NARCOTIC ANTAGONISTS FOR SEVERE PAIN | | |
| Morphine | 30 to 60 mg q3 to 4h | 5 to 10 mg q3 to 4h |
| Levorphanol | 2 to 4 mg q3 to 4h | 1 to 2 mg q3 to 4h |
| Methadone | 5 to 10 mg q8 to 12h | 2.5 to 5.0 mg q8 to 12h |
| Hydromorphone | 2.5 to 5 mg q4 to 6h | 1 to 2 mg q4 to 6h |

testinal irritation and bleeding and are contraindicated in patients with active gastrointestinal hemorrhage or peptic ulcer disease. These agents can be combined with acetaminophen for some improvement in mild pain. If anxiety plays a substantial role in the patient with mild pain, a mild benzodiazepam such as diazepam (5 to 10 mg PO twice a day) can be added, but these agents have little role in the relief of pain apart from reducing anxiety. If the pain is unresponsive to these agents, narcotic analgesics with a low likelihood of causing addiction such as codeine (15 to 30 mg every 4 to 6 hours) or oxycodone (5 mg every 4 to 6 hours) can be added. These agents are generally well tolerated but do cause nausea, vomiting, constipation, and drowsiness, especially in large doses.

As already described, in the patient with acute pain, narcotic analgesics are often underutilized by physicians fearful of the drugs' potential for addiction and their side effects despite their potent ability to relieve severe pain. Only rarely do patients hospitalized with severe acute pain from an organic cause become addicted to narcotic analgesics. The most common side effects of narcotic analgesics used in the short-term management of hospitalized patients with acute severe pain are constipation and somnolence. One can prevent and manage constipation by beginning a bowel care program when narcotics are first prescribed; one can manage somnolence by a reduction in the doses of narcotic analgesics and more frequent administration, or by the use of another narcotic agent. Used in the long term for the management of severe pain, analgesics induce both tolerance and physical dependence. Tolerance to narcotics means that larger and larger doses are required to achieve analgesia; physical dependence means that patients treated for long periods of time must have the drug gradually discontinued if the drug is withdrawn. Virtually all the narcotic analgesics can be administered parenterally as well as orally with varying potencies and duration of action. Morphine (2 to 5 mg IM or SC), for example, has good parenteral effectiveness and a relatively long duration of action (4 to 5 hours) compared with parenteral meperidine (75 mg IM), which has a brief duration of action (3 to 4 hours). Narcotics with good oral efficacy include levorphanol (2 to 4 mg; duration of action 4 to 6 hours) and methadone (10 to 20 mg PO; duration of action 3 to 10 hours). Again, physicians should familiarize themselves with the characteristics of one or two parenterally and orally effective narcotic analgesics; narcotic analgesics should never be used in combination. The introduction of patient-controlled analgesia for the management of acute postoperative pain in the last decade has improved pain control, patient satisfaction, and shortened postoperative stays. Narcotics are administered in small intravenous boluses from a pump controlled by the patient.[9]

# MANAGEMENT OF THE PATIENT WITH TERMINAL ILLNESS

In the patient with a terminal illness (defined as illness likely to cause death within 1 year) experiencing severe pain, pain control should be one of the central features in management.[10-12] The goal of management is indefinite pain control. Analgesics should be given on a regular dosing schedule for patients with continuous pain; as-needed dosing schedules should be avoided. For terminally ill patients who can tolerate oral medication, levorphanol (2 mg every 3 to 4 hours) or methadone (10 to 20 mg every 4 hours) are recommended. Several side effects of these medications should be anticipated. First, constipation is a universal side effect of these medications; a bowel care regimen that includes stool softeners, laxatives, and dietary bulk should be prescribed from the outset to avoid obstipation. Secondly, drug tolerance and the requirement for increasing doses during the first few weeks of therapy should be expected. Bedtime doses of pain medication should be increased two- to threefold to avoid the patient's waking with pain. Finally, patients experiencing sedation and somnolence with increasing doses of narcotic analgesics can take dextroamphetamine orally (5 to 20 mg daily in a single morning dose) to counter the sedative effects of the narcotic analgesics. In the presence of severe pain (as from bony metastases), intravenous infusions of morphine or the placement of an indwelling epidural catheter for morphine infusion may provide good pain relief. The physician should *not* be concerned about addiction and habituation to these drugs when caring for patients with a terminal illness.

## MANAGEMENT OF THE PATIENT WITH CHRONIC PAIN

Patients with chronic pain syndromes present for consultation with a physician, usually having seen several other specialists and having had extensive evaluations and often surgery. The diagnostic approach outlined previously should be followed carefully. We find it helpful when evaluating patients with chronic pain to keep in mind four major kinds of chronic pain syndromes. Although there is often overlap among these types of pain syndromes even in the same patient, they are nevertheless helpful in the structuring of a treatment plan.

First, patients with chronic organic diseases can suffer bouts of pain as part of their disease. Patients with rheumatoid arthritis, osteoarthritis, or sickle cell anemia may have intermittent periods of moderate to severe pain. Second, patients may have chronic pain from some injury to the central or peripheral nervous system that causes dysesthesia and causalgia. Patients with peripheral neuritis, postherpetic neuralgia, and phantom-limb pain after amputation are examples of patients with this kind of pain. Third, patients may have chronic pain initially caused by acute injury or trauma but that persists long after the original injury has healed, because of its psychologic significance for the patient. Such psychologic pain should be treated with a combination of physical treatment and psychiatric care that addresses the psychologic dimensions of the patient's pain. Fourth, patients have chronic pain as a manifestation of primary psychiatric or psychologic disturbances in the absence of any known structural or physiologic abnormality. Patients with hypochondriasis, psychotic depression, and somatization disorder are examples of these illnesses.

The management of patients with chronic pain syndromes usually involves multiple different modalities and collaboration with other specialists. In each hospital it is helpful if a pain committee or consortium (staffed by medicine, neurology, psychiatry, rehabilitation, anesthesia, and social service) is available. The general principles of management are similar to those for treating acute pain. Treatment should be the least complicated means of effectively reducing pain and suffering; every effort should be taken to ensure that the patient is pain free with a minimum of side effects. The initiation of therapy should be prompt in those patients not previously treated, since breaking the pain cycle early may prevent the development of psychologic pain behavior.

Although the management of chronic pain should be the least complicated, effective regimen, multiple different modalities should be used together, since many of the different therapies are synergistic. Evaluation by a psychiatrist is imperative in patients in whom a psychogenic component to their pain syndrome is suspected. When patients with both physical and psychologic components of the pain syndrome are managed, a good working relationship between the mental health therapist and the internist facilitates caring for the patient and may prevent unnecessary procedures and diagnostic testing. In patients whose pain is a manifestation of primary psychiatric disease, diagnosis and treatment require extended evaluation by a psychiatrist. The internist's role is to reassure the patient that no structural abnormality exists, to discourage repeated unnecessary evaluations, and to prevent unwarranted surgery. This often is a frustrating experience for both patient and physician.

The pharmacologic management of patients with chronic pain syndromes includes several different classes of drugs. Narcotics *should be avoided* in patients with chronic pain syndromes, since these drugs have only limited efficacy and the potential for tolerance and habituation is high in these patients. Antidepressants deserve a trial in almost all patients with chronic pain who have not responded to other interventions. Low doses of amitriptyline (25 to 75 mg at bedtime) have mild analgesic properties and are often helpful in alleviating the pain of chronic radiculopathy. Most chronic pain patients who have not responded to treatment deserve a supervised trial of antidepressants at levels used to treat major depression before any invasive treatments are considered. Drugs such as amitriptyline (150 to 250 mg at bedtime) or desipramine (75 to 125 mg at bedtime) should be tried; none of the antidepressants has been reported to be superior to any other in the treatment of chronic pain patients, and drug choice is empiric. Fluoxetine is less effective in patients with chronic pain than tricyclic antidepressants.[13] In patients with chronic pain in whom anxiety is an important feature, antipsychotic agents in small doses (such as haloperidol 1 to 2 mg twice a day) may be effective in controlling both pain and anxiety. In patients with chronic pain secondary to injuries to the central or peripheral nervous system, such as postherpetic neuralgia or phantom-limb syndrome, anticonvulsants may be helpful. Carbamazepine (300 to 1200 mg daily), phenytoin (300 mg daily), or clonazepam (1 to 3 mg daily) should be tried.

Nonpharmacologic therapy of chronic pain syndromes includes numerous different techniques. Nondestructive procedures should be tried first, and the choice of therapies should be dictated both by the cause of the patient's pain and the skill and experience of the physician in providing some of these techniques. For patients with intractable or severe pain syndromes, multidisciplinary pain clinics provide consultation and treatment from teams of physicians experienced in treating chronic pain.[14] Noninvasive techniques that attempt to increase central pain-inhibitory stimuli include hypnosis, biofeedback, and relaxation training. Hypnosis is more successful in the alleviation of acute rather than chronic pain. Biofeedback trains patients to control tension by teaching techniques to change physiologic parameters. Relaxation training, which involves progressive muscle relaxation, has become a popular and often successful adjunct to other therapies used in managing chronic pain.

Several neurologic techniques are available to interrupt the transmission of pain from peripheral nerves to the CNS. Some of these techniques are an attempt to stimulate large afferent nerve fibers that inhibit the transmission of signals along A-delta and smaller type C pain fibers. Simply rubbing the skin around a painful area excites these large afferent fibers and reduces pain. Battery-powered transcutaneous nerve stimulators (TENS) that apply continuous or intermittent stimuli to areas of injury to reduce pain are available. These stimulators are helpful in the management of phantom-limb pain, chronic radiculopathies, and other peripheral nerve injuries but have been shown to be ineffective in low back pain.[15] Acupuncture, introduced from Chinese medical practice, has been advocated for use in the management of chronic pain. Needles, placed into the skin, often at sites remote from the pain, provide stimulation when twirled or when an electrical impulse is applied through the needles. However, the mechanism of action and the effectiveness of acupuncture have not yet been definitively demonstrated in controlled trials. Peripheral nerve blocks, performed by anesthesiologists using injections of either anesthetic agents or neurolytic agents, can achieve short- and intermediate-term pain control. These techniques can also be used in ablating nerve root pain by injection into the subarachnoid space. These techniques should be performed only by physicians experienced in their use, since the injection of neurolytic agents such as phenol into the spinal column can result in serious permanent damage.

Finally several invasive neurosurgical procedures, including percutaneous spinothalamic cordotomy and cingulotomy—interruption of the cingulum bundle and its limb projections into the frontal lobe of the brain—have been used in the treatment of severe, intractable chronic pain that has not responded to any other therapies. Candidates for these neurosurgical procedures should have failed all other modalities and have had a full psychiatric evaluation to eliminate a psychogenic cause for the chronic pain.

## References

1. Fields HL: *Pain,* New York, 1987, McGraw-Hill.
2. Wall PD, Melzack RE: *Textbook of Pain,* ed 3, Edinburgh, 1994, Churchill Livingstone.
3. Rueler JB, Girard DE, Nardone DA: The chronic pain syndrome: misconceptions and management, *Ann Intern Med* 93:588-596, 1980.
4. Classification of chronic pain: descriptions of chronic pain syndromes and definitions of pain terms, *Pain,* suppl 3:S1-S225, 1986.
5. Marks RM, Sacher EJ: Undertreatment of medical inpatients with narcotic analgesics, *Ann Intern Med* 78:173, 1973.
6. Sriwatanakul K, Weis OF, Alloza JL, et al: Analysis of narcotic analgesic usage in the treatment of postoperative pain, *JAMA* 250:926, 1983.
7. Miller RR, Jick H: Clinical effects of meperidine in hospitalized patients, *J Clin Pharmacol* 18:180, 1978.
8. Cleeland CS, Gonin R, Hatfield AK, et al: Pain and its treatment in outpatients with metastatic cancer, *N Engl J Med* 330:592, 1994.
9. White PF: Use of patient-controlled analgesia for management of acute pain, *JAMA* 259:243, 1988.

10. McGivney WT, Crooks GM: The care of patients with severe chronic pain in terminal illness, *JAMA* 251:1182, 1984.
11. Foley KM: The treatment of cancer pain, *N Engl J Med* 313:84-95, 1985.
12. Jacox A, Carr DB, Payne R, et al: *Clinical practice guidelines number 9: Management of cancer pain*, U.S. Dept. of Health and Human Services Public Health Service, Agency for Health Care Policy and Research (AHCPR Publication No. 94-0592), 1994.
13. Max MB, Lynch SA, Muir J, et al: Effects of desipramine, amitriptyline, and fluoxetine on pain in diabetic neuropathy, *N Engl J Med* 296:712, 1992.
14. Hallett EC, Pilowsky I: Response to treatment in multidisciplinary pain clinic, *Pain* 12:365-374, 1982.
15. Deyo RA, Walsh NE, Martin DC, et al: A controlled trial of transcutaneous stimulation electrical nerve stimulation (TENS) and exercise for chronic low back pain, *N Engl J Med* 322:1627, 1990.

# Chapter 50

# *Diabetes*

Jennifer Daley
John T. Harrington

Diabetes mellitus afflicts approximately 2.5% of Americans. In addition, another 3% of the population has glucose intolerance without overt diabetes. Patients with diabetes mellitus may exhibit physiologic and metabolic abnormalities of glucose metabolism as well as chronic diabetic syndromes that affect numerous end organs. The common feature of all diabetic syndromes is abnormal glucose metabolism, characterized by the inability of the patient to dispose appropriately of a glucose load because of relative or absolute insulin deficiency. Protean in its clinical manifestations, diabetes mellitus ranges in severity from mild glucose intolerance during the stress of an infection or surgery to severe glucose intolerance with retinopathy, nephropathy, and advanced, premature atherosclerosis. In this chapter, we briefly review the two major types of diabetes, insulin-dependent diabetes mellitus (IDDM) and non–insulin dependent diabetes mellitus (NIDDM).[1] We then address in detail some of the more common questions for which we are consulted in our outpatient and inpatient practice.

## OVERVIEW OF THE TWO MAJOR FORMS OF DIABETES MELLITUS

Most patients with diabetes fall into one of two general categories. Patients with classic insulin-dependent diabetes mellitus (IDDM) are also known as juvenile-onset, ketosis-prone, or type I diabetics and constitute only 5% or so of all diabetics. Patients with non–insulin dependent diabetes mellitus (NIDDM), the most commonly encountered diabetics, constitute 85% to 90% of all diabetics.[2] Other terms for NIDDM include maturity-onset diabetes, type II, or stable diabetes. Insulin-dependent diabetes and non–insulin dependent diabetes have distinctly different causes, patterns of inheritance, age of onset, and typical clinical characteristics (Table 50-1).

Insulin-dependent diabetics typically present between 10 and 20 years of age with polydipsia, polyuria, rapid weight loss, occasionally a craving for sweets, and, not infrequently, acute diabetic ketoacidosis. The insulin-dependent diabetic develops an absolute lack of insulin

**Table 50-1.** *Comparison of insulin-dependent diabetes and non-insulin dependent diabetes*

| | Insulin-dependent diabetes | Non-insulin dependent diabetes |
|---|---|---|
| Age at onset | Childhood or adolescence 7 to 18 years | Midlife: 45 to 85 years |
| Symptoms at onset | Polydipsia, polyuria, weight loss, weakness, acute ketoacidosis | Polydipsia, polyuria, weight gain, usually obese |
| Pathophysiologic characteristics | Absolute lack of insulin from pancreatic beta-cell destruction | Decrease in pancreatic beta-cell function Peripheral insulin resistance |
| Causes | Autoimmune beta-cell destruction, genetic susceptibility, induced by viral infection | Genetic susceptibility |
| Treatment | Diet Insulin | Weight loss Diet Sulfonylureas Insulin |
| Ketoacidosis | Yes | No |
| Hyperosmolar states | Yes | Yes |

secretion within 12 to 18 months of onset of disease. Genetic susceptibility to IDDM is transmitted on chromosome 6 near the major histocompatibility complex; patients with this susceptibility appear to develop an autoimmune response, perhaps virally induced, to the insulin-producing beta cells of the pancreas. Because of their absolute lack of insulin secretion, patients with insulin-dependent diabetes require insulin therapy throughout their lives. Major chronic diabetic complications occur frequently. These patients are at substantial risk for development of blindness, premature aggressive atherosclerosis, and renal failure 20 to 30 years after the onset of disease.

Non-insulin dependent diabetes, a more heterogeneous disease, is characterized by impaired release of insulin from beta cells as well as peripheral tissue insensitivity to the action of insulin.[3] Prevalence for non-insulin dependent diabetes mellitus in this and subsequent decades is projected to be 10%. The typical non-insulin dependent diabetic is a 40- to 60-year-old overweight individual who has recently gained 10 to 30 pounds. Polydypsia and polyuria are common symptoms in the non–insulin dependent diabetic. Occasionally the patient may have experienced some weight loss after the onset of polydypsia and polyuria. Other common symptoms include an increase in soft-tissue infections, such as cellulitis or vulvovaginal candidiasis, that are refractory to therapy. Most non–insulin dependent diabetics never experience ketoacidosis and present with clinical manifestations of hyperglycemia or with one of the major chronic diabetic syndromes, such as microangiopathic peripheral vascular disease of the lower extremities, peripheral neuropathy, and "silent" myocardial infarction. These diabetics do not require insulin except during periods of stress (such as surgery, infection, acute myocardial infarction) and are best managed with a combination of diet, weight loss, and oral hypoglycemic agents.

Rarely, diabetes mellitus is caused by other problems or diseases, such as pancreatic resection for pancreatic pseudocyst or for carcinoma of the pancreas, severe pancreatic trauma, or infiltrative diseases such as hemochromatosis. Diabetes mellitus also may be found in association with other endocrine diseases that alter glucose homeostasis, such as Cushing's syndrome, acromegaly, or pheochromocytoma, or medications that unmask diabetes (such as thiazides, glucocorticoids).

## DIAGNOSIS OF DIABETES MELLITUS

A formal glucose tolerance test is rarely indicated to make the diagnosis of diabetes mellitus. Most insulin-dependent diabetics present with polydypsia and polyuria attributable to pronounced hyperglycemia and glucosuria. The patient with ketoacidosis, may complain of nausea or vomiting or may present with alterations in mental status and abdominal pain. The asymptomatic non–insulin dependent diabetic is most often detected by routine screening during an annual checkup. Although most multichannel screening is done in the fasting state, a screening blood glucose level is best obtained 2 hours after a large breakfast is eaten. Blood glucose levels of less than 120 mg/dL (2 hours post cibum) eliminate the presence of diabetes. A fasting blood glucose of greater than 140 mg/dL is diagnostic of diabetes.

Infrequently we are asked to pursue the diagnosis of diabetes in a patient with a normal fasting blood glucose level and some clinical syndrome suggestive of occult diabetes mellitus (such as lower-extremity microvascular ulcers). In these cases, a formal oral glucose tolerance test (75 to 100 g of glucose) may be indicated. The patient should have an oral intake of more than 200 g of carbohydrate daily for 3 days before the glucose tolerance test. Unstressed healthy individuals should have a blood glucose level below 110 mg/dL before glucose ingestion; blood glucose levels should be less than 160 mg/dL at 1 hour and less than 120 mg/dL at 3 hours. These criteria reflect normal glucose tolerance for young and middle-aged patients. Glucose tolerance decreases with age; a 1-hour value of 180 mg/dL and a 2-hour value of 150 mg/dL are normal for patients over 70 years of age.

Patients whose values are greater than the upper limits of normal but who do not have symptomatic hyperglycemia are designated as having impaired glucose tolerance. Glucose tolerance can be affected by stress, anxiety, infection, hypokalemia, and prior fasting or carbohydrate deprivation. The results of any formal glucose tolerance test should be interpreted in the light of these factors.

# INITIATING AND MONITORING THERAPY IN THE NONACUTE DIABETIC

By definition, insulin-dependent diabetics require therapy with insulin and diet. Occasionally in the insulin-dependent diabetic, a brief "honeymoon" of 3 to 18 months occurs after the initial episode of hyperglycemia. During this interval the patient may require little or no insulin, but ultimately the pancreatic beta cells cease functioning and the patient requires insulin. Many non–insulin dependent diabetics, most of whom are overweight, can be treated by diet alone. Many non–insulin dependent diabetics who are motivated to lose weight can achieve good control of their serum glucose with a weight loss of as little as 10 to 15 pounds. If they can't, oral hypoglycemic agents are available. New-onset non–insulin dependent diabetics who have lost a considerable amount of weight or in whom ketonuria is noted initially require therapy with insulin.

## Diet

Dietary therapy is the *cornerstone* of the treatment of all diabetics. The principles of dietary management for the non–insulin dependent diabetic are the same as for an insulin-dependent diabetic; given the increased risk of cardiovascular disease, a low-fat, low-cholesterol diet is important for both insulin-dependent and non–insulin dependent diabetics. Obese diabetics should be instructed in a reducing regimen. Weight loss of as little as 10 to 15 pounds may lead to a significant improvement in the control of blood glucose levels and the symptoms of hyperglycemia in the obese non–insulin dependent diabetic.[4] Caloric requirements for all diabetics must be determined by the level of daily activity. All diabetics require a meal schedule of three meals a day at fixed times as well as midafternoon and bedtime snacks. General dietary recommendations include a well-balanced diet that avoids concentrated sweets and beverages and that is high in polyunsaturated fats, rather than saturated animal fats. Caloric intake should be balanced so that 40% of the daily kilocalories allowed are in the noon meal and afternoon snack, 40% are in the dinner meal and bedtime snack, and 20% are at breakfast. A careful dietary history should be obtained from all diabetics to accommodate the patient's food preferences, activity levels, and eating habits. Extensive patient education by a trained dietician or nurse practitioner familiar with the principles of diabetic dietary management is extremely helpful in promoting patient management, education, and compliance. Principles of diabetic dietary management and meal planning guides are available from the American Diabetes Association.

## Insulin

Many insulin preparations are available for use in the treatment of insulin-dependent diabetics and non–insulin dependent diabetics who require insulin therapy. The use of single-component or single-peak insulin from both pork and beef reduces the induction of antibody-related insulin resistance as does the use of the human insulin (Humulin), a product of recombinant DNA technology. Near total transition to the use of human insulin has occurred in recent years.

Insulin regimens must be tailored to the individual patient's exercise level, caloric intake, and metabolic requirements. The goal of insulin therapy is to mimic a normal physiologic pattern of insulin secretion in response to diet and to exercise. Some non–insulin dependent diabetics require only a single injection of long-acting insulin in the morning before breakfast. Diabetics who have had the disease for several years require the addition of a small dose of regular (short-acting) insulin to intermediate- or long-acting insulin before breakfast and a second injection of an intermediate-acting insulin before dinner. This "split-dose" regimen better mimics the normal physiologic pattern of insulin secretion.

The management of diabetic patients, particularly those requiring split-dose insulin regimens, has been improved by the availability of blood glucose self-monitoring techniques. Physicians and patients had previously relied on urine testing to assess the adequacy of blood glucose control, but urinary levels do not always accurately reflect blood glucose levels. The use of blood glucose monitors (reflectometer) by the patient has made the adjustment of insulin doses much more accurate. When insulin doses are being adjusted initially or in response to a change in a diabetic's lifestyle, blood glucose levels can be monitored before each meal, at bedtime, and occasionally, in the middle of the night if hypoglycemia is suspected.

The major complication of insulin therapy is hypoglycemia. Minor hypoglycemic reactions, characterized by mood changes or by difficulty in mentation, may be followed by hunger and signs of sympathetic overactivity with sweating, tachycardia, and anxiety. Treatment is the oral administration of carbohydrate, such as candy or fruit juice. Severe hypoglycemic reactions include unconsciousness and convulsions. Subcutaneously or intramuscularly administered glucagon (1 mg) can be given by the patient, if conscious, or by family members. Hypoglycemia that occurs in an emergency room or office setting can be treated intravenously with 1 mg of glucagon or by the intravenous injection of 25 mL of 50% glucose (12.5 g). The major physiologic reaction to hypoglycemia is a rebound hyperglycemia known as the *Somogyi effect*.

Patients who experience nocturnal hypoglycemia may have rebound hyperglycemia in the morning with elevated blood glucose values and glycosuria. Physicians and patients unfamiliar with the Somogyi effect may unknowingly increase insulin to "cover" the rebound hyperglycemia, thus increasing the nocturnal hypoglycemia. Nocturnal hypoglycemia may be documented by obtaining a 3 AM blood glucose specimen, and the treatment of early morning rebound hyperglycemia is a reduction of the insulin dose. A gradual decrease of insulin activity in the early morning hours may also result in morning hyperglycemia. This "dawn" phenomenon is not preceded by hypoglycemia and again can be distinguished from the Somogyi effect by obtaining a 3 AM blood glucose specimen.

## Oral hypoglycemic agents

Oral hypoglycemic agents (sulfonylureas) stimulate the secretion of insulin from the pancreas and increase the number of peripheral insulin receptors. Because sulfonylureas work by increasing pancreatic secretion of insulin, they are not indicated in the treatment of insulin-dependent diabetics who no longer produce insulin endogenously. Treatment of non–insulin dependent diabetics with sulfonylureas has been controversial since 1970 when the University Group Diabetes Program (UGDP) reported a higher incidence of sudden death among diabetics treated with tolbutamide than among those treated with insulin or placebo.[5] Reexamination of this issue in recent years has indicated that treatment with sulfonylureas can be beneficial in some patients. Non–insulin dependent diabetics in midlife, either of normal weight or moderately obese, respond best to treatment with oral hypoglycemic agents. In contrast, non–insulin dependent diabetics who are underweight respond better to treatment with insulin.

Oral hypoglycemic agents always should be used with dietetic therapy and an exercise program. Obese non–insulin dependent diabetics should be encouraged to lose weight because the efficacy of sulfonylureas is enhanced by even a moderate amount of weight loss. Six sulfonylureas are currently available for use in the United States. Tolbutamide, chlorpropamide, acetohexamide, and tolazamide are first-generation sulfonylureas. The selection of one of these agents depends on several factors, including the patient's age, the use of other medications, and the presence of chronic liver or kidney disease. The drugs differ from each other in their duration of action and mechanism of drug elimination. Chlorpropamide (100 to 400 mg daily), for example, has a long duration of action (24 to 48 hours) and can be given on a once-a-day basis. Chlorpropamide is excreted unchanged by the kidneys and therefore is contraindicated in patients with chronic renal insufficiency. Patients receiving chlorpropamide should be monitored carefully for hypoglycemia (and hyponatremia as well). Tolbutamide (250 to 2000 mg daily), the most commonly used hypoglycemic agent, has a shorter duration of action (6 to 12 hours) and must be given twice a day to achieve tight control of glucose levels. Tolbutamide is excreted by the liver.

Glipizide (2.5 to 30 mg daily) and glyburide (2.5 to 20 mg daily), the two second-generation sulfonylureas, have durations of action of 24 hours or more and can be given in single or divided doses. Some of the drug interactions and complications of the first-generation sulfonylureas are not observed with these second-generation drugs, and they have become the first line of therapy for diabetics who are beginning oral therapy. Occasionally, patients who have shown no response to first-generation agents do respond to the second-generation drugs. Drug interactions with all the sulfonylureas are common in patients taking thiazide diuretics, barbiturates, and anticoagulants such as warfarin; diabetics receiving these drugs with oral hypoglycemic agents should be carefully monitored and drug doses adjusted appropriately. Sulfonylureas are contraindicated in diabetics who are allergic to sulfonamide compounds and in the pregnant diabetic. Non-insulin dependent diabetics with acute medical problems such as myocardial infarction or overwhelming infection usually require insulin therapy; oral hypoglycemic agents are of little value during the acute phases of these illnesses (Table 50-2). Metformin, a biguanide that acts by decreasing glucose production in the liver and increasing glucose uptake, has recently become available and may be used in conjunction with sulfonylureas. Acarbose, a recently approved intestinal $\alpha$-glucosidase inhibitor, delays glucose absorption, thus resulting in lower plasma glucose levels. It also can be used together with sulfonylureas.

One in five non-insulin dependent diabetics who begin therapy with oral agents will fail to respond at maximum doses (primary failures). Another 10% to 15% of diabetics treated with oral agents will fail to respond to oral agent therapy each year (secondary failures). These patients require insulin therapy. Insulin therapy may also be used as a first-line treatment of non-insulin dependent diabetics who fail to lose weight. Some patients prefer to use oral agents, however, and these may be tried first.

### The controversy over tight metabolic control
Debate over how tightly insulin-dependent diabetics should control their blood glucose levels has been lessened by the results of the

**Table 50-2.** *Orally administered hypoglycemic agents*

| Name | Daily dose | Duration of action |
|------|-----------|--------------------|
| **FIRST-GENERATION SULFONYLUREAS** | | |
| Chlorpropamide | 100-500 mg in single dose | 36 hours |
| Tobutamide | 0.5-3.0 g in divided doses | 6-12 hours |
| Tolazamide | 0.1-1.0 g in single or divided doses | 12-24 hours |
| Acetohexamide | 0.25-1.5 g in single or divided doses | 12-18 hours |
| **SECOND-GENERATION SULFONYLUREAS** | | |
| Glipizide | 5-40 mg in single or divided doses | 12-18 hours |
| Glyburide | 2.5-20 mg in single or divided doses | 18-24 hours |
| **BIGUANIDE** | | |
| Metformin | 500-850 mg b.i.d. | 6-12 hours |

publication of the results of the Diabetes Control and Complications Trial (DCCT).[6] Intensive therapy with multiple insulin injections (3 or more a day) and frequent self-monitoring (4 to 7 times a day) to achieve preprandial glucose levels and hemoglobin $A_{1c}$ levels in the nondiabetic range decreased the risk of development and progression of diabetic neuropathy, retinopathy, and nephropathy by 40% to 76% over 7 years. The major side effect, however, was a threefold increase in the incidence of hypoglycemia, and patients in the study did not achieve nondiabetic levels of hemoglobin $A_{1c}$. Current recommendations from the DCCT and the American Diabetes Association endorse intensive therapy for all insulin-dependent diabetics. Intensive patient education, support, and motivation are required to achieve the recommended levels of insulin administration, self-monitoring, and blood glucose levels.

The role of "tight" glycemic control for non–insulin dependent diabetics and the prevention of long-term complications is not clear, although definitive results of a controlled trial should be forthcoming.[7] We recommend maintaining blood glucose levels as close to normal as possible in the non–insulin dependent diabetic 40 to 55 years of age at the onset of diabetes. These patients should be carefully monitored for hypoglycemic reactions. Older, non–insulin dependent diabetics who have the onset of diabetes in the seventh or eighth decade do not require such vigorous control of blood glucose levels.

Hemoglobin $A_{1c}$, a glucose-conjugated hemoglobin in which approximatley 7% of hemoglobin is combined with carbohydrate at the N-terminal of the beta chain, can be used to monitor the overall efficacy of glucose control. Hemoglobin $A_{1c}$ levels are helpful in the assessment of the average blood glucose level for the previous 8 weeks of insulin therapy and diabetes management. Other commonly available tests such as the concentration of glycosylated albumin or serum protein (such as fructosamine) reflect glucose levels over a 20-day period.

The introduction of innovative insulin-delivery systems has changed the management of patients who are trying to achieve normal or near-normal levels of blood glucose. Insulin-infusion pumps that deliver insulin continuously subcutaneously or intravenously have been used in recent years in insulin-dependent diabetics to achieve near-normal glucose levels. The patient receives a low-dose continuous infusion of insulin and then increases insulin infusion in response to measured blood glucose levels or to meals. Diabetics with insulin-infusion pumps measure blood glucose levels frequently and adjust their insulin requirements as necessary. Complications of the infusion pump include frequent episodes of hypoglycemia, occasional episodes of ketoacidosis, and infection at the site of the infusion. Failure of the battery-driven infusion pumps often results in episodes of ketoacidosis. Insulin-infusion pumps are most appropriate for insulin-dependent diabetics who are highly motivated to control their blood glucose levels and are willing to measure their blood glucose levels frequently.

# DIABETIC EMERGENCIES

In addition to hypoglycemic coma from insulin, the diabetic may develop other acute diabetic emergencies. The first, diabetic ketoacidosis, is the result of insulin insufficiency. Fatty tissues, reacting as if in a prolonged fasting state, release free fatty acids, and the liver takes up circulating amino acids and free fatty acids, thereby generating maximal amounts of glucose and keto acids. Plasma levels of glucose and keto acids rise dramatically with resulting ketonuria and glucosuria. The osmotic load of glucose and ketones excreted in the urine leads to polyuria, intravascular volume depletion, ketoacidosis, and coma. Excessive lipolysis and the production of keto acids is avoided in the non-insulin dependent diabetic who still produces some insulin. However, if the patient becomes dehydrated in the face of profound hyperglycemia, intravascular volume depletion and hyperosmolarity occur. In the situation of the non-insulin dependent diabetic, typically the elderly, the resultant diabetic crisis is hyperglycemic hyperosmolar coma.

## Management of diabetic ketoacidosis

The primary concern in the management of a patient with acute diabetic ketoacidosis is the replacement of salt and water deficits,[8] though the underlying metabolic defect in diabetic ketoacidosis is insufficient insulin secretion. Patients with acute diabetic ketoacidosis present with hypovolemia, incipient or overt shock, dehydration, and Kussmaul's hyperventilation. Precipitating events include noncompliance with the prescribed regimen, poor patient education about the need to increase insulin dosages in the face of acute infection or stress, or the presence of previously unidentified sources of sepsis or infection, including cholecystitis, pneumonia, or urinary tract infection. Silent myocardial infarction also can precipitate diabetic ketoacidosis.

Management of diabetic ketoacidosis begins with a rapid assessment of the history and physical examination. Blood samples are obtained for the measurement of glucose, BUN, creatinine, electrolytes, and serum ketones, and urine samples are obtained for glucose and ketone measurements. At the same time these samples are being obtained, a large-bore intravenous line should be inserted. The patient should have isotonic saline solution administered immediately, and unless the patient is in definite congestive heart failure or is anuric (unusual in the patient with diabetic ketoacidosis), the isotonic saline should be administered rapidly (approximately 10 mL/min for the first hour). Average fluid deficits in patients with diabetic ketoacidosis are 4 to 6 liters. One of the goals of prompt treatment should be the administration of approximately 1 liter of normal saline per hour during each of the first 3 hours of therapy or until blood pressure has returned to normal.

In addition to being severely volume depleted, patients with diabetic ketoacidosis are also profoundly total body potassium depleted because of the accompanying metabolic acidosis and osmotic diuresis. The average potassium deficit is 300 mEq (range, 200 to 600 mEq). In acidosis, potassium shifts from intracellular fluid to extracellular fluid, thereby producing hyperkalemia despite this total body potassium deficit. Potassium, in the form of potassium chloride or potassium phosphate, should be administered unless the serum potassium level is greater than 5.0 mEq/L. Unless the patient has known renal insufficiency, 40 mEq of potassium should be given to the patient every hour until the deficit is repaired. We recommend administration of potassium chloride during the first hour and replacement with potassium phosphate during the second hour because diabetics also are typically phosphate depleted.

Patients with diabetic ketoacidosis also should have arterial blood gas measurements obtained on arrival in the emergency room. Once the arterial pH is known, consideration should be given to the administration of alkali. Although controversial, we recommend the administration of small amounts of sodium bicarbonate (1 ampule equals 50 mEq) in patients in whom the arterial pH is below 7.15 or in patients in whom the serum bicarbonate level is less than 8 mEq/L. The goal of treatment with alkali is not to completely correct the acidemia but to prevent further declines in pH and to return the arterial pH to approximately 7.2. Further administration of fluids, potassium, and insulin allows the metabolism of excess keto acids in the blood, thereby restoring serum bicarbonate to normal.

The continuous intravenous infusion of insulin, by use of an initial bolus of regular insulin (0.2 units/kg) followed by a constant infusion of 0.1 units/kg/hour, is both a safe and an easily controllable way of reducing blood glucose levels.[9] Intravenous infusion assures a constant rate of delivery and a gradual decrease in levels of glucose and keto acids. When the infusion of insulin is stopped, the patient should be given a subcutaneous injection of insulin to prevent rebound hyperglycemia and ketoacidosis. An effective response of blood glucose levels to the intravenous infusion of insulin is approximately a 10% to 15% decrease in blood glucose levels every hour. When blood glucose levels have fallen to the range of 200 to 300 mg/dL, glucose should be administered as a mixture of half normal saline and 5% dextrose in water to prevent hypoglycemia.

We cannot overemphasize the importance of constant observation of the patient in diabetic ketoacidosis and the use of a detailed flow chart that records the patient's clinical condition, vital signs, serum glucose, BUN, creatinine, electrolytes, arterial blood gases, infusion of intravenous fluids, potassium chloride, potassium phosphate, sodium bicarbonate, and insulin. Patients with diabetic ketoacidosis should have a physician in attendance and be examined on an hourly basis with a review of their laboratory values and clinical condition. The typical patient with diabetic ketoacidosis becomes stable over a period of 3 to 8 hours. An intensive search for precipitating causes should be begun as soon as the patient is hemodynamically stable.

## Hyperosmolar coma

Patients with hyperosmolar hyperglycemic coma are typically elderly, non-insulin dependent diabetics with severe intravascular volume depletion and an underlying acute stress such as pneumonia, urinary tract infection, stroke, or myocardial infarction. Blood glucose levels may range from 500 to 2000 mg/dL. The goal of therapy is replacement of critical intravascular fluid and restoration of extracellular fluid volume. Initial treatment should be 2 liters of isotonic saline infused over a period of 2 to 3 hours. Thereafter, hypotonic saline (½ normal saline) can be used if the patient remains significantly hyperosmolar. The patient's total body fluid deficit may be as much as 5 to 6 liters. Volume replacement should take place expeditiously over the first few hours. Thereafter, volume replacement should be carried out more slowly. In elderly patients, in whom fluid overload and congestive heart failure are concerns, careful monitoring of volume replacement may require the placement of central venous monitoring. Insulin requirements in hyperosmolar coma are generally quite small. In most patients, volume replacement with isotonic saline alone results in a prompt decrease in the blood glucose. Sometimes as little as 5 to 10 units of insulin administered subcutaneously results in a significant decrease in blood glucose levels; a low-dose continuous infusion of insulin is also effective. As in patients with diabetic ketoacidosis, potassium levels must be monitored and potassium replacement initiated if appropriate. A reduction in blood glucose levels to normal over 12 to 18 hours is the goal of therapy and avoids rapid shifts of fluid and glucose from extracellular to intracellular spaces.

# END-ORGAN DIABETIC COMPLICATIONS

The acute metabolic complications of diabetics (such as hyperglycemia and hyperosmolarity) reverse with the administration of fluids and insulin over a period of hours to a few days. Physiologic changes from hyperglycemia, such as the glycosylation of hemoglobin, gradually reverse with the control of hyperglycemia. Chronic end-organ changes of diabetes are less clearly attributable to hypoinsulinemia. We will review the major diabetic complications and address areas in which there have been recent advances in diagnosis or therapy.

## Atherosclerosis

Atherosclerosis of large and medium-sized vessels is much more common in diabetics who have had insulin-dependent diabetes for more than 20 years than in age- and sex-matched controls. Diabetics are much more susceptible to myocardial infarction, peripheral vascular disease, and stroke. The management of these common complications does not differ significantly from that of patients without diabetes. The physician, however, should be aware that diabetics who suffer stroke, myocardial infarction, and the consequences of large-vessel peripheral vascular disease have much higher levels of morbidity and mortality than patients without diabetes mellitus.

Microangiopathic changes of the capillaries of the eye, kidney, and skin are unique to diabetics. A growing body of evidence indicates that the extent and the severity of microangiopathy correlate with the extent and the duration of hyperglycemia. In addition to an increased incidence of cataracts and of glaucoma, diabetics develop exudative and proliferative retinopathy. Non–insulin dependent diabetics more typically develop exudative diabetic retinopathy. Proliferative retinopathy develops in both insulin-dependent and non–insulin dependent diabetics. Photocoagulation therapy can have dramatic results in diabetics with proliferative retinopathy, and both insulin-dependent and non–insulin dependent diabetics should be seen annually by an ophthalmologist. The majority of insulin-dependent diabetics with diabetes for longer than 20 years also develop microangiopathic changes in the renal glomerulus. The diabetic typically develops end-stage renal failure within 3 to 5 years after the development of overt proteinuria. Blood pressure control, low-protein diets, and treatment with angiotensin-converting enzyme inhibitors may slow the progression to end-stage renal disease.[10,11] Many insulin-dependent diabetics with end-stage renal disease have been successfully treated with hemodialysis and renal transplantation. We suggest transplantation if at all possible.

Almost all diabetics develop some involvement of the nervous system within 5 to 10 years of the diagnosis of clinical diabetes. The most common form of neurologic involvement is a peripheral neuropathy, usually confined to the lower extremities and characterized by painful paresthesias and nocturnal pain. Other manifestations of neurologic involvement include bladder dysfunction and autonomic nervous system involvement with delayed gastric emptying, malabsorption, impotence in males, and orthostatic hypotension. The treatment of the nervous system complications of diabetes is frustrating. Painful neuropathy of the lower extremities can be treated with amitriptyline (50 to 100 mg at bedtime) with some success.

# PERIOPERATIVE MANAGEMENT OF THE DIABETIC PATIENT

Frequently, surgical colleagues request consultation about the management of the diabetic patient around the time of surgery. Control of hyperglycemia in the perioperative period decreases the chance of infection in the diabetic. Careful attention should be given to the maintenance of blood glucose levels under 200 mg/dL. Insulin-dependent diabetics should receive half their usual morning dose of insulin before anesthesia is performed, and an infusion of 5% dextrose and water should be given throughout surgery. The balance of the morning insulin dose should be given after the procedure is completed, and blood glucose should be measured frequently in the 24 hours after surgery. We recommend obtaining a blood glucose level every 6 hours in the 24 hours after the surgery; elevations of blood glucose can be treated with appropriate intravenous doses of regular insulin. Once oral intake has been reinstituted, the patient's insulin can be adjusted for current metabolic needs, level of activity, and caloric intake.

# THE MANAGEMENT OF THE PREGNANT DIABETIC

Insulin-dependent diabetics who become pregnant have a higher rate of fetal loss and of congenital abnormalities in the fetus and are more susceptible to eclampsia, hydramnios, and premature delivery.[12,13] Strict maintenance of glucose levels in the normal range during the course of pregnancy considerably reduces the incidence of these complications. The goal of therapy of the diabetic during pregnancy is to maintain glucose levels as close as possible to that of the nondiabetic pregnant woman. Normal glucose levels in pregnant nondiabetics vary with each trimester of pregnancy, and the pregnant diabetic should be managed by a physician who is experienced in the management of such patients. Insulin requirements may decrease in the first trimester of pregnancy. Blood glucose levels become more variable in the second trimester of pregnancy, and ketoacidosis should be avoided. Most pregnant diabetics need multiple split-dose injections and daily frequent blood glucose levels measured during their pregnancy; pregnant diabetics have been successfully treated with insulin-infusion pumps. The primary goal of the treatment of the pregnant diabetic is to maintain the pregnancy until such a time as fetal lung maturity has been achieved. Physicians should keep in mind that insulin requirements drop greatly in the hours after delivery. Insulin dosages should be rapidly and greatly reduced to avoid hypoglycemia in the immediate postpartum period.

## References

1. National Diabetes Data Group: Classification and diagnosis of diabetes and other categories of glucose intolerance, *Diabetes* 28:1039 1056, 1979.
2. Harris MI, Haden WC, Knowler WC, et al: Prevalence of diabetes and impaired glucose tolerance and plasma glucose levels in U.S. population aged 20-74 yr, *Diabetes* 36:523, 1987.
3. Moller DE, Flier JS: Insulin resistance—mechanisms, syndromes, and implications, *N Engl J Med* 325:938, 1991.
4. Hadden DR, Montgomery DAD, Skelly RF, et al: Maturity onset diabetes mellitus: response to intensive dietary management, *Br Med J* 3:276, 1975.
5. University Group Diabetes Program: A study of the effects of hypoglycemic agents on vascular complications in patients with adult onset diabetes: supplementary report on nonfatal events in patients treated with tolbutamide, *Diabetes* 25:1129, 1976.
6. The Diabetes Control and Complications Trial Research Group: The effect of intensive treatment of diabetes on the development and progression of long-term complications in insulin-dependent diabetes mellitus, *N Eng J Med* 329:977, 1993.
7. Turner R, Cull C, Holman R: United Kingdom Prospective Diabetes Study 17: A 9-year update of a randomized controlled trial on the effect of improved metabolic control on complications in non–insulin dependent diabetes mellitus, *Ann Intern Med* 124:136, 1996.
8. Foster DW, McGarry JD: The metabolic derangements and treatment of diabetic ketoacidosis, *N Engl J Med* 309:159-169, 1983.

9. Page M, Alberti KGGM, Greenwood R, et al: Treatment of diabetic coma with continuous low-dose infusion of insulin, *Br Med J* 2:287, 1974.

10. Lewis EJ, Hunsicker LG, Bain RP, et al: The effect of angiotensin-converting-enzyme inhibition on diabetic nephropathy, *N Engl J Med* 329:1456, 1993.

11. Sano T, Kawamura T, Matsumae H, et al: Effects of long-term enalapril treatment of persistent micro-albuminuria in well-controlled hypertensive and normotensive NIDDM patients, *Diabetes Care* 17:420, 1994.

12. Freinkel N, Dooley SL, Metzger B: Care of the pregnant woman with insulin dependent diabetes mellitus, *N Engl J Med* 313:96-101, 1985.

13. Management of diabetes mellitus in pregnancy, *ACOG Technical Bull* 92:1, 1986 (American College of Obstetricians and Gynecologists).

# Chapter 51

# Hypertension

Jennifer Daley
John T. Harrington

Hypertension, the most significant risk factor for the development of cardiovascular disease and a leading cause of stroke, renal failure, and cardiac failure, affects 60 million Americans. Most patients with hypertension are evaluated and managed in office practices; the focus of this chapter, therefore, is on the ambulatory patient with hypertension. However, because a substantial minority of patients with newly diagnosed or poorly controlled hypertension is seen in hospital, the last section of this chapter is devoted to the management of hypertension in the hospitalized patient.

## HYPERTENSION IN THE OFFICE PRACTICE SETTING

### Evaluation

Patients with hypertension arrive at the internist's office by a variety of routes. They may be referred by surgical or subspecialty medical colleagues, or they may be referred from community or work related hypertension screening programs. Increasingly, patients who are aware through media campaigns of the long-term complications of untreated hypertension refer themselves for evaluation of hypertension.

**Confirming the presence of hypertension.** The first step in evaluating the patient with suspected hypertension is confirmation of the diagnosis and appropriate follow-up examinations of single measurements of elevated pressure. Blood pressure should be measured on a bared arm with the patient seated comfortably. Systolic and diastolic blood pressures should be recorded; a minimum of two measurements should be taken at each visit and the average recorded. A large-sized cuff must be used in obese individuals. Good evidence exists that casual blood pressure measurements are an accurate representation of a patient's true blood pressure and an accurate prediction of hypertensive complications. We do not use 24-hour blood pressure recordings routinely.

In adults the diagnosis of hypertension usually is confirmed when the average of at least two diastolic blood pressures on a minimum of two visits is 90 mm Hg or higher, or when the average of two or more

**Table 51-1.** *Classification of blood pressure*

| Range (mm Hg) | Category |
|---|---|
| **DIASTOLIC** | |
| <85 | Normal BP |
| 85-89 | High normal BP |
| 90-104 | Mild hypertension |
| 105-114 | Moderate hypertension |
| >115 | Severe hypertension |
| **SYSTOLIC (WHEN DIASTOLIC BP <90)** | |
| <140 | Normal |
| 140-159 | Borderline isolated systolic hypertension |
| >160 | Isolated systolic hypertension |

From The 1984 Report of the Joint National Committee on Detection, Evaluation, and Treatment of High Blood Pressure, *Arch Intern Med* 144:1045-1057, 1984.

systolic pressures is greater than 140 mm Hg. In fact, the World Health Organization (WHO) recommends three elevated blood pressure recordings over a 4-week period before making the diagnosis of hypertension.[1] The 1984 Joint National Committee on Detection, Evaluation, and Treatment of High Blood Pressure categorization of blood pressure is described in Table 51-1.[2] Recommendations for follow-up study of elevated blood pressures are presented in Table 51-2. Risk stratification

**Table 51-2.** *Recommended follow-up study for a single blood pressure measurement*

| Blood pressure (mm Hg) | Follow-up |
|---|---|
| **DIASTOLIC** | |
| 90-104 | Confirm within 2 months |
| 105-114 | Evaluate or refer for evaluation within 2 weeks |
| >115 | Evaluate or refer for evaluation immediately |
| **SYSTOLIC (WHEN DIASTOLIC BP <90)** | |
| 140-199 | Confirm within 2 months |
| >200 | Evaluate or refer for evaluation immediately |

Adapted from The 1984 Report of the Joint National Committee on Detection, Evaluation and Treatment of High Blood Pressure, *Arch Intern Med* 144:1045-1057, 1984.

for patients with hypertension also varies by age and sex. Highest risk groups are men younger than 45 years with blood pressures of 130/90 mm Hg or higher, men 45 years of age and older with blood pressures 140/95 mm Hg or higher, and all women with blood pressures of 160/95 mm Hg and higher. Patients whose diastolic blood pressures on repeat measurement are less than 85 mm Hg should have a blood pressure measurement repeated in 2 years; if the diastolic blood pressure is between 85 and 90 mm Hg, the blood pressure measurement should be repeated in 1 year, or sooner if the patient has an increased risk of developing further blood pressure elevations. Among the risk factors are a family history of hypertension or cardiovascular disease, obesity, black race, use of medications known to elevate blood pressure, or excessive alcohol consumption. Patients whose diastolic blood pressures are noted to be greater than 90 mm Hg on a subsequent measurement should be evaluated within 2 months; if the diastolic blood pressure is between 105 and 114 mm Hg, the patient should be evaluated within 2 weeks.

**Evaluation of the patient with confirmed diastolic hypertension.** Three questions must be answered in the patient with confirmed diastolic hypertension.

- Does the patient have evidence of end-organ damage from hypertension?
- Does the patient have additional risk factors for the development of cardiovascular disease?
- Does the patient have any evidence for reversible or secondary causes of hypertension?

More than 90% to 95% of patients with diastolic hypertension have primary, or essential, hypertension. A detailed medical history, physical examination, and a few judicious laboratory tests usually exclude or detect reversible or secondary causes of hypertension and also provide information to answer the first two questions.

The medical history should document any previous history of hypertension and its treatment, the severity and complications of hypertension (cardiovascular, renal, or cerebrovascular disease), and, as well, any history of other cardiovascular risk factors (obesity, smoking, hyperlipidemia, diabetes mellitus). Careful attention should be paid to clues to secondary hypertension. A careful drug history should be taken, since the leading cause of reversible hypertension is the use of medications, both prescription and over the counter. The physician should ask specifically about the use of oral contraceptives, thyroid hormones, nonsteroidal anti-inflammatory agents, estrogens, corticosteroids, nasal and oral decongestants, diet pills, tricyclic antidepressants, and over-the-counter medications containing nonsteroidal anti-inflammatory agents or adrenergic agonists. Other relatively important causes of secondary hypertension include renovascular disease, renal parenchymal disease, coarctation of the aorta, and primary hyperaldosteronism. Hypertension is more rarely caused by Cushing's syndrome, pheochromocytoma, hypothyroidism, or hyperthyroidism. The patient should be questioned carefully about sources of stress in the home or work-place, and a record should be made of personal habits, such as diet, excess sodium intake, weight gain, and alcohol or recreational drug use, that might have an influence on hypertension.

Physical examination of the hypertensive patient should focus on the search for end-organ damage and for clues to the presence of secondary hypertension. The examination should include the patient's weight, an examination of the fundi for evidence of hypertensive vascular changes, a neurologic examination, a detailed examination of the heart and lungs, an examination of the thyroid gland for evidence of enlargement, an examination of the abdomen for renal enlargement or abdominal bruits, and a vascular examination for evidence of peripheral vascular disease and coarctation of the aorta. Observation for the signs of Cushing's syndrome, hypothyroidism, hyperthyroidism, and pheochromocytoma also should be carried out.

Laboratory examination of the hypertensive patient has three purposes: (1) to exclude some of the secondary causes of hypertension, (2) to establish the presence or absence of other cardiovascular risk factors, and (3) to establish base-line values of the patient's biochemical profile that might be affected by hypertensive therapy. Controversy exists over the costs and benefits of diagnostic tests in the evaluation of the hypertensive patient, but we believe that complete blood count, serum potassium, serum creatinine or BUN, serum uric acid, fasting blood glucose, and total and high-density-lipoprotein (HDL) cholesterol should be measured; complete urinalysis should be performed; and an electrocardiogram (ECG) should be obtained. Further diagnostic evaluation must be tailored by the findings of significant end-organ damage, other cardiovascular risk factors, or possible secondary causes of hypertension found on initial evaluation.

## Treatment

**Involving the patient in the goals of therapy.** Once the presence of essential hypertension has been confirmed, the next critical step in the management of hypertension is to involve the patient in his or her own care. Patients need careful detailed explanations of the asymptomatic nature of most hypertension, the extent of their hypertension, and the risks associated with untreated hypertension. Involvement of the patient in making decisions regarding appropriate, convenient, and flexible schedules of treatment and follow-up exams for hypertension engages the patient as an ally in the long-term management of this asymptomatic chronic illness. Patients and physicians need constant reinforcement that the goal of therapy of hypertension is the reduction of the likelihood of serious cardiovascular disease by the reduction of elevated blood pressure while maintaining the patient's life and work as free of significant side effects of therapy as possible.

Asymptomatic patients often ask, "Why do I need my blood pressure lowered?" In patients with moderate (diastolic blood pressure, 105 to 114 mm Hg) or severe (DBP >115 mm Hg) hypertension, good evidence exists that drug therapy can reduce cardiovascular mortality and morbidity.[3,4] Several large studies have shown that patients with mild diastolic hypertension benefit from treatment, in reducing both cardiovascular morbidity and mortality.[5-8] We believe that all patients with sustained diastolic blood pressure greater than 100 mm Hg should be treated; usually we will treat patients with diastolic blood pressure levels greater than 95 mm Hg if other risk factors are present. We will return to this issue later. We will first discuss nondrug treatment and, subsequently, drug treatment of sustained diastolic hypertension.

Nonpharmacologic therapy of hypertension. Nonpharmacologic therapy of hypertension is used as sole treatment for mild hypertension and as an adjunct in patients who also take antihypertensive medications.[9] A variety of biofeedback and relaxation techniques have been shown to have a moderate sustained effect in the reduction of blood pressure in patients with mild hypertension.[10] These modalities have been used as initial steps in the management of patients with mild hypertension and no evidence of end-organ damages; however, these patients require frequent monitoring to assess the extent of blood pressure reduction and to anticipate the need for drug therapy if hypertension accelerates.

Obese hypertensive patients have been shown to have significant reductions in blood pressure with weight loss (approximately 2.3 mm Hg decrease in DBP per kilogram lost) independent of sodium restriction and regardless of whether ideal body weight is achieved.[11] Moderate salt restriction (daily intake of sodium of 2 to 4 g) may reduce blood pressure in some hypertensive patients, but this is not a universal phenomenon. Patients need to be monitored on an individual basis to assess their response to sodium restriction. Reduction of unsaturated fat in the diet may reduce cardiovascular risk by lowering serum cholesterol but has no antihypertensive effect. Similarly, hypertensive patients should be advised to avoid smoking to reduce further the risk of cardiovascular disease. Heavy or excessive alcohol use increases blood pressure in hypertensive patients and should be avoided.[12] Vigorous physical exercise and physical fitness, particularly in combination with weight reduction, has a beneficial effect on high blood pressure.

Drug therapy of hypertension. The ultimate goal of antihypertensive therapy is the prevention of cardiovascular morbidity and mortality: stroke, renal insufficiency, hypertensive cardiomyopathy, atherosclerotic cardiovascular disease, and peripheral vascular disease. More specifically, the strategic goal of treatment is to lower the diastolic blood pressure to 90 mm Hg or less in the absence of side effects with a drug regimen that is customized to the patient's lifestyle to encourage compliance.[13]

Drugs currently available for the treatment of hypertension include diuretics, sympatholytics, vasodilators, angiotensin-converting enzyme inhibitors, and calcium-channel blockers. Limitations of space prohibit a discussion of each drug currently available in each category. Physicians should be familiar with one or two drugs in each category for use in the hypertensive patient requiring drug therapy.

The availability of angiotensin-converting enzyme inhibitors and calcium-channel blockers in recent years has made the initial therapy for hypertension easier and reduced the incidence of side effects. Enalapril (5 to 40 mg/day) in single or twice a day doses is highly effective and well tolerated. Calcium-channel blockers such as diltiazem (60 to 120 mg/day) are also effective. Patients with evidence of autonomic hyperactivity are good candidates for single-drug therapy with beta-adrenergic receptor blockers (such as atenolol 50 to 100 mg daily). These drugs are also indicated in patients with concomitant symptomatic coronary artery disease and appear more successful in patients under 50 years of age. Thiazide diuretics in low or moderate doses (up to 50 mg per day of hydrochlorothiazide) are suitable for elderly patients, patients with asthma or peripheral vascular disease, black patients, and other patients with volume-dependent hypertension. Drug dosages should be increased over several weeks until the blood pressure goal is achieved, maximum drug dose is reached, or side effects occur.

If adequate blood pressure control is not achieved with single-drug therapy, two therapeutic possibilities exist. A diuretic may be combined with an angiotensin-converting enzyme inhibitor or beta-blocker therapy, or clonidine may be combined with a calcium-channel blocker. If blood pressure is not adequately controlled on these regimens, several questions must be asked before one progresses to another step. A careful review must be made for other factors that can result in poor blood pressure control. The patient should be questioned about suitability of, understanding of, and compliance with the drug regimen; a detailed drug history should be taken to look for drugs that may aggravate hypertension (see above). Reassessment of compliance with nonpharmacologic measures, in terms of excess sodium intake, weight gain, and excessive alcohol use, should be made. Lastly, a detailed review should be made of causes of secondary hypertension that may have emerged or been overlooked. This is especially true of patients with essential hypertension and atherosclerotic vascular disease whose hypertension may become suddenly refractory to an established regimen because of acquired atherosclerotic renovascular disease.

If none of these reversible problems is discovered, several options are available. If the patient's regimen includes a diuretic and a beta-blocker, the addition of modest doses of a vasodilator such as hydralazine 50 to 100 mg/day, or a calcium-channel blocker may bring the blood pressure under control. If therapy with a beta-blocker is contraindicated, a diuretic can be combined with high doses of an angiotensin-converting enzyme inhibitor (such as captopril 75 to 150 mg/day or enalapril 20 to 40 mg/day); an angiotensin-converting enzyme inhibitor can be combined with a calcium-channel blocker. If beta-blockers can be tolerated and the patient is already taking a diuretic and an angiotensin-converting enzyme inhibitor, a beta-blocker or an alternative sympathomimetic agent such as clonidine may be added.

If none of these regimens is successful at achieving adequate blood pressure control and if secondary causes of hypertension have been excluded, potent vasodilators such as minoxidil, 10 to 40 mg/day or high-dose angiotensin-converting enzyme inhibitors, a diuretic, and one or more sympathomimetic agents should be combined.

## Special situations

Mild hypertension. There is no question that aggressive therapy of hypertension in patients with a diastolic blood pressure of greater than 100 to 105 mm Hg results in reduced cardiovascular morbidity and mortality. Several studies of treatment of patients with blood pressures ranging from 90 to 104 mm Hg have been carried out. Four major studies—the Oslo study,[5] the Australian Management Committee Study,[6] the Hypertension Detection and Follow-up Program (HDFP) of the National Heart, Lung, and Blood Institute,[7] and the Medical Research Council Working Party[8]—demonstrated a significant reduction in stroke, heart failure and ventricular hypertrophy, and aortic dissection. The HDFP study also showed a significant decrease in cardiovascular morbidity and mortality from ischemic cardiac events. These studies confirm a decreased mortality in treated patients over 50 years of age and in patients with diastolic blood pressures ranging from 95 to 104 mm Hg. As stated earlier, we believe that mild hypertension (DBP 95 to 104 mm Hg) merits drug therapy, especially if the patient has any evidence of end-organ damage or additional risk factors for cardiovascular disease.

Controversy still exists over appropriate therapy for patients with diastolic blood pressures ranging from 90 to 94 mm Hg in whom nonpharmacologic therapy has not reduced blood pressure adequately. Young patients with blood pressures in this range may be committed to many years of drug therapy with diuretics and beta-blockers; in these patients the long-term side effects of raising serum lipid levels may outweigh the benefits of lowering the blood pressure. Many physicians postpone treating younger patients with mild hypertension (in the absence of evidence of end-organ damage) with drug therapy, preferring to continue nonpharmacologic treatment and to monitor blood pressure at frequent intervals. Physicians who elect to do so should have a clear follow-up plan for these patients; they should be informed about the possibility that they may require active drug therapy in the future.

Isolated systolic hypertension. Isolated systolic hypertension, predominantly a disease of the elderly, is defined as a systolic blood pressure greater than 140 mm Hg with a diastolic blood pressure less than 90 mm Hg in patients younger than 35 years of age and greater than 160 mm Hg in patients older than 60 years of age. In general, the risk of stroke and cardiovascular events is greater in patients with isolated systolic hypertension; treatment of systolic hypertension reduces the incidence of cardiovascular events, though not overall mortality.[14] Secondary causes of isolated systolic hypertension, including anemia, thyrotoxicosis, aortic regurgitation, and high-output congestive heart failure, should be specifically sought and excluded. The goal of treatment is to reduce the systolic blood pressure by 10% without precipitating serious side effects, especially orthostatic hypotension. Nonpharmacologic approaches are particularly effective in this group of patients and are the initial choice in therapy.[15] The initial treatment of choice is diuretic therapy (such as hydrochlorothiazide 25 mg daily), which is usually effective without major side effects. Angiotensin-converting enzyme (ACE) inhibitors or centrally acting adrenergic inhibitors can be added in small doses if diuretic therapy alone is not effective. Meticulous attention must be paid to the avoidance of symptomatic orthostasis because baroreceptor sensitivity is diminished in the elderly; the significant risk of orthostatic syncope should be seriously considered before any elderly patient is prescribed medical therapy for isolated systolic hypertension.

**Hypertension in pregnancy.** Hypertension in pregnancy usually results either from worsening of preexisting hypertension or from preeclampsia. Multigravida women in their thirties, with preexisting chronic hypertension, frequently develop an exacerbation of their hypertension in the second and third trimesters of pregnancy. Antihypertensive medications should be continued during pregnancy; methyldopa, hydralazine, and beta-blockers have been used safely and effectively in the management of established hypertension during pregnancy. Angiotensin-converting enzyme inhibitors, reported to cause fetal death in some animal species, are contraindicated during pregnancy.

The syndrome of preeclampsia—edema, proteinuria, and blood pressures of 140/90 mm Hg or higher—is seen most commonly in young primigravida women. All the findings resolve completely with delivery of the fetus. Treatment is with bedrest and judicious antihypertensive therapy. Several randomized controlled trials have demonstrated that low-dose aspirin (60 mg/day) administered to high-risk patients in the second and third trimester may reduce the incidence of eclampsia without harming the fetus.[16] A hypertensive crisis in eclampsia is best treated by prevention, that is, good prenatal care. Acute hypertension in eclampsia with diastolic blood pressures greater than 110 mm Hg can be treated with intramuscular or intravenous hydralazine.

**Hypertension in patients with renal parenchymal disease.** Most patients with renal parenchymal disease, especially glomerular disease, and with sufficient renal impairment to reduce glomerular filtration by 50% develop hypertension. This hypertension is in part secondary to the inability of the kidney to excrete sodium and the resultant salt retention and volume expansion. Therefore an important part of therapy of hypertension in patients with renal insufficiency is the use of potent loop diuretics such as furosemide and ethacrynic acid. Doses up to 500 mg/day may be required, but one must be careful not to produce volume depletion and worsening azotemia by the excessive use of diuretics. Calcium-channel blockers are very effective in these patients and are often required in addition to the diuretics. Thiazide diuretics are ineffective in patients with serum creatinines greater than 2 to 3 mg/dL. Further aggressive therapy of uncontrolled hypertension in patients with chronic renal impairment by the use of diuretics, calcium-channel blockers, and minoxidil is critical in the maintenance of residual renal function. ACE inhibitors have the added advantage of lowering intraglomerular pressure, but they do carry the risk of aggravating renal insufficiency.

# HYPERTENSION IN THE HOSPITALIZED PATIENT

## Management of the stable hypertensive patient undergoing surgery

The basic assessment of the stable hypertensive patient before routine surgery is similar to that already outlined. A detailed history, a physical examination, and a review of laboratory tests including an ECG should reveal any significant cardiac events that might increase the patient's risk of anesthetic complications. In general, patients with diastolic blood pressures less than 110 mm Hg whose hypertensive medications are continued through surgery tolerate routine surgery without complication. If the diastolic blood pressure is greater than 110 mm Hg, any nonemergent surgery should be postponed until the hypertension is controlled.

Perioperative management of antihypertensive medications deserves some attention. Medications such as guanethidine, guanadrel, and monoamine oxidase inhibitors used in the treatment of depression should be replaced by other agents several weeks before surgery. All the alpha-adrenergic inhibiting agents, if withdrawn suddenly, can result in rebound hypertension. Therefore, patients should be continued on these agents perioperatively and placed on parenteral forms of alpha-adrenergic inhibitors, such as intravenous methyldopa 250 mg three or four times a day, if the patient is unable to take medication orally. Beta-blockers can be continued safely through surgery and do not need to be discontinued or tapered perioperatively.

The goal of the perioperative management of hypertension is to attain and to maintain blood pressure at its preoperative level, rather than to achieve perfect control. The hospital environment and perioperative period are accompanied by numerous medications, stress, pain, and physiologic changes that make it nearly impossible to tailor a hypertensive regimen to patients and their lives outside the hospital. We are often consulted to recommend therapy for patients initially noted to be hypertensive in the postoperative period. If the patient has mild to moderate hypertension and no acute end-organ changes requiring immediate therapy, we prefer to see the patient in the office within a week or two after surgery and to begin the process of confirming and evaluating hypertension once the patient has returned to his or her usual work and surroundings.

## Management of hypertensive emergencies

Hypertensive emergencies include dissecting aortic aneurysm, acute left ventricular failure with pulmonary edema, intracranial hemorrhage, hypertensive encephalopathy, hypertension accompanying acute cardiac ischemia, and toxemia of pregnancy and these patients often present to emergency departments.[17] Accelerated or malignant-range hypertension may occur without devastating end-organ damage, but acute management of the blood pressure is required to ready the patient for any emergency surgery.

Patients with hypertensive crisis should be managed in an intensive care unit so that the blood pressure can be reduced rapidly to a level closer to normal range. We believe that the treatment of choice is the administration of intravenous sodium nitroprusside (50 to 100 mg in 500 mL of 5% dextrose in water ($D_5W$) at a rate of 0.5 to 1.0 $\mu g/kg/$ min initially to a maximum of 10 $\mu g/kg/min$) under carefully monitored conditions. Rapid reduction in blood pressure levels may also be achieved by the use of 10 to 20 mg of sublingual or oral nifedipine, parenteral labetolol, or intravenous diazoxide in situations where continuous invasive monitoring is not available.

Patients with malignant hypertension who require rapid control of their blood pressure to undergo emergency surgery can be managed with intravenous nitroprusside or sublingual nifedipine. Parenteral hydralazine can be used for less severely ill patients but should be avoided in patients with cardiac disease because of reflex tachycardia. Labetalol also can be used intravenously to reduce blood pressure acutely over a matter of hours. Esmolol, a beta-blocker released for control of supraventricular tachycardia, has been used intraoperatively to control hypertension rapidly; its half-life is only 9 minutes.

## References

1. 1986 guidelines for treatment of mild hypertension: a memorandum from a W.H.O./I.S.H. meeting, *J Hypertension* 4:383, 1986.
2. The 1984 report of the Joint National Committee on Detection, Evaluation, and Treatment of High Blood Pressure, *Arch Intern Med* 144:1045-1057, 1984.
3. Freis ED, Arias LA, Armstrong ML, et al: Veterans Administration Cooperative Study Group on Antihypertensive Agents: Effects of treatment on morbidity in hypertension: I. Results in patients with diastolic blood pressures averaging 115 through 129 mm Hg, *JAMA* 202:1028-1034, 1967.
4. Freis ED, Calabresi M, Castle CH, et al: Veterans Administration Cooperative Study Group on Antihypertensive Agents: Effects of treatment on morbidity in hypertension: II. Results in patients with diastolic blood pressures averaging 90 through 114 mm Hg, *JAMA* 213:1143-1152, 1970.
5. Helgelund A: Treatment of mild hypertension: a five year controlled drug trial, *Am J Med* 69:725-732, 1980.
6. The Management Committee: The Australian therapeutic trial in mild hypertension, *Lancet* 1:1261-1267, 1980.
7. Hypertension Detection and Follow-up Program Cooperative Group: Five year findings of the hypertension detection and follow-up program. Reduction in mortality of persons with high blood pressure, including mild hypertension; I. Mortality by race, sex and age; II. Reduction in stroke incidence among persons with high blood pressure; III, *JAMA* 242:2561-2562, 2572-2577, 1979; 247:633-638, 1982.
8. Medical Research Council Working Party: MRC trial of treatment of mild hypertension: principal results, *Br Med J* 291:97, 1985.
9. Trials of Hypertension Prevention Research Group: The effects of nonpharmacologic interventions on blood pressure of persons with high normal levels: results of the Trials of Hypertension Prevention, Phase I, *JAMA* 267:1213, 1992.

10. Patel C, Marmot MG, Terry DJ, et al: Decreased blood-pressure in pharmacologically treated hypertensive patients who regularly elicited the relaxation response, *Br Med J* 290:1103, 1985.

11. MacMahon SW, Wilcken DEL, Macdonald GJ: The effect of weight reduction on left ventricular mass: a randomized controlled trial in young, overweight hypertensive patients, *N Engl J Med* 314:334, 1986.

12. Maheswaran R, Gill JS, Davies P, et al: High blood pressure due to alcohol: a rapidly reversible effect, *Hypertension* 17:787, 1991.

13. Oparil S: Antihypertensive therapy — efficacy and quality of life (editorial), *N Engl J Med* 328:959, 1993.

14. SHEP Cooperative Research Group: Prevention of stroke by antihypertensive drug treatment in older persons with isolated systolic hypertension: final results of the Systolic Hypertension in the Elderly Program (SHEP), *JAMA* 265:3255, 1991.

15. The Fifth Report of the Joint National Committee on Detection, Evaluation, and Treatment of High Blood Pressure (JNC V), *Arch Intern Med* 153:154, 1993.

16. Imperiale TF, Petrulis AS: A meta-analysis of low-dose aspirin for the prevention of pregnancy-induced hypertensive disease, *JAMA* 266:260, 1991.

17. Zampaglione B, Pascale C, Marchisio M, et al: Hypertensive urgencies and emergencies. Prevalence and clinical presentation, *Hypertension* 27:144, 1996.

# Chapter 52

# Evaluation of a Patient with Polyarthritis

Don L. Goldenberg

Polyarthritis, defined as arthritis involving two or more joints, initially should be classified as acute or chronic (see box at the top of p. 589). Generally acute polyarthritis is defined as arthritis of less than 4 weeks in duration. Although less common than chronic polyarthritis, it is more likely to represent a condition that can be definitively diagnosed and treated. In contrast, chronic polyarthritis includes several idiopathic disorders that are more difficult to diagnose and to treat effectively. Chronic polyarthritis can be subdivided into inflammatory and noninflammatory types, based on the clinical and pathologic characteristics of the synovial reaction.

## ACUTE POLYARTHRITIS

### Disseminated gonococcal infection (DGI)

Infection is the most important cause of acute polyarthritis. Within this category, bacterial infection is the initial diagnosis that must be considered in any patient with acute polyarthritis. Disseminated gonococcal infection (DGI), the most common cause of acute arthritis at most urban medical centers, typically presents with multiple joint involvement. Patients are usually young, sexually active adults. DGI is five times more common in females who generally have no symptoms of current pelvic inflammatory disease. The most common rheumatic presentation is a migratory polyarthralgia with subsequent polyarthritis or tenosynovitis. Tendon inflammation is more common than that of joints; typical tendons or joints involved include knees, wrists, ankles, and fingers. Dermatitis, present in 60% of patients, may include macules, vesicles, or pustules. These skin lesions, often multiple and on the extremities, generally are not symptomatic.

The diagnosis of DGI is usually made by the clinical presentation and a rapid response to antibiotics (see the box at the bottom of p. 589). The clinicians should consider DGI as the most likely diagnosis in any young adult presenting with acute polyarthritis or tenosynovitis, particularly if associated with fever and skin lesions. As with any form of suspected joint infection, arthrocentesis should be performed

---

**Classification of Major Forms of Acute versus Chronic Polyarthritis**
..........................................................................

ACUTE

---

Gonococcal
Nongonococcal bacterial
Crystal-induced
Viral
Lyme disease

CHRONIC

---

Rheumatoid arthritis
Seronegative spondyloarthritis
Osteoarthritis

---

immediately with Gram stain and culture of the synovial fluid. The synovial fluid is typically inflammatory with greater than 30,000 leukocytes/mm$^3$, but this is not specific. Unfortunately, synovial fluid culture is positive in less than 50% and Gram stain in less than 25% of cases of presumed DGI. These results probably are related to the fastidious

---

**Acute Inflammatory Polyarthritis: Key Diagnostic Signs, Symptoms, and Tests**
..........................................................................

**Gonococcal arthritis:** Young, sexually active adult, migratory polyarthralgias or arthritis, tenosynovitis, dermatitis, positive culture of genitourinary site or synovial fluid (definitive), rapid response to antibiotics

**Nongonococcal bacterial arthritis:** Elderly or young child, often with preexisting chronic illness or arthritis, severely painful and swollen joints, positive synovial fluid culture (definitive)

**Viral arthritis:** History of upper respiratory infection, multiple small joint polyarthritis, rash, especially urticaria, positive serologic test, elevated liver function test values, self-limited arthritis

**Gout:** Prior acute attack of arthritis, arthritis that involves big toe or other foot or ankle joint, hyperuricemia, demonstration of monosodium urate crystals from synovial fluid (definitive), rapid response to colchicine or antiinflammatory drugs

**Pseudogout (CPPD disease):** Chondrocalcinosis on roentgenogram, calcium pyrophosphate dihydrate (CPPD) crystals demonstrated in synovial fluid (definitive)

**Lyme disease:** Spring or summer onset, rash characteristic of erythema chronicum migrans, history of tick bite, positive Lyme serologic test

---

growth requirements of *Neisseria gonorrhoeae.* Negative culture also could result from an immune cause, as in rheumatoid arthritis, rather than an infectious cause of the synovitis. Recently, polymerase chain reaction (PCR), which can detect minute amounts of gonococcal DNA, has been positive in culture-negative synovial fluid from patients with presumptive DGI and eventually may be a valuable diagnostic tool. Blood cultures and cultures of the skin lesions are rarely positive, whereas genitourinary cultures are usually positive. Thus the diagnosis is often presumptive, based on the typical clinical manifestations, a positive genitourinary culture and confirmed by a rapid response to antibiotics (see the box at the bottom of p. 589). Most patients respond dramatically, usually within 24 to 48 hours. Because of the emergence of penicillinase-producing strains of *N. gonorrhoeae,* a third-generation cephalosporin should be administered until culture results and antimicrobial sensitivities are completed.

## Nongonococcal bacterial arthritis

Nongonococcal bacterial arthritis is typically an acute monoarthritis, but in 20% of cases more than one joint is involved. The diagnosis in such cases is often delayed, possibly because the polyarticular presentation is atypical. Such a delay in diagnosis often results in a poor outcome. Nongonococcal bacterial arthritis is most common in neonates, young children, the elderly, or patients with chronic illness or chronic systemic arthritis. In some reports, 50% of patients with septic polyarthritis had coexistent rheumatoid arthritis.

As soon as the possibility of septic polyarthritis is considered, arthrocentesis of one or more than one joint must be performed immediately. In contrast to DGI, Gram-stain examination of the synovial fluid is positive in more than 50% and synovial fluid culture is positive in greater than 90% of cases of nongonococcal bacterial arthritis. Blood cultures are positive in 50% and cultures of skin, the urine, or sputum are often positive and will provide a clue as to identity of the organism in the joint. The synovial fluid is very inflammatory with a pronounced leukocytosis (often greater than 40,000 cells/mm³). Peripheral blood leukocytosis is common, and the erythrocyte sedimentation rate (ESR) is elevated, but these findings are nonspecific. *Staphylococcus aureus* is the most common bacteria recovered, but other gram-positive cocci as well as gram-negative bacilli and anaerobes are often the cause of nongonococcal bacterial arthritis.

The diagnosis of nongonococcal bacterial arthritis is based on the clinical manifestations and a positive synovial fluid culture (see box at the bottom of p. 589). A particularly confusing picture may occur in the patient with rheumatoid arthritis (RA) who presents with a possible exacerbation of polyarthritis in a few joints. The index of suspicion for concurrent infection should be high in this situation and joint aspiration must be performed quickly. The mortality approaches 50% in RA patients with septic polyarthritis, even with prompt treatment.

Once the diagnosis is made, patients with nongonococcal bacterial arthritis should be treated with appropriate parenteral antibiotics and joint drainage. Joint drainage, often accomplished by repeated needle aspiration, may require arthroscopy or open surgical drainage, particularly in hips or axial joints. Most patients become afebrile within a few days though joint effusions may persist for more than a week. Persistent joint effusions may be an indication of incomplete joint drainage.

## Viral polyarthritis

Many viruses have been associated with acute polyarthritis. Usually these are self-limited forms of acute joint and tendon inflammation, lasting 1 to 4 weeks. They present often as an acute serum sickness, with fever, urticaria, and polyarthritis. Viral polyarthritis most often develops in children and young adults. The joint manifestations may precede or occur together with typical signs of an upper respiratory infection, fever, lymphadenopathy, or rash. The dermatitis depends on the specific virus involved and is often urticarial as in hepatitis B infection. However, the typical rash of parvovirus, erythema infectiosum, or of rubella is strong evidence that the polyarthritis is related to that specific virus.

Viral polyarthritis usually involves multiple small joints, including fingers, wrists, ankles, and toes and mimics early RA. The synovial characteristics are usually less inflammatory than those of bacterial infection or of RA, with 1000 to 2000 leukocytes/mm$^3$, predominantly mononuclear cells, and the culture is negative. The arthritis usually responds well to nonsteroidal anti inflammatory drugs (NSAIDs) or low doses of corticosteroids, but treatment for the joint manifestations often is not necessary, since the polyarthritis is self limited.

The diagnosis of hepatitis-associated polyarthritis is aided by biochemical evidence of abnormal liver function and positive hepatitis serologic tests. Hepatitis B is the most common cause of viral polyarthritis though hepatitis A and C, rubella, mumps, and various enteroviruses may cause an acute polyarthritis. Certain viral antibody markers, such as IgM antibody to parvovirus, will be diagnostically helpful. However, the diagnosis of many forms of viral polyarthritis is based largely on the clinical presentation and the self-limited nature of the joint inflammation.

## Lyme disease

The arthritis associated with Lyme disease is most often a chronic, recurrent monoarthritis that occurs months after the initial infection. However, during the early stages of Lyme disease, polyarthralgias and less often polyarthritis may develop. During this stage, patients present with fever, headache, or a stiff neck and may have or have had the characteristic rash of erythema chronicum migrans. The diagnosis is made in patients with these symptoms, in geographic areas endemic with Lyme disease, or after a history of a tick bite, seasonal presentation typical of tick-borne infections, or a positive serologic test for infection by *Borrelia burgdorferi*. It is important that serologic confirmation be performed by western blot or specific immunoassays.

## Crystal-induced polyarthritis

Although gout and pseudogout (calcium pyrophosphate dihydrate crystal disease) generally present as a monoarthritis, both may also cause acute polyarthritis. Gout classically involves the first metatarsophalangeal joint, but polyarticular gout may involve a number of toes and the ankle or knees, wrists, or fingers. Polyarticular gout rarely occurs as the initial attack of gout, but 25% of cases of long-standing gout will present in a polyarticular fashion. Polyarticular gout is especially common in alcoholics and other patients with many risk factors for gout and who are not compliant with treatment. Patients with polyarticular gout tend to be systemically ill, with fever and a peripheral blood leukocytosis. Gout rarely occurs in premenopausal females, and patients often have a history of antecedent events such as joint trauma, surgery, significant alcohol intake, or use of drugs known to cause hyperuricemia, such as diuretics. Pseudogout less commonly affects more than one joint and usually involves the knees, wrists, or shoulders. Elevated serum calcium is, by itself, not associated with pseudogout, though pseudogout may first occur after rapid fluctuations in the serum calcium levels.

Crystal-induced arthritis should be considered in any patient presenting with a very painful, acute polyarthritis. Gout should be the initial diagnostic consideration in a patient who has had similar attacks of acute monoarthritis or polyarthritis, if the big toe is involved, or if there is hyperuricemia. However, 25% to 40% of patients will have a nomal serum uric acid at the time of acute gouty arthritis. Pseudogout should be considered in elderly patients presenting with an acute monoarthritis or polyarthritis, but, in particular, radiologic evidence of chondrocalcinosis is strong evidence for calcium pyrophosphate dihydrate (CPPD) crystal disease. Nevertheless, demonstration of either monosodium urate or CPPD crystals in the synovial fluid is the only definitive way to diagnose gout and pseudogout. Thus, whenever possible, joint aspiration with synovial fluid analysis that includes "compensated-polarization" microscopic examination for crystals should be performed. Treatment can also be helpful for diagnostic purposes, especially in gout where more than 75% of patients respond within 1 to 2 days to high-dose NSAIDs, or to colchicine, corticosteroids, or ACTH. These same medications are also quite effective in pseudogout, but the response to therapy is more erratic.

# CHRONIC POLYARTHRITIS

## Rheumatoid arthritis

Chronic polyarthritis is generally divided into inflammatory or noninflammatory forms based on the degree of synovial membrane and synovial fluid inflammation (Table 52-1). Rheumatoid arthritis (RA), the most prevalent inflammatory joint disease, is the prototype for chronic, idiopathic inflammatory polyarthritis. The synovial membrane is infiltrated by mononuclear cells, especially small lymphocytes and plasma cells, and pathologically as well as immunologically it behaves much like an activated lymph node. The synovia tends to contain acute inflammatory cells. Although the cause of RA is not known, there is

**Table 52-1.** *Important classification criteria used to distinguish inflammatory (RA) from noninflammatory (osteoarthritis) polyarthritis*

| Criteria | Inflammatory | Noninflammatory |
|---|---|---|
| Morning stiffness | Severe and for hours | Mild, minutes |
| Fatigue | Usually prominent | Rare |
| Pain | Generalized, at rest | Joint, with activity |
| Joint swelling | Feels soft, spongy | Feels hard, bony |
| Large joint effusions | Common | Rare |
| Extra-articular symptoms | Common | Rare |
| Synovial fluid | Inflammatory | Noninflammatory |
| Erythrocyte sedimentation rate | Elevated | Normal |
| Anemia | Common | Rare |
| Roentgenogram of joint | Erosions, osteoporosis | Osteophytes, osteosclerosis |

overwhelming evidence of abnormal immune activation as well as of a genetic predisposition.

RA classically presents as a symmetric polyarthritis, involving the small joints of the hands and feet, especially the proximal interphalangeal, metacarpophalangeal, and metatarsophalangeal joints. Knees, wrist, elbows, jaws, and sternoclavicular joints are commonly involved. Women are three times more often involved than men, and the peak age of onset is from 30 to 50. The arthritis seldom spontaneously remits completely though wide variations in disease activity are common. In general, more joint involvement with irreversible anatomic changes slowly progresses. Many patients also have systemic features, including fatigue, fever, weight loss, lymphadenopathy, and peripheral neuropathy, such as carpal tunnel syndrome. Less common, but more serious, nonarticular manifestations of RA include systemic vasculitis, pericarditis, pleurisy and pleural effusions, interstitial lung disease, and amyloidosis.

The diagnosis of RA is based primarily on the typical chronic, symmetric polyarthritis involving the hands, feet, and other joints. Subcutaneous nodules, usually best noted over the extensor surface of the elbows, are very suggestive of RA but present in only 25% and 35% of patients. The most helpful laboratory features are a positive rheumatoid factor, present in 40% to 70% of patients, and radiologic demonstration of an erosive, small joint polyarthritis that begins in the corners of articular cartilage and bone. Less specific but common laboratory features include anemia, thrombocytosis, an elevated erythrocyte sedimentation rate and C-reactive protein, and an inflammatory synovia. The presence of rheumatoid factor and of subcutaneous nodules is not only highly suggestive of RA but also associated with a poor outcome. The diagnosis, however, should never be made if the characterisitc polyarthritis is not present, no matter what laboratory tests are noted.

Treatment is with NSAIDs, physical therapy, appropriate exercise and medications, often called "disease-modifying anti-rheumatic drugs (DMARD)." Unfortunately, most drugs do not significantly alter the slow but progressive joint morbidity. Methotrexate may be an exception and has been the most effective DMARD. Patients have tolerated it longer than other antirheumatic drugs, which include other cytotoxic drugs, gold salts, and hydroxychloroquine. Methotrexate is generally given orally, once per week in doses that average 7.5 to 15 mg per week. Liver function tests and blood counts are followed at 3- to 8-week intervals. Hopefully, more targeted immune therapy that can indeed modify the usual course of RA will soon be developed.

## Juvenile rheumatoid arthritis (JRA)

JRA actually may be several different, unrelated forms of chronic polyarthritis that occur in children and in young adults. One form of JRA is identical to typical RA in adults, including its poor outcome. Still's disease is another variant that develops in children or in young adults, where it is often termed "adult onset JRA." In Still's disease the polyarthritis tends to be mild and not progressive but is overshadowed by the systemic features of striking fevers, a peripheral blood leukocytosis, generalized lymphadenopathy, and hepatosplenomegaly. JRA also may present as a spondyloarthropathy (see below).

Still's onset JRA tends to be the most difficult to diagnose because of the mild joint involvement and the striking systemic manifestations. In children and in young adults, these patients are often initially considered to have an infection or a malignancy and often wind up in the category of fever of unknown origin. A diagnosis of one of the variants of JRA, which is similar to RA or to the spondyloarthropathies, is based on the disease patterns described for their respective adult counterparts.

## Seronegative spondyloarthropathies

The seronegative spondyloarthropathies are a group of interrelated disorders that cause a chronic polyarthritis that usually affects both peripheral and axial joints. The peripheral joints most often involved are the ankles and feet, although virtually any joint may be affected. The axial joints involved include the sacroiliac joints but seronegative spondyloarthropathies also may affect the lumbar, thoracic, and cervical apophyseal spinal joints, producing a so-called bamboo spine. These seronegative spondyloarthropathies include psoriatic arthritis, Reiter's syndrome, ankylosing spondylitis, and the arthritis associated with inflammatory bowel disease.

Each of the seronegative spondyloarthropathies shares several clinical and diagnostic features, the most important being the pattern of a combined peripheral and axial chronic polyarthritis. In addition, they are each more common in males, there is often a family history of seronegative spondyloarthropathies, they are each rheumatoid factor negative, that is, "seronegative," and they are commonly associated with characteristic dermatitis and mucus membrane lesions. The seronegative spondyloarthropathies also often cause inflammation of tendons, such as the Achilles tendon. The exact pattern of the joint and extra-articular manifestations depends on the specific category of the seronegative spondyloarthropathies, but these disorders should be considered in any patient with sacroiliitis and an asymmetric polyarthritis. Psoriasis or psoriasis-like dermatitis, nail pitting or dystrophy, conjunctivitis, urethritis, oral sores, and decreased spinal range of motion are very suggestive of one of the seronegative spondyloarthropathies. The most helpful laboratory features include radiologic evidence of sacroiliitis, particularly with concurrent spinal joint involvement, a negative rheumatoid factor, and the presence of the HLA-B27 antigen, which is found in 70% to 90% of patients with seronegative spondyloarthropathies. These disorders tend to have spontaneous remissions and exacerbations, though ankylosing spondylitis often slowly progresses to involve the total spine and may cause significant morbidity. NSAIDs often are very helpful in controlling the peripheral arthritis but less so in altering the course of axial joint involvement. DMARDs are often used, but they tend to be less effective in this disorder than in RA.

## Osteoarthritis

The most common and important noninflammatory, chronic polyarthritis is osteoarthritis. Osteoarthritis is by far the most prevalent form of arthritis and affects most of the elderly population in one form or another. It is unusual for osteoarthritis to develop in patients under 50 years of age, but it may develop in patients with joints subject to repetitive trauma or in patients with a strong family history of osteoarthritis.

The diagnosis of osteoarthritis is based on clinical and radiologic features (see Table 52-1). Most patients present with an indolent, chronic polyarthritis, most often affecting the distal interphalangeal and proximal interphalangeal joints of the fingers, the carpometacarpal thumb joints, the knees and hips, and the spine. The fingers on palpation demonstrate bony enlargement and deformities with little tenderness, the so-called Heberden's nodes and Bouchard's nodes (for the distal and proximal interphalangeal joints, respectively). Bony crepitus is commonly noted on range of motion of the knees, which also may reveal a valgus or varus deformity. Loss of rotation of the hip is an early sign of hip osteoarthritis.

The most important diagnostic feature is radiologic demonstration of nonuniform joint-space narrowing, osteophytes, and periarticular osteosclerosis. In contrast to each of the inflammatory polyarthritis conditions described above, patients with osteoarthritis have no signs or symptoms of a systemic illness, have a normal ESR, and have synovial fluid that is noninflammatory with few leukocytes, the majority of which are mononuclear cells. Treatment with NSAIDs is marginally helpful, primarily for analgesia, and acetaminophen probably is just as effective. The major improvement in treating osteoarthritis of hips and knees in the last decade has been total joint replacement, which usually is very helpful in reducing or eliminating pain in that joint. At least 80% to 90% of patients report significant improvement in their lifestyle with total hip or knee replacement.

## References

1. Goldenberg DL, Reed JI: Bacterial arthritis, *N Engl J Med* 312:764-771, 1985.
2. Sharp JT, Calkins E, Cohen AS, et al: Observations on the clinical, chemical and serologic manifestation of rheumatoid arthritis based on the course of 154 cases, *Medicine* 43:41-58, 1964.
3. Pouchet J, Sampalis JS, Beaudet F, et al: Still's disease: manifestations, disease course, and outcome in 62 patients, *Medicine* 70:118-136, 1991.
4. Mau W, Zeidler H, Mau R, et al: Clinical features and prognosis of patients with possible ankylosing spondylitis: results of a 10-year follow-up, *J Rheumatol* 15:1109-1114, 1988.
5. Ryan LM, McCarty DJ: Calcium pyrophosphate crystal deposition disease: pseudogout, articular chondrocalcinosis. In McCarty DJ, Koopman WJ, editors: *Arthritis and allied conditions,* ed 12, Philadelphia, 1993, Lea & Febiger.
6. Steere AC: Lyme disease, *N Engl J Med* 321:586-596, 1989.
7. Altman R, Alarcon G, Appelrouth D: The American College of Rheumatology criteria for the classification and reporting of osteoarthritis of the hand, *Arthritis Rheum* 33:1601-1610, 1990.

# Index